H.K.F. van Saene
L. Silvestri
M.A. De La Cal
Infection Control in the Intensive Care Unit

H.K.F. van Saene (Editor)
L. Silvestri (Editor)
M.A. De La Cal (Editor)

Infection Control in the Intensive Care Unit

Second Edition

Series edited by
Antonino Gullo

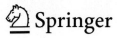 Springer

H.K.F. Van Saene, M.D.
Department of Medical Microbiology
University of Liverpool
Alder Hey Children's Hospital, NHS Trust
Liverpool, UK

L. Silvestri, M.D.
Emergency Department and Unit
of Anesthesia and Intensive Care
Presidio Ospedaliero of Gorizia
Gorizia, Italy

M.A. De La Cal, M.D.
Department of Critical Care Medicine
University Hospital of Getafe
Madrid, Spain

Series *Topics in Anaesthesia and Critical Care* edited by
Prof. A. Gullo
Department of Perioperative Medicine, Intensive Care and Emergency
Trieste University School of Medicine,
Trieste, Italy

Library of Congress Control Number: 2004114978

ISBN 88-470-0185-4 Springer Milan Berlin Heidelberg New York

Springer is a part of Springer Science+Business Media
springeronline.com
© Springer-Verlag Italia 2005
Printed in Italy

Cover design: Simona Colombo, Milan, Italy
Typesetting: Graphostudio, Milan, Italy
Printing: Grafiche Porpora, Cernusco S/N, Italy

Preface

Seven years have passed since the first edition of 'Infection Control in the Intensive Care Unit' was published. That book was a compilation of the lectures read at an intensive course on management of infection in the critically ill organised by Professor A. Gullo in Trieste, Italy, and has been completely rewritten by Italian, Spanish, South American, Dutch and Anglo-Canadian authors in this second edition. The book is up to date, with references to publications from 2004. We regard it as important that all statements are justified by the best available evidence. All authors have made efforts to avoid unsubstantiated expert opinion. Although prevention is not entirely separate from therapy, prevention rather than cure is pivotal in this publication.

There are five sections in this second edition. The first section deals with basics in microbiology specifically as they operate in supporting infection control. Surveillance cultures of throat and rectum are an integral part of the microbiological approach of this publication. Surveillance cultures are required to determine the carrier state. Carriage is indispensable for the classification of micro-organisms into low level, high level pathogens and potentially pathogenic micro-organisms. This distinction is crucial as prevention methods target only potentially pathogenic micro-organisms and high level pathogens. The front cover illustrates the usefulness of classifying infections occurring on the intensive care unit [ICU], again using carriage as detected by surveillance cultures. Primary endogenous pneumonias are the main infectious problem on the ICU, with an incidence of about 55%. Primary endogenous pneumonia caused by potential pathogens, both 'normal' and 'abnormal', usually occurs within a week of admission to ICU. Previously healthy individuals including trauma and surgical patients develop early endogenous pneumonias with the 'normal' potential pathogens such as *Streptococcus pneumoniae*, *Haemophilus influenzae*, *Moraxella catarrhalis* and *Staphylococcus aureus*. Patients with underlying chronic conditions such as diabetes, alcoholism and chronic obstructive pulmonary disease and who are referred to the ICU from home or from other wards and hospitals, may carry abnormal aerobic Gram-negative bacilli [AGNB] such as *Klebsiella*, *Acinetobacter* and *Pseudomonas* species in their admission flora. This type of patient may develop a primary endogenous pneumonia with abnormal flora. Fortunately, most patients recover from their primary endogenous pneumonia after intensive care treatment including antibiotic therapy. About one third of ICU admissions may develop a late pneumonia, usually after the first weeks' treatment on ICU. These patients invariably acquire abnormal AGNB, which are associated with the ICU-environment, in their oropharynx. This leads to secondary carriage and oropharyngeal over-

Contents

SECTION ONE
ESSENTIALS IN CLINICAL MICROBIOLOGY

Chapter 1
Glossary of Terms and Definitions
R.E. SARGINSON, N. TAYLOR, M.A. DE LA CAL, H.K.F. VAN SAENE   3

Chapter 2
Carriage
S. ROSSENEU, G. RIOS, P.E. SPRONK, J.J.M. VAN SAENE   15

Chapter 3
Colonization and Infection
L. SILVESTRI, G. MINO, H.K.F VAN SAENE   37

Chapter 4
Classification of Micro-Organisms According to their Pathogenicity
M.A. DE LA CAL, E. CERDÀ, A. ABELLA, P. GARCIA-HIERRO   49

Chapter 5
Classification of ICU Infections
L. SILVESTRI, M. VIVIANI, H.K.F. VAN SAENE   61

Chapter 6
**Gut Microbiology: Surveillance Samples for the Detection
of the Abnormal Carrier State**
H.K.F VAN SAENE, G. IZQUIERDO, P. GARCIA-HIERRO, F. FONTANA   73

SECTION TWO
ANTIMICROBIALS

Chapter 7
Systemic Antibiotics
A.R. DE GAUDIO, S. RINALDI, A. NOVELLI 91

Chapter 8
Systemic Antifungals
F. J. COOKE, T. ROGERS 155

Chapter 9
Enteral Antimicrobials
M. SANCHEZ, B.P. PIZER, S.R. ALCOCK 171

SECTION THREE
INFECTION CONTROL

Chapter 10
Evidence-Based Infection Control in the Intensive Care Unit
J. HUGHES, N. TAYLOR, E. CERDÀ, M.A. DE LA CAL 191

Chapter 11
Device Policies
A.R. DE GAUDIO, A. DI FILIPPO 213

Chapter 12
Antibiotic Policies in the Intensive Care Unit
H.K.F. VAN SAENE, N.J. REILLY, A. DE SILVESTRE, G. NARDI 231

Chapter 13
Outbreaks of Infection in Intensive Care Units-Usefulness of Molecular Techniques for Outbreak Analysis
V. DAMJANOVIC, X. CORBELLA, J.I. VAN DER SPOEL, H.K.F. VAN SAENE 247

Chapter 14
Prevention of Infection Using Selective Decontamination of the Digestive Tract
L. SILVESTRI, S. KERR, A. GULLO 297

SECTION FOUR
INFECTIONS ON ICU

Chapter 15
Lower Airway Infection
N. FÀBREGAS, A. ALCÓN, A. TORRES 315

Chapter 16
Bloodstream Infections Including Endocarditis and Meningitis
J. VALLÉS, R. FERRER, P. FERNÁNDEZ-VILADRICH 337

Chapter 17
Infections of the Peritoneum Including Pancreas, Mediastinum, Pleura,
Wounds, and Urinary Tract
G. SGANGA, G. BRISINDA, G. MARIA, M. CASTAGNETO 379

Chapter 18
Infection on the Neonatal and Pediatric Intensive Care Units
A.J. PETROS, V. DAMJANOVIC, A. PIGNA, J. FARIAS 415

Chapter 19
Immediate Adequate Antibiotics control Morbidity and Mortality
in Patients with Pancreatitis, Extensive Burns, Trauma, Exacerbated
Chronic Obstructive Pulmonary Disease, or Liver Transplantation
I. ALÍA, M.A. DE LA CAL, E. CERDÁ, H.K.F. VAN SAENE 429

Chapter 20
Intensive Care Unit Patients following Transplantation
A. MARTÍNEZ-PELLÚS, M. PALOMAR 455

Chapter 21
Clinical Virology in NICU, PICU and Adult ICU
W. TONG, S. SCHELENZ 469

Chapter 22
AIDS Patients in the Intensive Care Unit
L. ALVAREZ-ROCHA, P. RASCADO-SEDES, J. PASTOR-BENAVENT,
F. BARCENILLA-GAITE 495

Chapter 23
Therapy of Infection
J.H. ROMMES, A. SELBY, D.F. ZANDSTRA 515

SECTION FIVE
SPECIAL TOPICS

Chapter 24
SIRS, Sepsis, and MODS
G. BERLOT, A. TOMASINI, M. VIVIANI 537

Chapter 25
SIRS/Sepsis: Metabolic and Nutritional Changes and Treatment
F. ISCRA, A. RANDINO 549

Chapter 26
Gut Mucosal Protection in the Critically Ill Patient.
Towards an Integrated Clinical Strategy
D. F. ZANDSTRA, P.H.J. VAN DER VOORT, K. THORBURN, H.K.F. VAN SAENE 565

Chapter 27
Selective Decontamination of the Digestive Tract:
the Role of the Pharmacist
N.J. REILLY, A.J. NUNN, K. POLLOCK 575

Chapter 28
Antimicrobial Resistance: a Prospective 5-Year Study
H.K.F. VAN SAENE, N. TAYLOR, N.J. REILLY, P.B. BAINES 593

Chapter 29
ICU-Acquired Infection: Mortality, Morbidity, and Costs
J.C. MARSHALL, K.A.M. MARSHALL 605

Chapter 30
Evidence-Based Medicine in the Intensive Care Unit
A.J. PETROS, K.G. LOWRY, H.K.F. VAN SAENE, J.C. MARSHALL................... 621

Subject Index 635

Contributors

Abella A.
Department of Critical Care Medicine, Hospital Universitario de Getafe, Madrid, Spain

Alcock S.R.
Department of Bacteriology, Western Infirmary Glasgow, Glasgow, UK

Alcón A.
Anesthesiology Department, Surgical Intensive Care Unit, URSC, Hospital Clínic, Universitat de Barcelona, Barcelona, Spain

Alía I.
Department of Critical Care Medicine, Hospital Universitario de Getafe, Madrid, Spain

Alvarez-Rocha L.
Intensive Care Unit, Juan Canalejo Hospital, Coruña, Spain

Baines P.B.
Pediatric Intensive Care Unit, Alder Hey Children's Hospital, Liverpool, UK

Barcenilla-Gaite F.
Intensive Care Unit, Arnau de Vilanova Hospital, Lleida, Spain

Berlot G.
Department of Anaesthesia, Perioperative Medicine, Intensive Care and Emergency, University Hospital School of Medicine, Trieste, Italy

Brisinda G.
Surgery and Transplantation Unit, Policlinico Universitario Agostino Gemelli, Rome, Italy

Castagneto G.
Surgery and Transplantation Unit, Policlinico Universitario Agostino Gemelli, Rome, Italy

Cerda E.
Department of Critical Care Medicine, Hospital Universitario de Getafe,
Madrid, Spain

Cooke F.J.
Division of Microbiology, Hammersmith Hospital, London, UK

Corbella X.
Department of Intensive Care, University of Barcelona, Barcelona, Spain

Damjanovic V.
Department of Medical Microbiology, University of Liverpool,
Liverpool, UK

De Gaudio A.R.
Department of Anesthesia and Critical Care, University of Florence,
Florence, Italy

de la Cal M.A.
Department of Critical Care Medicine, Hospital Universitario de Getafe,
Madrid, Spain

de Silvestre A.
Department of Anaesthesia and Intensive Care, University Hospital of
S. Maria della Misericordia, Udine, Italy

Di Filippo A.
Section of Anesthesiology and Intensive Care, Department of Critical Care,
University of Florence, Florence, Italy

Fàbregas N.
Anesthesiology Department, Surgical Intensive Care Unit, URSC, Hospital Clínic,
Universitat de Barcelona, Barcelona, Spain

Farias J.
Pediatric Intensive Care Unit, Children's Hospital Ricardo Gutierrez,
Buenos Aires, Argentina

Ferrer R.
Intensive Care Department, Hospital Sabadell, Sabadell, Spain

Fernández-Viladrich P.F.
Infectious Diseases Department, Hospital Bellvitge,
Barcelona, Spain

Fontana F.
Department of Medical Microbiology, University Hospital of Gorizia,
Gorizia, Italy

Garcia-Hierro P.
Department of Medical Microbiology, University Hospital of Getafe,
Madrid, Spain

Gullo A.
Department of Perioperative Medicine, Intensive Care and Emergency, University
of Trieste, Cattinara Hospital, Trieste, Italy

Hughes J.
Department of Clinical Microbiology and Infection Control, University Hospital
Aintree, Liverpool, UK

Iscra F.
Department of Perioperative Medicine, Intensive Care and Emergency,
University of Trieste, Cattinara Hospital, Trieste, Italy

Izquierdo G.
Department of Medical Microbiology, University of Trujillo, Peru

Kerr S.
Department of Pediatric Intensive Care, Alder Hey Children's Hospital,
Liverpool, UK

Lowry K.G.
Intensive Care Unit, Royal Victoria Hospital, Belfast, Northern Ireland

Maria G.
Surgery and Transplantation Unit, Policlinico Universitario Agostino Gemelli,
Rome, Italy

Marshall J.C.
Department of Surgery, and Interdepartmental Division of Critical Care,
General Hospital and University of Toronto, Toronto, Canada

Marshall K.A.M.
Department of Surgery, and Interdepartmental Division of Critical Care,
General Hospital and University of Toronto, Toronto, Canada

Martínez-Pellús A.
Intensive Care Unit,Hospital Universitario Virgen de la Arrixaca,Murcia,Spain

Mino G.
Department of Bacteriology, University Hospital, Guayaquil, Ecuador

Nardi G.
Department of Anesthesia and Intensive Care, University Hospital of S. Camillo Forlanini, Rome, Italy

Novelli A.
Department of Pharmacology, Florence University, Florence, Italy

Nunn A.J.
Department of Pharmacy, Alder Hey Children's Hospital, Liverpool , UK

Palomar M.
Intensive Care Unit, Hospital Universitario Vall d'Hebrón, Barcelona, Spain

Pastor-Benavent J.
Intensive Care Unit, Juan Canalejo Hospital, Coruña, Spain

Petros A.J.
Pediatric Intensive Care Unit, Great Ormond Street Children's Hospital, NHS Trust, London, UK

Pigna A.
Neonatal Intensive Care Unit, San Orsola Hospital, Bologna, Italy

Pizer B.P.
Department of Oncology, Alder Hey Children's Hospital, NHS Trust, Liverpool, UK

Pollock K.
Department of Pharmacy, Western Infirmary, Glasgow, UK

Randino A.
Department of Perioperative Medicine, Intensive Care and Emergency, University of Trieste, Cattinara Hospital, Trieste, Ital

Rascado-Sedes P.
Intensive Care Unit, Juan Canalejo Hospital, Coruña, Spain

Reilly N.J.
Department of Pharmacy, Alder Hey Children's Hospital, Liverpool, UK

Rinaldi S.
Department of Anesthesia and Critical Care, Florence University, Florence, Italy

Rios G.
Department of Pediatric Intensive Care, Gustavo Fricke Children's Hospital,
Vina del Mar, Chile

Rogers T.
Department of Clinical Microbiology, Trinity Centre, Dublin, Ireland

Rommes J.H.
Department of Intensive Care, Gelre Ziekenhuizen, Apeldoorn, The Netherlands

Rosseneu S.
Department of Pediatric Gastroenterology, Barts and the London NHS Trust,
London, UK

Sanchez M.
Department of Intensive Care, University Hospital of Principe de Asturias,
Madrid, Spain

Sarginson R.E.
Department of Anaesthesia and Intensive Care, Alder Hey Children's Hospital,
NHS Trust, Liverpool, UK

Schelenz S.
Department of Infection, Guy's and St. Thomas' Hospital Trust and Department
of Infectious Disease, GKT School of Medicine, St. Thomas' Hospital,
London, UK

Selby A.
Department of Anaesthesia and Intensive Care, Alder Hey Children's Hospital
NHS Trust, Liverpool, UK

Sganga G.
Surgery and Transplantation Unit, Policlinico Universitario Agostino Gemelli,
Rome, Italy

Silvestri L.
Emergency Department and Unit of Anesthesia and Intensive Care, Presidio
Ospedaliero of Gorizia, Gorizia, Italy

Spronk P.E.
Department of Intensive Care, Gelre Ziekenhuizen, Apeldoorn, The Netherlands

Taylor N.
Department of Medical Microbiology, University of Liverpool, Liverpool, UK

Thorburn K.
Department of Pediatric Intensive Care, Alder Hey Children's Hospital, ,
Liverpool, UK

Tomasini A.
Department of Perioperative Medicine, Intensive Care and Emergency, University
of Trieste, Cattinara Hospital, Trieste, Italy

Tong C.Y.W.
Department of Infection, Guy's and St. Thomas' Hospital Trust and Department
of Infectious Disease, GKT School of Medicine, St. Thomas' Hospital,
London, UK

Torres A.
Institut Clínic de Pneumologia i Cirurgia Toràcica, Hospital Clínic,
Universitat de Barcelona, Spain

Vallés J.
Intensive Care Department, Hospital Sabadell, Sabadell, Spain

van der Spoel J.I.
Department of Intensive Care, OLV Gasthuis, Amsterdam, The Netherlands

van der Voort P.H.J.
Department of Intensive Care, Medical Center Leeuwarden,
Leeuwarden, The Netherlands

van Saene H.K.F.
Department of Medical Microbiology, University of Liverpool, Alder Hey
Children's Hospital, NHS Trust, Liverpool, UK

van Saene J.J.M.
Department of Pharmaceutical Technology, University of Groningen,
Groningen, The Netherlands

Viviani M.
Department of Perioperative Medicine, Intensive Care and Emergency, University
of Trieste, Cattinara Hospital, Trieste, Italy

Zandstra D.F.
Department of Intensive Care, Onze Lieve Vrouwe Gasthuis Hospital,
Amsterdam, The Netherlands

Authors' Index

ABELLA A., 49
ALCOCK S.R., 171
ALCÓN A., 315
ALÍA I., 429
ALVAREZ-ROCHA L., 495
BAINES P.B., 593
BARCENILLA-GAITE F., 495
BERLOT G., 537
BRISINDA G., 379
CASTAGNETO G., 379
CERDÀ E., 49, 191, 429
COOKE F.J., 155
CORBELLA X., 247
DAMJANOVIC V., 247, 415
DE GAUDIO A.R., 91, 213
DE LA CAL M.A., 3, 49, 191, 429
DE SILVESTRE A., 231
DI FILIPPO A., 213
FÀBREGAS N., 315
FARIAS J., 415
FERNÀNDEZ-VILADRICH P.F., 337
FERRER R., 337
FONTANA F., 73
GARCIA-HIERRO P., 49, 73
GULLO A., 297
HUGHES J., 191
ISCRA F., 549
IZQUIERDO G., 73
KERR S., 297
LOWRY K.G., 621
MARIA G., 379
MARSHALL J.C., 605, 621
MARSHALL K.A.M., 605
MARTÍNEZ-PELLÚS A., 455
MINO G., 37
NARDI G., 231
NOVELLI A., 91

NUNN A.J., 575
PALOMAR M., 455
PASTOR-BENAVENT J., 495
PETROS A.J., 415, 621
PIGNA A., 415
PIZER B.P., 171
POLLOCK K., 575
RANDINO A., 549
RASCADO-SEDES P., 495
REILLY N.J., 231, 575, 593
RINALDI S., 91
RIOS G., 15
ROGERS T., 155
ROMMES J.H., 515
ROSSENEU S., 15
SANCHEZ M., 171
SARGINSON R.E., 3
SCHELENZ S., 469
SELBY A., 515
SGANGA G., 379
SILVESTRI L., 37, 61, 297
SPRONK P.E., 15
TAYLOR N., 3, 191, 593
THORBURN K., 565
TOMASINI A., 537
TONG C.Y.W., 469
TORRES A., 315
VALLÉS J., 337
VAN DER SPOEL J.I., 247
VAN DER VOORT P.H.J., 565
VAN SAENE H.K.F., 3, 37, 61, 73, 231, 247, 429, 565, 593, 621
VAN SAENE J.J.M., 15
VIVIANI M., 61, 537
ZANDSTRA D.F., 515, 565

SECTION ONE
ESSENTIALS IN CLINICAL MICROBIOLOGY

Chapter 1

Glossary of Terms and Definitions

R.E. Sarginson, N. Taylor, M.A. de la Cal, H.K.F. van Saene

Introduction

Definitions of terms are important to avoid ambiguity, particularly in an era of global communication. Several words have often been used in an imprecise fashion in the past, including "sepsis", "nosocomial", "colonization", and even "infection". Although standardization in terminology is useful, frequent revisions will be needed in an era of rapid change in biomedical knowledge.

Definitions can be based on a variety of concepts, varying from abnormalities in patient physiology and clinical features to sophisticated laboratory methods. A thoughtful introduction to clinical terminology can be found in the extensive writings of A.R. Feinstein [1, 2], who made use of set theory and Venn diagrams to categorize clinical conditions. The choice of boundaries between sets or values on measurement scales can be difficult. In practice such boundaries, which are used to differentiate between the presence, the absence, and/or the severity of a condition, are often somewhat fuzzy, for example, in the diagnosis of ventilator-associated pneumonia [3].

The situation is further complicated by considering problems in measurement and the timing of assessments. An apparently simple criterion such as temperature measurement is subject to variation in time, site, and technique of measurement, together with errors from device malfunction, displacement, or misuse. Most definitions of infection at various sites include fever as a necessary criterion, typically temperature $\geq 38.3^{\circ}C$. Do we have good evidence that this criterion is a reliable discriminator, in conjunction with other "necessary" criteria, in distinguishing the presence or absence of a particular type of infection [4]?

Roger Bone raised some important issues a decade ago [5–8] for the terms "sepsis" and "inflammation", a debate that continues. Other interesting approaches in the fields of sepsis, the systemic inflammatory response, and multiple organ dysfunction are the use of "physiological state space" concepts by Siegel et al. [9] and ideas from "complex adaptive system" and network theory [10–13].

The glossary described here forms a basis for our clinical practice in various aspects of intensive care infection and microbiology. We advocate definitions that are usable in routine clinical practice and that emphasize the role of surveillance samples in classifying the origins of infection.

Terms and Definitions

Acquisition

A patient is considered to have acquired a micro-organism when a single surveillance sample is positive for a strain that differs from previous and subsequent isolates. This is a transient phenomenon, in contrast to the more-persistent state of carriage.

Carriage/Carrier State

The same strain of micro-organism is isolated from two or more surveillance samples in a particular patient. In practice, consecutive throat and/or rectal surveillance samples taken twice a week (Monday and Thursday) yield identical strains.

Normal carrier state. Surveillance samples yield only the indigenous aerobic and anaerobic flora, including *Escherichia coli* in the rectum. Varying percentages of people carry "community" or "normal" potential pathogens in the throat and/or gut. *Streptococcus pneumoniae* and *Hemophilus influenzae* are carried in the oropharynx by more than half of the healthy population. *Staphylococcus aureus* and yeasts are carried in the throat and gut by up to a third of healthy people.

Abnormal carrier state. Opportunistic "abnormal" aerobic Gram-negative bacilli (AGNB) or methicillin-resistant *S. aureus* (MRSA) are persistently present in the oropharynx and/or rectum. MRSA and AGNB are listed under "hospital or abnormal micro-organisms". *E. coli,* isolated from the oropharynx in high concentrations ($>3+$ or $>10^5$ CFU/ml), also represents an abnormal carrier state.

Supercarriage (secondary carriage). Commonly used antibiotics eliminate "community" or "normal" bacteria such as *S. pneumoniae* or *H. influenzae*, but promote the acquisition and subsequent carriage of abnormal AGNB and MRSA. This phenomenon is sometimes referred to as *super* or *secondary* carriage. Overgrowth with micro-organisms of low pathogenicity, such as coagulase-negative staphylococci and enterococci, can also occur during selective decontamination of the digestive tract (SDD). Such organisms are not targeted by SDD protocols.

Central Nervous System Infections

This important group includes the terms meningitis, meningo-encephalitis, encephalitis, and ventriculitis and shunt infection. These conditions have some overlap and may also co-exist with sinus or mastoid infections and septicemia. Microbiological diagnosis usually rests on culture of cerebrospinal fluid (CSF). Frequently, lumbar puncture is contraindicated in suspected meningitis [14]. For example, in meningococcal infection, contraindications include a coagulopathy or where computed tomography (CT) scan features suggest a risk of tentorial pressure coning where lumbar puncture is to be performed. Also empirical antibiotics have frequently been started prior to hospital admission. These issues are particularly important in pediatric practice, where meningococcal DNA detection in blood and/or CSF by polymerase chain reaction [PCR] assays, together with bacterial antigen tests, improves diagnostic yield [15]. The use of molecular techniques including PCR in the detection of septicaemia in critically ill patients is still in the development stage but shows great promise [16]. The usual non-specific criteria of fever or hypothermia, leukocytosis or leukopenia, and tachycardia are present, with specific symptoms that may include headache, lethargy, neck stiffness, irritability, fits, and coma. Cut-off values depend on age and should be defined at age-specific percentile thresholds for physiological variables, e.g., >90th percentile for heart rate. Detailed definitions would require a separate chapter!

Colonization

Micro-organisms are present in body sites that are normally sterile, such as the lower airways or bladder. Clinical features of infection are absent. Diagnostic samples yield ≤1+ leukocytes per high power field [17] and microbial growth is high <3+ or <10^5 CFU/ml.

"Community" or "Normal" Micro-Organisms

These are micro-organisms carried by varying percentages of healthy people. These include *S. aureus, S. pneumoniae, H. influenzae, Moraxella catarrhalis, E. coli*, and *Candida albicans*.

Defense

Against carriage. The defense mechanisms of the oropharynx and gastrointestinal tract to prevent abnormal carrier states, e.g., fibronectin, saliva, and gastric secretions.

Against colonization. The defense mechanisms of internal organs against microbial invasion, e.g., the muco-ciliary elevator in the airways and secreted immunoglobulins.

Against infection. The defense mechanisms of the internal organs, beyond skin and mucosa, include antibodies, lymphocytes, and neutrophils.

"Hospital" or "Abnormal" Micro-Organisms

These include micro-organisms carried by people with chronic disease or those admitted to the intensive care unit (ICU) from in-patient wards or other hospitals. These are typically AGNB or MRSA. AGNB include *Pseudomonas, Stenotrophomonas, Acinetobacter, Klebsiella, Enterobacter, Serratia, Proteus,* and *Morganella* spp. These organisms are rarely carried by healthy people.

Infection

This can be remarkably difficult to define in clinical circumstances. Patients have often received empirical antibiotics. In principle, infection is a microbiologically proven, clinical diagnosis of local and/or generalized inflammation. The microbiological criteria conventionally include $\geq 10^5$ CFU/ml of diagnostic sample from the infected organ and $\geq 2+$ leukocytes present per high-power field in the sample. The thresholds chosen for clinical features and laboratory measurements depend on the age of the patient and the timing of assessment. These may include temperature changes, heart rate, and changes in heart rate variability [10], white cell counts, C-reactive protein [18], and procalcitonin [19, 20].

Infections can be classified according to the concept of the *carrier state* [21]. Primary endogenous infection is caused by micro-organisms carried by the patient at the time of admission to the ICU, including both "normal" and "abnormal" micro-organisms.

Secondary endogenous infection is caused by micro-organisms acquired on the ICU and not present in the admission flora. These micro-organisms usually belong to the "abnormal" group. Potentially pathogenic micro-organisms are acquired in the oropharynx, followed by carriage and overgrowth in the digestive tract. Subsequently colonization and then infection of internal organs may occur following migration or translocation across the gut mucosa into the lymphatics or bloodstream is possible.

Exogenous infection is caused by micro-organisms introduced into the patient from the ICU environment. Organisms are transferred directly, omitting the stage of carriage, to a site where colonization and then infection occurs.

Inflammatory Markers

These are cells and proteins associated with the pro-inflammatory process. These include C-reactive protein [18], procalcitonin [19, 20], tumor necrosis factor-α, interleukins-1 and -6 [22], lymphocytes, and neutrophils. The onset, magnitude, and duration of changes in these factors vary with site and severity of infection.

ICU Infection

ICU infection refers to secondary endogenous and exogenous infections – infections due to organisms not carried by the patient at the time of admission to the ICU [23]. The term "nosocomial" (literally "related to the hospital") is in widespread use, but lacks a precise definition and should probably be abandoned!

Intra-Abdominal Infection

This is an infection of an abdominal organ and of the peritoneal cavity (peritonitis). Peritonitis can be a local or general inflammation of the peritoneal cavity. Local signs such as tenderness and guarding may be difficult to elicit in sedated ICU patients. Generalized, non-specific, features are fever (temperature $\geq 38.3^\circ C$), leukocytosis (WBC >12,000/mm^3) or leukopenia (WBC <4,000/mm^3). Ultrasonography and/or CT evaluation may contribute to the diagnosis. Isolation of micro-organisms from diagnostic samples at a concentration of $\geq 3+$ or $\geq 10^5$ CFU/ml, with $\geq 2+$ leukocytes confirms the diagnosis. Specific examples include fecal peritonitis due to colon perforation and peritonitis associated with peritoneal dialysis.

Isolation

Patients are nursed in separate cubicles or rooms, with strict hygiene measures, including protective clothing and hand washing, to control transmission of micro-organisms. These measures particularly apply to patients infected with high level pathogens or resistant micro-organisms and those with impaired immunity.

Micro-Organisms

Micro-organisms can be ranked by pathogenicity into three types.

Highly pathogenic micro-organisms can cause infection in an individual with a normal defense capacity, e.g., *Salmonella* spp.

Potentially pathogenic micro-organisms can cause infection in a patient with impaired defense mechanisms, e.g., *S. pneumoniae* in community practice and *Pseudomonas aeruginosa* in hospital practice. These two types of microbes cause both morbidity and mortality.

Microbes of low pathogenicity cause infection under special circumstances only, e.g., anaerobes can cause abscesses when tissue necrosis is present. Low level pathogens in general only cause morbidity.

Intrinsic pathogenicity refers to the capacity to cause infection. The intrinsic pathogenicity index (IPI) is defined as the ratio of the number of patients who develop an infection due to a particular micro-organism and the number of patients who carry the organism in throat and/or rectum. Indigenous flora, including anaerobes and *Streptococcus viridans*, rarely cause infections despite being carried in high concentrations. The IPI is typically in the range 0.01-0.03. Coagulase-negative staphylococci and enterococci are also carried in the oropharynx in high concentrations, but are unable to cause lower airway infections. High-level pathogens, such as *Salmonella* spp, have an IPI approaching 1 in the gut. Potentially pathogenic micro-organisms have an IPI in the range 0.1-0.3. These include the "community" or "normal" microbes and the "hospital" or "abnormal" AGNBs, which are the targets of SDD.

Migration

Migration is the process whereby micro-organisms carried in the throat and gut move to colonize and possibly infect internal organs. Migration is promoted by underlying chronic disease, some drugs, and invasive devices.

Outbreak

An outbreak is defined as an event where two or more patients in a defined location are infected by identical micro-organisms, usually within an arbitrary time period of 2 weeks. Such episodes often occur with multi-resistant micro-organisms such as *Pseudomonas*, MRSA, or vancomycin-resistant enterococci. In the pediatric ICU, viruses such as respiratory syncytial virus or rotavirus can also be a major problem. Outbreak of *carriage* of microbes may have considerable significance for infection control.

Overgrowth

Overgrowth is defined as the presence of a high concentration of potentially pathogenic micro-organisms, ≥3+ or $\geq 10^5$ CFU/ml, in surveillance samples from the digestive tract [24]. Overgrowth in the small intestine can induce a state of systemic immunoparalysis. Overgrowth is also a risk factor for the colonization and infection of internal organs, translocation into the blood stream, selection of resistant micro-organisms, and transmission of organisms between patients.

Pneumonia

Microbiologically confirmed pneumonia
1. Presence of new or progressive infiltrates on a chest X-ray for ≥48 h and
2. Fever ≥38.3ºC and
3. Leukocytosis (WBC >12,000/ml) or leukopenia (WBC <4,000/ml) and
4. Purulent tracheal aspirate containing ≥2+ WBC per high-power field and
5. Tracheal aspirate specimen yielding $\geq 10^5$ CFU/ml or
6. Protected brush specimen (PBS) yielding $>10^3$ CFU/ml or
7. Broncho-alveolar lavage (BAL) specimen yielding $>10^4$ CFU/ml

Clinical diagnosis only. This is when criteria 1-4 fulfilled, but tracheal aspirates, PBS, or BAL are sterile. Criteria for the diagnosis of pneumonias remain controversial [3]. The situation is sometimes complicated by viral etiologies and/or prior antibiotic treatment, particularly in infants and children. There is also overlap with other pathophysiological terms, such as pneumonitis and bronchiolitis.

Resistance

A micro-organism is considered to be resistant to a particular antimicrobial agent if:
1. The minimal inhibiting concentration of the antimicrobial agent against a colonizing or infecting microbial species is higher than the non-toxic blood concentration after systemic administration.
2. The minimum bactericidal concentration of the antimicrobial agent against microbes carried in throat and gut is higher than the non-toxic concentration achieved by enteral administration.

Samples

Diagnostic. Diagnostic or clinical samples are taken from sites that are normally sterile to diagnose infection or evaluate response to therapy. Samples are taken on clinical indication only from blood, lower airways, CSF, urinary tract, wounds, peritoneum, joints, sinuses, or conjunctiva.

Surveillance. Surveillance samples are taken from the oropharynx and rectum on admission and subsequently at regular intervals (usually twice weekly). These specimens are needed to:
1.   Evaluate the carriage of potentially pathogenic micro-organisms
2.   Assess the eradication of potential pathogens by non-absorbable antimicrobial regimens used in SDD protocols
3.   Detect the carriage of resistant strains

Selective Decontamination of the Digestive Tract

The full SDD protocol has four components [23, 25]:
1.   A parenteral antibiotic is administered for the first few days to prevent or control primary endogenous infection (e.g., cefotaxime)
2.   Non-absorbable antimicrobials are administered into the oropharynx and gastrointestinal tract, when surveillance cultures show abnormal carriage. The usual combination is polymyxin E (colistin), tobramycin, and amphotericin B (PTA).
3.   A high standard of hygiene is required to prevent exogenous infection episodes.
4.   Regular surveillance samples of throat and rectum are obtained to diagnose carrier states and monitor the efficacy of SDD.
      The policy at Alder Hey is to use SDD "à la carte", guided by the abnormal carrier state detected by surveillance samples. However, most ICUs that use SDD start the regimen on admission, irrespective of surveillance swab results.

Systemic Inflammatory Response Syndrome, Sepsis, Septic Shock

Definitions for systemic inflammatory response syndrome (SIRS), sepsis, severe sepsis, and septic shock have been extensively reviewed in the last decade, particularly in relation to the inclusion criteria for clinical trials [8, 26, 27]. Consensus definitions form categories based on cut-off points in a number of variables. Cut-off points based on indices of perfusion can be difficult to evaluate in practice. Furthermore, a patient's clinical state can change rapidly [28]. Microbiological confirmation or exclusion of infection may occur a considerable time after the clinical diagnosis of septic states. The cut-offs and thresholds have to be adjusted in the pediatric population [29].

Systemic inflammatory response syndrome is the systemic inflammatory response to a wide variety of clinical insults [8, 30, 31], manifested by two or more of the following
1.   Temperature >38 or <36°C
2.   Heart rate >90 beats per minute

3. Respiratory rate >20 breaths per minute
4. White blood cell count >12,000/mm^3 or <4,000mm^3, or >10% immature forms

Sepsis is defined as SIRS with a clear infectious etiology.

Septicaemia is sepsis with a positive blood culture. In contrast, bacteraemia is defined as a positive blood culture exhibiting no clinical symptoms.

Severe sepsis is defined as sepsis with organ dysfunction, hypoperfusion, or hypotension. Manifestations of hypoperfusion may include, but are not limited to, lactic acidosis, oliguria, and acute alterations in mental state.

Septic shock is sepsis-induced hypotension, persisting despite adequate fluid resuscitation, together with manifestations of hypoperfusion. Hypotension is defined as a systolic blood pressure <90 mmHg or a reduction of >40 mmHg from baseline in the absence of other causes of hypotension.

Sinusitis

Sinusitis is infection of the paranasal sinuses - maxillary, ethmoidal, frontal, or sphenoidal. Symptoms and signs such as localized tenderness and purulent discharge may be absent in the sedated ICU patient. Fever (temperature ≥38.3°C) and leukocytosis (WBC >12,000/mm^3) or leukopenia (WBC <4,000/mm^3) are the main clinical features. Plain radiographs or CT imaging may show fluid levels of obliteration in the sinus air spaces. Surgical drainage is performed to obtain microbiological confirmation (≥3+ or ≥10^5 CFU/ml of pus, together with ≥2+ leukocytes).

Tracheitis, bronchitis

In the absence of pulmonary infiltrates on the chest X-ray tracheitis/bronchitis is defined as:
1. Purulent tracheal aspirate and
2. Fever >38.3°C and
3. Leukocytosis (WBC >12,000/mm^3) or leukopenia (WBC <4,000/mm^3)
4. ≥10^5 CFU/ml of tracheal aspirate

Translocation (Transmural Migration)

Translocation is defined as the passage of viable micro-organisms from the throat and gut through mucosal barriers to regional lymph nodes and internal organs, including the blood.

Transmission

Transmission is defined as the spread of micro-organisms between patients, by means of "vectors" such as the hands of carers. Measures to control transmission include isolation, hand washing, protective clothing, and care of equipment.

Urinary Tract Infection

Urinary tract infection is defined as infection of the urinary tract, most frequently the bladder. The common clinical features of dysuria, suprapubic pain, frequency, and urgency are often absent in the sedated ICU patient. The diagnosis rests on a freshly voided catheter urine specimen or suprapubic sample containing $\geq 10^5$ bacteria or yeasts/ml of urine and ≥ 5 WBC per high-power field.

Wound Infection

Wound infection is defined as purulent discharge from wounds, signs of local inflammation, and a culture yielding $\geq 3+$ or $\geq 10^5$ CFU/ml. The isolation of skin flora in the absence of these features is considered contamination.

References

1. Feinstein AR (1967) Clinical judgment. Williams and Wilkins, Baltimore
2. Feinstein AR (1994) Clinical judgment revisited: the distraction of quantitative models. Ann Intern Med 120:799-805
3. Bonten M (1999) Controversies on diagnosis and prevention of ventilator-associated pneumonia. Diagn Microbiol infect Dis 34:199-204
4. Toltzis P, Rosolowski B, Salvator A (2001) Etiology of fever and opportunities for reduction of antibiotic use in a pediatric intensive care unit. Infect Control Hosp Epidemiol 22:499-504
5. Bone RC (1991) Let's agree on terminology: definitions of sepsis. Crit Care Med 19:973-976
6. Canadian Multiple Organ Failure Study Group (1991) "Sepsis" – clarity of existing terminology…or more confusion? Crit Care Med 19:996-998
7. Bone RC, Grodzin CJ, Balk RA (1997) Sepsis: a new hypothesis for pathogenesis of the disease process. Chest 112:235-243
8. Levy MM, Fink MP, Marshall JC et al (2003) 2001 SCCM/ESICM/ACCP/ATS/SIS International Sepsis Definitions Conference. Crit Care Med 31:1250-1256
9. Rixen D, Siegel JH, Friedman HP (1996) "Sepsis/SIRS," physiologic classification, severity stratification, relation to cytokine elaboration and outcome prediction in post-trauma critical illness. J Trauma 41:581-598
10. Seeley AJE, Christou NV (2000) Multiple organ dysfunction syndrome: exploring the

paradigm of complex non-linear systems. Crit Care Med 28:2193-2200

11. Toweill DL, Goldstein B (1998) Linear and nonlinear dynamics and the pathophysiology of shock. New Horiz 6:155-168

12. Aird WC (2002) Endothelial cell dynamics and complexity theory. Crit Care Med 30 [Suppl]:S180-S185

13. Strogatz SH (2001) Exploring complex networks. Nature 410:268-276

14. Smith TL, Nathan BR (2002) Central nervous system infections in the immune-competent adult. Curr Treat Options Neurol 4:323-332

15. Carrol ED, Thomson AP, Shears P et al (2000) Performance characteristics of the polymerase chain reaction assay to confirm clinical meningococcal disease. Arch Dis Child 83:271-273

16. Cursons RTM, Jeyerajah E, Sleigh JW (1999) The use of the polymerase chain reaction to detect septicemia in critically ill patients. Crit Care Med 27:937-940

17. A'Court CHD, Garrard CS, Crook D et al (1993) Microbiological lung surveillance in mechanically ventilated patients, using non-directed bronchial lavage and quantitative culture. Q J Med 86:635-648

18. Reny JL, Vuagnat A, Ract C et al (2002) Diagnosis and follow up of infections in intensive care patients: value of C-reactive protein compared with other clinical and biological variables. Crit Care Med 30:529-535

19. Claeys R, Vinken S, Spapen H et al (2002) Plasma procalcitonin and C-reactive protein in acute septic shock: clinical and biological correlates. Crit Care Med 30:757-762

20. Christ-Crain M, Jaccard-Stolz D, Bingisser R et al (2004) Effect of procalcitonin-guided treatment on antibiotic use and outcome in lower respiratory tract infections: cluster-randomised, single-blinded intervention trial. Lancet 363:600-607

21. van Saene HKF , Damjanovic V, Murray AE, de la Cal MA (1996) How to classify infections in intensive care units – the carrier state, a criterion whose time has come? J Hosp Infect 33:1-12

22. Dinarello CA (2000) Pro-inflammatory cytokines. Chest 118:503-508

23. Sarginson RE, Taylor N, Reilly N et al (2004) Infection in prolonged pediatric critical illness: a prospective four-year study based on knowledge of the carrier state. Crit Care Med 32:839-847

24. Husebye E (1995) Gastrointestinal mobility disorders and bacterial overgrowth. J Intern Med 237:419-427

25. Baxby D, van Saene HKF, Stoutenbeek CP, Zandstra DF (1996) Selective decontamination of the digestive tract: 13 years on, what it is, what it is not. Intensive Care Med 22:699-706

26. Brun-Buisson C (2000) The epidemiology of the systemic inflammatory response. Intensive Care Med 26 [Suppl]:S64-S74

27. Cohen J, Guyatt G, Bernard GR et al (2001) New strategies for clinical trials in patients with sepsis and septic shock. Crit Care Med 29:880-886

28. Rangel-Frausto MS, Pittet D, Costigan M et al (1995) The natural history of the systemic inflammatory response syndrome (SIRS). A prospective study. JAMA 273:117-123

29. Watson RS, Carcillo JA, Linde-Zwirble WT et al (2003) The epidemiology of severe sepsis in children in the United States. Am J Respir Crit Care Med 167:695-701

30. Marik PE (2002) Definition of sepsis: not quite time to dump SIRS. Crit Care Med 30:706-708

31. Zahorec R (2000) Definitions for the septic syndrome should be re-evaluated. Intensive Care Med 26:1870

Chapter 2

Carriage

S. Rosseneu, G. Rios, P.E. Spronk, J.J.M. van Saene

Host Defence Against Microbial Carriage Guarantees a Normal, Stable Flora

What is Normal Flora?

Only healthy people carry normal flora in throat and gut [1]. Normal flora comprises mainly of anaerobic bacteria requiring a low oxygen tension. These indigenous micro-organisms are present in high concentrations, 10^8 anaerobes per ml of saliva and 10^{12} per g of feces. Aerobic micro-organisms grow easily in the presence of oxygen and are also present in the human body. However, their concentrations are 10^4 lower than the anaerobic concentrations. Everybody carries their own indigenous aerobic Gram-negative bacillus (AGNB), *Escherichia coli*, in a concentration of 10^3–10^6/g of feces. It is remarkable that over time the throat and gut flora does not change either qualitatively or quantitatively, illustrating the unique stability of this microbial organ system [1, 2]. Normal flora represents a living tissue that covers the inside of the digestive tract as wallpaper. The size of this bacterial tissue is enormous in terms of both numbers and weight. It has been estimated that microbial cells outnumber the human cells by a factor 10 [2], and bacteria account for 30%–50% of the volume of the contents of the human colon, this equals 41%–57% of the dry weight of colonic contents [3].

Mechanisms of Protection Against Abnormal Carriage

AGNB, including *Klebsiella, Proteus, Morganella, Enterobacter, Citrobacter, Serratia, Acinetobacter,* and *Pseudomonas,* do not belong to the normal flora. Healthy individuals efficiently clear the abnormal AGNB from the oropharyngeal cavity and the digestive tract. This clearing property is called carriage defense [4]. Individuals are continuously exposed to AGNB. Healthy people acquire AGNB in the oropharynx via food intake, whilst unconscious patients acquire the AGNB in the oropharynx from the environment, e.g., the intensive care (ICU). The source of AGNB may be the inanimate environment, such as equipment, or the animate environment, but in general the other long-stay patients represent the major source. Acquisition of AGNB by such patients generally results in carriage, as the critically ill patient is unable to clear these abnormal bacteria due to underlying disease. Conversely, the healthy individual effectively clears the non-indigenous AGNB by means of seven mechanisms (Table 1).

Table 1. Mechanisms protecting against abnormal carriage

Intact anatomy of throat and gut

Physiology: gastric pH and fibronectin

Intestinal motility

Epithelial renewal

Gut immunity: gut-associated lymphoid tissue (GALT)

Secretions: saliva, bile, and mucus

Indigenous anaerobic flora

Intact anatomy. The alimentary canal is an 8-m long tube-like structure starting at the lips and ending at the anus; several layers compose the gut wall (Fig. 1). The structure of the intestinal wall differs according to the anatomical position in the intestinal canal. The relative stasis at the oropharyngeal level is responsible for the large number of indigenous bacteria in the saliva. The esophagus, stomach, and small intestine are free from microbes, mainly as a result of gut motility. The even more-pronounced stasis at the colonic level explains the higher concentrations of the indigenous flora in the feces compared with saliva. The inner surface of the gut is covered with a sticky mucus layer in which the indigenous flora is embedded [5]. The mucus layer also contains the glycoprotein fibronectin. Beneath the mucus layer there are the extended fields of villi that, with a surface of about 500 m^2, are responsible for absorption. The terminal ileum, the last part of the small intestine, functions as a window through which nutrition can be brought in. However, that terminal ileum also represents a leak through which micro-organisms and their toxic products gain access to the body. A tissue called gut-associated lymphoid tissue (GALT) surrounds the small intestine. The GALT, a huge and potent organ, aims to control both local and systemic inflammation. Inflammation would invariably occur as a consequence of microbial invasion. A layer of muscle required for the gut motility surrounds the GALT. Motility is the main factor that determines the expulsion of food and abnormal bacteria from the body [6]. Any impairment of

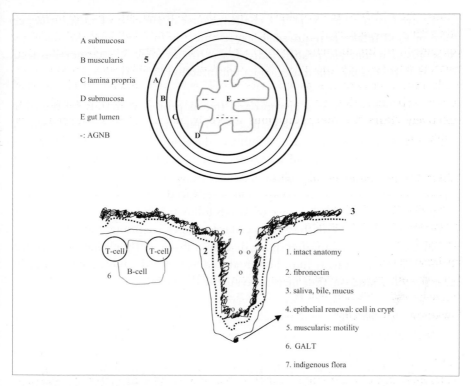

Fig. 1. This figure represents the seven factors providing anatomy and carriage defence

anatomical integrity may result in abnormal AGNB carriage. As long as clearing mechanisms, including chewing, swallowing, and intestinal motility, are intact, bacterial overgrowth, defined as the presence of $\geq 10^5$ AGNB/ml of saliva or g of feces [7], is unlikely to develop.

Physiology: gastric acid barrier. There are specialized cells in the antral wall of the stomach, called the parietal cells, that produce acid, i.e., hydrochloride. Hydrochloride promotes the digestion of food and contributes to the control of micro-organisms present in food and beverages. The pH of the empty stomach is 2; the pH increases to 6.7 following a meal and returns to the pH of an empty stomach within 2 h [8]. Microbes, in particular the abnormal AGNB, are killed by pH values of less than 4, the contact time required being a minimal of 15 min [9]. Any severe underlying disease may impair the exocrine function of the stomach; such as in the critically ill patient who requires ventilation [10]. Patients who require at least 3 days of ventilation invariably have a pH over 4. Thus, the gastric acid barrier fails and may lead to bacterial overgrowth [11]. Patients who take acid inhibitors all have a gastric pH of more than 4 and hence an impaired gastric barrier [12]. A challenge dose of 10^2 cells of *Salmonella* per gram of food intake is required to cause enteritis in a patient who takes H_2 antagonists. In contrast, healthy individuals with an intact gastric barrier need minimally 10^5 *Salmonella* to develop a gut infection [13, 14].

Physiology: fibronectin is a glycoprotein that is produced mainly by the liver and found in plasma and on cell surfaces. Fibronectin is excreted via saliva, bile, and mucus and covers the mucosal lining of the alimentary canal [15]. Digestive tract mucosa is hypothesized to express receptors for abnormal AGNB, and under normal conditions the fibronectin layer covers these receptors in order to prevent adherence of AGNB [16]. Thus, a reduced fibronectin concentration results in an increased adherence of AGNB following the increased availability of AGNB receptor sites on the mucosa. Macrophages are thought to release elastase in the presence of an underlying disease. Subsequently, elastase is excreted by saliva, bile, and mucus into the throat and gut, and denudes the fibronectin layer from the mucosa, thus making available the AGNB receptor sites [17].

Secretions: saliva, bile, and mucus. Large quantities of secretions are daily excreted into the oropharynx and the intestine, e.g., 1 l of saliva and 0.5 l of bile per day. Although several antibacterial substances are present in saliva and in bile, the "gliding" factor is primarily responsible for the inability of bacteria to adhere to a wet gut surface [18]. Patients who receive total parenteral nutrition (TPN) do not use their gut, the gall bladder does not contract, and the concentration of bile in feces is significantly lower [19]. Paralysis of the gut by its non-use is thought to be an important factor contributing to AGNB overgrowth in TPN [20]. The gastrointestinal mucosal lining excretes mucus that—as a sticky layer—covers and protects the gut mucosa [5]. Mucin is the most-important component of mucus and is responsible for the viscosity and the elasticity of the gel-like mucus. The "stickiness" of mucus makes it ideal for trapping AGNB. The mucus secretion with the trapped AGNB are effectively and continually removed and replaced by fresh secretions. Animals who were parenterally fed [21], or received endotoxin challenge [22], had less mucus in the gut lumen and there was less mucin in the mucus layer. The bacterial adherence was enhanced and translocation of *E. coli* was demonstrated.

Motility. In the digestive tract there is ongoing motility even while fasting. During meals, the motility pattern ensures adequate mixing of the ingested food with digestive enzymes and secretions, and allows a prolonged contact between the food and the intestinal mucosa, optimizing digestion and nutrient absorption. After the meal this "feeding motility pattern" is disrupted and replaced by the "fasting motility pattern". During the fasting state, the gastrointestinal tract is characterized by a regular, cyclical and contractile activity, characterized by the interdigestive migrating motor complex (MMC) [6]. The MMC is a typical cycling complex of myo-electrical activity and associated contractile activity, the aim being the flushing out of food remnants, cell debris, and bacteria [6]. In humans the MMC occurs every 100 min and migrates along the upper digestive tract at a speed of about 6–8 cm/min [23]. This moving band of intense contractions has been called the intestinal housekeeper. This housekeeper function, through the clearance of luminal contents including bacteria, is the most important factor in the carriage defense against overgrowth of abnormal flora [6]. When intestinal motility is impaired, bacteria accumulate, leading to overgrowth [24]. Depending on the severity of the underlying disease, gut paralysis is associated with overgrowth of either normal [25] or abnormal flora [26, 27].

Epithelial renewal. The intestinal epithelial layer constitutes an interface of immense proportions lying between the host and the environment, an interface that simultaneously serves as a barrier and as a selective portal of entry. The epithelial mucosal cells have a rapid turnover, which explains why these cells are highly dependent on adequate nutritional supply and oxygen availability [28]. The most important stimulus for intestinal epithelial growth and functioning is the presence of nutrients in the gut lumen [29]. The direct presence of nutrients creates a mechanical stimulus and provides local substrate for increased growth of enterocytes. Indirectly, the presence of nutrients mediates an effect through production of trophic gastrointestinal hormones. The single cell layer of epithelial cells covering the mucosa is in a continuous state of turnover [30]. Undifferentiated epithelial cells proliferate in the crypts of Lieberkuhn and travel up onto the villus, differentiating and maturing as they proceed, until functional mature cells are found on the top of the villus. After a short but usually active life, the cells are lost into the lumen of the intestine. The turnover time for normal intestinal epithelium is 2–5 days, and it has been calculated that 250 mg in weight of epithelial cells is shed into the lumen each day. A uniform finding in a number of animal species has been that in the absence of the indigenous flora the epithelial renewal process is slowed down [31]. The mitotic index of epithelial cells is lower, the generation cycle is prolonged, and the pool of proliferating cells is smaller. Also, the transit time of the cells moving along the villous surface is prolonged and the average age of epithelial cells correspondingly increased. This condition in the germ-free host is rapidly shifted towards normalization of mucosal renewal during recolonization with indigenous, anaerobic flora [31].

The gut-associated lymphoid tissue. The AGNB encounter their host via the mucosal surface of the digestive tract. Once carried at this site, the AGNB may migrate into the normally sterile internal organs of the body, causing inflammation of lungs and bladder. Consequently, the human being has evolved sophisticated immune tissues and mechanisms for controlling microbial replication on, and spread from, these digestive tract surfaces. The mucosa-associated immune tissue of the digestive tract is called the GALT (Fig. 2) and is the largest lymphoid tissue in the body, 20% of body lymphoid tissue is found in the bone marrow and 80% in the GALT [32]. The GALT protects the gut against the continuing exposure to the ingested AGNB. The GALT includes: (1) the follicle-associated gut epithelium or dome epithelium, (2) aggregated lymphoid follicles or the patches of Peyer containing T and B lymphocytes, (3) solitary lymphoid follicles, (4) the lamina propria with its lymphoid cells, and (5) the liver. The small intestine of a young adult contains around 250 Peyer's patches. However, there are at least 10-20 times as many solitary follicles [33]. The dome epithelium that covers the patches of Peyer contains Microfold cells (M cells) and lymphocytes. Of 5 gut epithelial cells, 1 cell is a lymphocyte, in general a T lymphocyte. These intra-epithelial T lymphocytes form a front against the AGNB and control the immune response both locally at gut level and generally at the systemic level. The first step in the induction of an immune response involves the uptake of the AGNB. The M cells, albeit few in number, are crucial in eliciting the immune response: they recognize and transport the AGNB through the mucosal lining towards the underlying macrophages. The

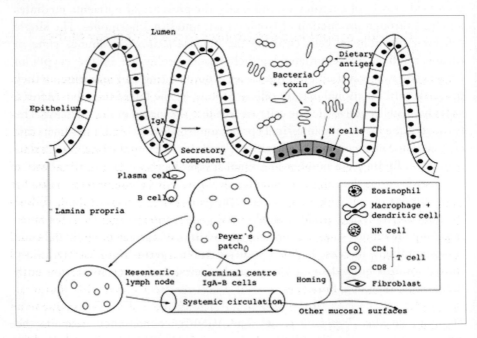

Fig. 2. Gut-associated lymphoid tissue

macrophages and dendritic cells process and present the AGNB to a T lymphocyte in the Peyer's patches. The T cells activated by the AGNB release cytokines, which stimulate the B lymphocytes, present in the center of the Peyer's patches, into the release of IgA. An adult produces on average 4.5 g of IgA per day in order to control these AGNB [34]. The B cells primed by the T lymphocytes are in an activated state. They migrate from the Peyer's patches via the lymph, thoracic duct, vena subclavia, and systemic circulation, returning or homing to the lamina propria of the digestive tract that is exposed to the incoming AGNB (Fig. 2). Secretory IgA (s-IgA), released during this migration, is the most-common immunoglobulin in saliva, bile, and mucus. Every day, intestinal B lymphocytes produce more immunoglobulins than do all other lymphoid organs. The s-IgA excreted into the gut lumen functions as an "antiseptic paint," hence enhancing the relative impermeability of the mucosa. The protective effect of s-IgA is due to its ability to inhibit AGNB adherence to the epithelium through coating of the micro-organisms [35]. There is more immune activity in the gut than in the rest of the body combined. The challenge facing the mucosal immune regulatory processes is to discriminate between pathogens and benign antigenic material by stimulating protective immunity without excessive amounts of inflammation that would disrupt the integrity or function of the fragile mucosa. The extensive immune activity in the absence of disease has been termed physiological inflammation of the gut [33].

The Indigenous Flora Contributes to the Physiology of the Human Body

The indigenous flora comprises mainly anaerobes and the indigenous E. coli. One-third of healthy people also carries Staphylococcus aureus and Candida albicans. The indigenous flora, embedded in the mucus layer covering the gut epithelium, plays an important role in the physiology of both alimentary canal and the whole body (Table 2) [36]. There is also a close interaction between the indigenous flora and the defense mechanisms of the host. The intestinal wall of germ-free animals is thinner and lighter in weight in comparison with the intestine of animals with normal flora. This is due to a decreased GALT following reduced or absent stimuli. Without indigenous micro-organisms, the intestinal villi are shorter and flatter, leading to a loss of surface of about 30% and subsequent absorption capacity. The epithelial turnover is significantly delayed in the absence of anaerobes. The anaerobic bacteria have an important enzymatic activity, e.g., in degrading mucin. One of the most-remarkable characteristics of germ-free rodents is a pronounced enlargement of the cecum due to an accumulation of a great deal of mucin not being degraded following the absence of the indigenous flora in these germ-free animals. Hydrolysis and fer-

Table 2. Role of the indigenous flora in the physiology of the digestive tract and the whole body

---

Digestive tract

Anatomy of the intestinal wall

Morphology and renewal of the mucosa

Metabolic well-being of the mucosa by the production of volatile fatty acids, necessary for the metabolism of the intestinal cell

β-Lactamase in feces protects against the harmful side effects of antibiotics

Functioning of the endocrine intestinal cells

The whole body

Water balance

Motility of the digestive tract

Production of vitamin K

Hemodynamic balance

Conservation of cecal anatomy

Enterohepatic cycle

---

mentation of carbohydrates by indigenous flora results in the release of volatile fatty acids that are the most important source of energy for the gut epithelium, e.g., butyrate. Deconjugation of bile salts by the indigenous flora is crucial for the enterohepatic circulation. The fluid balance is impaired in animals without indigenous flora. Anaerobes produce β-lactamases that neutralize the β-lactam antibiotics following excretion via bile. Thus, the body is protected against the harmful side effects of antibiotics, including diarrhea, overgrowth of *Clostridium difficile*, yeast, AGNB, enterococci, and *S. aureus*. The indigenous flora releases biopeptides that play a role in the gastro-endocrine metabolism. The indigenous flora also plays a role in gut motility. The indigenous bacteria promote the physiological MMC. In germ-free animals, peristalsis is delayed; this is the so-called lazy-gut syndrome. Vitamins, including folate, biotin, and riboflavin, are produced by the normal flora. *Bacteroides fragilis* and *E. coli* release vitamin K in quantities sufficient to fulfil the body requirement. There is also a close interaction between the normal flora and the immunity of the host. The migration of white blood cells towards the infected peritoneal cavity is more pronounced in animals with normal flora than germ-free animals. In germ-free animals the cardiac output is reduced, hemoconcentration occurs due to reduced water absorption, and the heart contractility decreases as soon as the normal anaerobic flora is destroyed.

Normal Flora as the Microbial Factor of the Defense Against Carriage

The physiological phenomenon of the normal indigenous flora controlling the abnormal AGNB is termed "ecology". Ecology constitutes the seventh component of the carriage defense [37]. The indigenous, mainly anaerobic, flora contributes to the control of the development of carriage of acquired AGNB. This microbial factor is active at four levels: (1) the normal flora acts as a living wallpaper covering the mucosal receptor sites and in that way prevents the adherence of AGNB to those receptors; (2) the highly concentrated anaerobes require huge quantities of nutrients, resulting in the starving of incoming AGNB; (3) normal flora produces bacteriocines that are bactericidal for AGNB and release volatile fatty acids that create a growth-inhibiting environment. Finally, (4) the presence of normal flora is required for the stimulation of peristalsis in order to wash out the AGNB. Antimicrobial agents that are active against the indigenous anaerobic flora and that are excreted in lethal concentrations in saliva and feces may suppress the indigenous flora. Diarrhea and candidiasis are well-known side effects of commonly used antibiotics. The use of antimicrobial agents that disregard ecology leads to an impaired microbial factor of the carriage defense. Under these circumstances, only 10^2 *Salmonella* cells are required to cause enteritis. In contrast, for *Salmonella* to cause enteritis in an individual with normal flora, 10^5 cells are required. In addition, overgrowth of abnormal AGNB and MRSA often occurs following the impairment of the microbial factor of the carriage defense, i.e., disregard for ecology [37].

Throat and Gut Flora in the Healthy and Diseased Individual

Definition: Normal Versus Abnormal Flora

"Community" or normal potentially pathogenic micro-organisms (PPM) are distinguished from "hospital" or abnormal PPM using the criterion of severity of underlying disease [37]. The community PPM include *Haemophilus influenzae, S. aureus, Streptococcus pneumoniae,* and *E. coli.* Varying percentages of healthy people carry them. Hospital PPM are the typical opportunistic AGNB, including *Klebsiella, Enterobacter, Acinetobacter,* and *Pseudomonas* species. Only individuals with underlying pathology, both acute and chronic, are abnormal carriers of the AGNB. The healthy individual uncommonly carries AGNB in the oropharynx. Individuals in good health only carry their indigenous *E. coli* in the gut besides the physiological and low pathogenic anaerobic flora. Illness severity is hypothesized to be the most-important risk factor for AGNB receptors expressed on the mucosa of the alimentary canal [4].

Underlying Disease Is the Most Important Risk Factor

Chronic underlying pathologies. The three most common chronic diseases in adults are alcoholism, diabetes, and chronic obstructive pulmonary diseases (COPD) (Table 3). One third of patients with each of these three chronic pathologies carry abnormal flora in the throat and gut [17, 38, 39]. In COPD, there is a correlation between abnormal carriage and the severity of COPD. Of three COPD patients, one carries abnormal flora as soon as the forced expiratory volume within 1 s is less than 50% [17]. The abnormal carriage in postoperative neonates requiring TPN was 40% [25].

Table 3. Illness severity as independent risk factor for abnormal carriage of aerobic Gram-negative bacilli

	AGNB carriage	
	oropharynx	gut
A. Chronic underlying disease		
Chronic obstructive pulmonary disease [17]	30 %	
Diabetes mellitus [38]	36 %	
Alcohol abuse [39]	35 %	
Parenteral nutrition [25]		42 %
B. Acute illness		
Artificial ventilation in ICU patients		
APACHE 15 [40]	30 %	
APACHE 27 [41]	57 %	
Acute long failure [42]	64 %	
Post surgical ICU patients [43]	86 %	61 %
Severe acute pancreatitis [44, 45]		92 %
Post cardiac surgery ICU patients [46]		67 %
Medical ICU patients [47]		33 %

AGNB= aerobic Gram-negative bacilli
APACHE II= acute physiology and chronic health evaluation II score

Acute diseases. Two studies in critically ill patients on ICU show a correlation between the severity of illness and abnormal AGNB carriage [40, 41]. The severity of underlying disease can be estimated using the acute physiology and chronic health evaluation score (APACHE II). One-third of ICU patients with an APACHE II score >15 carried AGNB [40]. Abnormal carriage increased to 50% as soon as the score was >27 [41]. Another study evaluated abnormal carriage in patients requiring an ICU stay for lung failure [42]. Of these patients, 64% were still carrying abnormal AGNB on discharge from the hospital. Following recovery, the carriage of 64% returned to 16%. A literature search reveals that there are only a few prospective studies that have analyzed throat and gut flora using the criteria of normal versus abnormal flora. In surgical ICU patients, the abnormal oropharyngeal carriage was 23% in patients requiring ventilation. Abnormal gut carriage was 20% following exclusion of the indigenous *E. coli* [43]. After 10 days of ICU stay, the abnormal carriage was 86% and 61% in throat and gut, respectively. Abnormal carriage reached 100% and 69% in throat and gut after 2 weeks of ICU stay. The infectious morbidity was 74% and mortality was 25%. In a randomized multicenter study in adult patients with severe acute pancreatitis, the risk of developing an infection of the pancreas was significantly higher in the subset of patients who carried abnormal AGNB in the gut compared with patients without AGNB or who carried only their indigenous *E. coli* [44]. Abnormal AGNB carriage was associated with a 3.7 higher risk of mortality [45]. Abnormal carriage of *Enterobacter* species was evaluated in post-operative cardiac patients. In the subset of post-cardiac surgery patients who required 4 days or more of intensive care and who were identified as abnormal carriers, there were significantly more post-operative complications compared with the group of patients who did not carry *Enterobacter* (85% versus 45.5%). In addition, the abnormal carriers stayed significantly longer on the ICU, 12.2 days versus 6.9 days [46]. Another study evaluated the acquisition and subsequent carriage of abnormal AGNB in patients who only carried their own *E. coli* on admission on the ICU. Multi-resistant *Klebsiella* and *Acinetobacter* were used in this study as markers of abnormal carriage; 30% of the patients developed abnormal carriage, and again a high score of underlying disease was the independent risk factor [47]. Abnormal carriage occurs early in the 1st week following ICU admission, when the illness is more severe and the immune depression often maximal. These observations support the concept of critical illness being the most important factor in the conversion of the normal to the abnormal carrier state.

Throat and Gut Endotoxin in Health and Disease

Endotoxin or lipopolysaccharide (LPS) is a component of the cell wall of both aerobic and anaerobic Gram-negative bacteria. Both killed and living bacteria release LPS. The digestive tract is an immense reservoir of endotoxin-producing bacteria and represents the major source of endotoxin. Endotoxin, once in the bloodstream, causes all symptoms of the acute-phase reaction of generalized inflammation: fever, leukocytosis, and a change in vascular permeability. However, there are major differences in intrinsic endotoxicity [48]: LPS released by AGNB, whether *E. coli* or abnormal hospital AGNB, is over 1,000 times more potent compared with endotoxins derived from anaerobes such as *Bacteroides*, *Fusobacterium*, and *Veillonella* species. For example, a septicemia due to

Bacteroides species is likely to have a better clinical outcome than a septicemia caused by the aerobes *E. coli* or *Klebsiella* species [49]. Following absorption from the gut, endotoxins arrive in the lungs via the thoracic duct, venous circulation, and heart. Alveolar macrophages—as immune cells—function as targets for the endotoxins and cytokines generated by the AGNB. Anaerobic endotoxins are unable to stimulate the alveolar macrophages to release cytokines such as tumor necrosis factor (TNF) [50]. Moreover, the interaction between macrophages and anaerobic *Bacteroides* LPS of low endotoxicity inhibits further stimulation by aerobic *E. coli* endotoxin of high endotoxicity [51].

Normal Values

Salivary and fecal endotoxin has been measured in healthy volunteers [52, 53]. None of the volunteers carried AGNB in the throat and gut, apart from the indigenous *E. coli* in the feces at a concentration of 10^4 colony-forming units (CFU) per gram of feces. Endotoxin levels were 1 mg/ml of saliva and 1 mg/g of feces. The salivary endotoxin was released by solely oropharyngeal anaerobes, whilst fecal endotoxin was produced by the aerobic indigenous *E. coli* characterized by a 1,000 times higher endotoxicity.

Abnormal Values

Intestinal endotoxin was measured in both adults and neonates who were carriers of abnormal AGNB [54]. All were admitted to the ICU and required mechanical ventilation. The fecal endotoxin concentrations were 10 times higher than normal values.

Mechanisms Controlling Endotoxin

The same factors that constitute the defense against carriage are responsible for the control of salivary and fecal endotoxin. In particular, (1) the integrity of anatomy, physiology, and motility of the digestive tract is the first line of defense against intestinal endotoxin [55], (2) the liver has an enormous capacity for the neutralization of endotoxin [56], and (3) the last barrier: blood [57]. Bacterial endotoxin may cross the gut mucosa through tight junctions of the mucosal lining and cause portal endotoxemia. The macrophages of the liver or the Kupffer cells attempt to clear the blood of the gut endotoxin. White blood cells, platelets, and proteins neutralize the small amounts of the gut endotoxins that enter the systemic circulation. Under normal physiological conditions, the indigenous *E. coli* is thought to regulate bone marrow activity following intermittent endotoxemias [58]. This physiological function is considered one of the roles of the indigenous *E. coli*. Following absorption of small amounts of gut endotoxin, macrophages are induced to release mediators and cytokines with a regulating impact on the bone marrow.

Bacterial Overgrowth Harms the Patient

Definition

Overgrowth is defined as the presence of $\geq 3+$ or $\geq 10^5$ CFU of PPM per ml of saliva and/or g of stool [7]. It differs from low-grade carriage, which means $\leq 2+$ or $\leq 10^3$ PPM per ml of saliva and/or g of feces. During overgrowth of abnormal opportunistic AGNB in the terminal ileum, clinical consequences, including liver disease and systemic immunoparalysis, may develop [59, 60].

Risk Factors for Translocation

Translocation or transmural migration is defined as the passage of micro-organisms from the gut lumen via the gut wall to the GALT and subsequently the bloodstream [61]. Microbial overgrowth, increased intestinal wall permeability, and systemic immunoparalysis are the three key factors necessary for the development of translocation [62]. The highly concentrated micro-organisms migrate through the intact or damaged intestinal wall. One of the primary functions of the GALT is a powerful and efficient local defense system for the prevention of spill-over into the bloodstream after the transmural passage of micro-organisms. The micro-organisms that escape from the GALT can still be destroyed by the white blood cells as soon as they reach the systemic circulation. However, sterility of the mesenteric lymph nodes and blood does not imply that translocation does not occur. Using immunofluorescence, bacteria have been detected in lymph nodes [63] and bacterial fragments, including LPS, can be detected after polymerase chain reaction [64].

Bacterial Overgrowth and the Liver

Animal and human studies show evidence that bacterial overgrowth can cause liver damage [59, 65, 66]. The degree of liver damage varies from a mild elevation of liver enzymes, to cholestasis, fibrosis, steatosis, and ultimately necrosis of the liver. The Kupffer cells, the resident liver macrophages, constitute 80%–90% of the fixed tissue mononuclear cell population. Positioned at the interface between the portal and systemic circulation, Kupffer cells are continuously exposed to AGNB and their endotoxins from the portal circulation. Endotoxin, cleared by Kupffer cells, is associated with the release of inflammatory mediators. The direct effect of endotoxins on the liver cells, together with the highly concentrated mediators, is responsible for the liver cell damage [67]. Experimental small bowel overgrowth in rats was associated with hepatobiliary injury [65]. When AGNB overgrowth was prevented by enteral polymyxin B, an antimicrobial agent with bactericidal activity and a neutralizing effect on endotoxin, liver steatosis was significantly reduced [68].

Bacterial Overgrowth Impairs Systemic Immunity

Bacterial overgrowth may also impair systemic immunity [60, 69]. Bacterial overgrowth of *E. coli* diminishes T cell activity, leading to an increased risk for infection in animals. After injection of LPS or endotoxins derived from AGNB into the portal vein of rats, pulmonary macrophage activity was reduced [70]. Once absorbed from the gut lumen, bacterial endotoxin stimulates the macrophages in the Peyer's patches to produce cytokines such as TNF. Cytokinemia is thought to result in a down-regulation of macrophage activity in the gut and in the liver, abdomen, and lungs [70, 71].

The Non-use of the Gut Invariably Leads to Overgrowth, Translocation, and Sepsis

Sepsis during long-term TPN. Liver disease is common in patients receiving long-term parenteral nutrition [72]. The wide spectrum of clinical, biochemical, and pathological manifestations of the liver disease varies from a benign, transient rise in liver enzymes to extensive liver damage with signs of cholestasis, fibrosis, steatosis, necrosis, and death as a result of liver failure. Despite intensive investigation, no clear pathophysiological mechanism has been demonstrated for these changes. All components of TPN have been held responsible for causing liver damage. However, liver failure has never been induced by TPN alone in animal models [72]. The non-use of the gut leads to a paralysis of the intestinal canal, subsequently followed by a reduced production of intestinal hormones, neuropeptides, bile, pancreatic enzymes, and mucus. Most importantly, the non-use of the gut leads to AGNB overgrowth [73]. AGNB overgrowth in the terminal ileum is associated with liver disease [59, 65, 66] and systemic immunoparalysis [60, 69, 74]. Several studies in animals and humans support this concept. Healthy volunteers maintained on TPN for 7 days show a higher inflammatory response after endotoxin injection than enterally fed volunteers. Translocation of bacteria and endotoxins follows systemic endotoxin injection [75]. In the case of AGNB overgrowth, gut endotoxin has been shown to stimulate the Kupffer cells via the portal vein, causing generalized inflammation. Healthy, enterally fed, individuals did not show overgrowth and there was neither translocation nor immunoparalysis. Infections only occur if systemic immunity is impaired. Trauma is associated with impaired immunity. If TPN is administered during trauma, the systemic immunity further decreases and translocation will occur following overgrowth. Septic morbidity in enterally fed trauma patients was 3% compared with 20% in TPN fed trauma patients [76]. Remarkably, liver injury generally preceded infection [25]. This supports the concept that AGNB overgrowth, and not TPN, is the most likely cause of the development of liver damage. Therapeutic studies were only performed in animal models. Rats receiving TPN have AGNB overgrowth, which was cleared following the administration of polymyxin B. Rats receiving polymyxin B showed less liver damage than those without polymyxin B [68]. The reintroduction of enteral feeding restores peristalsis and subsequent clearance of AGNB. The non-use of the gut during long-term TPN leads to AGNB overgrowth, high gut endotoxin levels, and bacterial translocation and absorption, leading to liver damage and suppressed systemic immunity. The degree of the immunoparalysis parallels the degree of liver damage.

Control of Throat and Gut Bacterial Overgrowth

Parenteral Antimicrobial Agents

Antimicrobial agents that are administered intravenously reach concentrations high enough in the blood, lower airways, and urine to be bactericidal for the AGNB that colonize/infect the internal organs. The aim of systemically administered antimicrobial agents is the return to the normal physiological state, i.e., blood, lower airways, and urine should be sterile. The intensivist should be aware that practically all parenteral antimicrobials are excreted in the throat and gut via saliva, bile, and mucus. However, the antimicrobial levels in saliva, bile, and mucus are generally not high enough for the eradication of the abnormal AGNB that are carried in the alimentary canal of individuals with underlying disease. The commonly used antimicrobial agents, including β-lactams, aminoglycosides, and fluoroquinolones, are invariably excreted into the digestive tract. However, the fecal levels of these antibiotics are in general not lethal for the AGNB, thus failing to clear the AGNB carrier state [77]. However, the levels achieved in the feces are often lethal for the indigenous mainly anaerobic micro-organisms. Hence, systemic antimicrobials impair the microbial carriage defense, subsequently leading to the overgrowth of the surviving abnormal AGNB [78]. Well-known examples include *Candida* species that are naturally resistant to antibiotics [79], AGNB such as *Klebsiella* species resistant to β-lactam antibiotics and aminoglycosides [78], and *Enterobacter*, *Citrobacter*, and *Pseudomonas* species that are induced to release β-lactamases following contact with β-lactam antibiotics [80]. This process practically always occurs in the gut, as the conditions for inducible β-lactamases are optimal in the alimentary canal. In the gut, (1) there is overgrowth of abnormal flora, (2) the concentrations of antimicrobial agents are in general not lethal for the AGNB present in high numbers, and (3) the white blood cells required for clearing the microorganisms are not present in saliva and feces. There are only a few studies evaluating abnormal flora in throat and gut of ICU patients during the administration of systemic antibiotics. Practically all those studies were performed on neonatal units and ICUs, where regular surveillance samples were an essential part of the infection control protocol. These reports suggest that almost all systemic antibiotics fail to eradicate abnormal carriage of AGNB from the throat and gut. In addition, the abnormal flora became resistant to the parenteral antibiotics, making successful eradication impossible. On a neonatal ICU, *Enterobacter cloacae* was endemic [80]: almost all critically ill neonates acquired the organism and readily developed carriage. Initially, the organism was sensitive to all β-lactam antibiotics. The first-line β-lactam, cefuroxime, was immediately given to all neonates when their surveillance cultures were found to be positive for *Enterobacter cloacae*. Within 3 days, *Enterobacter cloacae* carried in the gut at a concentration of >3+ released β-lactamases that neutralized cefuroxime. Cefuroxime was stopped and replaced by cefotaxime, which was still reported to be active against the organism. The subsequent surveillance samples showed that cefotaxime was also neutralized by the β-lactamases induced in *Enterobacter cloacae*. Aminoglycosides are almost completely cleared from the body via the kidneys. These pharmacokinetics explain why aminoglycosides are difficult to detect in saliva and feces [77]. Therefore, parenterally administered aminoglycosides cannot be expected to eradicate AGNB from the throat and gut. In two pediatric ICUs, in London (UK) [78] and Cleveland (USA) [81], ceftazidime was replaced by a potent combination of piperacillin/tazobactam and amikacin. Even this potent combination failed to reduce/clear abnormal carriage of AGNB. Systemic vancomycin has never been shown to be effective in the eradication of abnormal carriage of methicillin-resistant *S. aureus* (MRSA), although MRSA is still invariably sensitive to vancomycin [82]. The first-line combination of amoxicillin and clavulanic acid/gentamicin not only failed in clearing AGNB and MRSA from the throat and gut but also had a negative impact on the patient's ecology, i.e., the microbial factor of carriage defense was impaired with subsequent endemicity of *Candida parapsilosis* [79]. Interestingly, parenteral anti-fungal agents were not effective in the eradication of carriage of *Candida parapsilosis*. In conclusion, systemic antimicrobials uncommonly reach lethal levels in the digestive tract. AGNB overgrowth is impossible to clear with systemic antibiotics and hence is a contra-indication for the administration of parenteral and oral absorbable antibiotics.

Enteral Antimicrobial Agents

The administration of enteral non-absorbable antibiotics is a technique termed selective decontamination of the digestive tract (SDD) [83]. SDD is based on the fact that critical illness almost invariably causes abnormal carriage of AGNB. The main aim of the administration of enteral antibiotics is the eradication of AGNB, as the patients themselves are unable to clear the abnormal AGNB due to their underlying disease. SDD aims at the reconversion of abnormal carriage into the normal carrier state using enteral antimicrobial agents. Enterally administered antibiotics are chosen carefully to selectively decontaminate the digestive tract, i.e., AGNB are eradicated whilst the indigenous anaerobic flora is left undisturbed. The ongoing impaired immunity combined with high concentrations of PPM in the oropharynx of ventilated patients often leads to pneumonia. In the small intestine, the combination of PPM overgrowth and systemic immunoparalysis promotes translocation of PPM with subsequent septicemia. Enteral administration of polymyxin E/tobramycin is necessary to successfully decontaminate the gut. The AGNB-free condition gives the critically ill patient a chance for recovery from the systemic immunoparalysis [84]. A recovering immunity combined with an effective SDD in the throat and gut is the result of a properly administered SDD. The best-evaluated SDD combination for the elimination of AGNB overgrowth is the combination of polymyxin E and tobramycin [83](Chapters 9,14).

Control of the Throat and Gut Endotoxins

Enteral polymyxin E/tobramycin is the most-potent SDD protocol available [83]. Both polymyxin E and tobramycin interact with the microbial cell membrane and a neutralizing effect on endotoxin has been shown in vitro [85, 86]. Experimental models support these observations [87, 88]. This antibiotic combination was tested in human and animal studies. A significant reduction in endotoxin per gram of feces was observed in rats on enteral polymyxin E/tobramycin [89]. In healthy volunteers and in patients, the AGNB-free state paralleled a decrease in fecal endotoxin [90, 91]. In both populations there was significant decrease of 10^4 in gut endotoxin after enteral treatment with polymyxin E/tobramycin.

References

1. Lee A(1985) Neglected niches. The microbial ecology of the gastro-intestinal tract. Adv Microb Ecol 8:115–162
2. Savage DC (1977) Microbial ecology of the gastro-intestinal tract. Annu Rev Microbiol 3:107–133

3. Stephen A, Cummings J (1980) The microbial constitution of human faecal mass. J Med Microbiol 13:45–51
4. Mobbs K, van Saene HKF, Sunderland D, Davies PDO (1999) Oropharyngeal Gram-negative bacillary carriage. A survey in 120 healthy individuals. Chest 115:1570–1575
5. Savage DC (1979) Introduction to mechanisms of association of indigenous microbes. Am J Clin Nutr 32:113–118
6. Vantrappen G, Janssens J, Hellemans J, Ghoos Y (1977) The interdigestive motor complex of normal subjects and patients with bacterial overgrowth of the small intestine. J Clin Invest 59:1158–1166
7. Husebye E (1995) Gastrointestinal motility disorders and bacterial overgrowth. J Intern Med 237:419–427
8. Walker H, Durie K et al (2000) Pediatric gastro-intestinal diseases, 3rd edn. Decker
9. Giannella RA, Broitman SA, Zamsheck N (1972) Gastric-acid barrier to ingested micro-organisms in man: studies in vivo and in vitro. Gut 13:251–256
10. Stannard VA, Hutchinson A, Morris DL, Byrne A (1988) Gastric exocrine failure in critically ill patients: incidence and associated features. BMJ 296:155–156
11. Hillman KM, Riordan T, O'Farrell SM, Tabaqchali S (1982) Colonization of the gastric content in critically ill patients. Crit Care Med 10:444–447
12. Thorens J, Froelich F et al (1996) Bacterial overgrowth during treatment with omeprazole compared with cimetidine: a prospective randomised double blind study. Gut 39:54–59
13. Howden CW, Hunt RH (1987) Relationship between gastric secretion and infection. Gut 28:96–107
14. Peterson WL, Mackowiak PA, Barnett CC et al (1989) The human gastric bactericidal barrier. J Infect Dis 159:979–983
15. Proctor RA (1987) Fibronectin: a brief overview of its structure, function and physiology. Rev Infect Dis 9:S317–S321
16. Dal Nogare AR, Toews GB, Pierce AK (1987) Increased salivary elastase precedes Gram-negative bacillary colonisation in post-operative patients. Am Rev Respir Dis 135:671–675
17. Mobbs KJ, van Saene HKF, Sunderland D, Davies PDO (1999) Oropharyngeal Gram-negative bacillary carriage in chronic obstructive pulmonary disease: relation to severity of disease. Respir Med 93:540–545
18. Clamp JR (1984) The relationship between the immune system and mucus in the protection of mucous membranes. Biochem Soc Trans 12:754–756
19. Balistreri WF, Bove KE (1990) Hepatobiliary consequences of parenteral alimentation. Prog Liver Dis 9:567–601
20. Pierro A, van Saene HKF, Jones MO, Nunn et al (1998) Clinical impact of abnormal gut flora in infants receiving parenteral nutrition. Ann Surg 227:547–552
21. Libosni Y, Nezu R, Kennedy M et al (1994) Total parenteral nutrition decreases luminal mucous gel and intestinal permeability of small intestine. J Parenter Enteral Nutr 18:346–350
22. Katayama M, Xu D, Specian RD, Deitch EA (1997) Role of bacterial adherence and the mucus barrier on bacterial translocation. Ann Surg 225:317–326
23. Bosscha K, Nieuwenhuijs VB, Vos A et al (1998) Gastrointestinal motility and gastric tube feeding in mechanically ventilated patients. Crit Care Med 26:1510–1517
24. Holte K, Kehlet H (2000) Postoperative ileus: a preventable event. Br J Surg 87:1480–1493
25. Donnell SC, Taylor N, van Saene HKF et al (2002) Infection rates in surgical neonates and infants receiving parenteral nutrition: a five-year prospective study. J Hosp Infect 52:273-280

26. Zietz B, Lock G, Straub RH et al (2000) Small-bowel bacterial overgrowth in diabetic subjects is associated with cardiovascular autonomic neuropathy. Diabetes Care 23:1200–1201

27. Skar V, Skar AG, Osnes M (1989) The duodenal flora in the region of papilla of Vater in patients with and without duodenal diverticula. Scand J Gastroenterol 24:649–656

28. Ikeda H, Suzuki Y, Koike M et al (1998) Apoptosis is a major mode of cell death caused by ischaemia and ischaemia/reperfusion injury to the rat intestinal epithelium. Gut 42:530–537

29. Sasaki M, Fitzgerald AJ, Grant G et al (2002) Lectins can reverse the distal atrophy associated with elemental diets in mice. Aliment Pharmacol Ther 16:633–642

30. Leblond CP, Walker BE (1956) Absorption. Physiol Rev 36:255–290

31. Gordon HA, Bruckner-Kardoss E (1961) Effect of normal microbial flora on intestinal surface area. Am J Physiol 201:175–178

32. Targan SR, Kognoff MF, Brogan MD et al (1987) Immunologic mechanisms in intestinal diseases. Ann Intern Med 106:853–870

33. MacDonald TT (2001) Introduction. Semin Immunol 13:159–161

34. Conley ME, Delacroix DL (1987) Intravascular and mucosal immunoglobulin A: two separate but related systems of immune defense? Ann Intern Med 106:892–899

35. Mestecky J, Russell M, Elson CO (1999) Intestinal IgA, novel views on its function in the defence of the largest mucosal surface. Gut 44:2–5

36. van Saene HKF, Zandstra DF (2004) Selective decontamination of the digestive tract: rationale behind evidence-based use in liver transplantation. Liver Transpl 10:828–833

37. van Saene HKF, Damjanovic V, Alcock SR (2001) Basics in microbiology for the patient requiring intensive care. Curr Anaesth Crit Care 12:6–17

38. Mackowiak PA, Martin RM, Jones SR et al (1978) Pharyngeal colonisation by gram-negative bacilli in aspiration-prone persons. Arch Intern Med 138:1224–1227

39. Fuxench-Lopez Z, Ramirez-Ronda CH (1978) Pharyngeal flora in ambulatory alcoholic patients: prevalence of gram-negative bacilli. Arch Intern Med 138:1815–1816

40. Kerver AJH, Rommes JH, Mevissen-Verhage EAE et al (1988) Prevention of colonization and infection in critically ill patients: a prospective randomized study. Crit Care Med 16:1087–1093

41. Sanchez Garcia M, Cambronero Galache JA, Lopez Diaz J et al (1998) Effectiveness and cost of selective decontamination of the digestive tract in critically ill intubated patients. Am J Respir Crit Care Med 158:908–916

42. Ketai LH, Rypka G (1993) The course of nosocomial oropharyngeal colonisation in patients recovering from acute respiratory failure. Chest 103:1837–1841

43. Kerver AJH, Rommes JH, Mevissen-Verhage EAE et al (1987) Colonization and infection in surgical intensive care patients: a prospective study. Intensive Care Med 13:347–351

44. Luiten EJT, Hop WCJ, Endtz HP, Bruining HA (1998) Prognostic importance of gram-negative intestinal colonization preceding pancreatic infection in severe acute pancreatitis. Intensive Care Med 24:438–445

45. Luiten EJT, Hop WCJ, Lange JF, Bruining HA (1995) Controlled clinical trial of selective decontamination for the treatment of severe acute pancreatitis. Ann Surg 222:57–65

46. Flynn DM, Weinstein RA, Nathan C, Gaston MA, Kabins SA (1987) Patients' endogenous flora as the source of "nosocomial" *Enterobacter* in cardiac surgery. J Infect Dis 156:363–368

47. Garrouste-Orgeas M, Marie O, Rouveau M, Villiers S, Arlet G, Schlemmer B (1996) Secondary carriage with multi-resistant *Acinetobacter baumannii* and *Klebsiella pneumoniae* in an adult population: relationship with nosocomial infections and mortality. J Hosp Infect 34:279–289

48. Sveen K, Hofstad T, Milner KC (1977) Lethality for mice and chick embryos, pyogenicity in rabbits and ability to gelate lysate from amoebocytes of *Limulus polyphemus* by polysaccharides from *Bacteroides, Fusobacterium* and *Veillonella*. Acta Pathol Microbiol Scand 85:388–3986

49. Simon GL, Gelfland JA, Conolly RA et al (1985) Experimental *Bacteroides fragilis* bacteremia in a primate model: evidence that *Bacteroides fragilis* does not promote the septic shock syndrome. J Trauma 25:1156–1162

50. Maier RV, Hahnnel GB, Pohlman TH (1990) Endotoxin requirements or alveolar macrophage stimulation. J Trauma 30 [Suppl 2]:S49–S57

51. Magnuson DK, Weintraub A, Pohlman TH, Maier RV (1989) Human endothelial cell adhesiveness for neutrophils, induced by *E. coli* lipopolysaccharide in vitro, is inhibited by *Bacteroides fragilis* lipopolysaccahride. J Immunol 143:3025–3030

52. Leenstra TS, van Saene JJM, van Saene HKF et al (1996) Oral endotoxin in healthy adults. Oral Surg Oral Med Oral Pathol 82:637–643

53. van Saene JJM, Stoutenbeek CP, van Saene HKF (1992) Faecal endotoxin in human volunteers: normal values. Microb Ecol Health Dis 5:179–184

54. van Saene HKF, Stoutenbeek CP, Faber-Nijholt R, van Saene JJM (1992) Selective decontamination of the digestive tract contributes to the control of disseminated intravascular coagulation in severe liver impairment. J Pediatr Gastroenterol Nutr 14:436–442

55. Rombeau JL, Takala (1997) Gut dysfunction in critical illness. Intensive Care Med 23:476–479

56. Sheth K, Bankey P (2001) The liver as an immune organ. Curr Opin Crit Care 7:99-104

57. Das J, Schwartz AA, Folkman J (1973) Clearance of endotoxin by platelets: role in increasing the accuracy of the *Limulus* gelation test and in combatting experimental endotoxemia. Surgery 74:235–240

58. Quesenberry P, Morley A, Stohlman F et al (1972) Effect of endotoxin on granulopoiesis and colony stimulating factor. N Engl J Med 286:227–232

59. Wigg AJ, Roberts-Thomson IC, Dymock RB et al (2001) The role of small intestinal bacterial overgrowth, intestinal permeability, endotoxaemia, and tumor necrosis factor alpha in the pathogenesis of non-alcoholic steatohepatitis. Gut 48:206–211

60. Marshall JC, Christou NV, Meakins JL (1988) Small-bowel bacterial overgrowth and systemic immunosuppression in experimental peritonitis. Surgery 104:404–411

61. Schweinburg FB, Seligman AM, Fine J (1950) Transmural migration of intestinal bacteria. N Engl J Med 242:747–751

62. Feltis BA, Wells CL (2000) Does microbial translocation play a role in critical illness? Curr Opin Crit Care 6:117–122

63. Brathwaite CEM, Ross SE, Nagole R et al (1993) Bacterial translocation occurs in humans after traumatic injury: evidence using immunofluorescence. J Trauma 34:586–590

64. Kane TD, Wesley Alexander J, Johannigman JA (1998) The detection of microbial DNA in the blood. Ann Surg 227:1–19

65. Lichtman SN, Sartor RB, Keku J, Schwab JH (1990) Hepatic inflammation in rats with experimental small intestinal bacterial overgrowth. Gastroenterology 93:234–237

66. Riordan SM, McIver CJ, Williams R (1998) Liver damage in human small intestinal bacterial overgrowth. Am J Gastroenterol 93:234–237

67. Nolan JP (1989) Intestinal endotoxins as mediators of hepatic injury—an idea whose time has come again. Hepatology 10:234–237

68. Pappo I, Becovier H, Berry EM et al (1991) Polymyxin B reduces cecal flora, TNF production and hepatic steatosis during parenteral nutrition in the rat. J Surg Res 51:106–112

69. Deitch E, Xu D, Lu Q, Berg R (1991) Bacterial translocation from the gut impairs systemic immunity. Surgery 104:269–276

70. Mason C, Dobard E, Summer W et al (1997) Intraportal lipopolysaccharide suppress pulmonary antibacterial defense mechanisms. J Infect Dis 176:1293–1302

71. Nathens AB, Rotstein OR, Dackiw APB, Marshall JC (1995) Intestinal epithelial cells down-regulate macrophage tumor necrosis factor-alpha secretion: a mechanism for immune homeostasis in the gut associated lymphoid tissue. Surgery 118:343–351

72. Sondheimer JM, Asturias E, Cadnapaphornchai M (1998) Infection and cholestasis in neonates with intestinal resection and long-term parenteral nutrition. J Pediatr Gastroenterol Nutr 27:131–137

73. van Saene HKF, Taylor N, Donnell SC et al (2003) Gut overgrowth of abnormal flora: the missing link in parenteral nutrition-related sepsis in surgical neonates. Eur J Clin Nutr 57:548–553

74. Alverdy JC, Burke D (1992) Total parenteral nutrition: iatrogenic immunosuppression. Nutrition 8:359–365

75. Fong Y, Marano MA, Barber A et al (1989) Total parenteral nutrition and bowel rest modify the metabolic response to endotoxin in humans. Ann Surg 210:449–457

76. Moore FA, Moore EE, Jones TN et al (1989) TEN versus TPN following major abdominal trauma—reduced septic morbidity. J Trauma 29:916–923

77. van Saene HKF, Percival A (1991) Bowel micro-organisms—a target for selective antimicrobial control. J Hosp Infect 19 [Suppl C}:19–41

78. Petros AJ, O'Connell, Roberts C et al (2001) Systemic antibiotics fail to clear multi-resistant *Klebsiella* from a pediatric ICU. Chest 119:862–866

79. Damjanovic V, Connelly CM, van Saene HKF et al (1993) Selective decontamination with nystatin for control of a *Candida* outbreak in a neonatal intensive care unit. J Hosp Infect 24:245–249

80. Modi V, Damjanovic V, Cooke RWI (1987) Outbreak of cephalosporin-resistant *Enterobacter cloacae* infection in a neonatal intensive care unit. Arch Dis Child 62:148–151

81. Toltzis P, Yamashita T, Vilt L et al (1998) Antibiotic restriction does not alter endemic colonization with resistant Gram-negative rods in a pediatric intensive care unit. Crit Care Med 26:1893–1899

82. Silvestri L, Milanese M, Oblach L et al (2002) Enteral vancomycin to control methicillin-resistant *Staphylococcus aureus* outbreak in mechanically ventilated patients. Am J Infect Control 30:391–399

83. Baxby D, Saene HKF van, Stoutenbeek CP, Zandstra DF (1996) Selective decontamination of the digestive tract: 13 years on, what it is and what it is not. Intensive Care Med 22:699–706

84. Yao YM, Lu LR, Yu Y et al (1997) Influence of selective decontamination of the digestive tract on cell-mediated immune function and bacteria-endotoxin translocation in thermally injured rats. J Trauma 42:1073–1079

85. Artenstein AW, Cross AS (1989) Inhibition of endotoxin reactivity by aminoglycosides. J Antimicrob Chemother 24:826–828

86. Crosby HA, Bion JF, Penn CW, Elliott TSJ (1994) Antibiotic-induced release of endotoxin from bacteria in-vitro. J Med Microbiol 40:23–30

87. Rifkind D (1967) Pevention by polymyxin B of endotoxin lethality in mice. J Bacteriol 93:1463–1464

88. Foca A, Matera G, Ianello D et al (1991) Aminoglycosides modify the in-vitro metachromatic reactions and murine generalized Shwartzman phenomenon induced by *Salmonella minnesota* R595 lipopolysaccharide. Antimicrob Agents Chemother 35:2161–2164

89. Rosman C, Wubbels GF, Manson LW, Bleichrodt RP (1992) Selective decontamination of the digestive tract prevents secondary infections of the abdominal cavity, and endotoxemia and mortality in sterile peritonitis in laboratory rats. Crit Care Med 20:1699–1704
90. van Saene JJM, Stoutenbeek CP, van Saene HKF, Matera G, Martinez-Pellus AE, Ramsay G (1996) Reduction of the intestinal endotoxin pool by three different SDD regimens in human volunteers. J Endotoxin Res 3:337–343
91. Conraads VM, Jorens PG, de Clerck LS et al (2004) Selective intestinal decontamination in advanced chronic heart failure: a pilot trial. Eur J Heart Fail 6:483-491

Chapter 3

Colonization and Infection

L. SILVESTRI, G. MINO, H.K.F VAN SAENE

Introduction

Physiologically, internal organs such as lower airways and bladder are sterile. However, colonization of lower airways and bladder by potentially pathogenic micro-organisms (PPMs) is common in critically ill patients on the intensive care unit (ICU) [1]. Colonization of the internal organs generally follows the impaired carriage defense of the digestive tract, which promotes carriage and overgrowth of PPMs (see Chapter 2), and the impaired defenses of the host against colonization, due to illness severity. Failure to clear colonizing micro-organisms from the internal organs invariably leads to high concentrations of PPMs, predisposing to invasion. The host mobilizes both humoral and cellular defense systems to hinder the invading micro-organisms. However, infection will require not only invasion, but also severity of the underlying disease, which jeopardizes immunocompetence.

The aims of this chapter are to define the concepts of colonization/infection and to describe the defense mechanisms of the host and the interventions for control of colonization/infection.

Definitions

Colonization

Colonization is defined as the presence of a micro-organism in an internal organ that is normally sterile (e.g., lower airways, bladder), without an inflammatory response of the host (Fig. 1). Diagnostic samples such as lower airway secretions, wound fluid, and urine generally yield $<10^5$ colony forming units (CFU) of potential pathogens per milliliter of diagnostic sample. In general,

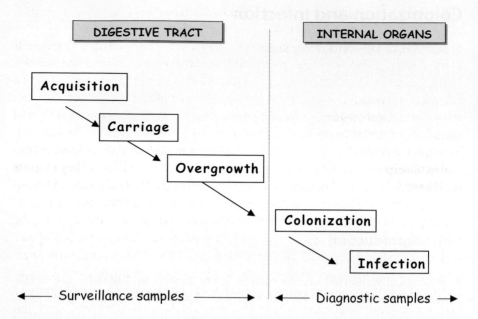

Fig. 1. The slippery slope of the pathogenesis of infection in critically ill patients (from Silvestri L, Lenhart FP, Fox MA (2001) Prevention of intensive care unit infections. Curr Anaesth Crit Care 12:34-40, with permission)

Acquisition develops if only one surveillance sample is positive for a potentially pathogenic micro-organism (PPM) that differs from the previous and following isolates. Acquisition refers to the transient presence of a micro-organism (usually in the oropharynx and gut), whilst carriage is a persistent phenomenon

Carriage or carrier state is the patient's state where the same bacterial strain is isolated from at least two surveillance samples (saliva, gastric fluid, feces, throat and rectal swabs) in any concentration over a period of at least 1 week

Overgrowth is defined as $\geq 10^5$ CFU/ml of saliva, gastric fluid, or g of feces, and is nearly always present in the critically ill ICU patient with impaired gut motility

Colonization is the presence of a PPM in an internal organ that is normally sterile (e.g,. lower airways, bladder) without an inflammatory host response. The diagnostic sample yields $<10^5$ CFU/ml of diagnostic sample

Infection is a microbiologically proven clinical diagnosis of inflammation. Apart from the clinical signs of infection the diagnostic sample obtained from the internal organ contains $\geq 10^5$ CFU/ml or is positive in the case of blood, cerebrospinal and pleural fluid

Surveillance samples are samples from body sites where PPMs are carried, such as digestive tract, and skin lesions (tracheotomy, wounds, pressure sores). A surveillance set comprises throat and rectal swabs taken on admission and afterwards twice weekly, e.g., on Monday and Thursday. The purpose of surveillance samples is the determination of the microbiological endpoint of the level of carriage of PPMs

Diagnostic samples are samples from internal organs that are normally sterile such as lower airways, blood, and bladder. The aim of diagnostic samples is clinical, i.e., to microbiologically prove a diagnosis of inflammation, both generalized or local

only a few leukocytes are present in colonized internal organs on a semiquantitative scale of +=few, 2+=moderate, and 3+=many leukocytes [2, 3].

The term colonization should be distinguished from carriage. Carriage is defined when the same strain is isolated from at least two surveillance samples (saliva, gastric fluid, feces, throat and rectal swabs) in any concentration over a period of at least 1 week (Fig. 1). Carriage and colonization are two different stages in the pathogenesis of endogenous infection in ICU patients. The first stage is almost always the oropharyngeal and gastrointestinal carrier state followed by overgrowth. Once the PPMs are present in high concentrations, in general $\geq 10^5$ of potential pathogens per ml of saliva and/or g of feces, they migrate into the sterile internal organs in order to colonize the lower airways and bladder. Unfortunately the term colonization is often used to cover both stages of carriage and colonization. Grouping together carriage and colonization may be misleading in interpreting the efficacy of antimicrobial interventions and risk factors for infection in ICU patients. For example, oral fluconazole was compared with oral nystatin in liver transplant patients to evaluate the impact on bladder colonization and rectal carriage [4]. Fluconazole is absorbable and hence sterilizes the bladder, whilst nystatin, which is not absorbed, does not have any impact on bladder colonization. However, fluconazole was no better in reducing carriage than nystatin. The authors reported that *Candida* colonization was significantly reduced in the fluconazole group following the inclusion of the data of the urine cultures. The Geneva group developed a colonization index to predict candidemia [5]. Both surveillance (throat and stomach) and diagnostic (lower airways, bladder, and wound) samples were considered to identify patients at high risk of severe *Candida* infections. When half the samples yielded *Candida* in heavy growth density, the chance of severe *Candida* infection was significantly higher than in patients who only had 20% of samples positive for *Candida* in high concentrations. We believe that this index is not very useful from a clinical point of view, as the authors were unable to recommend the timing of antifungal therapy. The normal physiological condition of tracheal aspirate, urine, and wound fluid is sterility. These diagnostic samples can only be kept free of yeasts if those microorganisms are absent or present in low concentration in throat, stomach, and gut. From a prevention point of view, enteral antifungals should be started as soon as possible, particularly if throat and rectal swabs show yeast in overgrowth.

Infection

Infection is a microbiologically proven clinical diagnosis of inflammation, local and/or generalized. This includes not only clinical signs, but also the presence of at least a moderate (2+) number of leukocytes and micro-organisms of $\geq 10^5$ CFU/ml in diagnostic samples obtained from an internal organ, or the isolation of a micro-organism from blood, cerebrospinal fluid, or pleural fluid. Sepsis is defined as clinical signs of generalized inflammation caused by micro-organisms and/or their products. Septicemia is sepsis combined with a positive blood culture (Fig. 1) [2]. In some studies of infection rates in liver transplant patients, microbiological proof was not even required, and vague terms, including "a positive culture from a T tube" [6] or "infected bile" [7], were used to define infections of wounds and bile.

Samples

Diagnostic samples are samples from internal organs that are normally sterile, such as the lower airways, bladder, and blood. They are obtained when clinically indicated and allow the diagnosis of colonization and infection [2].

Surveillance samples are samples from body sites where the potential pathogens are carried, i.e., the digestive tract, and skin lesions (tracheotomy, wounds, pressure sores). Generally, a set of surveillance samples consists of throat and rectal swabs taken on admission of the patient to the ICU and twice weekly, thereafter. The purpose of surveillance samples is the determination of the microbiological endpoint of the level of carriage of PPMs. They are not useful for diagnosing infection of internal organs, as diagnostic samples are required for this purpose [2].

Internal Organs in Health and Disease

Carriage

Micro-organisms are carried in the oropharynx, gut, and vagina. Micro-organisms present in healthy people belong to the "normal flora". They are mainly anaerobes and aerobes of the indigenous flora, together with "community" micro-organisms, such as *Streptococcus pneumoniae, Staphylococcus aureus, Haemophilus influenzae, Moraxella catarrhalis, Escherichia coli,* and *Candida albicans.* The "opportunistic" or hospital micro-organisms are uncommon in healthy people, and may be only transiently present [8], whilst disease promotes oropharyngeal and gastrointestinal carriage of these abnormal micro-organisms. They include eight aerobic Gram-negative bacilli (AGNB) (e.g., *Klebsiella, Proteus, Morganella, Enterobacter, Citrobacter, Serratia, Acinetobacter, and Pseudomonas spp.*), and methicillin-resistant *S. aureus* (MRSA). Approximately one-third of patients with an underlying chronic condition such as diabetes, alcoholism, or chronic obstructive pulmonary disease (COPD) are likely to demonstrate abnormal bacteria in their oropharynx and gut [8]. Moreover, previously healthy patients admitted to the ICU and requiring long-term ventilatory support due to an acute insult, such as (surgical) trauma, pancreatitis, or acute liver failure, may become carriers of abnormal hospital flora in their digestive tract (Chapter 2).

Colonization and Infection

Secretions from internal organs such as the lower airways, sinuses, middle ear, lachrymal gland, and urinary tract of healthy individuals are normally sterile. Colonization of internal organs can occur with the two types of PPMs, community, including *S. pneumoniae* and *H. influenzae*, and "abnormal" opportunistic PPMs such as *Klebsiella* and *Pseudomonas* species. Three examples illustrate the concept of colonization followed by infection.

1. Elderly people cared for in a nursing home carry *S. pneumoniae* and *H. influenzae* in their oropharynx. During winter months elderly people are at high risk of developing the flu. The flu virus destroys the cilia and causes systemic immunosuppression. Colonization of the lower airways with *S. pneumoniae* and *H. influenzae* invariably occurs in this population during the flu epidemic. If these patients do not receive a short course of commonly used antibiotics, colonization of the lower airways often progresses to pneumonia associated with high mortality. A similar pattern has been described for trauma patients [9, 10].

2. COPD patients with a forced expiratory volume in 1 s (FEV$_1$) <50% are oropharyngeal carriers of both types of flora, including *H. influenzae* and AGNB [11]. The severity of their underlying lung disease promotes colonization of the lower airways with oral flora, including "community" and "hospital" bacteria. The presence of bacteria in the lower airways or colonization is proinflammatory and may result in a range of important effects on the lung. These include activation of host defenses with release of inflammatory cytokines, such as interleukin-8 [12] and subsequent neutrophil recruitment, mucus hypersecretion, impaired mucociliary clearance, and respiratory cell damage [13]. Bacterial colonization of lower airways in COPD patients modulates the character and frequency of exacerbations [14], and is associated with greater airway inflammation and an accelerated decline in FEV$_1$ [15]. An acute exacerbation of their underlying condition may require intubation and ventilation on the ICU. The immediate administration of an adequate antimicrobial that is active against *H. influenzae* and AGNB such as *Klebsiella* species is required in order to prevent infection of the lower airways (see Chapter 19).

3. A patient who is transferred from another hospital or ward into the ICU needing ventilatory support often carries abnormal flora, including MRSA or *Pseudomonas* species, due to the underlying disease. The acute deterioration of their underlying disease requires intubation leading to colonization

of the lower airways with hospital flora. Colonization may develop into infection depending on the level of the immunosuppression of the patient. The experience that a delay in immediate adequate antimicrobial treatment increases mortality prompted the American Thoracic Society to advocate empirical treatment, including vancomycin and ciprofloxacin, to cover MRSA and *Pseudomonas* [16].

Patient's Defenses Against Colonization and Infection

Defense Against Colonization of the Internal Organs [17]

The first line of defense against carriage of PPMs in the digestive tract has been described in detail in Chapter 2. "Abnormal" carriage of AGNB and MRSA inevitably leads to overgrowth of these bacteria in a patient who requires mechanical ventilation following deterioration of the underlying disease. The multiple factors and interventions that promote overgrowth are discussed in Chapter 2. Intestinal overgrowth of abnormal flora promotes and maintains systemic immunoparalysis via liver macrophage activation [18], and is considered an independent risk factor for colonization and infection of internal organs [19–21]. PPMs may migrate from the digestive tract towards lower airways or bladder (endogenous colonization) or may be introduced directly into the internal organ from an "external" source, both animate or inanimate (exogenous colonization). Six clearing factors are present in these internal organs. In the lower airways these are the following [22] (Fig. 2).

Integrity of anatomy. The endotracheal tube damages the mucosa and promotes adherence of micro-organisms.

Intactness of physiology. Inhaled particles or micro-organisms have to survive and penetrate the aerodynamic filtration system of the tracheobronchial tree. The airflow is turbulent, causing micro-organisms to affect the mucosal surfaces. Humidification also causes hygroscopic organisms to increase in size, thereby aiding trapping. Mucosal surface adhesins are known to mediate adherence of bacteria to host extracellular matrix components, such as collagen, fibrinogen, and fibronectin [23–25]. Fibronectin covers the cell surface receptors and thereby blocks the attachment of many micro-organisms. The mucociliary blanket transports the invading micro-organism out of the lung, and coughing aids this expulsion. In addition, the bronchial secretions contain various antimicrobial substances, such as lysozyme, and defensins. Once the micro-organism reaches the alveoli, the alveolar macrophages and tissue histiocytes play an important role in protecting the host.

Motility of cilia in conjunction with *mucus* mechanically removes micro-organisms reaching its surface. Airway hygiene depends largely on mucociliary

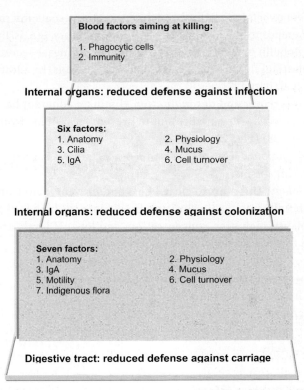

Blood factors aiming at killing:

1. Phagocytic cells
2. Immunity

Internal organs: reduced defense against infection

Six factors:
1. Anatomy   2. Physiology
3. Cilia   4. Mucus
5. IgA   6. Cell turnover

Internal organs: reduced defense against colonization

Seven factors:
1. Anatomy   2. Physiology
3. IgA   4. Mucus
5. Motility   6. Cell turnover
7. Indigenous flora

Digestive tract: reduced defense against carriage

Fig. 2. Three hurdles of defense against carriage, colonization, and infection

clearance, which in turn depends upon the movement of viscoelastic mucus along the airway [26]. Cilia are small cell appendices aligned in the direction of the effective beat of the cilia, which move with a metachronal wave form. At the tip of each cilium there are protuberances that hook in the overlying mucus so as to propel it along the airway. Aspirated or breathed material sticks to this mucus, and it is thus cleared from the respiratory tract. A thin periciliary fluid made by products of alveolar and bronchial epithelium moves centrally, undergoing modifications in ion content and volume. Mucociliary clearance can be impaired by (1) genetic defects, e.g., primary ciliary dyskinesia, cystic fibrosis; (2) secondary ciliary dyskinesia due to artificial ventilation or toxins released by micro-organisms producing cytotoxic damage of epithelial cells (in this situation, micro-organisms may remain longer in the airways, causing colonization and infection); (3) abnormal physico-chemical properties of mucus, making it difficult to move it along the airway. A persistent host inflammatory response driven by cytokines fails to eliminate micro-organisms, which maintain the inflammatory process.

Secretory immunoglobulin A in bronchial secretions coats micro-organisms to prevent adherence to mucosal cell receptors. Secretory IgA is the predominant immunoglobulin present in the respiratory tract, nasal secretions, saliva, tears, gastrointestinal fluids, and other mucous secretions. In addition IgA can neutralize toxin activity [27].

Mucosal *cell turnover* and *desquamation* eliminate adherent bacteria.

Similarly, six mechanisms are present to prevent fecal PPMs from colonizing the urinary tract [28] (Fig. 2).

Integrity of anatomy. The bladder mucosa acts as a barrier to eliminate invading micro-organisms.

Intact physiology. This aims to clear PPMs and prevent them from migrating form the rectal cavity into the urethra and finally into the bladder [29]. Extreme levels of osmolality, high urea concentration, and low pH levels are inhibitory for the growth of some bacteria causing urinary tract infection.

Urinary flow and *micturition* mechanically remove PPMs unless they are capable of adhering to epithelial cells of the urinary tract.

Mucus covers the bladder mucosa.

Secretory IgA present in the mucus prevents adherence of fecal bacteria.

Mucosal cell turnover promotes the elimination of PPMs already adhering to bladder mucosal cells.

Defense Against Infection

Failure to eliminate colonizing micro-organisms from the internal organs invariably leads to high concentration of $\geq 10^5$ PPMs, predisposing to invasion. The host mobilizes both humoral and cellular defense systems to hinder the invading micro-organisms. However, infection requires not only invasion but also critical illness, which jeopardize immunocompetence, and the treatment of which facilitates crossing the physical barriers (Fig. 2).

Mechanisms of Colonization and Infection in ICU Patients

There are two basic mechanisms of colonization and infection in ICU patients: migration and translocation, or transmural migration. Migration is the movement of live PPMs from one place, e.g., throat and gut where they are present in overgrowth, to other sites, in particular normally sterile internal organs. Migration is the main mechanism by which micro-organisms cause *endogenous* colonization/infection in ICU patients. The migration of micro-organisms contained in contaminated secretions from the oropharynx into the lower airways within few days of mechanical ventilation is considered to be the most-common route by which PPMs enter the lung and cause colonization and infection [19, 30, 31]. The severity of the underlying disease causing impairment of clearance of PPMs is the main factor promoting colonization of the lower airways. The presence of the plastic endotracheal tube is invariably associated with mucosal lesions, which further enhance colonization. Finally, the progress towards infection depends on the immune status or defense capacity of the patient.

Potential pathogens may also cause colonization and subsequent infection, bypassing the stage of carriage and overgrowth, i.e., *exogenous* colonization/ infection. An example is a lower respiratory tract colonization/infection in a tracheotomized patient due to micro-organisms not previously carried in the throat and/or gut, but directly introduced into the internal organ following breaches of hygiene [32, 33].

Translocation (or transmural migration) is defined as the ingress of oropharyngeal or gut PPMs through the mucosal lining of the alimentary canal into gut-associated lymphoid tissue (GALT), which includes macrophages in the mesenteric lymph nodes, liver, spleen, and blood. The GALT macrophages are generally effective in killing intestinal micro-organisms translocating from the gut in normally healthy people. In the case of impairment of gut function, such as in the critically ill patient, either with an anatomically intact gastrointestinal tract or altered intestinal mucosa, bacterial translocation can be followed by spreading into the systemic bloodstream, leading to sepsis and multiple organ failure [34]. Gut overgrowth of PPMs, in particular in the terminal ileum, is required for transmural migration or translocation [35]. The phenomenon of translocation has been described in surgical patients [21, 36], patients with pancreatitis [20] and neutropenia [37], in surgical neonates and infants receiving parenteral nutrition [38], and in patients requiring intensive care, including mechanical ventilation [39].

Control of Colonization/Infection

Parenteral antimicrobials are required to sterilize internal organs such as lower airways, bladder, and blood. In patients who are successfully decontaminated, i.e., the throat and gut are free from potential pathogens including AGNB, S. *aureus,* and yeasts following selective decontamination of the digestive tract (SDD) [40], the diagnostic samples of lower airway secretions, blood, and urine are almost always sterile within 3 days of systemic antimicrobials [41]. The eradication of overgrowth in the throat and gut using SDD promotes sterilization of the internal organs, as the microbial load responsible for migration and translocation is reduced/lifted. Some micro-organisms, such as S. *aureus* sensitive and resistant to methicillin, P. *aeruginosa,* and yeasts, have an affinity for plastic devices, including the ventilation tube, the indwelling vascular devices, and the bladder catheter. Adhering micro-organisms may interfere with the sterilization process of the intravenously administered antimicrobials. If the lower airway secretions, blood, and urine are not sterile after 3 days of systemic administration of antimicrobials, removal and/or replacement of the foreign body is indicated. An additional step to control colonization/infection of the lower airways includes nebulization of the antimicrobials to increase the antimicrobial levels in the lower airways [42] (Chapter 23).

Table 1. Diagnostic samples: normal and abnormal values

	Normal values	Abnormal values
Blood	Sterile	Any growth
Lower airway secretions	Sterile	Any growth whether colonization or infection, except viridans streptococci, enterococci, coagulase-negative staphylococci and yeasts
Urine	Sterile	Any growth whether colonization or infection, except enterococci, coagulase-negative staphylococci
Wound	Sterile	Any growth whether colonization or infection, except coagulase-negative staphylococci
Cerebrospinal fluid	Sterile	Any growth

References

1. Kerver AJH, Rommes JH, Mevissen-Verhage EAE et al (1987) Colonization and infection in surgical intensive care patients: a prospective study. Intensive Care Med 13:347–351
2. Sarginson RE, Taylor N, van Saene HKF (2001) Glossary of terms and definitions. Curr Anaesth Crit Care 12:2–5
3. A'Court CHD, Garrard CS, Crook D et al (1993) Microbiological lung surveillance in mechanically ventilated patients using non-directed bronchial lavage and quantitative culture. Q J Med 86:635–648
4. Lumbreras C, Cuervas-Mons V, Jara P et al (1996) Randomized trial of fluconazole versus nystatin for the prophylaxis of Candida infection following liver transplantation. J Infect Dis 174:583–588
5. Pittet D, Monod M, Suter PM, Frenk E, Auckentaler R (1994) Candida colonization and subsequent infections in critically ill surgical patients. Ann Surg 220:751–758

6. Rayes N, Seehofer D, Hansen S et al (2002) Early enteral supply of *Lactobacillus* and fiber versus selective bowel decontamination: a controlled trial in liver transplant patients. Transplantation 74:123–128

7. Zwaveling JH, Maring JK, Klompmaker IJ et al (2002) Selective decontamination of the digestive tract to prevent postoperative infection: a randomized placebo-controlled trial in liver transplant patients. Crit Care Med 30:1204–1209

8. Mobbs KJ, van Saene HKF, Sunderland D, Davies PDO (1999) Oropharyngeal Gram-negative bacillary carriage. A survey of 120 healthy individuals. Chest 115:1570–1575

9. Sirvent JM, Torres A, Vidaur L et al (2000) Tracheal colonisation within 24 h of intubation in patients with head trauma: risk factor for developing early-onset ventilator-associated pneumonia. Intensive Care Med 26:1369–1372

10. Ewig S, Torres A, El-Ebiary M et al (1999) Bacterial colonization patterns in mechanically ventilated patients with traumatic and medical injury. Incidence, risk factors and association with ventilator-associated pneumonia. Am J Respir Crit Care Med 159:188–198

11. Mobbs KJ, van Saene HKF, Sunderland D, Davies PDO (1999) Oropharyngeal Gram-negative bacillary carriage in chronic obstructive pulmonary disease: relation to severity of disease. Respir Med 93:540–545

12. Yamamoto C, Yoneda T, Yoshikawa M et al (1997) Airway inflammation in COPD patients assessed by sputum levels of interleukin-8. Chest 112:505–510

13. Sethi S, Murphy TF (2001) Bacterial infection in chronic obstructive pulmonary disease in 2000: state of the art. Clin Microbiol Rev 14:336–363

14. Patel IS, Seemungal TA, Wilks M et al (2002) Relationship between bacterial colonisation and the frequency, character, and severity of COPD exacerbations. Thorax 57:753–754

15. Wilkinson TMA, Patel IS, Donaldson GC, Wedzicha JA (2003) Airway bacterial load and FEV1 decline in patients with chronic obstructive pulmonary disease. Am J Respir Crit Care Med 167:1090–1095

16. Anonymous (1996) Hospital-acquired pneumonia in adults: diagnosis, assessment of severity, initial antimicrobial therapy, and preventing strategies. A consensus statement, American Thoracic Society. Am J Respir Crit Care Med 153:1711–1725

17. van Saene HKF, Damjanovic V, Alcock SR (2001) Basics in microbiology for the patient requiring intensive care. Curr Anaesth Crit Care 12:6–17

18. Marshall JC, Christou NV, Meakins JL (1988) Small-bowel bacterial overgrowth and systemic immuno-suppression in experimental peritonitis. Surgery 104:404–411

19. van Uffelen R, van Saene HKF, Fidler V et al (1984) Oropharyngeal flora as a source of colonizing the lower airways in patients on artificial ventilation. Intensive Care Med 10:233–237

20. Luiten EJT, Hop WCJ, Endtz HP et al (1988) Prognostic importance of Gram-negative intestinal colonization preceding pancreatic infection in severe acute pancreatitis. Intensive Care Med 24:438–445

21. de la Cal MA, Cerdà E, van Saene HKF et al (2004) Effectiveness and safety of enteral vancomycin to control endemicity of methicillin-resistant Staphylococcus aureus in a medical/surgical intensive care unit. J Hosp Infect 56:175-183

22. Manson CM, Summer WR, Nelson S (1992) Pathophysiology of pulmonary defence mechanisms. J Crit Care 7:42–56

23. Beachey EH (1981) Bacterial adherence. Adhesin-receptor interactions mediated the attachment of bacteria to mucosal surfaces. J Infect Dis 143:325–345

24. Peacock SJ, Foster TJ, Cameron BJ, Berend R (1999) Bacterial fibronectin-binding proteins and endothelial cell surface fibronectin mediate adherence of *Staphylococcus aureus* to resting human endothelial cells. Microbiology 145:3477–3486

25. Mongodin E, Bajolet O, Cutrona J et al (2002) Fibronectin-binding proteins of *Staphylococcus aureus* are involved in adherence to human airway epithelium. Infect Immun 70:620–630
26. Cole P (2001) Pathophysiology and treatment of airway mucociliary clearance. Minerva Anestesiol 67:206–209
27. Hienzel FP (2000) Antibodies. In: Mandell GL, Bennett JE, Dolin R (eds) Mandell, Douglas and Bennett's Principles and practice of infectious diseases. Churchill Livingstone, Philadelphia, pp 45–67
28. Kass EH, Schneiderman LJ (1957) Entry of bacteria into the urinary tract of patients with implying catheters. N Engl J Med 256:556–557
29. Kunin CM, Evans C, Bartholomew D, Bates DG (2002) The antimicrobial defense mechanism of the female urethra: a reassessment. J Urol 168:413–419
30. Johanson WG Jr, Pierce AK, Sandford JP et al (1972) Nosocomial respiratory tract infections with Gram-negative bacilli: the significance of colonization of the respiratory tract. Ann Intern Med 77:701–706
31. Estes RJ, Meduri GU (1995) The pathogenesis of ventilator associated pneumonia. I. Mechanisms of bacterial transcolonization and airway inoculation. Intensive Care Med 21:365–383
32 de Latorre JF, Pont T, Ferrer A, Rossello J, Palomar M, Planas M (1995) Pattern of tracheal colonization during mechanical ventilation. Am J Respir Crit Care Med 152:1028-1033
33. Morar P, Makura Z, Jones A et al (2000) Topical antibiotics on tracheostoma prevent exogenous colonization and infection of lower airways in children. Chest 117:513–518
34. Sganga G, van Saene HKF, Brisinda G, Castagneto M (2001) Bacterial translocation. In: van Saene HKF, Sganga G, Silvestri L (eds) Infection in the critically ill: an ongoing challenge. Springer, Milan, pp 35–45
35. Husebye E (1995) Gastro-intestinal motility disorders and bacterial overgrowth. J Intern Med 237:419–427
36. Kane TD, Wesley Alexander J, Johannigman JA (1998) The detection of microbial DNA in the blood. A sensitive method for diagnosing bacteremia and/or bacterial translocation in surgical patients. Ann Surg 227:1–9
37. Tancrede CH, Andremont AO (1985) Bacterial translocation and Gram-negative bacteremia in patients with hematological malignancies. J Infect Dis 152:99–103
38. van Saene HKF, Taylor N, Donnell SC et al (2003) Gut overgrowth with abnormal flora: the missing link in parenteral nutrition-related sepsis in surgical neonates. Eur J Clin Nutr 57:548–553
39. Feltis BA, Wells CL (2000) Does microbial translocation play a role in critical illness? Curr Opin Crit Care 6:117–122
40. Baxby D, van Saene HKF, Stoutenbeek CP, Zandstra DF (1996) Selective decontamination of the digestive tract: 13 years on, what it is and what it is not. Intensive Care Med 22:699–706
41. Stoutenbeek CP, van Saene HKF, Miranda DR, Zandstra DF, Langrehr D (1986) Nosocomial Gram-negative pneumonia in critically ill patients. Intensive Care Med 12:419–423
42. Brown RB, Kruse JA, Counts GW (1990) Double-blind study of endotracheal tobramycin in the treatment of Gram-negative pneumonia. Antimicrob Agents Chemother 34:269–272

Chapter 4

Classification of Micro-Organisms According to Their Pathogenicity

M.A. de la Cal, E. Cerdà, A. Abella, P. Garcia-Hierro

Introduction

Isenberg wrote in 1988: "A modern clinical microbiologist who asks what is a pathogen and what is meant by virulence will meet with derision and probably be declared heretic, bereft of his or her senses" [1]. He expressed the difficulties in defining the concepts of pathogenicity and virulence that have changed, and are still changing, with the growing number of infectious diseases in the hospital setting and in the immunocompromised host.

It is accepted that infection is the result of the interaction between the host, the micro-organism, and the environment. Pathogenicity (Table 1) is not only an intrinsic quality of micro-organisms but the consequence of some properties of the micro-organisms and the host. For example, coagulase-negative staphylococcus has been considered an avirulent, opportunistic organism and not a true pathogen [5], but the increasing number of bacteremias due to this organism in the past decades has emphasized its pathogenicity and virulence. The ability of coagulase-negative staphylococcus to induce disease increases when a patient's defence mechanisms are altered. Freeman et al. [6] emphasized that the fivefold increase of coagulase-negative staphylococcus bacteremia found in a neonatal care unit from 1975 to 1982 was mainly attributed to an increase in the number of children with a birth weight less than 1,000 g. Thus, the separation of pathogenicity, defence mechanisms, and type of infection is only justified for didactic reasons. Some terms routinely used by physicians working in intensive care units (ICUs) describe many aspects involved in pathogenicity.

1. Intrinsic characteristics of bacteria, i.e., Gram's stain, aerobic-anaerobic requirements for growth, antibiotic sensitivity-resistance patterns.
2. Quantitative criteria for defining some infections, i.e., pneumonia associated with mechanical ventilation or urinary tract infection. For instance, the probability of having pneumonia is higher if the quantitative culture of a

Table 1. Glossary of terms [2, 3]

Pathogenicity: The ability of micro-organisms to induce disease, which may be assessed by disease-carriage ratios

Virulence[a]: The severity of the disease induced by micro-organisms. In epidemiological studies virulence may be assessed by mortality or morbidity rates and the degree of communicability

Reservoir: The place where the organism maintains its presence, metabolizes, and replicates

Source: The place from which the infectious agent passes to the host. In some cases the reservoir and the source are the same, but not always

Infection: A microbiologically proven clinical diagnosis of inflammation

Carriage[b]: Permanent (minimally 1 week) presence of the same strain in any concentration in body sites normally not sterile (oropharynx, external nares, gut, vagina, skin)

Abnormal carrier state: The abnormal carrier state exists when the isolated micro-organisms is not a constituent of normal flora (i.e., enterobacterial or pseudomonal strains) [3]

Colonization[b]: The presence of micro-organisms in an internal organ that is normally sterile (e.g., lower airways, bladder). The diagnostic sample yields less than a predetermined level of cfu/ml of diagnostic sample [3]

---

[a]Some authors [4] consider virulence as a synonym of pathogenicity
[b]Some authors [2] define colonization as the permanent presence of a micro-organism in or on a host without clinical expression. Carrier state is the condition of an individual colonized with a specific organism. These definitions do not take the sterility of colonized sites in normal subjects into consideration

protected brush catheter sample yields 10^4 colony forming units (cfu) instead of 10^3 cfu. Even the significance of the quantitative culture is different if the patient is neutropenic. These criteria are related to the classic concept of infective dose, which is the estimated dose of an agent necessary to cause infection.

3. Sites of isolation when evaluating the clinical significance of a culture. For instance, *Staphylococcus aureus* may colonize the external nares without any evidence of disease but its presence in a fresh surgical wound may indicate colonization or infection.

4. "Community" versus "hospital" versus ICU-acquired flora, which recognizes that the relationship between the different species, the host, and the environment induces changes in the microbial habitat.

5. Carriage, colonization, and infection, which defines some possible host states according to the significance of the presence of micro-organisms in different organs.

6. Exogenous, primary endogenous, and secondary endogenous infections, which describe a pathogenetic model based on some epidemiological criteria.

In this chapter we will address the concept of pathogenicity and the epidemiological aspects of micro-organisms in clinical practice.

The Magnitude of the Problem

The surveillance of micro-organisms in the oropharynx, respiratory and digestive tracts in ICU patients has provided an essential basis for our present understanding of infectious diseases in the ICU:

- Patients' flora change after hospital admission and this process is time dependent [7–9].
- In a high percentage of cases, from 70% to 100% [7, 8, 10], infections were preceded by oropharyngeal or gut carriage with the same potentially pathogenic micro-organism (PPM).
- Digestive tract is usually the reservoir of antibiotic-resistant strains.
- Different micro-organisms found in the same patient show different abilities to induce infection, i.e., they have a different pathogenicity.

Those observations imply two questions: Where is the flora and which types of flora can be differentiated on an epidemiological basis?

The Habitat

It is estimated that the human body consists of approximately 10^{13} cells and hosts 10^{14}–10^{15} individual micro-organisms [1]. These micro-organisms can be divided into two groups: those that usually remain constant in their normal habitat (indigenous flora) and those that are accidentally acquired and after their adherence to epithelial or mucosal surfaces have to compete with other micro-organisms and host defences. The final outcome could be clearance or colonization of the new organisms.

Body areas that usually harbor micro-organisms (Tables 2, 3) are skin, mouth, nasopharynx, oropharynx and tonsils, large intestine and lower ileum, external genitalia, anterior urethra, vagina, skin, and external ear. Nevertheless, the various anatomical sites suitable for microbiological habitats display overlapping boundaries and are subject to variation. Temporary habitats include larynx, trachea, bronchi, accessory nasal sinuses, esophagus, stomach and upper portions of the small intestine, and distal areas of the male and female genital organs [12], and permanent colonization is often found in patients with some risks factors, i.e., chronic bronchitis [13].

Table 2. Micro-organisms commonly found in healthy human body surfaces [11]

Surface	Micro-organism	Frequency of isolation
Skin	*Staphylococcus epidermidis*	4+
	Diphtheroids	3+
	Staphylococcus aureus	2+
	Streptococcus spp.	+
	Acinetobacter spp.	±
	Enterobacteriaceae	±
Mouth and throat	Anaerobic Gram-negative spp.	4+
	Anaerobic cocci	+
	Streptococcus viridans	4+
	Streptococcus pneumoniae	2+
	Streptococcus pyogenes	+
	Staphylococcus epidermidis	4+
	Neisseria meningitidis	+
	Haemophilus spp.	+
	Enterobacteriaceae	±
	Candida spp.	2+
Nose	*Staphylococcus epidermidis*	4+
	Staphylococcus aureus	2+
	Streptococcus pneumoniae	+
	Streptococcus pyogenes	+
	Haemophilus spp.	+
Large intestine (95% or more of species are obligate anaerobes)	Anaerobic Gram-negative spp.	4+
	Anaerobic Gram-positive spp.	4+
	E. coli	4+
	Klebsiella sp	3+
	Proteus spp.	3+
	Enterococcus spp.	3+
	Group B streptococci	+
	Clostridium spp.	3+
	Pseudomonas spp.	+
	Acinetobacter spp.	+
	Staphylococcus epidermidis	+
	Staphylococcus aureus	+
	Candida spp.	+
External genitalia and anterior urethra	"Skin flora"	4+
	Gram-negative anaerobic spp.	+
	Enterococcus spp.	+
	Enterobacteriaceae	±

cont. →

Table 2. *cont.*

Surface	Micro-organism	Frequency of isolation
Vagina	*Lactobacillus spp.*	4+
	Gram-negative anaerobic spp.	2+
	Enterococcus spp.	3+
	Enterobacteriaceae	1+
	Acinetobacter spp.	±
	Staphylococcus epidermidis	1+
	Candida spp.	1+

Relative frequency of isolation: 4+ almost always present; 3+ usually present; 2+ frequently present; + occasionally present; ± rarely present

Table **3.** Quantitative cultures of healthy human surfaces [3]

Surface	Micro-organism	% Carriers	cfu
Skin (per cm)	*Staphylococcus epidermidis*	100	10^5
	Anaerobes (*Propionibacterium acnes*)	100	10^3
Mouth and throat	Anaerobic micro-organisms	100	10^8
(per ml of saliva)	*Streptococcus viridans*	100	10^6
	Streptococcus pneumoniae	30–60	10^3–10^5
	Haemophilus influenzae	30–80	10^3–10^5
	Moraxella catarrhalis	5	10^3–10^5
	Staphylococcus aureus	30	10^3
Large intestine	Anaerobic spp.	100	10^{12}
(per g of feces)	*E. coli*	100	10^3–10^6
	Enterococcus	100	10^3–10^6
	Staphylococcus aureus	30	10^3–10^5
	Candida spp.	30	10^3–10^5
Vagina	Aerobic spp.	100	10^8
(per ml of vaginal fluid)	Anaerobic spp.	100	10^7

The Flora

The indigenous flora is very dynamic and reflects changes induced by environmental settings, medical treatments, and host and microbial characteristics. It is well accepted that normal subjects have a flora called normal indigenous flora (Tables 2, 3) that represents the equilibrium reached between the normal hosts and the organisms. The quantitative estimation of different micro-organisms found in human body surfaces helps us to understand the pathogenicity because it is often obvious that predominantly isolated micro-organisms rarely

induce disease. Anaerobes are a good example of organisms of low pathogenicity. They represent the highest percentage of micro-organisms isolated per surface area but they are only involved in a small proportion of infections.

Surveillance cultures performed in patients after hospital or ICU admission
[7–9] have demonstrated that flora changes over time. The carriage of aerobic
Gram-negative bacilli (AGNB) *Pseudomonas spp., Klebsiella spp., Enterobacter
spp., Acinetobacter spp., Serratia spp., Morganella spp.* and yeasts *Candida spp.*
increases. This process of acquisition of new organisms is time dependent. For
example, Kerver et al. [7] studied 39 intubated patients admitted to the ICU for
more than 5 days, obtaining samples three times a week from the oropharynx,
tracheal aspirate, urine, and feces. The prevalence of AGNB in the oropharyngeal cavity on admission was 23% and increased to 80% after 10 days. Similar
figures were found for yeasts. In feces, the prevalence of AGNB other than *E. coli*
was 20% and reached 79% on day 15. Yeasts were found in 13% of rectal swabs
on admission and in 61% of samples on day 15. In 75.6% of infections, the same
PPM was found in previous surveillance cultures [10].

This new flora comes into the human body from different animate (mostly
patients and uncommonly health personnel) or inanimate (e.g., food, furniture)
sources through different vehicles (e.g., hands, respiratory equipment). After
being introduced, the new organisms adhere to surfaces and have to compete
with pre-existing flora and host defence barriers before a permanent carriage
state is achieved. Apart from the severity of the underlying disease, parenteral
antibiotic administration is the main mechanism that favors the acquisition of
hospital flora through selective pressure exerted against indigenous flora [14].

The boundaries between normal, community, and hospital flora are not
always strict. Some groups of patients admitted to the hospital carry organisms,
usually constituents of hospital flora. Alcoholism, diabetes, and chronic bronchitis have been regarded as risk factors for carrying aerobic Gram-negative
bacilli [13, 15] in the oropharynx and in the tracheobronchial tree, respectively.

Classification of Micro-Organisms According to their Pathogenicity

Leonard et al. [16] attempted to quantitatively estimate intrinsic pathogenicity
in a population of 40 infants admitted for at least 5 days to a neonatal surgical
unit. The intrinsic pathogenicity index (IPI) for a *y* species was defined as:

$$IPI_y = \frac{\text{Number of patients infected by y}}{\text{Number of patients carrying y in throat/rectum}}$$

The range of this index is 0–1. The highest IPI found was for *Pseudomonas spp* (0.38). Other potential pathogens isolated had an IPI of less than 0.1 (*Enterobacter spp.* 0.08, *S. aureus* 0.06, *Klebsiella spp.* 0.05, *E. coli* 0.05, *S. epidermidis* 0.03, and *Enterococcus spp.* 0). This index provides useful information about the relative pathogenicity of different micro-organisms in a specific population and could be used to design antibiotic policies, both prophylactic and therapeutic, in selected groups of patients in which microbiological surveillance could be indicated (e.g., burns, severe trauma patients).

There are inherent limitations related to the small number of studied patients and the small number of infections (i.e., *S. aureus* 1 infection over 17 colonizations), which can give an unreliable estimation of the IPI. Furthermore, the authors suggested that the results should be interpreted taking into account technical aspects (definitions used, sites chosen for surveillance, microbiological techniques, interpretation of results) and population characteristics, because IPI does not differentiate between the organism's intrinsic pathogenicity and other factors (host and environment) that allow their expression. The extreme alterations in host defence mechanisms in immunosuppressed patients is a good example of the different pathogenicity of micro-organisms depending on the specific type of systemic immunosuppression, i.e., neutropenia or cellular (T-lymphocyte) immune defect [17].

In general the classification of micro-organisms according to their pathogenicity is based on scales with few categories. Isenberg and D' Amato [12] classify organisms as commonly involved, occasionally involved, and rarely involved in disease production. Murray et al. [3] classify the pathogenicity of organisms as high, potential, and low. Categories in both classifications are not always equivalent.

We found that the classification of Murray et al. [3] (Table 4) is useful in ICU practice because it is best adapted to flora isolated in ICU patients and is more discriminatory between organisms of interest in the ICU. Another possible advantage is that this classification integrates other concepts of clinical epidemiology, such as "community" or "normal" and hospital or "abnormal" flora.

Antimicrobial Resistance as a Virulence Factor

The evaluation of the influence of antimicrobial resistance on mortality is difficult because of the requirement for adjustment for underlying disease and illness severity. Recent literature suggests that the factor of immediate, adequate treatment plays an important role in the evaluation of the contribution of antimicrobial resistance to mortality [18–21]. Fagon et al. [22] found that in patients suspected of having ventilator-associated pneumonia an invasive strat-

Table 4. Classification of micro-organisms based on their intrinsic pathogenicity [3] (MRSA methicillin-resistant *Staphylococcus aureus*)

	Intrinsic pathogenicity	Flora
Indigenous flora		
Oropharynx: peptostreptococci, *Veillonella* spp., *Streptococcus viridans*		
Gut: *Bacteroides* spp., *Clostridium* spp., enterococci, *Escherichia coli*	Low pathogenic	Normal
Vagina: peptostreptococci, *Bacteroides* spp., lactobacilli		
Skin: *Propionibacterium acnes*, coagulase-negative staphylococci		
Community or normal micro-organisms		
Oropharynx: *Streptococcus pneumoniae*, *Haemophilus influenzae*, *Moraxella catarrhalis*		
Gut: *Escherichia coli*	Potentially pathogenic	Normal
Oropharynx and gut: *Staphylococcus aureus*, *Candida* spp.		
Hospital or abnormal micro-organisms		
Klebsiella spp., *Proteus* spp., *Enterobacter* spp., *Morganella* spp., *Citrobacter* spp., *Serratia* spp., *Pseudomonas* spp., *Acinetobacter* spp., MRSA	Potentially pathogenic	Abnormal
Epidemic micro-organisms		
Neisseria meningitidis, *Salmonella* spp.	Highly pathogenic	Abnormal

egy based on the use of fiberoptic bronchoscopy improved the survival rate at day 14 (p=0.02); 16.2% died in the invasive management group and 25.8% in the clinical management group, i.e., a difference of 9.6%. This survival benefit can be explained by the fact that significantly more patients who did not undergo bronchoscopy received early, inadequate antimicrobial therapy (1 patient died in the invasive group versus 24 in the control group, $p<0.001$). The survival benefit was only transient as the difference in mortality was not significant anymore at day 28 (p=0.10). Only a few of the evaluable studies have adjusted the mortality data for appropriate antimicrobial treatment, underlying disease, and illness severity.

Methicillin-Resistant *S. aureus* versus Methicillin-Sensitive *S. aureus*

Of 31 bacteremia studies comparing mortality due to methicillin-resistant *S. aureus* (MRSA) and methicillin-sensitive *S. aureus* MSSA [23], only 6 adjusted for confounding factors including adequate antibiotic therapy [24–29]. Three studies involving 401 patients did find a significantly increased mortality with odds ratios varying between 3 and 5.6. The other 3 studies with a total of 1,385 patients did not show a significant difference. Only one study compared mortality due to MRSA in 86 bacteremic pneumonia patients without a significant difference [30].

Vancomycin-Resistant Enterococci versus Vancomycin-Sensitive Enterococci

Three studies in patients with positive blood cultures and adjusted for appropriate antibiotic treatment are available [31–33]. Only one study in 106 patients reports a significantly higher mortality due to vancomycin-resistant enterococci (VRE) with an odds ratio of 4.0 (1.2–13.3). The other two studies in a total of 467 patients failed to show a mortality difference.

Aerobic Gram-Negative Bacilli Including *Acinetobacter spp.* and *Pseudomonas aeruginosa*

One study in 135 patients compared mortality in patients with infections due to piperacillin-resistant *P. aeruginosa* and mortality in patients with infections due to sensitive *P. aeruginosa* [34]. Mortality data were not adjusted for immediate, adequate antimicrobial therapy, as there was no difference in crude mortality. There are no data on *Acinetobacter* mortality, whether sensitive or resistant.

These data show that the association of antimicrobial resistance to mortality has not yet been appropriately evaluated. The present evidence supports the concept that antibiotic resistance does not contribute to mortality.

Conclusions

Although the properties of the different micro-organisms fail to explain completely their pathogenicity, it is clear that some characteristics determine the different pathogenicity, for example encapsulated pneumococci are more virulent than non-encapsulated pneumococci. Advances in molecular biology make it possible to characterize some virulence factors that allow micro-organisms to overcome the set of obstacles to accomplish infection. These include selection of the niche and adherence to human body surfaces or medical devices (i.e., adhesins), competition with pre-existing organisms in some cases, impairment of the host defence mechanism (i.e., antiphagocytic capsules, toxins), and production of tissue damage (i.e., toxins, enzymes). A recent paper discusses the impact of critical illness on the expression of virulence in gut flora [35]. It has been hypothesized that gut bacteria change and become more virulent as the micro-organisms sense that the host's capacity to control them is severely impaired. Identification of the virulent genes also provides a better understanding of the relationship between virulence factors and their clinical expression [36] and can be helpful in epidemiological studies, such as in the determination of transmission, carriage, colonization, and infection routes with specific micro-organisms and the investigation of outbreaks [37].

References

1. Isenberg HD (1988) Pathogenicity and virulence: another view. Clin Microbiol Rev 1:40–53
2. Brachman PS (1992) Epidemiology of nosocomial infections. In: Bennett JV, Brachman PS (eds) Hospital infections, 3rd edn. Little Brown, Boston, pp 3–20
3. Murray AE, Mostafa SM, van Saene HKF (1991) Essentials in clinical microbiology. In: Stoutenbeek CP, van Saene HKF (eds) Infection and the anaesthetist, vol 5. Bailliere Tindall, London, pp 1–26
4. McCloskey RV (1979) Microbial virulence factors. In: Mandell GL, Douglas RG, Bennett IE (eds) Principles and practice of infectious diseases, 1 st edn, vol 1. Wiley, NewYork, pp 3–11
5. Pfaller MA, Herwald LA (1988) Laboratory, clinical, and epidemiological aspects of coagulase-negative staphylococci. Clin Microbiol Rev 1:281–299
6. Freeman I, Platt R, Sidebottom DG et al (1987) Coagulase-negative staphylococcal bacteremia in the changing neonatal intensive care unit population. JAMA 258:2548–2552
7. Kerver AIH, Rommes IH, Mevissen-Verhage EAE et al (1987) Colonization and infection in surgical intensive care patients. Intensive Care Med 13:347–351
8. Leonard EM, van Saene HKF, Shears P, Walker I, Tam PKH (1990) Pathogenesis of colonization and infection in a neonatal surgical unit. Crit Care Med 18:264–269
9. van Saene HKF, Stoutenbeek CP, Zandstra DF, Gilberston A, Murray A, Hart CA (1987) Nosocomial infections in severely traumatized patient: magnitude of problem, pathogenesis, prevention and therapy. Acta Anaesthesiol Belg 38:347–356
10. van Saene HKF, Damjanovic V, Murray AE, de la Cal MA (1996) How to classify infections in intensive care units—the carrier state, a criterion whose time has come? J Hosp Infect 33:1–12

11. Tramont EC (1979) General or nonspecific host defense mechanisms. In: Mandell GL, Douglas RG, Bennett IE (eds) Principles and practice of infectious diseases, lst edn, vol 1. Wiley, NewYork, pp 13–21

12. Isenberg HD, D' Amato RF (1990) Indigenous and pathogenic micro-organisms of humans. In: Mandell GL, Douglas RG, Bennett IE (eds) Principles and practice of infectious diseases, 3rd edn, vol 1. Churchill Livingstone, New York, pp 2–14

13. Jordan GW, Wong GA, Hoeprich PB (1976) Bacteriology of the lower respiratory tract as determined by fiberoptic bronchoscopy and transtracheal aspiration. J Infect Dis 134:428–435

14. van der Waaij D (1992) Selective gastrointestinal decontamination: history of recognition and measurement of colonization of the digestive tract as an introduction to selective gastrointestinal decontamination. Epidemiol Infect 109:315–326

15. Mackowiak PA, Martin RM, Smith LW (1979) The role of bacterial interference in the increased prevalence of oropharyngeal Gram-negative bacilli among alcoholics and diabetics. Am Rev Respir Dis 120:289–593

16. Leonard EM, van Saene HKF, Stoutenbeek CP, Walker I, Tam PKH (1990) An intrinsic pathogenicity index for micro-organisms causing infection in a neonatal surgical unit. Microb Ecol Health Dis 3:151–157

17. Shelhamer IH, Toews GB, Masur H et al (1992) Respiratory disease in the immuno-suppressed patient. Ann Intern Med 117:415–443

18. Alvarez-Lerma F (1996) Modification of empiric antibiotic treatment in patients with pneumonia acquired in the intensive care unit. ICU-Acquired Pneumonia Study Group. Intensive Care Med 22:387–394

19. Luna CM, Vujacich P, Niederman MS et al (1997) Impact of BAL data on the therapy and outcome of ventilator-associated pneumonia. Chest 111:676–685

20. Iregui M, Ward S, Sherman G, Fraser VJ, Kollef MH (2002) Clinical importance of delays in the initiation of appropriate antibiotic treatment for ventilator associated pneumonia. Chest 122:262–268

21. Valles J, Rello J, Ochagavia A, Garnacho J, Alcala MA (2003) Community-acquired bloodstream infection in critically ill adult patients: impact of shock and inappropriate antibiotic therapy on survival. Chest 123:1615–1624

22. Fagon JY, Chastre J, Wolff M et al (2000) Invasive and noninvasive strategies for management of suspected ventilator associated pneumonia. A randomized trial. Ann Intern Med 132:621–630

23. Cosgrove SE, Sakoulas G, Perencevich EN, Schwaber MJ, Karchmer AW, Carmeli Y (2003) Comparison of mortality associated with methicillin-resistant and methicillin-susceptible *Staphylococcus aureus* bacteremia: a meta-analysis. Clin Infect Dis 36:53–59

24. Conterno LO, Wey SB, Castelo A (1998) Risk factors for mortality in *Staphylococcus aureus* bacteremia. Infect Control Hosp Epidemiol 19:32–37

25. Romero-Vivas J, Rubio, M Fernández C, Picazo JJ (1995) Mortality associated with nosocomial bacteremia due to methicillin-resistant *Staphylococcus aureus*. Clin Infect Dis 21:1417–1423

26. Harbarth S, Rutschmann O, Sudre P, Pittet D (1998) Impact of methicillin resistance on the outcome of patients with bacteremia caused by *Staphylococcus aureus*. Arch Intern Med 158:182–189

27. Soriano A, Martínez JA, Mensa J et al (2000) Pathogenic significance of methicillin resistance for patients with *Staphylococcus aureus* bacteremia. Clin Infect Dis 30:368–373

28. Mylotte JM, Tayara A (2000) *Staphylococcus aureus* bacteremia: predictors of 30-day mortality in a large cohort. Clin Infect Dis 31:1170–1174

29. Topeli A, Unal S, Akalin HE (2000) Risk factors influencing clinical outcome in *Staphylococcus aureus* bacteraemia in a Turkish University Hospital. Int J Antimicrob Agents 141:57–63

30. González C, Rubio M, Romero-Vivas J, González M, Picazo JJ (1999) Bacteremic pneumonia due to *Staphylococcus aureus*: a comparison of disease caused by methicillin-resistant and methicillin-susceptible organisms. Clin Infect Dis 29:1171–1177

31. Garbutt JM, Ventrapragada M, Littenberg B, Mundy LM (2000) Association between resistance to vancomycin and death in cases of *Enterococcus faecium* bacteremia. Clin Infect Dis 30:466–472

32. Vergis EN, Hayden MK, Chow JW et al (2001) Determinants of vancomycin resistance and mortality rates in enterococcal bacteremia. A prospective multicenter study. Ann Intern Med 135:484–492

33. Lodise TP, McKinnon PS, Tam VH, Rybak MJ (2002) Clinical outcomes for patients with bacteremia caused by vancomycin-resistant enterococcus in a level 1 trauma center. Clin Infect Dis 34:922–929

34. Trouillet JL, Vuagnat A, Combes A, Kassis N, Chastre J, Gibert C (2002) *Pseudomonas aeruginosa* ventilator-associated pneumonia: comparison of episodes due to piperacillin-resistant versus piperacillin-susceptible organisms. Clin Infect Dis 34:1047–1054

35. Alverdy JC, Laughlin RS, Wu L (2003) Influence of the critically ill state on host-pathogen interactions within the intestine: gut-derived sepsis redefined. Crit Care Med 31:598–607

36. Relman DA, Falkow S (1990) A molecular perspective of microbial pathogenicicty. In: Mandell GL, Douglas RG, Bennett IE (eds) Principles and practice of infectious diseases, 3rd edn, vol 1. Churchill Livingstone, New York, pp 25–32

37. Emori TG, Gaynes RG (1993) An overview of nosocomial infections, including the role of the microbiology laboratory. Clin Microbiol Rev 6:428–442

Chapter 5

Classification of ICU Infections

L. Silvestri, M. Viviani, H.K.F. van Saene

Introduction

Classifying infections is crucial in any infection surveillance program, in particular in the intensive care unit (ICU). From the practical point of view, time cut-offs, generally 48 h, have been accepted to distinguish community and hospital-acquired infections from infections due to micro-organisms acquired during the patient's stay on the ICU (i.e., ICU-acquired infections) [1]. However, many clinicians have appreciated that an infection developing after 48 h of ICU stay, due to a micro-organism carried by the patient on admission to the ICU, can not be considered as "true" ICU acquired. Obviously, this infection is nosocomial, i.e., the infection occurs in the ICU because the patient required intensive care treatment for her/his underlying disease associated with the immuno-paralysis. However, the causative micro-organism does not belong to the ICU microbial ecology, as the patient imported the micro-organism in her/his admission flora.

A new classification of ICU infections, based on knowledge of the patient's carrier state, has been proposed [2]. This approach allows the distinction between imported, or primary, and secondary carriage of potentially pathogenic micro-organisms (PPMs), in addition to endogenous and exogenous infections. The aim of this chapter is to compare the traditional approach with the novel concept of the use of the carrier state for classifying infection developing in critically ill patients requiring intensive care treatment.

Traditional and Novel Classifications of ICU Infections

The Traditional Approach

There are two standard means of traditionally classifying infections occurring in the ICU: the Gram staining technique, which groups both micro-organisms and infections into Gram-negative and Gram-positive categories, and the incubation time, which distinguishes community from nosocomial infections (Table 1).

The in vitro staining method, described 120 years ago, is still used to distinguish Gram-positive from Gram-negative bacteria, and to classify micro-organisms causing infection in the ICU. In the European prevalence study of infection in ICU (EPIC) [3], bacterial isolates were almost equally divided between Gram-positive and Gram-negative micro-organisms. However, there is no correlation between the Gram reaction of a particular micro-organism and its pathogenicity (see Chapter 4). For example, amongst five Gram-positive cocci present in the oropharynx of critically ill ICU patients, such as enterococci, coagulase-negative staphylococci (CNS), viridans streptococci, *Staphylococcus aureus*, and *Streptococcus pneumoniae*, only *S. aureus* and *S. pneumoniae* generally cause lower airway infections, suggesting a different pathogenicity amongst Gram-positive bacteria. Similarly, mortality is higher in ICU patients with a lower airway infection due to *Pseudomonas aeruginosa* than with *Haemophilus influenzae*, both aerobic Gram-negative bacilli (AGNB). Additionally, a worse outcome for septicemia due to AGNB has been reported compared with Gram-positive bacteria. However, bloodstream catheter-related infections due to CNS, which is associated with low mortality, are frequently included in these reports, artificially lowering the mortality due to Gram-positive bacteria. No difference in mortality was shown in a South African study between Gram-positive or Gram-negative community acquired septicemia due to high-level and potential pathogens [4]. We prefer to classify micro-organisms causing ICU infections according to their intrinsic pathogenicity index into low-level pathogens, high-level pathogens, and PPMs. Only high-level and potential pathogens cause mortality, whilst low-level pathogens only result in morbidity.

Studies on the prevalence of infections in ICU have included the usual definition of hospital-acquired infections (i.e., nosocomial) issued by the Centers for Disease Control and Prevention (CDC) [5], "for an infection to be defined as

Table 1. Classification of ICU infection using the time criterion of 48 h

Type of infection	Micro-organisms	Timing	Incidence
Community-acquired		Within 48 h of ICU stay[b]	About 15%–50%[c]
Hospital acquired	Gram-positive and/or Gram-negative[a]		
ICU acquired		After 48 h of ICU stay	About 50%–85%

[a]for community, hospital and ICU-acquired infections
[b]only for community and hospital-acquired infection
[c]the percentage includes both community and hospital-acquired infections

nosocomial there must be no evidence that the infection was present or incubating at the time of hospital admission". Based on this definition, the EPIC study, which enrolled 10,038 patient-cases with a total of 4,501 infected patients, distinguished each infection as one of the following (Table 1) [3]:

1. Community acquired: an infection occurring in the community and manifest on admission to the ICU
2. Hospital acquired: an infection manifest on admission to the ICU and deemed to be related to the present hospital admission
3. ICU acquired: an infection originating in the ICU, but not clinically manifest at the time of ICU admission.

This study showed that approximately 45% of enrolled patients were infected; nearly half (46%) of these patients acquired their infection in the ICU. The vagueness of this definition has prompted investigators to adopt "incubation times" in order to improve the distinction between infections acquired in the community and/or hospital/ward from those acquired during the patient's treatment on the ICU. Arbitrary time cut-offs varying between 24 h and 7 days [6–14] were chosen to distinguish ICU from non-ICU infections, because the CDC failed to specify a particular time cut-off [5]. The 48 h threshold has been applied in most epidemiological studies on infection rates in ICU, reflecting the firm assumption that all infections occurring after 2 days of ICU stay are nosocomial and due to micro-organisms transmitted via the hands of carers, and substantially magnifying the "ICU-acquired" infectious problem.

The Novel Approach

The traditional approach can now be challenged by the carrier state [2]. Carriage or carrier state exists when the same strain is isolated from at least two consecutive surveillance samples (e.g., throat and rectal swabs) from an ICU patient, at any concentration, over a period of at least 1 week [15]. Surveillance samples are samples obtained from body sites where PPMs are carried, i.e., the oropharynx and the digestive tract [15]. A surveillance set comprises throat and rectal swabs taken on admission and afterwards twice weekly (e.g., Monday and Thursday). Diagnostic or clinical samples are samples from internal organs that are normally sterile, such as lower airways, blood, bladder, and skin lesions; they are only taken on clinical indication with the aim of microbiologically proving a diagnosis of inflammation, either generalized or local [15].

Knowledge of the carrier state, together with diagnostic cultures, allows the distinction between the three types of infection occurring in the ICU (Table 2):

1. *Primary endogenous* infections are the most-frequent infections in the ICU; the incidence varies between 50% and 85%, depending on the population studied and the degree of immunosuppression [16–21]. They are caused by both normal and abnormal PPMs imported into the ICU by the patient in

Table 2. Three different types of infection due to 15 potentially pathogenic micro-organisms (PPMs)

Type of infection	PPM	Timing	Incidence
Primary endogenous	Normal/abnormal	<1 week	55%
Secondary endogenous	Abnormal	>1 week	30%
Exogenous	Abnormal	Any time during ICU treatment	15%

the admission flora. These episodes of infection generally occur early, during the 1st week of ICU stay. The main infection problem in ventilated patients is lower airway infection occurring during the 1st week of ICU stay. *S. pneumoniae, H. influenzae,* and *S. aureus* are the etiological agents in previously healthy individuals requiring intensive care following an acute event, such as (surgical) trauma, pancreatitis, acute hepatic failure, and burns. Abnormal hospital AGNB, such as *Klebsiella spp.*, can cause primary endogenous infections in patients with previous chronic underlying disease, such as severe chronic obstructive pulmonary disease, following acute deterioration of the underlying disease. Adequate parenteral antibiotics given immediately on admission to the ICU reduce the incidence of primary endogenous infection [22].

2. *Secondary endogenous* infections are invariably caused by eight abnormal AGNB and methicillin-resistant *S. aureus* (MRSA), accounting for one-third of all ICU infections [16–21]. This type of infection, in general, occurs after 1 week on the ICU. These PPMs are first acquired in the oropharynx, and subsequently in the stomach and gut. The topical application of non-absorbable antimicrobials polymyxin E/tobramycin/amphotericin B has been shown to control secondary endogenous infection [23].

3. *Exogenous infections* (approximately 15%) are caused by abnormal hospital PPMs, and may occur at any time throughout the patient's stay in the ICU. Typical examples are *Acinetobacter* lower airway infection following the use of contaminated ventilation equipment, or cystitis caused by *Serratia* associated with urinometers, or a MRSA tracheobronchitis in a tracheostomized patient. Surveillance samples are negative for micro-organisms that readily appear in diagnostic samples. High levels of hygiene are required to control these infections [24].

According to this criterion, only secondary endogenous and exogenous infections are labeled ICU-acquired infections, whilst primary endogenous infections are considered to be imported infections. Figure 1 enables clinicians to classify infections based on knowledge of the carrier state.

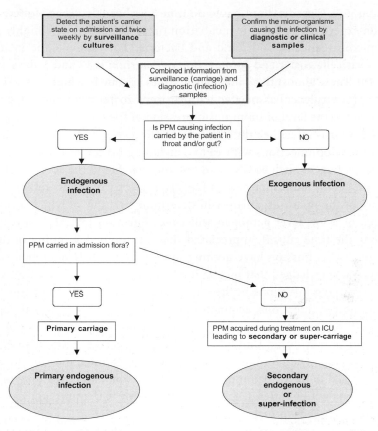

Fig. 1. Flowchart for classifying infections in the ICU using knowledge of the carrier state (*PPM* potentially pathogenic microorganism)

Evidence Behind the Time and the Carriage Classification of ICU Infections

There is no evidence that infections occurring on, or at a specific time after ICU admission, are attributable solely to micro-organisms transmitted via the hands of carers and, hence, acquired during the ICU stay [25]. It also still remains uncertain from the literature whether the given time cut-off refers to the number of days on the ICU or the number of days following intubation. The failure of the CDC guidelines to specify a time cut-off has led to the introduction of arbitrary and different time cut-offs, and to the use of the type of micro-organism causing the infections to distinguish between community, hospital-, and ICU-acquired infections. For example, *H. influenzae* is assumed to cause only community-acquired infections [26], *P. aeruginosa* must be nosocomial [16], and CNS are by definition the low-level pathogens causing catheter-related infections [27]. Classifications based on time have been developed following the common experience of specific incubation times associated with highly pathogenic micro-organisms, both viral and bacterial. For example, the incubation time for varicella zoster and *Salmonella typhimurium* is 12 and 3 days, respectively [28]. These almost fixed incubation times are due to a high intrinsic pathogenicity (or virulence) associated with varicella zoster virus and *S. typhimurium*, and not to the level of immunosuppression of the host. *S. typhimurium* and influenza A virus infect healthy individuals. However, patients requiring intensive care develop infections with PPMs, including MRSA and AGNB, and with low-level pathogens such as CNS and enterococci, due to the severity of illness and associated immunosuppression [29]. The severity of illness rather than the virulence of the micro-organism will determine the time at which a potential pathogen or a low-level pathogen will cause infection [30, 31]. Clinicians, in extending the time cut-off, appreciated that infections developing in the first days after ICU admission have nothing to do with the ICU microbial ecology, and hence acknowledged that incubation time represents an inaccurate criterion for classifying infections in the critically ill. According to the pathogenesis of ICU-acquired infections, acquisition of a PPM is followed by carriage and overgrowth of that micro-organism before colonization and infection of an internal organ may occur. Undoubtedly, this process takes more than 2, 3, or 4 days to develop. Therefore, a low respiratory tract infection due to a PPM already carried in the throat and/or gut on admission and developing in a ventilated trauma patient after 3, 4, or even 10 days of ICU admission, can not be considered as ICU acquired.

In contrast, knowledge of the carrier state at the time of admission and throughout the ICU stay is indispensable in distinguishing infections due to "imported" PPMs (i.e., primary endogenous) from infections due to bacteria acquired on the unit (i.e., secondary endogenous and exogenous). Only secondary endogenous and exogenous infections are "true" ICU-acquired infections, as the origin of the causative bacteria is outside the ICU patient, the ICU environment. In the case of the secondary endogenous infections, the micro-organism acquired on the unit goes through a digestive tract phase, but this does not apply to the exogenous infections.

Over the last 5 years, seven studies have prospectively evaluated the accuracy of the 48 h time cut-off using carriage as the gold standard (Table 3) ([16–21]; M. Viviani, personal communication). These studies included more than 2,700 patients with more than 1,500 infection episodes. Five studies in adult ICUs showed that 65%–80% of infections were classified as ICU acquired by the use of the 48 h time cut-off ([16, 17, 19, 20]; M. Viviani, personal communication). Conversely, when the carriage method was used, up to 50% of those ICU-acquired infection episodes were re-classified as primary endogenous. This figure was similar, or even higher, in the pediatric population [18, 20,

Table 3. Summary of studies on classification of infections (*PE* primary endogenous, *SE* secondary endogenous)[a]

Author	No. of patients	No. of infection episodes	Classification of infection episodes				
			PE	SE	Exogenous	ICU-acquired*	Nosocomial (48 h cut-off)
Murray et al. [16]	21	12	6 (50)	6 (50)	0	6 (50)	9 (75)
Silvestri et al. [17]	117	74	44 (60)	17 (23)	13 (17)	30 (40)	59 (80)
Petros et al. [18]	52	18	15 (85)	2 (10)	1 (5)	3 (15)	15 (83)
de la Cal et al. [19]	56	37	21 (57)	14 (38)	2 (5)	16 (43)	30 (81)
Silvestri et al. [20]							
Adult	130	27	14 (52)	10 (37)	3 (11)	13 (48)	19 (70)
Pediatric	400	40	32 (80)	4 (10)	4 (10)	8 (20)	26 (65)
Sarginson et al. [21]	1,214	792	480 (61)	42 (5)	270 (34)	312 (39)	547 (69)
Viviani M.[b]	778	573	292(51)	173 (30)	108 (19)	281 (49)	379 (66)
Total	2,795	1,573	904 (58)	268 (17)	401 (25)	669 (42)	705 (71)

[a]For each study, the same episodes of infection are classified both with the carrier state concept and with the traditional 48 h cut-off. ICU-acquired, *total of secondary endogenous and exogenous infections based on the knowledge of the carrier state; nosocomial, the infection episodes of the previous columns are re-classified using the traditional 48 h time cut-off. Values in parentheses are percentages. [b]Viviani M., personal communication

21]. Moreover, two cohort studies assessed the time cut-off that was most in line with the carrier state concept [17, 20]. A period ranging from 7 to 10 days (depending on the population studied) was found to identify more accurately ICU-acquired infections than the 48 h cut-off, although time was found to be a less-reliable method for identifying imported and ICU-acquired infections.

Impact of the Time and Carrier State Classification of ICU Infections

The main message of the traditionalists, who use a time cut-off of 48 h for classifying infection, is that the ICU-acquired infectious problem is a huge early phenomenon involving about two-thirds (up to 85%) of all ICU infections. Their approach implies that most infections occurring on the ICU are nosocomial, due to micro-organisms transmitted via the hands of carers, except those established in the first 2 days. The 48 h time cut-off is also responsible for blaming staff for almost all infections occurring in the ICU and for initiating expensive transmission investigations. Therefore, hand washing is highly recommended by influential authorities [32, 33] as the most important measure to control the exaggerated nosocomial problem due to an overestimated level of transmission. Community and hospital-acquired infections, which are present or incubating at the time of ICU admission, cannot be prevented by hand washing.

These concepts are in sharp contrast to the data from the seven previous studies. Table 3 and Figs. 2 and 3 show that more than 60% of all ICU infections are primary endogenous, i.e., due to micro-organisms not related to the ICU ecology, and develop during the 1st week of ICU stay. The remaining 40% are "true" ICU-acquired infections and develop after 1 week. Hand washing cannot be expected to control primary endogenous infections because it fails to clear oropharyngeal and gastrointestinal carriage of PPMs present on arrival. Being inherently active solely on transmission, hand hygiene cannot reduce the major infection problem of primary endogenous infection, as transmission is not involved in this type of infection. Additionally, as an ex vivo maneuver, hand washing does not influence the immune status of the patient. [34]. Detection of primary endogenous infection as the major infection problem in the ICU avoids blaming health carers for misclassified infections after 48 h, for which they are not responsible, and prevents unnecessary expensive cross-infection investigations. Finally, in strictly identifying the primary endogenous and the nosocomial problem of secondary endogenous and exogenous infections, the surveillance of both infection and carriage allows the intensivist to start with the appropriate prevention measures, including the selective decontamination of the digestive tract (SDD) [35–38].

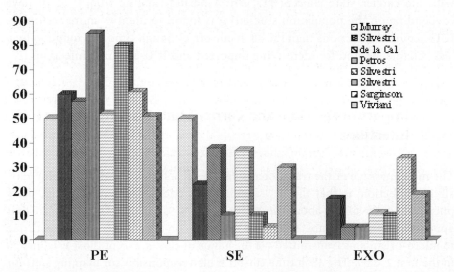

Fig. 2. Histogram showing the three types of infections in the seven different studies (*PE* primary endogenous, *SE* secondary endogenous, *EXO* exogenous)(data from table 3)

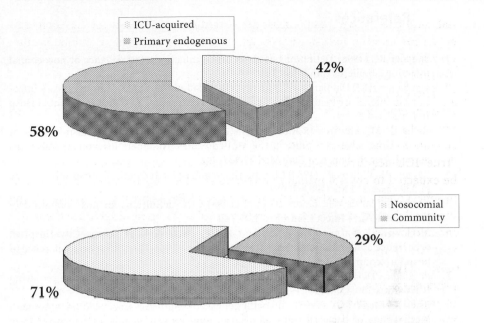

Fig. 3. ICU-acquired infections using the 48 h time cut-off versus the criterion of carriage (data from Table 3). The pie charts represent the ICU-acquired infection rate using the time and the carriage classification and mirror each other

Conclusion

Most ICU infections are due to micro-organisms that are carried by the patient on admission to the ICU. The difference in philosophy between the traditionalists and those who advocate the carriage state method for classifying ICU infections is that the former focus on the prevention of transmission of all micro-organisms via the hands of carers in order to control all Gram-positive and Gram-negative infections occurring after 2 days of ICU stay. However, we believe that ICU patients may benefit from an infection control program that includes surveillance of both carriage and infection. In detecting abnormal carriage and overgrowth, surveillance cultures are indispensable for the identification of a subset of patients at high risk of infection. Awareness of carriage in long-stay patients can provide more insights into the epidemiology of infection. The "true" nosocomial infection problem (i.e., secondary endogenous and exogenous infections) is easily and early detected. A monthly report of patients with only nosocomial infections may be useful, as the combination of secondary endogenous and exogenous infections may highlight a transmission problem in the ICU.

References

1. Spencer RC (1996) Definitions of nosocomial infections. Surveillance of nosocomial infections. Bailieres Clin Infect Dis 237–252
2. van Saene HKF, Damjanovic V, Murray AE, de la Cal MA (1996) How to classify infections in intensive care units–the carrier state, a criterion whose time has come? J Hosp Infect 33:1–12
3. Richards MJ, Edwards JR, Culver DH, Gaynes RP (1999) Nosocomial infections in medical intensive care units in the United States. National Nosocomial Infections Surveillance System. Crit Care Med 27:887–892
4. Rayner BL, Willcox PA (1988) Community acquired bacteraemia: a prospective survey of 239 cases. Q J Med 69:907–919
5. Garner JS, Jarvis WR, Emori TG et al (1988) CDC definitions for nosocomial infections, 1988. Am J Infect Control 16:128–140
6. McGowan JE, Barnes MW, Finland M (1975) Bacteremia at Boston City Hospital: occurrence and mortality during 12 selected years (1965-72), with special reference to hospital-acquired cases. J Infect Dis 132:316–335
7. Potgieter PD, Hammond JMJ (1992) Etiology and diagnosis of pneumonia requiring ICU-admission. Chest 101:199–203
8. Estes RJ, Meduri GV (1995) The pathogenesis of ventilator-associated pneumonia. I. Mechanisms of bacterial transcolonization and airway inoculation. Intensive Care Med 21:365–383
9. Pugin J, Auckenthaler R, Lew DP, Suter PM (1991) Oropharyngeal decontamination decreases incidence of ventilator-associated pneumonia. A randomized, placebo-controlled, double-blind clinical trial. JAMA 265:2704–2710
10. Chevret S, Hemmer M, Carlet J, Langer M (1993) Incidence and risk factors of pneumonia acquired in intensive care units. Results from a multicenter prospective study on 996 patients. Intensive Care Med 19:256–264
11. Rolando N, Gimson A, Wade J et al (1993) Prospective controlled trial of selective parenteral and enteral antimicrobial regimen in fulminant liver failure. Hepatology 17:196–201
12. Korinek AM, Laisne MJ, Nicolas MH et al (1993) Selective decontamination of the digestive tract in neurosurgical intensive care units patients—a double-blind, randomized, placebo-controlled study. Crit Care Med 21:1466–1473
13. Langer M, Cigada M, Mandelli M et al (1987) Early onset pneumonia: a multicenter study in intensive care units. Intensive Care Med 13:342–346
14. Trouillet JL, Chastre J, Vuagnat A et al (1998) Ventilator-associated pneumonia caused by potentially drug-resistant bacteria. Am J Respir Crit Care Med 157:531–539
15. Sarginson RE, Taylor N, van Saene HKF (2001) Glossary of terms and definitions. Curr Anaesth Crit Care 12:2–5
16. Murray AE, Chambers JJ, van Saene HKF (1998) Infections in patients requiring ventilation in intensive care: application of a new classification. Clin Microb Infect 4:94–102
17. Silvestri L, Monti-Bragadin C, Milanese M et al (1999) Are most ICU infections really nosocomial? A prospective observational cohort study in mechanically ventilated patients. J Hosp Infect 42:125–133
18. Petros AJ, O'Connell M, Roberts C et al (2001) Systemic antibiotics fail to clear multiresistant *Klebsiella* from a pediatric intensive care unit. Chest 119:862–866
19. de la Cal MA, Cerda E, Garcia-Hierro P et al (2001) Pneumonia in severe burns: a classification according to the concept of the carrier state. Chest 119:1160–1165

20. Silvestri L, Sarginson RE, Hughes J et al (2002) Most nosocomial pneumonias are not due to nosocomial bacteria in ventilated patients. Prospective evaluation of the accuracy of the 48 h time cut-off using carriage as the gold standard. Anaesth Intensive Care 30:275–282

21. Sarginson RE, Taylor N, Reilly N et al (2004) Infection in prolonged pediatric critical illness: a prospective four year study based on knowledge of the carrier state. Crit Care Med 32:839-847

22. Stoutenbeek CP (1989) The role of systemic antibiotic prophylaxis in infection prevention in intensive care by SDD. Infection 17:418–421

23. van Saene HKF, Petros AJ, Ramsay G, Baxby D (2003) All great truths are iconoclastic: selective decontamination of the digestive tract moves from heresy to level 1 truth. Intensive Care Med 29:677–690

24. Larson EL. Association for Professionals in Infection Control and Epidemiology 1992-1993, 1994 APIC Guidelines Committee (1995) APIC guideline for handwashing and hand antisepsis in health care settings. Am J Infect Contr 23:251–269

25. European Task Force on Ventilator-Associated Pneumonia (2001) Ventilator-associated pneumonia. Eur Respir J 17:1034–1046

26. Miller EH, Caplan ES (1984) Nosocomial *Haemophilus* pneumonia in patients with severe trauma. Surg Gynecol Obstet 159:153–156

27. Das I, Philpott C, George RH (1997) Central venous catheter-related septicaemia in paediatric cancer patients. J Hosp Infect 36:67–76

28. Gorbach SL, Bartlett JG, Blacklow NR (1998) Infectious diseases, 2nd edn. Saunders, Philadelphia

29. Leonard EM, van Saene HKF, Stoutenbeek CP et al (1990) An intrinsic pathogenicity index for microorganisms causing infection in a neonatal surgical unit. Microbiol Ecol Health Dis 3:151–157

30. Girou E, Pinsard M, Auriant I, Canonne M (1996) Influence of the severity of illness measured by the Simplified Acute Physiology Score (SAPS) on occurrence of nosocomial infections in ICU patients. J Hosp Infect 34:131–137

31. Bueno-Cavanillas A, Rodriguez-Contreras R, Lopez-Luque A et al (1991) Usefulness of severity indices in intensive care medicine as a predictor of nosocomial infection risk. Intensive Care Med 17:336–339

32. Liberati A, D'Amico R, Pifferi et al (2004) Antibiotic prophylaxis to reduce respiratory tract infections and mortality in adults receiving intensive care (Cochrane Review). In: The Cochrane Library, Issue 1. John Wiley and Sons, Chichester, UK

33. Larson E (1988) A causal link between handwashing and risk of infection? Examination of the evidence. Infect Control Hosp Epidemiol 9:28–36

34. van Saene HKF, Silvestri L, de la Cal MA (2000) Prevention of nosocomial infection in the intensive care unit. Curr Opin Crit Care 6:323–329

35. Silvestri L, Mannucci F, van Saene HKF (2000) Selective decontamination of the digestive tract: a life saver. J Hosp Infect 45:185–190

36. Liberati A, D'Amico R, Pifferi et al (2004) Antibiotic prophylaxis to reduce respiratory tract infections and mortality in adults receiving intensive care (Cochrane Review). In: The Cochrane Library, Issue 1. John Wiley and Sons, Chichester, UK

37. Krueger WA, Lenhart F-P, Neeser G et al (2002) Influence of combined intravenous and topical antibiotic prophylaxis on the incidence of infections, organ dysfunctions, and mortality in critically ill surgical patients. A prospective, stratified, randomized, double-blind, placebo-controlled clinical trial. Am J Respir Crit Care Med 166:1029–1037

38. de Jonge E, Schultz MJ, Spanjaard L, Bossuyt PMM, Vroom MB, Dankert J (2003) Effects of selective decontamination of the digestive tract on mortality and acquisition of resistant bacteria in intensive care: a randomised trial. Lancet 362:1011–1016

Gut Microbiology: Surveillance Samples for the Detection of the Abnormal Carrier State

H.K.F. van Saene, G. Izquierdo, P. Garcia-Hierro, F. Fontana

Introduction

Critical illness impacts all organ systems such as lungs, heart, and gut. The gut also includes the vast living microbial tissue of the indigenous, mainly anaerobic, flora. This enormous bacterial tissue is embedded in the mucous layer and covers the inner wall of the gut. Amongst the aerobic Gram-negative bacilli (AGNB) only the indigenous *Escherichia coli* is carried by healthy people in the gut. Critical illness converts the normal carrier state of *E. coli* into carriage of abnormal AGNB, including *Klebsiella, Enterobacter, Pseudomonas* species, and methicillin-resistant *Staphylococcus aureus* (MRSA) [1]. It is hypothesized that receptors for AGNB and MRSA are constitutively expressed on the mucosal lining, but are covered by a protective layer of fibronectin in the healthy mucosa. Significantly increased levels of salivary elastase have been shown to precede AGNB carriage in the oropharynx in post-operative patients and the elderly [2, 3]. It is probable that in individuals suffering both acute and chronic underlying illness, activated macrophages release elastase into mucosal secretions, thereby denuding the protective fibronectin layer. It is thought that this possible mechanism is a deleterious consequence of the inflammatory response encountered during and after illness. This shift towards abnormal flora due to underlying disease is aggravated by most iatrogenic interventions in the patient requiring intensive care including mechanical ventilation. Gut protection using H_2 antagonists and antimicrobials are commonly applied in the critically ill. H_2 antagonists increase gastric pH, thereby impairing the gastric acidity barrier [4]. Antimicrobials that are active against the indigenous mainly anaerobic flora, and that are excreted via bile into the gut, may disturb the gut ecology [5]. Integrity of both physiology and flora is essential for the individual's defense against carriage of AGNB. The impairment of these two factors promotes the overgrowth of abnormal potentially pathogenic micro-organisms (PPM), such as AGNB in concentrations of $>10^5$ colony forming units (CFU) per milliliter or gram of feces [6].

Gut overgrowth of abnormal flora is not only a marker of critical illness, but harms the patient as it is a disease in itself. In addition, gut overgrowth of abnormal flora has a major epidemiological impact on the other patients in the intensive care unit (ICU) and on the ICU environment.

Clinical Impact of Gut Overgrowth

Intestinal overgrowth with AGNB causes systemic immuno-paralysis [7]. Together with the depressed immunity, high concentrations of AGNB and MRSA in the throat and gut may result in pneumonia [8] and septicemia [9] following aspiration into the lower airways and translocation in the terminal ileum. Gut overgrowth guarantees amongst the AGNB population the presence of antibiotic-resistant strains producing enzymes that neutralize the antimicrobials [10]. The salivary and fecal concentrations of the parenterally administered antimicrobials are in general not bactericidal for the PPM present in high numbers in the gut, and create an environment in which antibiotic-resistant strains readily survive.

Epidemiological Impact of Gut Overgrowth

The higher the salivary and fecal concentrations of AGNB and MRSA, the higher the possibility of PPM transmission via the hands of carers [11–13]. Acquisition of PPM invariably leads to carriage, as the critically ill are unable to clear the acquired AGNB and MRSA. Carriers of abnormal bacteria in overgrowth shed these micro-organisms into the environment and determine the contamination level of the inanimate environment, including beds, tables, telephones, and floors [14].

Definitions

Surveillance Samples

Surveillance samples are defined as samples obtained from body sites where PPM may potentially be carried, i.e., the digestive tract comprising the oropharyngeal and rectal cavities [15]. Surveillance cultures should be distinguished from surface and diagnostic samples.

Surface Samples

Surface samples are taken from the skin, such as axilla, groin, and umbilicus, and from the nose, eye, and ear. They do not belong to a surveillance sampling protocol because positive surface swabs merely reflect the oropharyngeal and rectal carrier states.

Diagnostic Samples

Diagnostic samples are from internal organs that are normally sterile, such as lower airways, blood, bladder, and skin lesions. They are only taken on clinical indication. The endpoint of diagnostic samples is clinical, as they aim to prove microbiologically a clinical diagnosis of inflammation, both generalized and/or local.

Endpoints

The aim of obtaining surveillance cultures is the determination of the microbiological endpoint of the carrier state of PPM [16]. Carriage or a carrier state exists when the same bacterial strain is isolated from at least two consecutive surveillance samples of the ICU patient in any concentration over a period of at least 1 week. Carriage implies persistence of a PPM, and is distinguished from acquisition or transient presence. Surveillance samples are not useful for diagnosing infection of lungs, blood, bladder, or wounds. Diagnostic samples are required for this purpose.

Sampling for Surveillance purposes

Which Patients?

Only the most critically ill patients require intensive microbiological monitoring using surveillance samples for the detection of the abnormal carrier state of AGNB and MRSA. Due to the severity of their illness they require intensive care, including mechanical ventilation, for a minimum of 3 days. In general they have impaired gut motility and, hence, are at high risk of developing throat and gut overgrowth.

What Samples?

A surveillance program for this type of patient includes samples from both the oropharynx and gut. Potential pathogens carried in the throat and gut cause pneumonia [8] and septicemia [9], respectively. These two serious infections are responsible for a high rate of mortality. Potential pathogens present in overgrowth in the throat and gut are implicated in transmission via the hands of carers, in particular in outbreak situations. A throat and rectal swab are taken to detect the oropharyngeal and gut carriage of AGNB and MRSA. Rectal swabs must be coated with stool. As MRSA has an affinity for the skin, skin is sampled only if lesions are present.

When?

Surveillance sets are obtained on admission and thereafter twice weekly (e.g., Monday, Thursday) throughout the ICU stay, in order to distinguish carriage due to PPM imported in the admission flora ("import") from carriage due to ICU-associated PPM acquired in the oropharynx and gut during the ICU stay ("nosocomial", "secondary" or "super" carriage).

Microbiological Procedures

Throat and rectal swabs are processed qualitatively and semi-quantitatively, including an enrichment broth, to detect the level of carriage of the three types of target micro-organisms, AGNB, *S. aureus* sensitive and resistant to methicillin, and yeasts [1, 17].

Three solid media, MacConkey (AGNB), staphylococcal, and yeast agar, are inoculated using the four-quadrant method, and a brain-heart infusion broth culture to detect low-grade carriage is included (Fig. 1). Each swab is streaked onto the three solid media, then the tip is broken off into 5 ml of enrichment broth. All cultures are incubated aerobically at 37°C. The MacConkey plate is examined after 1 night, the plates for staphylococci and yeasts after 2 nights. In addition, if the enrichment broth is turbid after 1 night's incubation, it is then inoculated onto the three media. A semi-quantitative estimation is made by grading growth density on a scale of 1+ to 5+, as follows (Table 1): growth in broth only=1+ (approximately 10 micro-organisms/ml), growth in the first quadrant of the solid plate=2+ ($>10^3$ CFU/ml), in the second quadrant=3+ ($>10^5$ CFU/ml), in the third quadrant=4+ ($>10^7$ CFU/ml), and on the whole plate=5+ ($>10^9$ CFU/ml). Macroscopically distinct colonies are isolated in pure culture. Standard methods for identification, typing, and sensitivity patterns are used for all micro-organisms. All data are entered into the computer. A simple program enables the intensive care specialist to view the microbiological overview chart of each long-stay patient at the bedside. Tables 2 and 3 show typical examples.

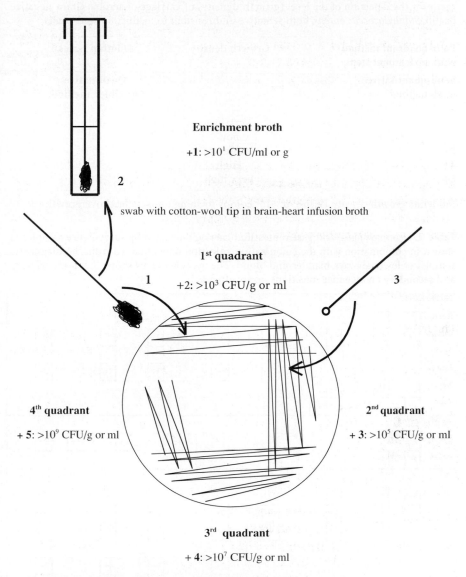

Enrichment broth

+1: $>10^1$ CFU/ml or g

swab with cotton-wool tip in brain-heart infusion broth

1st quadrant

+2: $>10^3$ CFU/g or ml

4th quadrant

+ 5: $>10^9$ CFU/g or ml

2nd quadrant

+ 3: $>10^5$ CFU/g or ml

3rd quadrant

+ 4: $>10^7$ CFU/g or ml

1. inoculation of solid medium (1st quadrant)

2. cotton-wool tip in liquid medium to detect low concentrations

3. diluting using different loops

Fig. 1. Processing surveillance swabs using the four-quandrant method and enrichment step

Table 1. Comparison of the surveillance (throat/rectal) swabs and (salivary/fecal) specimens for the detection of the level (growth density) of carriage of aerobic Gram-negative bacilli, *Staphylococcus aureus*, both sensitive and resistant to methicillin, and yeasts

Four-quadrant method with enrichment step	Growth density	Dilution series
Semi-quantitative swab method		Quantitative specimen method
1+	Very low	10^1
2+	Low	10^3
3+	Moderate	10^5
4+	High	10^7
5+	Very high	10^9

Moderate growth density, i.e., >3 or >10^5 colony forming units, reflects overgrowth

Table 2. Oropharyngeal and gastrointestinal carriage detected by surveillance samples is shown in combination with the colonization/infection data obtained from the diagnostic samples of lower airways, bladder, and blood. The overview chart shows that both primary and secondary endogenous infections occur after 48 h

	1	2	3	4	5	6	7	8	9	10	11	12	13	14	15	16	17	18	19	20	21	22	23	24	25	26
OROPHARYNX																										
S. aureus	1+		2+					--			--			--			--			--						--
Candida	1+		3+				4+		1+			2+					2+				1+					2+
P. aerug												1+		3+			3+				2+					2+
E. cloac			1+				2+																			
E. coli	1+																									
LOWER AIRWAYS																										
P. aerug														1+			2+	3+			1+			1+		2+
S. pneu	1+		3+					--																		
GUT																										
S. aureus	3+		2+				2+				--			--			--				--					--
Candida	2+		2+				3+		2+			3+					2+				1+					2+
E. coli	4+		3+				4+		4+			2+					3+				2+					4+
P. aerug												3+					3+				4+					3+
Klebsiella												1+					1+				2+					3+
E. cloac									1+			3+					3+				2+					3+
BLADDER																										
Candida	--											1+								--						
BLOOD																										
P. aerug																	+									+
S. pneu			+																							

penicillin G   ceftazidime/amikacin

Table 3. This microbiological chart shows the pattern of a trauma patient who received the full protocol of selective decontamintion of the digestive tract, immediately on admission. Cefotaxime controlled primary endogenous infection developing within the 1st week, and the enteral polymyxin E/tobramycin/amphotericin B (PTA) prevented the development of supercarriage and subsequent supercolonization and infection

	1	2	3	4	5	6	7	8	9	10	11	12	13	14	15	16	17	18	19	20	21	22	23	24	25	26
OROPHARYNX																										
S. aureus	1+		2+		--			--			--				--			--		--		--				
Candida	2+		1+		--			--			--	1+			--			--		--		1+				
	--		--		--			--			--				--			--		--		--				
LOWER AIRWAYS																										
S. aureus	1+	1+	1+	--	--			--			--				--					--						
GUT																										
S. aureus	3+		3+		2+			--			--				--			--		--						
Candida	1+		--		--			2+		1+		--			1+			--		1+						
E. coli	2+		3+		2+			2+		3+		2+			--			--		--						
	--		--		--			--			--				--			--		--						
BLADDER																										
	--																									
BLOOD																										
		--	--	--				--																		

```
        |----------------|
           cefotaxime
|------------------------------------------------------------------|
        polymyxin E/tobramycin/amphotericin B (PTA)
```

Interpretation of Surveillance Samples

Surveillance cultures allow the intensive care specialist to distinguish the normal from the abnormal carrier state, overgrowth from low-level carriage, and endogenous from exogenous infections in combination with diagnostic samples.

Normal versus Abnormal Carriage

Surveillance swabs processed for one group of target micro-organsims, AGNB, using an inexpensive MacConkey agar plate yield a positive or negative result after 18 h of incubation. AGNB, including *E. coli,* are uncommon in the oropharynx, whilst healthy people carry their own indigenous *E. coli* in the intestine in concentrations varying between 10^3 and 10^6 CFU/ml or g of feces [16] (Table 4). There are no other AGNB, including *Klebsiella, Proteus, Morganella, Enterobacter, Citrobacter, Serratia, Acinetobacter,* and

Table 4. Surveillance cultures: normal and abnormal values (*CFU* colony forming units, *AGNB* aerobic Gram-negative bacilli, *MRSA* methicillin-resistant *Staphylococcus aureus*)

	Normal Values	Abnormal Values
1. Throat	*S. aureus/C. albicans* (30% carriage)	*S. aureus/C. albicans* (30% carriage)
- Swab	< 3+ CFU/ml	>3+ CFU/ml
- Saliva	< 10^5 CFU/ml	>10^5 CFU/ml
		E. coli, AGNB, MRSA in any concentration
2. Rectum	Indigenous *E. coli* (100% carriage)	Indigenous *E. coli* (100% carriage)
	S. aureus/C. albicans (30% carriage)	*S. aureus/C. albicans* (30% carriage)
- Swab	<3+ CFU/g	>3+ CFU/g
- Feces	< 10^5 CFU/g	>10^5 CFU/g
		AGNB/MRSA in any concentration
3. Vagina	See rectum	See rectum

Pseudomonas species, in either the throat or gut. Interpreting the staphylococcal plate requires 2 nights of incubation. About one-third of the healthy population carries methicillin-sensitive *S. aureus*. The isolation of MRSA is always abnormal [1]. Yeasts also require 48 h of incubation, and can be carried by approximately 30% of the healthy adult population in concentrations of <3+ or <10^5 CFU/ml of saliva and per gram of feces. However, yeast overgrowth promotes translocation and fungemia.

Low-Grade Carriage versus Overgrowth

Oropharyngeal and intestinal overgrowth is defined as >3+ or >10^5 micro-organisms per ml of saliva and/or g of feces and is distinguished from low-grade carriage of <3+ or <10^5 micro-organisms [1, 6, 17]. Individuals with a chronic disease, such as chronic obstructive pulmonary disease, generally carry

Table 5. Strengths and weaknesses of both surveillance methods of infection only and of infection combined with carriage

Strengths	Weaknesses
Surveillance of infection (solely diagnostic samples)	Surveillance of infection (solely diagnostic samples)
• Already routine • Easy to fulfil • Number of infections per 1,000 device-days: useful to know the trends in infection rates in one unit	• Substantial delay between the detection of a problem and the implementation of the appropriate measures to control it, because of the extra work required to identify the pathogenesis of the problem • Cost-effectiveness: has to be tested • Time cut-off of 48 h: not accurate for the estimation of infection due to ICU micro-organisms • Value of method for interhospital comparison: limited • Detection of resistance, transmission and outbreaks: late
Surveillance of infection/carriage (diagnostic samples combined with surveillance samples)	Surveillance of infection/carriage (diagnostic samples combined with surveillance samples)
• More accurate estimation of infections due to ICU-acquired micro-organisms • Early implementation of the appropriate preventive measures according to the pathogenesis of the infections • Detection of resistance at an early stage • Detection of transmission at an early stage • Indispensable in control of an outbreak • Monitoring the efficacy of selective digestive decontamination	• Workload for laboratory is higher • Cost-effectiveness: has to be tested • Value of method for interhospital comparison: has to be tested • Surveillance cultures: unpopular amongst traditional microbiologists

abnormal flora in low concentrations once the forced expiratory volume in 1 s is <50% [18]. The low-level carrier status is mainly due to the presence of clearing mechanisms such as swallowing, chewing, and peristalsis. However, patients who require mechanical ventilation for a minimum of 3 days generally have impaired gut motility and readily develop overgrowth [19]. Gut overgrowth is an independent risk factor for (1) colonization/infection of internal organs [8, 9], (2) the expression of an antibiotic-resistant mutant among the microbial population [10], and (3) transmission of (often antibiotic-resistant) micro-organisms [11–13].

'Imported' versus 'Nosocomial' Carriage

Knowledge of the carrier state, at the time of admission and subsequently, is crucial to the management of infection on the ICU. Hygiene measures will only have an impact on infections due to externally transmitted micro-organisms. A primary endogenous infection caused by a PPM imported by the patient into the ICU in the admission flora can only be managed effectively with knowledge of the carrier state. It is obvious that hand hygiene fails to eradicate carriage in the throat and gut detected by surveillance samples on admission. However, that information enables the intensivist to implement isolation and to reinforce hygiene measures as soon as possible following admission. Two recent studies show that MRSA and ceftazidime-resistant AGNB were identified in 23.8% and 52.1% of patients within the first 72 h of admission to the ICU [20, 21].

Interaction between Carriage and Infection

With the structured approach, which combines data from surveillance and diagnostic samples (Tables 2 and 3), infection can be categorized into three different groups [22].

1. Primary endogenous infections are the most frequent; the incidence is ca 15% and varies between 60% and 85%, depending on the severity of illness of the patient population studied [23–26]. They are caused by both "community" and "hospital" micro-organisms carried in the throat and gut on admission. These episodes typically occur within the 1st week of the ICU stay. Examples include lower airway infection in a previously healthy individual caused by *Streptococcus pneumoniae*, or "hospital"-type organisms such as *Klebsiella pneumoniae* in patients with underlying disease. The incidence of primary endogenous infection is reduced by adequate parenteral antibiotics, e.g., cefotaxime, given immediately on admission, for 4 days [27–29].

2. Secondary endogenous infections are caused by ICU-associated micro-organisms appearing late in the ICU stay, in general after 1 week [23]. These ICU micro-organisms are acquired first in the oropharynx, followed by the stomach and gut. One-third of ICU infections are secondary endogenous infections [23–26]. Significantly, in patients not taking antibiotics on admission, almost all such infections develop only in patients who have previously had a primary endogenous infection, i.e., a subset of critically ill patients who develop more than one infection during their ICU stay [25]. Only the topical application of non-absorbable antimicrobials polymyxin E/tobramycin/amphotericin B (PTA) throughout the ICU stay has been shown to control secondary endogenous infection [11–13].

3. Exogenous infections are less common (approximately 15%) [23–26], but may occur throughout the patient's ICU stay and are caused by "hospital" bacteria, in particular *Acinetobacter* spp., *Pseudomonas* spp., and MRSA

without previous carriage. Typical examples are lower airway infections caused by *Acinetobacter* spp. in patients with a tracheostomy whether they receive PTA or not [30, 31]. A high level of hygiene is required to control exogenous infections [32].

To control the three types of infection that may occur on the ICU, the enteral PTA antimicrobials are added to the parenteral cefotaxime, whilst a high level of hygiene is maintained at all times. Surveillance samples of throat and rectum are an integral part of this infection control program for the ICU patient, for the following reasons: (1) to monitor the compliance and efficacy of PTA, (2) to detect any exogenous problems on the ICU, and (3) to detect the emergence of resistant micro-organisms at an early stage. The full four-component strategy is termed selective decontamination of the digestive tract (SDD) [33–35].

Role of Surveillance Samples in Infection Control in the ICU Patient

Recent studies using surveillance cultures of throat and rectum to detect the carrier state demonstrate that only infections occurring after 1 week of ICU stay are due to microbes transmitted via the hands of health care workers [23–26]. The incidence varies between 15% and 40%, depending on the severity of the illness. Micro-organisms related to the ICU environment are first acquired in the oropharynx. In the critically ill, oropharyngeal acquisition invariably leads to secondary or super-carriage. The subsequent build up to digestive tract overgrowth, which can then result in colonization of normally sterile internal organs, takes a few days. Finally, it is the degree of immunosuppression of the ICU patients that determines the day of colonization leading to an established secondary endogenous or super-infection. The other type of ICU infection is the exogenous infection [30–32] due to breaches of hygiene. The causative bacteria are also acquired on the unit but are never present in the throat and/or gut flora of patients. For example, long-stay patients, particularly those who receive a tracheostomy on respiratory units, are at high risk of exogenous lower airway infections. Purulent lower airway secretions yield a micro-organism that has never been previously carried by the patients in the digestive tract flora, or indeed in their oropharynx. Although both the tracheostomy and the oropharynx are equally accessible for bacterial entry, the tracheotomy tends to be the entry site for bacteria that colonize/infect the lower airways. However, the major infection problem is primary endogenous and the micro-organisms involved do not bear any relation to the ecology of the ICU. A recent study compared the traditional 48-h cut-off and the criterion of the carrier state to find that the time cut-off significantly over-estimated the magnitude of the nosocomial problem [26]. This approach to the carrier state may be more useful for interhospital comparison, as only infections due to micro-organisms acquired on the different units are compared, independent of the severity of illness.

In identifying the right population with primary endogenous infections, the classification using the carrier state avoids blaming staff for all infections occurring after 48 h for which they are not responsible. Knowledge of the carrier status thus prevents fruitless investigation of apparent cross-infection episodes. Secondly, without surveillance samples, exogenous infections are impossible to recognize, at least at an early stage when only diagnostic samples such as tracheal aspirate, urine, and blood have been tested. Finally, knowledge of the carrier state using surveillance cultures on admission and twice weekly is an effective strategy for early identification of carriers of multi-resistant micro-organisms, including AGNB such as *Acinetobacter baumannii* [36], MRSA [21, 23, 25, 37], and vancomycin-resistant enterococci [38], both on admission and during the ICU stay. Surveillance cultures, in particular of the oropharynx, that become positive for a PPM during the ICU stay reveal ongoing transmission and an impending outbreak long before the diagnostic samples yield the outbreak strain [39]. This surveillance strategy optimizes targeted infection control interventions, including (1) hand hygiene, (2) isolation, (3) personal protective equipment, and (4) the care of the patient's equipment to control transmission from one patient-carrier to another via hands of the carers.

Future Lines of Research on Surveillance Samples in the ICU Patient

Most infection surveillance programs include all patients admitted to the ICU whether they stay a few days or 2 weeks [40, 41]. The inclusion of a large number of relatively short-stay patients with a low risk of infection tends to dilute the total rates of infection by increasing the size of the denominator. However, low percentages look good to the manager of the hospital, but do not allow room for improvement, i.e., the detection of a significant reduction in infection rate following the introduction of an intervention [24]. We believe that critically ill patients benefit from a surveillance program of both infection and of carriage [42, 43], in particular in combination with SDD [33–35].

References

1. van Saene HKF, Damjanovic V, Alcock SR (2001) Basics in microbiology for the patient requiring intensive care. Curr Anaesth Crit Care 12:6–17

2. Dal Nogare AR, Toews GB, Pierce AK (1987) Increased salivary elastase precedes Gram-negative bacillary colonization in post operative patients. Am Rev Respir Dis 135:671–675
3. Palmer LB, Albulak K, Fields S et al (2001) Oral clearance and pathogenic oropharyngeal colonization in the elderly. Am J Respir Crit Care Med 164:464–468
4. Hillman KM, Riordan T, O'Farrell SM, Tabaqchali S (1982) Colonization of the gastric contents in critically ill patients. Crit Care Med 10:444–447
5. Vollaard EJ, Clasener HAL (1994) Colonization resistance. Antimicrob Agents Chemother 38:409–414
6. Husebye E (1995) Gastro-intestinal motility disorders and bacterial overgrowth. J Intern Med 237:419–427
7. Marshall JC, Christou NV, Meakins JL (1988) Small-bowel bacterial overgrowth and systemic immuno-suppression in experimental peritonitis. Surgery 104:404–411
8. van Uffelen R, van Saene HKF, Fidler V et al (1984) Oropharyngeal flora as a source of bacteria colonizing the lower airways in patients on artificial ventilation. Intensive Care Med 10:233–237
9. Luiten EJT, Hop WCJ, Endtz HP et al (1998) Prognostic importance of gram-negative intestinal colonization preceding pancreatic infection in severe acute pancreatitis. Intensive Care Med 24:438–445
10. Modi V, Damjanovic V, Cooke RWI (1987) Outbreak of cephalosporin-resistant *Enterobacter cloacae* infection in a neonatal intensive care unit. Arch Dis Child 62:145–151
11. Taylor ME, Oppenheim BA (1991) Selective decontamination of the digestive tract as an infection control measure. J Hosp Infect 71:271–278
12. Damjanovic V, Connolly CM, van Saene HKF et al (1993) Selective decontamination with nystatin for control of a *Candida* outbreak in a neonatal intensive care unit. J Hosp Infect 24:245–259
13. Silvestri L, Milanese M, Oblach L et al (2002) Enteral vancomycin to control methicillin-resistant *Staphylococcus aureus* outbreak in mechanically ventilated patients. Am J Infect Control 30:391–399
14. Go ES, Urban C, Burns J et al (1994) Clinical and molecular epidemiology of *Acinetobacter* infections sensitive only to polymyxin B and sulbactam. Lancet 344:1329–1332
15. Damjanovic V, van Saene HKF, Weindling AM (1994) The multiple value of surveillance cultures: an alternative view. J Hosp Infect 28:71–78
16. Mobbs KJ, van Saene HKF, Sunderland D, Davies PDO (1999) Oropharyngeal Gram-negative bacillary carriage. A survey of 120 healthy individuals. Chest 115:1570–1575
17. Crossley K, Solliday J (1980) Comparison of rectal swabs and stool cultures for the detection of gastro-intestinal carriage of *Staphylococcus aureus*. J Clin Microbiol 11:433–434
18. Mobbs KJ, van Saene HKF, Sunderland D, Davies PDO (1999) Oropharyngeal Gram-negative bacillary carriage in chronic obstructive pulmonary disease: relation to severity of disease. Respir Med 93:540–545
19. van der Spoel JI, Oudemans-van Straaten HM, Stoutenbeek CP et al (2001) Neostigmine resolves critical illness-related colonic ileus in intensive care patients with multiple organ failure–a prospective, double-blind, placebo-controlled trial. Intensive Care Med 27:822–827
20. Toltzis P, Yamashita T, Vilt L et al (1997) Colonization with antibiotic-resistant Gram-negative organisms in a pediatric intensive care unit. Crit Care Med 25:538–544
21. Viviani M, van Saene HKF, Dezzoni R et al (2005) Control of imported and acquired

methicillin-resistant *Staphylococcus aureus* [MRSA] in mechanically ventilated patients: a dose response study of oral vancomycin to reduce absolute carriage and infection. Anaesth Intensive Care (in press)

22. van Saene HKF, Damjanovic V, Murray AE, de la Cal MA (1996) How to classify infections in intensive care units—the carrier state, a criterion whose time has come? J Hosp Infect 33:1–12

23. Silvestri L, Monti Bragadin C, Milanese M et al (1999) Are most ICU-infections really nosocomial? A prospective observational cohort study in mechanically ventilated patients. J Hosp Infect 42:125–133

24. Petros AJ, O'Connell M, Roberts C et al (2001) Systemic antibiotics fail to clear multidrug-resistant *Klebsiella* from a pediatric ICU. Chest 119:862–866

25. de la Cal MA, Cerda E, Garcia-Hierro P et al (2001) Pneumonia in patients with severe burns. A classification according to the concept of the carrier state. Chest 119:1160–1165

26. Silvestri L, Sarginson RE, Hughes J et al (2002) Most nosocomial pneumonias are not due to nosocomial bacteria in ventilated patients. Evaluation of the accuracy of the 48h time cut-off using carriage as the gold standard. Anaesth Intensive Care 30:275–282

27. Stoutenbeek CP (1989) The role of systemic antibiotic prophylaxis in infection prevention in intensive care by SDD. Infection 17:418–421

28. Sirvent JM, Torres A, El-Ebiary M et al (1997) Protective effect of intravenously administered cefuroxime against nosocomial pneumonia in patients with structural coma. Am J Respir Crit Care Med 155:1729–1734

29. Alvarez-Lerma F, and the ICU-pneumonia study group (1996) Modification of empiric antibiotic treatment in patients with pneumonia acquired in the intensive care unit. Intensive Care Med 22:387–394

30. Hammond JMJ, Potgieter PD, Saunders GL et al (1992) Double blind study of selective decontamination of the digestive tract in intensive care. Lancet 340:5–9

31. Morar P, Singh V, Makura Z et al (2002) Differing pathways of lower airway colonization and infection according to mode of ventilation (endotracheal versus tracheostomy). Arch Otolaryngol Head Neck Surg 128:1061–1066

32. Morar P, Makura Z, Jones AS et al (2000) Topical antibiotics on tracheostoma prevents exogenous colonization and infection of lower airways in children. Chest 117:513–518

33. Baxby D, Saene HKF van, Stoutenbeek CP et al (1996) Selective decontamination of the digestive tract: 13 years on, what it is and what it is not. Intensive Care Med 22:699–706

34. de Jonge E, Schultz MJ, Spanjaard L et al (2003) Effects of selective decontamination of the digestive tract on mortality and acquisition of resistant bacteria in intensive care: a randomised controlled trial. Lancet 362:1011-1016

35. Liberati A, D'Amico R, Pifferi S et al (2004) Antibiotic prophylaxis to reduce respiratory tract infections and mortality in adults receiving intensive care (Cochrane Review) In: The Cochrane Library, Issue 1. John Wiley & Sons, Ltd, Chichester, UK

36. Corbella X, Pujol M, Ayats J et al (1996) Relevance of digestive tract colonization in the epidemiology of nosocomial infections due to multiresistant *Acinetobacter baumannii*. Clin Infect Dis 23:329–334

37. de la Cal MA, Cerda E, van Saene HKF et al (2004) Effectiveness and safety of enteral vancomycin to control endemicity of methicillin-resistant *Staphylococcus aureus* in a medical/surgical intensive care unit. J Hosp Infect 56:175-183

38. Hendrix CW, Hammond JMJ, Swoboda SM et al (2001) Surveillance strategies and impact of vancomycin-resistant enterococcal colonization and infection in critically ill patients. Ann Surg 233:259–265

39. Chetchotisakd P, Phelps CL, Hartstein AI (1994) Assessment of bacterial cross-transmission as a cause of infections in patients in intensive care units. Clin Infect Dis 18:929–937
40. Kollef MH, Sherman G, Ward S, Fraser VJ (1999) Inadequate antimicrobial treatment of infections. Chest 115:462–474
41. Richards MJ, Edwards JR, Culver DH et al (1999) Nosocomial infections in medical intensive care units in the United States. Crit Care Med 27:887–892
42. Langer M, Carretto E, Haeusler EA (2001) Infection control in ICU: back (forward) to surveillance samples? Intensive Care Med 27:1561–1563
43. Silvestri L,van Saene HKF (2002) Surveillance of carriage. Minerva Anestesiol 68 [Suppl 1]:S179–S182

SECTION TWO
ANTIMICROBIALS

Chapter 7

Systemic Antibiotics

A.R. De Gaudio, S. Rinaldi, A. Novelli

Introduction

Over recent years growing interest about systemic antibiotic therapy in critically ill patients has been observed. This chapter aims to provide a clinical review of the main antibiotics available for systemic administration. The pharmacological and microbiological factors involved in the antimicrobial activity of these drugs are also discussed. Moreover, anytime an antibacterial regimen is used in patients already exposed to antibiotics and to the hospital environment, the issue of antibiotic resistance challenges the intensivist. As new drugs have been developed to overcome this problem, bacteria acquired new kinds of resistance in the endless war for their survival. Probably, the development of new antibiotics is not the definitive answer to infectious diseases, and the correct use of the drugs available today may limit many problems linked to the antibiotic therapy.

Bacteria have the capacity to adapt to a wide range of conditions. Any strategy aimed at the destruction of the bacterial flora resulted in a dramatic failure. The goal of the intensivist challenged with an infectious disease is to turn the relationship between bacterial flora and the host from infection back to symbiosis. In this effort antibiotic drugs play a significant role that waits to meet drugs modulating the reaction of the host.

Main Antibiotics

Main antibiotics include drugs of common use in the intensive care units (ICU) like β-lactams, drugs to be used under specific indications like aminoglycosides, glycopeptides, fluoroquinolones and macrolides, and drugs used only for multiresistant micro-organisms including streptogramins, linezolid and polymyxin E or colistin (Table 1).

of the drug to reach its site of action. Aerobic Gram-negative bacilli (AGNB) have an outer membrane that is an impenetrable barrier for some antibiotics while other antibiotics (i.e. broad spectrum penicillins and cephalosporins) diffuse through aqueous channels in the outer membrane termed *porins*. Their number and size are variable among different AGNB, for example *Pseudomonas aeruginosa* lacks some porins. Another mechanism of resistance to β-lactams includes their enzymatic disruption by β-lactamases that may be conveniently classified from a clinical point of view according to their substrate specificity in penicillinases or cephalosporinases. Gram-positive bacteria produce and secrete extracellularly large amounts of β-lactamase encoded in a plasmid that may be transferred to other bacteria. AGNB produce less β-lactamases but they are strategically located in the periplasmic space between the inner and outer cell membranes, and are more efficient [5, 6].

Side-effects. Hypersensitivity reactions are the most common adverse effects to penicillins. Manifestations of allergy to penicillins include maculopapular rash, urticarial rash, fever, bronchospasm, vasculitis, serum sickness, exfoliative dermatitis. The overall incidence of such reactions to the penicillins varies from 0.7% to 10%.

Allergy to one penicillin exposes the patient to a greater risk of reaction if another is given, even if the occurrence of the side effect does not imply repetition on subsequent exposures. Hypersensitivity reactions may appear in the absence of a previous known exposure to the drug because of unrecognized prior exposure to penicillin. Exfoliative dermatitis and exudative erythema multiforme of either the erythematopapular or vesiculobullous type constitute the characteristic Stevens-Johnson syndrome [2, 3].

Apparent toxic effects of penicillins include bone marrow depression, granulocytopenia, and hepatitis.

Classification. Penicillins are usually classified according to their spectrum of antimicrobial activity (Table 3).

Table 3. Classification of penicillins

Penicillin G and penicillin V
Penicillinase-resistant penicillins
Aminopenicillins
Carboxypenicillins
Ureidopenicillins

Penicillin G and Penicillin V

Spectrum of activity and clinical use. Penicillin G is still useful for streptococcal pharyngitis caused by *Streptococcus pyogenes* and for infections caused by other streptococci like the *viridans* streptococci and enterococci. Syphilis, actinomycosis and anthrax can be treated successfully with penicillin G. It is still useful also in meningococcal and clostridial infections. *Corynebacterium diphtheriae, Streptobacillus moniliformis, Pasteurella multocida,* and *Listeria monocytogenes* are *in vitro* sensitive to penicillin G. Most anaerobic micro-organisms, except *Bacteroides fragilis,* are sensitive to penicillin. One of the most exquisitely sensitive micro-organisms is *Treponema pallidum. Borrelia burgdorferi,* causing Lyme disease, is also susceptible [1–3].

Pharmacological properties. After intramuscular injection, peak concentrations in plasma are reached within 15 to 30 minutes. This value declines rapidly, since the half-life of penicillin G is within 30 minutes. Under normal conditions, penicillin G is rapidly eliminated from the body, mainly by the kidney but in small part in the bile and by other routes. Approximately 60% to 90% of an intramuscular dose of penicillin G is eliminated in the urine, largely within the first hour after injection. The half-time for elimination is about 30 minutes in normal adults. Approximately 10% of the drug is eliminated by glomerular filtration and 90% by tubular secretion. The international unit of penicillin is the specific penicillin activity contained in 0.6 μg of the crystalline sodium salt of penicillin G. One mg of pure penicillin G sodium equals 1667 units; 1.0 mg of pure penicillin G potassium represents 1595 units [1, 2].

Penicillinase-resistant Penicillins

Spectrum of activity and clinical use. They are resistant to staphylococcal penicillinase and remain useful despite the increasing incidence of methicillin-resistant micro-organisms, term that denotes resistance to all of the penicillinase-resistant penicillins and cephalosporins. MRSA contains a high molecular weight PBP (PBP 2') with a very low affinity for β-lactams. Between 40% and 60% of strains of *Staphylococcus epidermidis* also are resistant to the penicillinase-resistant penicillins by the same mechanism.

Pharmacologic properties. The penicillinase-resistant penicillins include: isoxazolyl penicillins and nafcillin.

The isoxazolyl penicillins include oxacillin, cloxacillin, and dicloxacillin. Dicloxacillin is the most active. These agents are, in general, less effective against micro-organisms susceptible to penicillin G, and they are not useful against AGNB. The daily oral dose of oxacillin for adults is 2 to 4 g, divided into

tive than mezlocillin against *Pseudomonas*. Ureidopenicillins are important agents for the treatment of patients with serious infections including bacteremia, pneumonia, and burns caused by AGNB.

Pharmacologic properties. Regarding mezlocillin the usual dose for adults is 6 to 18 g per day, divided into four to six doses. Mezlocillin and piperacillin are excreted in bile to a significant degree. In the absence of biliary tract obstruction, high concentrations of mezlocillin in bile are achieved by intravenous administration. Regarding piperacillin, the usual doses are 6 to 18 g per day, given in three to six equal doses [1–3].

Cephalosporins

Mechanism of action. The mechanism of action of cephalosporins is the inhibition of the bacterial cell-wall synthesis similar to that of penicillin. It is important to realise that cephalosporins are not active against the following microorganisms: MRSA, methicillin-resistant CNS, *Enterococcus spp.*, *L. monocytogenes*, *Legionella pneumophila*, *L. micdadei*, *C. difficile*, *Stenotrophomonas maltophilia*, *P. putida*, *Campylobacter jejuni*, and *Acinetobacter* species.

Mechanism of resistance. Resistance to the cephalosporins may be related to the inability of the antibiotic to reach its sites of action, to alterations in the PBPs, or to β-lactamases. Alterations in two PBPs (1A and 2X) is enough for the pneumococcus to become resistant to third-generation cephalosporins. The cephalosporins have variable susceptibility to β-lactamase: cefazolin is more susceptible than cephalothin, cefoxitin, cefuroxime, and the third-generation cephalosporins are more resistant than the first-generation cephalosporins. However, third-generation cephalosporins are susceptible to hydrolysis by inducible, chromosomally encoded (type I) β-lactamases [1, 2, 7].

Side-effects. Hypersensitivity reactions to the cephalosporins are the most common side effects. Among these, the development of a macupapular rash after several days of therapy is the most common. Immediate reactions including anaphylaxis, bronchospasm, and urticaria may be observed. Patients who are allergic to penicillins may manifest cross-reactivity to cephalosporins. There are no skin tests that can reliably predict whether a patient will manifest an allergic reaction to cephalosporins [1, 2].

Cephalosporins may be nephrotoxic agents, but less than the aminoglycosides or the polymyxins. High doses of cephalothin have produced acute tubular necrosis. The concurrent administration of cephalothin and gentamicin or tobramycin acts synergistically to cause nephrotoxicity. Diarrhea and intolerance of alcohol can result from the administration of cephalosporins. Serious bleeding related to either hypoprothrombinemia, thrombocytopenia, and/or platelet dysfunction has been reported with several β-lactam antibiotics.

Clinical use. Cephalosporins have an important role in many infectious diseases: ceftriaxone is the therapy of choice for gonorrhea, cefotaxime or ceftriaxone are the drugs of choice for meningitis in nonimmunocompromised patients, cefoxitin and cefotetan are useful for anaerobic infections and ceftriaxone or cefotaxime are the treatment of choice for Lyme disease. Severe infections with *Pseudomonas* should be treated with ceftazidime plus an aminoglycoside. Moreover, the spectrum of activity of cefuroxime, cefotaxime, ceftriaxone, and ceftizoxime appears to be excellent for the treatment of community acquired pneumonia caused by pneumococci, *H. influenzae*, or staphylococci. Before surgery a single dose of cefazolin is the preferred prophylaxis for procedures in which skin flora are the likely pathogens [1, 2, 7].

Classification. The classification of cephalosporins by "generations" is based on general features of antimicrobial activity (Table 4).

First-generation cephalosporins include *cephalothin, cefazolin, cephalexin, cephradine and cefadroxil.* They have good activity against Gram-positive bacteria and relatively modest activity against Gram-negative micro-organisms. Most Gram-positive cocci with the exception of enterococci, MRSA, and CNS are susceptible. Most oropharyngeal anaerobes are sensitive, but the *B. fragilis* group is usually resistant. Activity against *Moraxella catarrhalis, E. coli, K. pneumoniae,* and *P. mirabilis* is good.

Cephalothin is not well absorbed orally and is available only for parenteral administration. Because of the pain following intramuscular injection, it is usually given intravenously. Cephalothin has a half-life of 30-40 minutes and is metabolized in addition to being excreted. This derivative does not enter the CSF to a significant extent, and it should not be used for meningitis. Among the cephalosporins, cephalothin is the most resistant to staphylococcal β-lactamase, and is effective in severe staphylococcal infections.

Table 4. Classification of cephalosporins by generations:

First-generation cephalosporins: cephalotin, cefazolin, cephalexin, cephradine, cefadroxil

Second-generation cephalosporins: cefamandole, cefoxitin, cefaclor, loracarbef, cefuroxime, cefotetan, cefprozil

Third-generation cephalosporins: cefotaxime, ceftizoxime, ceftriaxone, cefoperazone and ceftazidime

Fourth-generation cephalosporins: cefepime, cefpirome

Cefazolin has an antimicrobial spectrum similar to that of cephalothin but is more active against *E. coli* and *Klebsiella* species. Cefazolin is relatively well tolerated after either intramuscular or intravenous administration. The half-life is 1.8 hours. 85% of cefazolin is bound to plasma proteins.

Cephalexin, cephradine and cefadroxil are available for oral administration, and they have the same antibacterial spectrum as the other first-generation cephalosporins [2, 7].

Second-generation cephalosporins, including cefamandole, cefoxitin, cefaclor, loracarbef, cefuroxime, cefotetan and cefprozil, have somewhat increased activity against AGNB (*Enterobacter* species, *Proteus* species, and *Klebsiella* species), but are less active than the third-generation agents. A subset of second-generation agents including cefoxitin and cefotetan are active against *B. fragilis.*

Cefamandole has a half-life of 45 minutes, and is excreted unchanged in the urine. Strains of *H. influenzae* containing the plasmid β-lactamase TEM-1 are resistant to cefamandole. Most Gram-positive cocci are sensitive to cefamandole.

Cefoxitin is less active than cefamandole against *Enterobacter* species, *H. influenzae* and Gram-positive bacteria. However cefoxitin is more active than other first- or second-generation agents (except cefotetan) against anaerobes, especially *B. fragilis* so it has a special role in the treatment of anaerobic infections such as pelvic inflammatory disease and lung abscess. The half-life is approximately 40 minutes.

Cefaclor, cefprozil and *loracarbef* are used orally.

Cefuroxime is very similar to cefamandole in *in vitro* antibacterial activity and it is more resistant to β-lactamases. Its half-life is 1.7 hours and it can be used every 8 hours. The prodrug cefuroxime axetil can be used orally.

Cefotetan has good activity against *B. fragilis,* like cefoxitin. It also is effective against several other species of *Bacteroides,* and it is more active than cefoxitin against AGNB. It has a half-life of 3.3 hours. Hypoprothrombinemia with bleeding has occurred in malnourished patients receiving cefotetan; this is preventable if vitamin K is also administered [1, 2, 7].

Third-generation cephalosporins include cefotaxime, ceftizoxime, ceftriaxone, cefixime, cefpodoxime, cefoperazone and ceftazidime. They are less active than first-generation agents against Gram-positive cocci, but they are much more active against the *Enterobacteriaceae*, including β-lactamase-producing strains. A subset of third-generation agents (*ceftazidime* and *cefoperazone*) also is active against *P. aeruginosa,* but less active than other third-generation agents against Gram-positive cocci.

Cefotaxime has a plasma half-life of about 1 hour, and the drug should be administered every 4 to 8 hours for serious infections.

Ceftizoxime has a half-life of 1.8 hours and it can be given every 8-12 hours for serious infections. Ceftizoxime is not metabolized, and 90% is recovered in urine.

Ceftriaxone has a half-life of about 8 hours so it can be used once or twice daily. More than half the drug can be recovered from the urine; the remainder appears to be eliminated by biliary secretion. Ceftriaxone is effective in the treatment of meningitis and gonorrhea.

Cefoperazone is less active than cefotaxime against Gram-positive micro-organisms and many species of AGNB. It may be active against *P. aeruginosa,* but less than ceftazidime. The half-life is about 2 hours. Most of the drug is eliminated by biliary excretion and the dose of cefoperazone should be modified in patients with hepatic dysfunction or biliary obstruction but not in those with renal insufficiency. Cefoperazone can cause bleeding due to hypoprothrombinemia; this can be reversed by the administration of vitamin K. A disulfiram-like reaction has been reported in patients who drink alcohol while taking cefoperazone.

Ceftazidime is less active than cefotaxime against Gram-positive micro-organisms, while its activity against AGNB is very similar. Its advantage is a good activity (better than cefoperazone or piperacillin) against *Pseudomonas.* Its half-life in plasma is about 1.5 hours, and the drug is not metabolized [2, 7].

Fourth-generation cephalosporins, such as *cefepime,* have an extended spectrum of activity compared to the third generation and have increased resistance to β-lactamases. Fourth-generation agents may prove to have particular therapeutic usefulness in the treatment of infections due to AGNB resistant to third-generation cephalosporins.

Cefepime has greater activity than cefotaxime against the Gram-negative bacteria (*H. influenzae, N. gonorrhoeae,* and *N. meningitidis*). Regarding *P. aeruginosa,* cefepime is as active as ceftazidime, although it is less active than ceftazidime for other *Pseudomonas* species and *Stenotrophomonas maltophilia.* Cefepime has higher activity than ceftazidime against streptococci and *S. aureus.* It is not active against MRSA, penicillin-resistant pneumococci, enterococci, *B. fragilis, L. monocytogenes.* The serum half-life of cefepime is 2 hours and it is renally excreted. Doses should be adjusted for renal failure. Cefepime has excellent penetration into CSF. Dosage for adults is 2 g intravenously every 12 hours [1, 2, 7].

Carbapenems

Imipenem is useful for the treatment of serious infections due to ICU-acquired AGNB. Imipenem is active against aerobic and anaerobic micro-organisms: streptococci, enterococci (excluding *E. faecium* and non-β-lactamase-producing penicillin-resistant strains), staphylococci, *Listeria, Enterobacteriaceae,* many strains of *Pseudomonas* and *Acinetobacter* and all anaerobes, including *B. fragilis.* On the other hand many strains of MRSA and methicillin-resistant CNS as well as *S. maltophilia* are resistant to imipenem.

Mechanism of action. The mechanism of action of imipenem is similar to that of other β-lactam antibiotics. In fact imipenem binds to penicillin-binding proteins, disrupts bacterial cell-wall synthesis, and causes death of susceptible micro-organisms. It is very resistant to hydrolysis by most β-lactamases. Imipenem is not absorbed orally. The drug is hydrolyzed rapidly by a dipeptidase found in the proximal renal tubule. Imipenem is used in association with cilastatin that inhibits the degradation of imipenem by this dipeptidase. 70% of administered imipenem is recovered in the urine using this combination. Both imipenem and cilastatin have a half-life of about 1 hour. Dosage should be modified for patients with renal insufficiency. The intravenous dose is 500 mg.

Side-effects. Nausea and vomiting are the most common adverse reactions. Seizures have been noted, especially when high doses are given to patients with CNS lesions and to those with renal insufficiency. Patients who are allergic to other β-lactam antibiotics may have hypersensitivity reactions when given imipenem [1, 8, 9].

Meropenem does not require co-administration with cilastatin because it is not sensitive to renal dipeptidase. Its antimicrobial activity is similar to that of imipenem, with activity against some imipenem-resistant *P. aeruginosa,* but less activity against Gram-positive cocci [1].

Monobactams

Aztreonam interacts with PBP of susceptible micro-organisms and induces the formation of long filamentous bacterial structures. The compound is resistant to many of the β-lactamases that are elaborated by most AGNB. The antimicrobial activity of aztreonam differs from those of other β-lactam antibiotics: Gram-positive bacteria and anaerobic organisms are naturally resistant. On the other hand, activity against *Enterobacteriaceae, P. aeruginosa, H. influenzae* and gonococci is good. Aztreonam is administered either intramuscularly or intravenously at the usual dose of 2 g every 6 to 8 hours. The half-life is 1.7 hours, and most of the drug is recovered unaltered in the urine. The dosage should be reduced in patients with renal insufficiency. Aztreonam generally is well tolerated; patients who are allergic to penicillins or cephalosporins seem not to react to aztreonam [1, 2, 10].

β-Lactams Combined with β-Lactamase Inhibitors

They can bind to β-lactamases and inactivate them, preventing the destruction of β-lactam antibiotics. β-lactamase inhibitors are most active against plasmid-encoded β-lactamases including the extended-spectrum ceftazidime- and cefotaxime-hydrolyzing enzymes, ESBL, but are inactive against the type I chromosomal β-lactamases induced in AGNB by second- and third-generation cephalosporins. β-lactamase inhibitors include clavulanic acid, sulbactam and tazobactam [1, 2].

Clavulanic acid is a "suicide" inhibitor that binds irreversibly β-lactamases produced by a wide range of both Gram-positive and Gram-negative micro-organisms. Clavulanic acid is well absorbed by mouth and also can be given parenterally. It has been combined with amoxicillin and ticarcillin. This combination extends the antimicrobial activity to β-lactamase-producing strains of staphylococci, *H. influenzae,* gonococci, and *E. coli*. The combination of ticarcillin and clavulanic acid is especially useful for mixed nosocomial infections and is often used with an aminoglycoside.

Sulbactam is similar to clavulanic acid. It is combined with ampicillin. The usual dose for adults is 1 to 2 g of ampicillin plus 0.5 to 1 g of sulbactam every 6 hours. Dosage must be adjusted for patients with impaired renal function. The combination has good activity against Gram-positive cocci, including β-lactamase-producing strains of *S. aureus,* AGNB (except *Pseudomonas*), and anaerobes.

Tazobactam has been combined with *piperacillin*. This combination does not increase the activity of piperacillin against *P. aeruginosa,* as resistance is due to either chromosomal β-lactamases or decreased permeability of piperacillin into the periplasmic space due to either loss of the porin protein OprD or upregulation of multi-drug efflux systems [1, 2, 11].

Aminoglycosides

Aminoglycosides are polycations containing amino-sugars linked to an aminocyclitol ring. The aminoglycosides are used primarily to treat infections caused by AGNB [1, 2, 12] (Table 5).

Mechanism of action. The aminoglycosides interfere with protein synthesis and are rapidly bactericidal. Bacterial killing is concentration-dependent: the higher the concentration, the greater the rate at which bacteria are killed. Aminoglycosides have a concentration-dependent postantibiotic effect, in fact residual bactericidal activity persists after the serum concentration has fallen below the minimum inhibitory concentration. The mechanism of action of

Table 5. Aminoglycosides

Streptomycin

Gentamicin

Tobramycin

Amikacin

Netilmicin

Kanamycin

Neomycin

aminoglycosides is the inhibition of protein synthesis and the decrease in the translation of mRNA at the ribosome, though these effects do not explain completely the rapidly lethal effect of aminoglycosides. Aminoglycosides diffuse through aqueous channels in the outer membrane of AGNB and then they cross the cytoplasmic membrane. This phase of transport has been termed *energy-dependent phase I*. It can be inhibited by divalent cations (Ca^{2+} and Mg^{2+}), hyperosmolarity, acidosis, and anaerobiosis. This is the reason why the antimicrobial activity of aminoglycosides is reduced markedly in the anaerobic environment of an abscess and in hyperosmolar acidic urine. Following transport across the cytoplasmic membrane, the aminoglycosides bind to polysomes and interfere with protein synthesis. The aberrant proteins produced may be inserted into the cell membrane, leading to altered permeability and further stimulation of aminoglycoside transport. This phase of aminoglycoside transport is termed *energy-dependent phase II* and is associated with the disruption of the cytoplasmic membrane that results in bacterial death. The primary intracellular site of action of the aminoglycosides is the 30 S ribosomal subunit. Aminoglycosides alter ribosomal function interfering with the initiation of protein synthesis and inducing the misreading of the mRNA template [1, 2, 13].

Mechanism of resistance. Mutations affecting proteins in the bacterial ribosome can confer resistance to aminoglycosides. Resistance can result from impaired transport of the drug into the cell and mainly from the acquisition of plasmids that contain genes that code for aminoglycoside-metabolizing enzymes such as phosphoryl, adenyl, or acetyl transferases. These enzymes are the most important mechanism for the acquired microbial resistance to aminoglycosides. The metabolites of the aminoglycosides may compete with the unaltered drug for intracellular transport, but they are incapable of binding effectively to ribosomes. The genetic information for these enzymes is acquired primarily by conjugation and the transfer of DNA as plasmids. The semi-synthetic derivatives amikacin, netilmicin and isepamicin are less vulnerable to these inactivating enzymes because of protective molecular side chains [2, 13, 14].

Spectrum of activity. The antibacterial activity of aminoglycosides includes AGNB. Kanamycin, like streptomycin, has a more limited spectrum compared with other aminoglycosides, and should not be used against *Serratia* species or *P. aeruginosa*. Aminoglycosides have little activity against anaerobic microorganisms or facultative bacteria under anaerobic conditions. Their action against most Gram-positive bacteria is limited. *Streptococcus pneumoniae* and *S. pyogenes* are resistant. Both gentamicin and tobramycin are active against *S. aureus* and *S. epidermidis*. However, staphylococci become rapidly gentamicin-resistant during exposure to the drug. Tobramycin and gentamicin exhibit similar activity against most AGNB, although tobramycin usually is more active against *P. aeruginosa* and against some strains of *Proteus* species. When bacteria are resistant to gentamicin and tobramycin, amikacin and netilmicin may have retained their activity [1, 2].

Pharmacologic properties. The aminoglycosides are very poorly absorbed from the gastrointestinal tract. Except for streptomycin, there is negligible binding (less than 5%) of aminoglycosides to plasma albumin. They have poor penetration in most cells, in the central nervous system and into respiratory secretions. High concentrations are found only in the renal cortex and in the endolymph and perilymph of the inner ear; this may contribute to the nephrotoxicity and ototoxicity. Inflammation increases the penetration of aminoglycosides into peritoneal and pericardial cavities.

   The aminoglycosides are excreted almost entirely by glomerular filtration, though they are partially reabsorbed (15%). Their half-lives in plasma are similar and vary between 2 and 3 hours in patients with normal renal function. A linear relationship exists between the concentration of creatinine in plasma and the half-life of aminoglycosides. Because of the risk of nephrotoxicity and ototoxicity, the dosage of these drugs should be reduced in patients with impaired renal function. Aminoglycosides are removed from the body by either hemodialysis or peritoneal dialysis. Newborn infants have half-lives for aminoglycosides ranging from 5 to 11 hours [1, 12].

Side effects. All aminoglycosides may produce vestibular, cochlear, and renal toxicity. These drugs accumulate in the perilymph and endolymph of the inner ear. Ototoxicity is more evident in patients with elevated concentrations of drug in plasma (mainly high through values) and it is largely irreversible resulting from the progressive destruction of vestibular or cochlear sensory cells. Streptomycin and gentamicin produce predominantly vestibular effects, whereas amikacin, kanamycin, and neomycin primarily affect auditory function; tobramycin affects both equally. Patients receiving aminoglycosides should be monitored for ototoxicity, since the initial symptoms may be reversible. Tinnitus is often the first symptom, then auditory impairment may develop.

Moderately intense headache may precede the onset of labyrinthine dysfunction. This is immediately followed by nausea, vomiting, and difficulty with equilibrium. This stage is followed by the appearance of chronic labyrinthitis, with difficulty in walking [1, 15].

Patients treated with aminoglycosides are at risk of mild renal impairment that is almost always reversible. The nephrotoxicity is the result of marked accumulation of aminoglycosides in the proximal tubular cells. They produce a defect in renal concentrating ability and mild proteinuria, after several days the glomerular filtration rate is reduced. The non-oliguric phase of renal insufficiency seems to be due to a decreased sensitivity of the collecting-duct to anti-diuretic hormone. Acute tubular necrosis may occur rarely, but a rise in plasma creatinine is common. Toxicity correlates with the total amount of drug administered. Continuous infusion is more nephrotoxic than intermittent dosing. Once daily administration reduces nephrotoxicity with no reduction in efficacy. Neomycin is highly nephrotoxic and should not be administered systemically [1, 2, 12].

Aminoglycosides may rarely cause neuromuscular blockade. Most episodes have occurred in association with the administration of other neuromuscular blocking agents. Patients with myasthenia gravis are particularly susceptible to neuromuscular blockade by aminoglycosides. Aminoglycosides inhibit prejunctional release of acetylcholine and reduce the postsynaptic sensitivity to the transmitter. The intravenous administration of calcium is the preferred treatment for this toxicity [1].

Clinical use. Aminoglycosides include streptomycin, gentamicin, tobramycin, amikacin, netilmicin and isepamicin.

Gentamicin, tobramycin, amikacin, and netilmicin can be used interchangeably for the treatment of AGNB infections including urinary tract infections, bacteremia, infected burns, osteomyelitis, pneumonia, peritonitis, and otitis caused by *P. aeruginosa, Enterobacter, Klebsiella, Serratia,* and other species resistant to less toxic antibiotics. Penicillins and aminoglycosides must never be mixed in the same flask because penicillin inactivates the aminoglycoside to a significant degree. An aminoglycoside in combination with a β-lactam antibiotic is indicated for empirical therapy of pneumonia acquired on the ICU. Combination therapy is also recommended for the treatment of pneumonia caused by *P. aeruginosa.* Aminoglycosides are ineffective for the treatment of pneumonia due to *S. pneumoniae.* Meningitis caused by AGNB are a therapeutic challenge usually requiring third-generation cephalosporins, though rare isolates such as *Pseudomonas* and *Acinetobacter* are resistant to β-lactam antibiotics and require aminoglycosides. They are very useful also in cases of enterococcal endocarditis. In granulocytopenic patients infected by *P. aerugi-*

nosa the administration of an anti-pseudomonal penicillin in combination with aminoglycosides is recommended [1, 2, 12].

Streptomycin is in general less active than other aminoglycosides against AGNB. Therefore gentamicin has almost entirely replaced streptomycin. Anyway streptomycin is still very effective in the treatment of tularemia, even if tetracyclines are preferred by some physicians. Streptomycin may be one of the few agents to which multiple-drug-resistant strains of *Mycobacterium tuberculosis* are susceptible. The dose is 15 mg/kg per day as a single intramuscular injection [1, 2].

Gentamicin is the aminoglycoside of first choice because of its reliable activity against all but resistant AGNB. However, emergence of resistant microorganisms in some hospitals has become a serious problem. The recommended dose of gentamicin is a 2 mg/kg loading dose then 3 to 5 mg/kg per day, one third being given every 8 hours. A once daily dosing regimen given as a single 30 to 60 minute infusion may also be used and may be preferred. Routine monitoring of the plasma concentration of aminoglycosides are strongly recommended to confirm that drug concentrations are in the therapeutic range. Gentamicin is very slowly absorbed when applied in an ointment, but absorption may be more rapid when a cream is used topically [1, 2, 12].

Tobramycin. The antimicrobial activity and pharmacokinetic properties of tobramycin are very similar to those of gentamicin. Dosages are identical to those for gentamicin. The superior activity of tobramycin against *P. aeruginosa* makes it desirable in the treatment of bacteremia, osteomyelitis, and pneumonia caused by *Pseudomonas* species. In contrast to gentamicin, tobramycin shows poor activity in combination with penicillin against enterococci. Tobramycin is ineffective against mycobacteria [1, 2, 12].

Amikacin is a semi-synthetic derivative of kanamycin. The spectrum of antimicrobial activity of amikacin is the broadest of the group, and because of its unique resistance to the aminoglycoside-inactivating enzymes, it has a special role in hospitals where gentamicin- and tobramycin-resistant micro-organisms are prevalent. Amikacin is active against nearly all strains of *Klebsiella, Enterobacter,* and *E. coli* that are resistant to gentamicin and tobramycin. Most resistance to amikacin is found among strains of *Acinetobacter, Providencia,* and strains of non-aeruginosa *Pseudomonas* species. It is effective against *M. tuberculosis.* The recommended dose of amikacin is 15 mg/kg per day, as a single daily dose or divided into two or three equal doses [1, 2, 12].

Netilmicin is a derivative of sisomicin and it is similar to gentamicin and tobramycin in its pharmacokinetic properties and dosage. Its antibacterial activity is broad against AGNB. Like amikacin, it is not metabolized by the majority of the aminoglycoside-inactivating enzymes, and it may be active against certain bacteria that are resistant to gentamicin, except enterococci. The recommended dose of netilmicin is 4 to 6.5 mg/kg administered as a single dose or divided into two or three doses [1, 2].

Isepamicin is a relatively recent semisynthetic derivative of gentamicin. This aminoglycoside is as effective as amikacin against AGNB, including *P. aeruginosa*, and has better activity against strains producing type I 6' acetyl transpherase. Isepamicin is administered as a daily dose of 15 mg/kg usually in one or two doses [16].

Fluoroquinolones

Fluorinated quinolones have broad antimicrobial activity, and are effective in the treatment of a wide variety of infectious diseases. These compounds are divided on the basis of a generational classification: first generation comprises not fluorinated compounds including nalidixic acid, pipemidic acid, cinoxacin, second generation compounds include norfloxacin, enoxacin, pefloxacin, ofloxacin, lomefloxacin and ciprofloxacin, while levofloxacin, gatifloxacin and moxifloxacin are third-generation fluoroquinolones (Table 6).

Mechanism of action. The mechanism of action of fluoroquinolones is the inhibition of two enzymes involved in bacterial DNA synthesis: DNA gyrase and topoisomerase IV. The first enzyme introduces negative supercoiling into DNA, while the latter is responsible for decatenation. Fluoroquinolones interact with either the DNA-DNA gyrase complex or the DNA-topoisomerase IV complex, producing conformational changes which lead to the inhibition of normal enzyme activity, blocking the progression of the replication fork with rapid inhibition of DNA synthesis and bacterial cell death [17]. Fluoroquinolones bind the A subunits of the bacterial DNA gyrase, which carry out the strand-cutting function of the gyrase. The bacterial DNA gyrase is responsible for the continuous introduction of negative supercoils into DNA.

Table 6. Generational classification of quinolones

First generation	Second generation	Third generation
Nalidixic acid	Norfloxacin	Levofloxacin
Cinoxacin	Enoxacin	Gatifloxacin
Oxolinic acid	Pefloxacin	Moxifloxacin
Pipemidic acid	Ofloxacin	
Piromid acid	Lomefloxacin	
	Ciprofloxacin	

This is an ATP-dependent reaction that requires both strands of the DNA to be cut to permit passage of a segment of DNA through the break; the break is then resealed [1, 18].

Mechanism of resistance. Fluoroquinolone resistance seems to be only chromosomally mediated and it develops through two main mechanisms: alterations in the drug target enzymes (DNA gyrase or topoisomerase mutations, according to the primary target) and reduced access due to the expression of multidrug resistant membrane-associated efflux pumps. Alterations in DNA gyrase (mainly Gyr A subunit) occur most commonly in AGNB, and cause resistance through decreased drug affinity for the altered gyrase-DNA complex. Topoisomerase IV mutations commonly occur in ParC1 subunit (Grl A in *S. aureus*) and reduce drug affinity. Efflux pumps reduce quinolone access to cell targets and contribute to low-level resistance [1, 19].

Side-effects. The most common adverse reactions are nausea, abdominal discomfort, headache, and dizziness. Rarely, hallucinations, delirium, and seizures have occurred, predominantly in patients who were also receiving theophylline or a nonsteroidal antiinflammatory drug. Rashes, including photosensitivity reactions, can also occur. Arthralgias and joint swelling have developed in children receiving fluoroquinolones; therefore, these drugs are not generally recommended for the use in prepubertal children or pregnant women. Ciprofloxacin and enoxacin inhibit the metabolism of theophylline, and toxicity from elevated concentrations of the methylxanthine may occur. Concurrent administration of some nonsteroidal antiinflammatory drugs mainly propionic acid derivatives may potentiate the central nervous system stimulating effects of the quinolones, resulting in seizures [1, 18].

Pharmacologic properties. Quinolones are well absorbed after oral administration and are widely distributed in body tissues. Peak serum levels of fluoroquinolones are obtained within 1 to 3 hours of an oral dose. The relatively low serum levels of norfloxacin limit its usefulness for the treatment of infections. Oral doses in adults are 200 to 400 mg every 12 hours for ofloxacin, 400 mg every 12 hours for pefloxacin, 400 mg every 24 hours for lomefloxacin, moxifloxacin and gatifloxacin, 500 to 750 mg every 12 hours for ciprofloxacin, 500 mg every 12-24 hours or 750 mg every 24 hours for levofloxacin. The serum half-life ranges from 3 to 5 hours for norfloxacin and ciprofloxacin to 7-8 hours for gatifloxacin and levofloxacin, to 10 to 12 hours for pefloxacin and moxifloxacin. The volume of distribution of quinolones is high, with concentrations of quinolones in urine, kidney, lung and prostate tissue, stool, bile, and macrophages and neutrophils higher than serum levels. Quinolone concentrations in cerebrospinal fluid and prostatic fluid are lower than in serum. Routes of elimination differ among the quinolones. Renal clearance predominates for ofloxacin, lomefloxacin, levofloxacin and gatifloxacin; pefloxacin and nalidixic acid are predominantly eliminated non-renally. Dose adjustments in patients with renal insufficiency are required for norfloxacin, ciprofloxacin, ofloxacin, enoxacin, lomefloxacin, levofloxacin and gatifloxacin but not for pefloxacin and moxifloxacin. None of the agents is efficiently removed by peritoneal or hemodialysis [1, 2, 18].

Spectrum of activity. Second-generation quinolones are rapidly bactericidal and are effective against *E. coli* and various species of *Salmonella, Shigella, Enterobacter, Campylobacter,* and *Neisseria.* Ciprofloxacin and levofloxacin have good activity against *P. aeruginosa.* Third-generation quinolones are highly active against pneumococci and enterococci, though they have low activity against *P. aeruginosa* strains. Several intracellular bacteria are inhibited by fluoroquinolones at concentrations that can be achieved in plasma; these include species of *Chlamydia, Mycoplasma, Legionella, Brucella,* and *Mycobacterium.* Most anaerobic micro-organisms are resistant to quinolones, while sensitive to third-generation compounds [18, 20].

Clinical use. Nalidixic acid and cinoxacin are useful only for urinary tract infections caused by susceptible micro-organisms. Fluoroquinolones are significantly more potent and have a much broader spectrum of antimicrobial activity. Norfloxacin is useful only for urinary tract infections. Norfloxacin, ciprofloxacin, and ofloxacin are effective for the treatment of prostatitis caused by sensitive bacteria. Second-generation quinolones have activity against *N. gonorrhoeae, C. trachomatis,* and *H. ducreyi.* A single oral dose of ofloxacin or ciprofloxacin is an effective treatment for gonorrhea and is an alternative to ceftriaxone. Pelvic inflammatory disease has been treated effectively with ofloxacin combined with an antibiotic with activity against anaerobes (clindamycin or metronidazole). For traveler's diarrhea due to enterotoxigenic *E. coli,* the quinolones are very effective. Norfloxacin, ciprofloxacin, and ofloxacin are effective in the treatment of patients with shigellosis. Norfloxacin is superior to trimethoprim-sulfamethoxazole in decreasing the duration of diarrhea in cholera. Ciprofloxacin and ofloxacin cure most patients with enteric fever caused by *S. typhi,* as well as bacteremic non-typhoidal infections in AIDS patients. The major limitation of the use of second-generation quinolones for the treatment of community-acquired pneumonia and bronchitis is their poor activity against *S. pneumoniae.* For these infections third generation derivatives are highly effective. However, fluoroquinolones have *in vitro* activity against other common respiratory pathogens, including *H. influenzae, M. catarrhalis, S. aureus, M. pneumoniae, C. pneumoniae,* and *Legionella pneumophila.* Mild to moderate respiratory exacerbations due to *P. aeruginosa* in patients with cystic fibrosis have responded to oral fluoroquinolone therapy. Third-generation quinolones are indicated for infections caused by *L. pneumophila, C. pneumoniae,* and *M. pneumoniae.* Fluoroquinolones may be appropriately used in some cases of chronic osteomyelitis because they are active against *S. aureus* and AGNB. Quinolones mainly third-generation derivatives are being used as part of multiple-drug regimens for the treatment of multidrug-resistant tuberculosis, and for the treatment of atypical mycobacterial infections [18, 20]. MRSA is resistant to fluoroquinolones.

Macrolides

Macrolides were introduced in the early 1950s. Advantages over existing drugs included their efficacy in patients with β-lactam intolerance and activity against penicillin-resistant pathogens. Drawbacks were rapidly evolving resistance, instability of the drug in an acid environment, poor absorption by the oral route and gastrointestinal side-effects.

Given the progressive developments regarding macrolides, a generational classification has been advocated for this class of antibiotics (Table 7).

Mechanism of action. MLS$_B$ antimicrobials, including macrolides, lincosamides and streptogramin B, have antimicrobial activity acting on the bacterial ribosomes, which consist of two subunits, 30S and 50S. The 30S ribosomal subunit interacts with the messenger RNA (mRNA) and translates in conjunction with transfer RNAs (tRNAs) the genetic code on the mRNA. The large subunit (50S) provides the peptidyl transferase centre where the amino acid binds to the peptide chain previously synthesized. The growing peptide passes through a peptide exit channel within the 50S subunit to emerge on the back of the ribosome [21, 22].

Table 7. Generational classification of macrolides

First generation: erythromycin

Second generation: spiramycin

Third generation: clarithromycin, azithromycin

Fourth generation: ketolides

The peptidyl transferase centre in the 50S subunit is the site of interaction of MLS$_B$ antibiotics. MLS$_B$ drugs bind to closely related sites on the 50S ribosomal subunit and interact with an internal loop structure within domain V of bacterial 23S rRNA in the upper portion of the peptide exit channel close to the peptidyl transferase centre. Macrolides and ketolides bind to the same region of 23S rRNA. But the strength of interaction is different. The binding affinity for ketolides seems to be 10-fold stronger than that for the other macrolides [1, 2, 23].

Mechanism of resistance. The main mechanisms of acquired resistance to MLS$_B$ antimicrobials are target site modification, reduced intracellular accumulation due to decreased influx or increased efflux of the drug, and production of inactivating enzymes.

Erythromycin is most effective against aerobic Gram-positive cocci and bacilli. Some staphylococci are sensitive to high concentrations of erythromycin, but resistant strains of *S. aureus* are frequently encountered in hospitals, and resistance may emerge during treatment. Erythromycin-resistant strains of *S. aureus* also are resistant to clarithromycin and azithromycin. Many other Gram-positive bacilli including *Clostridium perfringens, Corynebacterium diphtheriae* and *Listeria monocytogenes* are sensitive. Erythromycin is not active against most AGNB. However, it retains activity against other Gram-negative organisms, including *N. meningitidis*, and *N. gonorrhoeae*. Useful antibacterial activity is also observed against *Pasteurella multocida, Borrelia* spp., and *Bordetella pertussis*. Resistance is common for *B. fragilis*. Erythromycin is effective against *M. pneumoniae, L. pneumophila* and *C. trachomatis*. Some of the atypical mycobacteria are sensitive to erythromycin [1, 2, 23].

This macrolide derivative is available for oral and intravenous administrations, though oral bioavailability is rather low (≤20%) and the derivative has to be administered as an esther pro-drug. It diffuses readily into intracellular fluids, and antibacterial activity can be achieved at all sites except the brain and CSF. Concentrations in middle ear exudate may be too low for the treatment of otitis media caused by *H. influenzae,* since this bacterial strain usually shows only moderate or very low sensitivity to the macrolide. Protein binding of erythromycin is approximately 70% to 80%. Erythromycin penetrates the placental barrier, and concentrations in breast milk also are significant. Only 2% to 5% of orally administered erythromycin is excreted in active form in the urine. The antibiotic is concentrated in the liver and is excreted as the active form in the bile. The plasma elimination half-life of erythromycin is approximately 1.6 hours. The drug is not removed significantly by either peritoneal or traditional hemodialysis. The usual oral dose of erythromycin ranges from 1 to 2 g per day, divided in four doses. Intravenous administration is used infrequently and is reserved for the therapy of severe infections, such as legionellosis [1, 2].

Clinically erythromycin is useful in pneumonia caused by *M. pneumoniae*, *L. pneumophila* and *Chlamydia pneumoniae*. Erythromycin is the drug of choice against *Bordetella pertussis*. Pharyngitis, scarlet fever, and erysipelas caused by *S. pyogenes* respond to macrolides. Pneumococcal pneumonia responds to erythromycin that is a valuable alternative for the treatment of streptococcal infections in patients who are allergic to penicillin. However, in recent years, the increasing incidence of antibiotic resistance among *S.pneumoniae* strains (20-40%) both in the United States and in different European countries has reduced the role of macrolides for the treatment of respiratory tract infections due to this organism [24].

Serious side-effects are rare. Among the allergic reactions observed are fever, eosinophilia, and skin eruptions. Cholestatic hepatitis is the most striking side effect. The administration of erythromycin is frequently accompanied by epigastric distress with abdominal cramps, nausea, vomiting, and diarrhea. It has been shown that erythromycin acts as a motilin receptor agonist to stimulate gastrointestinal motility. Rarely, erythromycin has been reported to cause cardiac arrythmias, including QT prolongation with ventricular tachycardia [1, 2].

Drug interactions between macrolide antibiotics and several compounds is based on their inhibitory activity on cytochrome P450 (CYP) system [25]. Macrolides have been reported to cause clinically significant drug interactions, potentiating the effects of astemizole, carbamazepine, corticosteroids, cyclosporine, digoxin, ergot alkaloids, terfenadine, theophylline, triazolam, valproate, and warfarin, probably by interfering with mediated metabolism of these drugs [1, 2, 23, 25].

However, some differences were found between the different macrolide derivatives in the incidence and magnitude of these effects and not all the members of this class are potential sources for drug interaction.

Spiramycin has a spectrum of antimicrobial activity that is similar to that of erythromycin. In particular spiramycin is active against all streptococci including *S. pneumoniae* and most anaerobic strains, *N. meningitidis*, *M. catarrhalis*, *B. pertussis*, *Corynebacterium diphtheriae*, *Listeria monocytogenes*, *Clostridium* species, *L. pneumophilia*, *Chlamydia* and *Mycoplasma pneumoniae*. Good activity has been demonstrated against *Toxoplasma gondii in vivo* and *in vitro*. Enterococci and *H. influenzae* are less sensitive.

Spiramycin accumulates in the tissues where it persists for long periods more than any other macrolide. This property probably accounts for its unpredictably good *in vivo* activity. The large volume of distribution is indicative of the particularly high tissue affinity of spiramycin. Concentrations many times higher than those found in serum have been reported in lung, liver, kidney, spleen, prostate, placenta, muscle, bone and tonsillar tissue. High levels may persist for as long as 72 hours following a single oral dose. High concentrations of spiramycin have been found in bile, saliva and lacrimal fluid. Intracellular concentrations in phagocytic cells are markedly elevated over prolonged periods and this is likely to account for the efficacy of spiramycin against intracellular organisms. Placental transfer is poor and only 9-16 % of maternal blood concentration appear in the amniotic fluid. Spiramycin binds poorly to serum proteins (15%). Spiramycin is extensively biotransformed in tissues, with only 14% of the dose excreted unchanged in urine. It is indicated for upper respiratory tract, broncho-pulmonary, cutaneous and genital infections. It is the drug of choice for toxoplasmosis in pregnancy where the treatment with spiramycin decreased the frequency of certain fetal abnormalities, although it has only moderate activity against established infections because the penetration into the fetal circulation is poor. Spiramycin does not cross the blood brain barrier and is ineffective against neurotoxoplasmosis.

Clarithromycin is more potent than erythromycin against streptococci and staphylococci, but has a lower activity than azithromycin against *N. gonorrhoeae,* and *H. influenzae.* However, for the latter strain a synergism has been demonstrated between the parent compound and the 14-OH metabolite with MIC_{90} values of 1-2mg/l. Clarithromycin has good activity against *M. catarrhalis, Chlamydia* spp., *L. pneumophila, B. burgdorferi,* and *M. pneumoniae.* This semi-synthetic macrolide is rapidly absorbed after oral administration (55% bioavailability). After absorption, clarithromycin undergoes rapid first-pass metabolism to the active 14-OH metabolite. It distributes widely throughout the body and achieves high intracellular concentrations. Concentrations in middle ear fluid are high. Protein binding of clarithromycin ranges from 40% to 70%. Clarithromycin is also eliminated by renal and non-renal mechanisms. It is metabolized in the liver to several metabolites. The elimination half-lives of clarithromycin is 3 to 7 hours. Although the pharmacokinetics of clarithromycin are altered in patients with either hepatic or renal dysfunction, dosage adjustment is not necessary unless a patient has severe renal dysfunction. Clarithromycin is usually given at a dose of 250 mg or 500mg twice daily.

This macrolide derivative is used in combination regimens for *H. pylori* infection associated with peptic ulcer disease and in multidrug regimens for the treatment of disseminated *Mycobacterium avium* complex infection [1, 2, 23].

Azithromycin generally is less active than erythromycin against Gram-positive organisms (*Streptococcus* spp. and enterococci) and is more active than either erythromycin or clarithromycin against *H. influenzae* and

Campylobacter spp. Azithromycin is very active against *M. catarrhalis, Pasteurella multocida, Chlamydia* spp., *Mycoplasma pneumoniae, L. pneumophila, B. burgdorferi, Fusobacterium* spp., and *N. gonorrhoeae* [1, 2, 23].

Azithromycin is absorbed rapidly (37% bioavailability) and distributes widely throughout the body, except to cerebrospinal fluid. It reaches high concentrations within cells including phagocytes. It appears that tissue fibroblasts act as the natural reservoir for the drug, and the transfer of drug to phagoctyes is easily accomplished. Protein binding is low (51%) and the antibiotic shares a very high volume of distribution (almost 5-10l/Kg) [26]. Azithromycin undergoes some hepatic metabolism to inactive metabolites, but biliary excretion is the major route of elimination. Only 6.5% of drug is excreted unchanged in the urine. The elimination half-life was reported to be 68 hours and is prolonged because of extensive tissue sequestration and binding.

A once-daily regimen is used, with a loading dosage of 500 mg on the first day followed by 250 mg per day thereafter usually in the United States, while in Europe the antibiotic is given 500mg daily for a 3-day regimen.

Chlamydial infections can be treated effectively with any of the macrolides. Azithromycin is specifically recommended as an alternative to doxycycline in patients with uncomplicated urethral, endocervical, rectal, or epididymal infections [1, 2, 23].

Telithromycin is the first antibiotic belonging to a new class of macrolides, named ketolides, to reach clinical use for the treatment of community-acquired respiratory tract infections.

The microbiological profile of telithromycin is characterized by high *in vitro* activity against many common and atypical/intracellular respiratory pathogens, including MLS$_B$-resistant strains. Telithromycin has more *in vitro* activity against Gram-positive aerobes than the other macrolides. It has high activity against atypical respiratory pathogens (*Bordetella* spp., *Legionella* spp., *Chlamydia pneumoniae, Mycoplasma pneumoniae*). Its potency against community pathogens such as *M. catarrhalis* and *H. influenzae* appeared similar to that of azithromycin. Telithromycin was found to be active against several Gram-positive and -negative anaerobic bacteria such as *Clostridium* spp., *Peptostreptococcus* spp. and *Bacteroides* spp.

The ketolide is inactive against *Enterobacteriaceae*, non-fermentative Gram-negative bacilli, *Acinetobacter baumanii* and constitutively MLS$_B$-resistant *S. aureus*.

Telithromycin displays significant *in vitro* activity against *S. pneumoniae* isolates.

As shown with macrolides, telithromycin lacks activity in an acid environment. Macrolides are not active against MRSA.

Telithromycin displays good *in vitro* activity against intracellular pathogens, such as *Rickettsia* spp. and *Bartonella* spp. At concentrations of 0.25–8 mg/L, telithromycin was ineffective against *Ehrlichia chaffensis*.

In humans telithromycin proved to be as effective as fluoroquinolones and macrolides in the treatment of community-acquired pneumonia. Its efficacy is retained in pneumonia caused by penicillin- or erythromycin-resistant pneumococci.

Intracellular accumulation of telithromycin has been detected mainly in the granule fraction of polymorphonuclear neutrophils. The slow efflux from human phagocytic cells suggested that these cells could act as transport vehicles for the antibiotic to the site of infection. The concentration of telithromycin in alveolar macrophages exceeded that in plasma up to 146 times 8 h after dosing. Good penetration of telithromycin into respiratory tissues was reported after administration of multiple oral doses of 800 mg. Mean MIC_{90}s for common respiratory pathogens *S. pneumoniae*, *M. catarrhalis* and *M. pneumoniae* (0.12, 0.03 and 0.001 mg/L) were exceeded for 24 h by concentrations of telithromycin in bronchial mucosa and epithelial lining fluid.

Telithromycin undergoes hepatic metabolization and is eliminated primarily through the feces.

Telithromycin is an inhibitor of CYP3A4 and *in vitro* of CYP2D6. Telithromycin should be used cautiously in combination with simvastatin, midazolam, cisaprid, theophylline, digoxin and levonorgestrel. An increase in QTc interval in special patients has been described.

Diarrhea has been the most common adverse event occurring in patients treated with 800 mg once daily. Other adverse reactions include nausea, headache, dizziness and vomiting [21].

Glycopeptides

Glycopeptides are antimicrobial agents based on their peptide and carbohydrate content.

Mechanism of action. They inhibit the synthesis of the cell wall in bacteria by binding with high affinity to the D-alanyl-D-alanine terminus of cell wall precursor units. The bound antibiotic inhibits transglycosylase and transpeptidase enzymes. They are rapidly bactericidal for dividing bacteria [1, 2, 27].

Mechanisms of resistance. Mechanisms of resistance to glycopeptides have been widely studied. Enterococcal resistance to vancomycin is due to the expression of an enzyme that modifies the cell wall precursor so that it no longer binds vancomycin. Three clinically important types of resistance have been described for vancomycin. The Van A phenotype confers resistance to both teicoplanin and vancomycin. The trait is inducible and has been identified in *E. faecium* and *E. faecalis*. The Van B phenotype, which tends to be a lower level of resistance, also has been identified in *E. faecium* and *E. faecalis*. The trait is inducible by vancomycin but not teicoplanin, and, consequently, many strains remain susceptible to teicoplanin. The Van C phenotype, the least important clinically and least well characterized, confers resistance only to vancomycin, is constitutive, and is present in no species of enterococci other than *E. faecalis* and *E. faecium* [1, 2].

Spectrum of activity and clinical use. Glycopeptides are primarily active against Gram-positive bacteria. *S. aureus* and *S. epidermidis,* including strains resistant to methicillin, are usually sensitive. Synergism between vancomycin and gentamicin or tobramycin has been demonstrated *in vitro* against *S. aureus,* including methicillin-resistant strains. *S. pyogenes, S. pneumoniae,* and viridans streptococci are highly susceptible, as are most strains of *Enterococcus* spp. Glycopeptides are not generally bactericidal for *Enterococcus* spp., and the addition of a synergistic aminoglycoside might be necessary to produce a bactericidal effect. *Corynebacterium* spp, *Actinomyces* spp. and *Clostridium* spp are sensitive. Several strains of *S. haemolyticus* and enterococci with high-level resistance to glycopeptides have now been isolated [27–29].

Drugs in clinical use. Glycopeptides include vancomycin and teicoplanin.

Vancomycin is available for enteral and parenteral administration. The drug has a serum elimination half-life of about 6 hours. Approximately 55% of vancomycin is bound to plasma protein. Vancomycin appears in various body fluids, including the CSF when the meninges are inflamed, bile and pleural, pericardial, synovial, and ascitic fluids. More than 90% of an injected dose is excreted by glomerular filtration. Dosage adjustments must be made in cases of renal failure. The drug can be cleared from plasma with hemodialysis. The dose of vancomycin for adults is 30 mg/kg per day divided every 6 to 12 hours. Vancomycin can be administered orally to eradicate carriage of *S. aureus* both sensitive and resistant to methicillin, and to treat *C. difficile* enteritis [1, 2, 27].

Hypersensitivity reactions produced by vancomycin include macular skin rashes and anaphylaxis. Chills, rash, and fever may occur. Rapid intravenous infusion may cause a variety of symptoms, including erythematous or urticarial reactions, flushing ("red-neck" or "red-man" syndrome), tachycardia, and hypotension. The most significant untoward reactions have been ototoxicity and nephrotoxicity. Nephrotoxicity was formerly quite common but has become an unusual side effect when appropriate doses are used [1, 2].

Teicoplanin is a mixture of six closely related compounds. The primary differences between vancomycin and teicoplanin are that teicoplanin can be administered safely by intramuscular injection; it is highly bound by plasma proteins (90% to 95%); and it has an extremely long serum elimination half-life (up to 100 hours). The dose of teicoplanin in adults is 6 to 30 mg/kg per day. A unique loading dose regimen may be required and once-daily dosing is possible for the treatment of most infections. As with vancomycin, teicoplanin doses must be adjusted in patients with renal insufficiency [1, 30, 31].

The main side effect reported for teicoplanin is skin rash, which is more common in higher dosages. Hypersensitivity reactions, drug fever, and neutropenia have also been reported. Ototoxicity has occurred rarely.

Polymyxins

There are two polymyxins in clinical use: polymyxin E or colistin and polymyxin B. These drugs, which are cationic detergents, are peptides with molecular masses of about 1000 Da [1, 2].

Mechanism of action. Polymyxins are surface-active, amphipathic agents containing both lipophilic and lipophobic groups. They interact with phospholipids and penetrate into cell membranes disrupting their structure. The permeability of the bacterial membrane changes following contact with polymyxins. Sensitivity to polymyxins apparently is related to the phospholipid content of the cell wall-membrane complex. The cell wall of certain resistant bacteria may prevent access of the drug to the cell membrane. The binding of polymyxins to the lipid A portion of endotoxin inactivates this molecule [1, 2].

Spectrum of activity. The antimicrobial activity of polymyxin B and colistin is restricted to AGNB, including *Enterobacter, E. coli, Klebsiella, Citrobacter, A. baumanii* and *P. aeruginosa* [1, 32]. *Proteus, Morganella, Serratia* are intrinsically resistant.

Clinical use. Colistin has been used until the early 1970 for treatment of infections due to AGNB, afterward the use of this antibiotic decreased because of its toxicity following parenteral administration. The emergence of multiresistant AGNB causing nosocomial infections has promoted a revival of intravenous colistin that may play an important role in this setting. Infections of the skin, mucous membranes, eye, and ear due to polymyxin-sensitive micro-organisms respond to topical application of the antibiotic in solution or ointment. Aerosol administration of the parenteral preparation also has been used as an adjuvant in patients with severe *Pseudomonas* and *Acinetobacter* pneumonia [1, 32, 33].

Pharmacologic properties. Polymyxin B and colistin are not absorbed when given orally and form an integral component of the SDD protocols. They may cause nephrotoxicity if used parenterally. Colistin is used by intravenous administration for the treatment of multi-resistant AGNB including *P. aeruginosa* and *A. baumannii*. Polymyxin B is available for ophthalmic, otic, and topical use [1, 2, 33].

Oxazolidinones

Linezolid is the first member of a new class of antibiotics known as oxazolidinones.

Mechanism of action. Linezolid inhibits the initiation of protein synthesis at the level of ribosomes. It prevents the formation of the fmet- tRNA:mRNA:30S subunit ternary complex. It also binds to the 50S ribosomal subunit. Linezolid is bacteriostatic in most cases and should not be used for the treatment of endocarditis [34, 35].

There have been reports of linezolid-resistant VRE in immunosuppressed patients including liver transplant recipients. However, in these special populations resistance needs to be checked before commencing treatments with linezolid [34, 35].

Side-effects. The main side effects include: thrombocytopenia, elevated liver and pancreatic enzymes, pseudomembraneous colitis, diarrhea, nausea and vomiting, headache, and dizziness. Linezolid has a relatively weak monoamine oxidase inhibitor action. Therefore, MAOI precautions should be followed to avoid potentially serious food-drug or drug-drug interactions [34].

Pharmacologic properties. Absorption of the oral form of linezolid is rapid and complete. It is widely distributed in the respiratory tract with plasma protein binding equal to 30%. About one third of dose is eliminated unchanged in the urine. Linezolid undergoes oxidation and opening of its morpholino ring resulting in the formation of two inactive metabolites. The elimination half life of the parent compound is about 6.5 hours [34, 35].

Dosage for most indications is 600 mg (iv or po) every 12 hours. There appears to be no need for renal dose adjustment [34, 35].

Clinical use. Linezolid is a bacteriostatic agent indicated for the treatment of nosocomial infections involving Gram-positive organisms including MRSA, multi-resistant strains of *S. pneumoniae*, and vancomycin-resistant *Enterococcus faecium* (VRE) [29, 34, 35].

Streptogramins

They include streptogramin A (dalfopristin) and streptogramin B (quin-upristin). Streptogramins were discovered over 40 years ago. Streptogramin A and Streptogramin B are structurally distinct compounds, they are bacteriostatic separately, but bactericidal in appropriate ratios. They are available in an injectable combination (Synercid®) in a ratio of 70:30 [36, 37].

Mechanism of action. These compounds inhibit protein synthesis binding to 23 S RNA of the 50 S ribosomal subunit where they cause the dissociation of pep-tidyl-tRNA from the ribosome [36, 37].

Mechanism of resistance. Resistance to streptogramins can occur by several mechanisms, including enzymatic modification through virginiamycin acetyl-transferases, efflux pump, and alteration of the target site. Resistance is rare in isolates of staphylococci and *E. faecium* from humans, while common in isolates from meat, in correlation with the use of virginiamycin as a feed additive [36, 37].

Untoward reactions. Main side effects include reversible arthralgias, myalgias, and peripheral venous irritation. A potential for drug interactions exists because quinupristin-dalfopristin significantly inhibits the cytochrome P450-3A4 enzyme system [36, 37].

Pharmacologic properties. Quinupristin/dalfopristin are metabolized by liver enzymes, including CYP450. The postantibiotic effect of streptogramins and their pharmacokinetic characteristics allow dosing at eight- to 12-hour intervals. An intravenous infusion of diluted drug during at least 1 hour is suggested to avoid venous irritation [36, 37].

Clinical use. Streptogramins are bactericidal against a variety of Gram-positive bacteria and are synergistic. Streptogramins may be effective for the treatment of infections caused by multi-resistant strains of staphylococci, pneumococci, and enterococci. Quinupristin-dalfopristin is inactive against *E. faecalis* but is effective against vancomycin-resistant *E. faecium*. Experimental data demonstrate that streptogramins are bactericidal *in vivo* and that they are as active as vancomycin against MRSA. In cases of infection localized in difficult-to-treat sites, the combination with other drugs, such as cefepime, glycopeptide or line-zolid, is able to potentiate the action of the streptogramins with good clinical results [37–39].

Bactericidal Activity

The knowledge gained over the last 10-15 years overruled the old classification into bacteriostatic and bactericidal compounds, since the final result of the antimicrobial activity depends on many factors including: the antimicrobial drug, the specific bacterial strain, and the setting in which the antimicrobial drug challenges the micro-organism [1, 2]. The pharmacological action of antimicrobial drugs is actually considered to be *concentration dependent* or *time dependent*, although this classification might depend on the specific antibiotic inside a class and, possibly on the bacterial pathogen involved [40, 40a].

Concentration-dependent antibiotics kill at a greater rate and to a greater extent with increasing antibiotic concentrations, whereas time-dependent antibiotics kill bacteria at the same rate and to the same extent once an appropriate threshold concentration has been achieved. Increasing the antibiotic concentration beyond this value typically does not augment the antibacterial activity. Aminoglycosides, fluoroquinolones, clarithromycin, azalides, ketolides and metronidazole are considered concentration-dependent antimicrobial drugs, whereas glycopeptides, clindamycin, natural macrolides, β-lactams, linezolid and quinupristin-dalfopristin are considered time-dependent drugs. Predictors of clinical and microbiological performance of a specific antibiotic against a specific bacterium include important pharmacodynamic parameters, like the ratio of the area under the concentration vs time curve during a 24-hour dosing period to minimum inhibitory concentration (AUC_{0-24}/MIC), the ratio of maximum serum antibiotic concentration to the minimum inhibitory concentration (C_{max}/MIC), and the duration of time that antibiotic concentrations exceed the minimum inhibitory concentration (T>MIC). As only free drug is therapeutically active, these parameters should be adjusted for the protein binding of the considered antibiotics [40, 41].

The most important characteristic of time-dependent antibiotics is that their antimicrobial activity is mainly dependent on the T>MIC parameter, while the antimicrobial activity of concentration-dependent antibiotics depends on the C_{max}/MIC and/or the AUC_{0-24}/MIC ratios. These differences in pharmacodynamic activity should result in different dosing regimens for time- and concentration-dependent antibiotics [40] (Table 8).

Beside these pharmachodynamic considerations, the bactericidal activity of antimicrobial agent is influenced by several factors correlated with the site of infection, including pH, bacterial load, phase of bacterial growth, and oxygen tension. Several studies, regarding the inoculum effect, considered the effect of the bacterial load on the MIC of several antibiotics [42]. Standard inoculum for

Time-Dependent Antibiotics

Antimicrobial agents with time-dependency include β-lactams, vancomycin, clindamycin, streptogramins, and natural macrolides [41, 44, 47–53] (Table 9).

β-lactams They exhibit time-dependent activity, correlated to T>MIC. Since 1950 penicillin activity against pneumococci has been correlated to the amount of time during which the drug concentration remained above minimally effective levels. Larger doses increase the efficacy of these antibiotics extending the time during which the drug remains above the effective concentration, rather than increasing its absolute concentration. The results of further studies in both *in vitro* and *in vivo* models confirm the importance of T>MIC in optimizing β-lactam activity. These pharmachodynamic studies led to a shift of dosage regimens towards more fragmented doses or even continuous infusion. For example, *in vivo* data from animal and human studies suggest that continuous infusion of ceftazidime may be useful, especially when host defenses are impaired. The importance of T>MIC has been demonstrated for ticarcillin against *P. aeruginosa,* ceftazidime against *E. coli,* cefazolin against *E. coli* and *S. aureus.* While the T>MIC should be 100% of the dosage interval for ticarcillin against *P. aeruginosa*, and for cefazolin against *E. coli* in order to achieve maximum efficacy, cefazolin activity against *S. aureus* needs a T>MIC of at least 55% of the dosing interval [44, 52–55].

Beside T>MIC, AUC_{0-24} and C_{max} are also important in predicting optimal β-lactam activity in certain types of infection. Higher doses of ampicillin against *H. influenzae* seem to achieve stronger bactericidal activity compared with continuous infusion [41].

Table 9. Time-dependent antibiotics

β-lactams

Glycopeptides

Clindamycin

Streptogramins

Natural macrolides

Linezolid

The pharmacodynamic parameter predicting the performance of time-dependent antibiotics is: T>MIC, that is the duration of time that antibiotic concentrations exceed the minimum inhibitory concentration

Clinical data regarding the bactericidal activity of β-lactam antibiotics in severe infections support the efficacy of very high doses, continuous infusion, or multiple-dose administration. Most of these studies have found that continuous infusion is at least as effective as more conventional intermittent dosing, and that very high doses do not increase efficacy. The results of these clinical studies recommend to exceed the MIC by 2-5 times for between 40% and 100% of the dosage interval when using β-lactams antibiotics. This time should probably be extended when using β-lactams that are highly protein bound (> 90%).

Strategies to keep drug concentrations above the MIC for a long time include: multiple doses given frequently, the administration of the antibiotics in a continuous infusion, the use of agents with long serum half-lives, the use of repository dosage forms, the use of agents with active metabolites, the choice of agents with the lowest MIC towards the causative micro-organism, and the concomitant administration of inhibitors of antibiotic elimination (probenecid) [55, 56].

Glycopeptides have a time-dependent bactericidal activity against Gram-positive pathogens. Experiments in rats with endocarditis due to *S. aureus* concluded that, increasing the administration frequency of vancomycin, the number of bacteria isolated from the valve vegetations decreased. *In vitro* studies evaluating vancomycin against *S. aureus* demonstrated that bolus doses achieving different C_{max} values resulted in not significantly different time-kill curves. Time-dependent bactericidal activity of vancomycin is slower in an anaerobic environment than in an aerobic one. Other animal studies considering peritonitis caused by *S. pneumoniae* and *S. aureus* concluded that the total dose that protected 50% of lethally infected animals was higher when administered as a single dose and that, using multiple doses, the pharmacodynamic parameters that correlate with the bactericidal activity are not only T>MIC, but also C_{max}/MIC, and AUC_{0-24}/MIC [57–59].

Clindamycin shows time-dependent antibacterial activity against *S. aureus* and *S. pneumoniae* in *in vitro* pharmacodynamic models.

Natural macrolides. With regards to macrolides, debate is ongoing about their classification as concentration-dependent or independent antibiotics. Results from different animal models (acute mouse pneumococcal pneumonia, mouse peritonitis and *M. pneumoniae* infection in hamsters) clearly demonstrate that erythromycin has a time-dependent activity [47, 48]. Therefore, though this macrolide has a consistent postantibiotic effect, its activity seems to correlate better with the exposure time of bacteria to this agent than to actual serum or tissue concentrations, thus classifying it in the group of time-dependent drugs [47, 48].

Streptogramins have been studied regarding their bactericidal activity. The combination has been administered by continuous and different intermittent infusions against *S. aureus* in several *in vitro* studies concluding that the bactericidal activity of quinupristin-dalfopristin shows different features, depending on the methicillin and erythromycin susceptibility of *S. aureus* strain. Against methicillin-erythromycin-sensitive isolates streptogramins act as concentration-dependent antimicrobials, against methicillin-erythromycin-resistant isolates quinupristin-dalfopristin show time-dependency. Streptogramins seem to act as concentration-dependent antibiotics against vancomycin-resistant *E. faecium* [60–64].

Linezolid is a new oxazolidinone with time dependent antimicrobial activity against Gram-positive cocci. In animal models increasing doses of linezolid produced minimal concentration-dependent antibacterial activity. Linezolid seems to be associated with a poor PAE with penicillin-susceptible *S. pneumoniae*, while the PAE with methicillin-susceptible *S. aureus* is around 3 hours. The AUC_{0-24}/MIC ratio and the time above the MIC seem to be the best parameters to determine the clinical efficacy of linezolid.

Concentration-Dependent Antibiotics

They include aminoglycosides, fluoroquinolones, clarithromycin, azalides and ketolides (Table 10).

Aminoglycosides. These antibiotics have demonstrated concentration-dependent activity against AGNB, even if, when they are used as adjunctive therapy for *S. aureus* or enterococci, they may have concentration-independent antimicro-

Table 10. Concentration-dependent antibiotics

Aminoglycosides

Fluoroquinolones

New macrolides (clarithromycin, azalides, ketolides).

The pharmacodynamic parameter predicting the performance of concentration-dependent antibiotics are:

AUC_{0-24}/MIC that is the ratio of the area under the concentration vs time curve during a 24-hour dosing period to minimum inhibitory concentration

C_{max}/MIC that is the ratio of maximum serum antibiotic concentration to the minimum inhibitory concentration

bial activity. In experimental studies a C_{max}/MIC ratio above at least eight to ten was required to optimize bactericidal activity and for aminoglycosides to prevent regrowth of *P. aeruginosa, K. pneumoniae, E. coli,* and *S. aureus.* In case of regrowth the MICs were much higher than those for the original isolates, therefore a proper therapeutic strategy may have important consequences also on the development of antibiotic resistance [65, 66]. In animal models that closely resemble infections in the human host, AUC_{0-24} and C_{max} have been found to be more important predictors of antimicrobial efficacy than time above the MIC [67]. Constant exposure to an aminoglycoside at concentration below or equal to MIC leads to decreased bacterial killing of *P. aeruginosa* because of adaptive resistance and refractoriness to bactericidal activity. Longer dosing intervals may preserve the bactericidal activity of subsequent doses of aminoglycosides introducing a drug free period. Animal studies demonstrated equal or greater effectiveness of once-daily aminoglycosides with less nephro and oto toxicity. Human studies concluded that increasing aminoglycoside concentrations kill bacteria more rapidly and that the concentration-dependent activity of aminoglycosides can be optimized using once-daily dosing [68, 69]. Clinical studies demonstrated a correlation between higher aminoglycoside peak levels and improved clinical outcome [68]. Increasing C_{max}/MIC ratios strongly correlated with the clinical response in a study considering patients with documented AGNB infection. Moreover, C_{max}/MIC ratio is a parameter easy to monitor and interpret. Prospective studies with a target of a C_{max}/MIC ratio of 10 concluded that this strategy is successful in terms of efficacy and toxicity. In this regard, single daily dosing of aminoglycosides takes advantage of the concentration-dependency of this class of antibiotics [70, 71]. Clinical studies in a variety of patient populations concluded that the efficacy of once-daily dosing with aminoglycosides is at least equal to that of multiple daily dosing with equal or less toxicity. Once-daily aminoglycoside therapy has still not been widely investigated in Gram-positive infections, meningitis, osteomyelitis and burn patients [70, 71]. The dosage of aminoglycosides in case of once-daily strategy should be 5-7 mg/Kg for gentamicin and tobramycin and 15-30 mg/Kg for amikacin. These dosages have been selected to reach a C_{max}/MIC ratio of ten considering the usual MIC for susceptible *P. aeruginosa* strains. With this causative pathogen tobramycin is preferred because usually it has a lower MIC. In case of patients with decreased renal function the interval between the doses should be lengthened, but the doses should not be decreased in order to maintain a high C_{max}/MIC ratio and allow an appropriate drug free period [70, 71].

Fluoroquinolones. They show concentration-dependent bactericidal activity. Many studies confirmed the importance of a C_{max}/MIC ratio above 10 as an important predictor of antimicrobial effect and clinical outcome. C_{max}/MIC ratios above eight prevent the regrowth of isolates of *P. aeruginosa, K. pneumo-*

niae, E. coli, and *S. aureus,* and the development of antimicrobial resistance. More recently, the research has considered the effect of the AUC_{0-24}/MIC ratio on the antimicrobial activity of fluoroquinolones. A ratio above 100 seems to optimize the activity of fluoroquinolones against *P. aeruginosa,* while a lower AUC_{0-24}/MIC ratio is associated with an increased risk of development of antimicrobial resistance [72, 73]. In clinical studies an AUC_{0-24}/MIC ratio above 175 was associated with an optimal antibacterial response, though lower AUC_{0-24}/MIC ($\approx$50) ratios might be sufficient in the treatment of Gram-positive infection. In fact many studies show a concentration-independent activity for fluoroquinolones against some Gram-positive pathogens, mainly *S. pneumoniae* and anaerobes. Probably this feature relies on differences in antibiotic uptake and bacterial topoisomerase II and IV. In humans, the maximal antimicrobial effect of fluoroquinolones has been demonstrated at 15-40 times MIC for Gram-positive organisms and 20-50 times MIC for AGNB [66, 67, 68].

Improper dosing regimens of fluoroquinolones that do not produce AUC_{0-24}/MIC ratios greater than 100 or C_{max}/MIC ratios > 8-10 may increase the risk of resistance in AGNB [74]. Underexposure to one fluoroquinolone can confer resistance to the entire class. Theoretically, the most potent agent should be used to treat an infection, but other bacterial populations including intestinal, vaginal, and oropharyngeal flora will be also challenged with the antimicrobial drugs used to treat the infection and the best agent or dosage strategy for the infecting pathogen may not be the best for the other bacterial flora resulting in the production of resistant flora [75-77].

New macrolides (clarithromycin, azalides, ketolides). All these antibiotics have a concentration-dependent activity. However, for the evaluation of macrolides many studies have been targeted to demonstrate the comparative efficacy of newer and older compounds, using escalating but generally single doses, without any relationship to different regimens or intervals of administration. The typical pharmacodynamic analyses appropriate for β-lactams, fluoroquinolones and aminoglycosides are probably not sufficient to explain their pharmacodynamic activity [47-50].

Different authors demonstrated that peak/MIC ratio or AUC/MIC ratio are the best predictors for azithromycin activity [47-49, 78].

There are few published studies for clarithromycin used in animal models. Some authors conclude that AUC/MIC is the most reasonable predictor of efficacy for clarithromycin, while other authors consider that clarithromycin C_{max} is a better predictor of success, indicating that a high dose given infrequently is more effective than the same amount divided into multiple administrations with short dosing intervals for this drug [47-50, 78].

One possible explanation for the different pharmacodynamic behavior observed between molecules of the same class might be related to their different kinetic properties, since clarithromycin and azithromycin have a non-linear pharmacokinetics outlined by the disproportionate increases in AUC with increasing doses and a possible concentration dependent uptake in cells [47].

Finally, ketolides express concentration- and inoculum-dependent killing. Telithromycin exhibited a significant PAE ranging from 1.2 to 8.2 h. A PAE up to several hours at 2 x and 4 x MIC was demonstrated against both erythromycin-susceptible and -resistant strains of *S. pneumoniae* and *S. aureus*, and both β-lactamase-negative and -positive strains of *H. influenzae* and *M. catarrhalis* [21].

Narrow vs Broad

In addition to treating infections, antibiotic use contributes to the emergence of resistance among potentially pathogenic micro-organisms. Therefore, avoiding unnecessary antibiotic use and optimizing the administration of antimicrobial agents will help to improve patient outcomes while minimizing further pressures for resistance. The widespread and often inappropriate use of broad spectrum antibiotics in the outpatient setting is recognized as a significant contributing factor to the spread of bacterial resistance [79]. A rational and strict antibiotic policy is thus of great importance for the optimal use of these agents. Antibiotic administration guidelines/protocols developed locally or by national societies potentially avoid unnecessary antibiotic administration and increase therapeutic effectiveness. However, locally developed guidelines often have the best chance of being accepted by local health care providers and hence of being implemented [79, 80].

There is an international trend toward a decline in the use of narrow-spectrum and older penicillins and prescribing more broad-spectrum and new antibiotics. However, inappropriate antibiotic prescribing should be avoided, the selection of antibiotic class should be appropriate and the prescription of antibiotics should be reduced. Often there is no rational basis for the therapeutic choices of antibiotics and no microbiological evidence to support the frequent use of broad-spectrum antibiotics. No difference in clinical efficacy has been often found between narrow and broad-spectrum antibiotics. Therefore, a simple management protocol, using a narrow-spectrum antibiotic initially, would be as effective, more logical and cheaper [79, 80].

Each hospital should have a program in place which monitors antibiotic utilization and its effectiveness in order to evaluate the impact of interventions aimed at improving antibiotic use. Preventing nosocomial infections is important to reduce the use of antibiotics [81, 82].

However, severe infections, including pneumonia and bacteremia, can be due to several potential pathogens and remain a major cause of morbidity and mortality among hospitalized patients. Clinical evidence suggests that failure to initially treat these infections with an adequate initial antibiotic regimen is associated with greater patient morbidity and mortality, therefore antibiotic therapy should be instituted as soon as sepsis is suspected in critically patients. Delays of 24–48 h in the initiation of adequate antibiotic treatment can be associated with increased patient mortality. Indeed, over the last decades the types of pathogens have significantly changed under selective pressure of broad-spectrum antimicrobial therapy. Shifts from AGNB to Gram-positive organisms and outbreaks of resistant pathogens address the need for appropriate empirical regimens. Inappropriate antimicrobial treatment is usually defined as either the absence of antimicrobial agents directed against a specific class of microorganisms (e.g. absence of therapy for fungemia) or the administration of antimicrobial agents to which the micro-organism responsible for the infection is resistant. Although early appropriate therapy results in improved outcomes, the micro-organism causing infection is frequently not known at the time antimicrobial therapy is initiated. This has led to the development of a novel paradigm guiding the administration of empirical antimicrobial therapy for patients with serious infections in the hospital setting named **antibacterial de-escalation**. It is an approach to antibacterial utilisation that attempts to balance the need to provide appropriate, initially broad antibacterial treatment, while limiting the emergence of antibacterial resistance. Antibacterial resistance is minimised by narrowing the antibacterial regimen once the pathogens and their susceptibility profiles are known, and by employing the shortest course of therapy [83] (Table 11).

The most common pathogens associated with the administration of inadequate antimicrobial treatment in patients with hospital-acquired pneumonia include potentially antibiotic-resistant AGNB *P. aeruginosa, Acinetobacter* species, *Klebsiella* species, *Enterobacter* species and MRSA. For patients with

Table 11. Measures to optimize the administration of antimicrobial drugs

Avoid unnecessary antibiotic use

In the hospital setting use programs to monitor antibiotic utilization, nosocomial infections, and effectiveness of antibiotic therapy

In serious infections likely to be due to antibiotic-resistant micro-organisms use antibacterial de-escalation with a broad coverage at the beginning that is narrowed when the pathogen is isolated

hospital-acquired bloodstream infections, antibiotic-resistant Gram-positive bacteria (MRSA, vancomycin-resistant enterococci and coagulase-negative staphylococci), *Candida* species and, less commonly, antibiotic-resistant AGNB account for most cases of inadequate antibiotic treatment. All these species should be covered with an initial broad antibiotic therapy that will be narrowed once the microbiological results are obtained.

De-escalation antimicrobial chemotherapy should be tailored to critically ill patients according to their clinical status, severity of illness and suspicion of sepsis or nosocomial pneumonia. Risk stratification should be employed to identify those patients at high risk of infection with antibiotic-resistant bacteria. These risk factors include prior treatment with antibiotics during the hospitalization, prolonged lengths of stay in the hospital, and the presence of invasive devices (e.g. central venous catheters, endotracheal tubes, urinary catheters). Patients at high risk for infection with antibiotic-resistant bacteria should be treated initially with a combination of antibiotics providing coverage for the most likely pathogens to be encountered in that specific intensive care unit setting. Such an approach to initial antibiotic treatment can be potentially modified if specific micro-organisms are excluded based on examination of appropriate clinical specimens. Such empiric therapy should, however, always be modified once the agent of infection is identified or discontinued altogether if the diagnosis of infection becomes unlikely. De-escalation of antibiotic therapy can be thought of as a strategy to balance the need to provide adequate initial antibiotic treatment in **high-risk patients** with the avoidance of unnecessary antibiotic utilization, which promotes resistance. Delays in the de-escalation of unnecessary antibiotic treatment are harmful promoting the emergence of patient colonization and infection with resistant bacterial pathogens. Decreasing the overall duration of empirical and potentially unnecessary antibiotic use reduces the incidence of hospital-acquired superinfections attributed to antibiotic-resistant micro-organisms. Therefore, it is important to minimize patient exposure to any unnecessary empirical antibiotic treatment [83, 84].

An appropriate choice of the antibiotic therapy is also important when the antibiotics are used with prophylactic purposes like the prevention of surgical site infections. In these cases the antimicrobial drug used for the prophylaxis against surgical site infections must be effective against pathogens associated with infection after a given procedure. The first generation cephalosporin, cefazolin, given about 30 minutes before incision (at induction of anesthesia) has been considered as the prophylactic drug of choice. A single dose of antimicrobial drugs before the operation is sufficient prophylaxis for most surgical procedures. The development of bacterial resistance is associated with antimicrobial use, and therefore prophylactic antibiotics should be used as little as possible; in addition, the spectrum of activity of drugs used should be as narrow as possible. Overconsumption of drugs with too broad a spectrum of activity should be avoided [85].

Respect for Ecology: a Prerequisite for Antibiotic Therapy

The effects of antibiotic drugs on the microbial ecology may be analysed from an individual or a global perspective because antibiotics cause alterations either in the individual microbial population and in the global bacterial population [86].

From an *individual perspective* it is noteworthy that the relationship between the microbes and the host is not just a fight between two contenders [87] (Table 12) (Chapters 2, 12).

Ecological studies have shown symbiosis in the microbial communities of the skin and mucous membranes. In these ecosystems, the resident micro-organisms play an important physiological role with mutualistic relationships. An important effect of this mutualistic relationship between humans and their microbiota is protection from infections. The normal microflora acts as a barrier against carriage of potentially pathogenic micro-organisms and against overgrowth of opportunistic micro-organisms (colonization resistance) [88]. For this protective effect to occur, a great stability of these ecosystems is fundamental, that is a composition of microbial communities as constant as possible. Administration of antimicrobial agents, either therapeutically or as prophylaxis, interferes with the ecological balance between the host and the normal microflora. The impact of antibiotics on the normal intestinal flora has been widely studied. The gastrointestinal tract is a complex ecosystem host to a diverse and highly evolved microbial community composed of hundreds of different microbial species [88]. Analysis of the indigenous anaerobes and aerobes has shown that

Table 12. Respect for the individual's microbial ecology

The normal microflora prevents carriage of potentially pathogenic micro-organisms and the overgrowth of opportunistic micro-organisms (colonisation resistance).

The use of probiotics may preserve the normal microflora and may potentiate colonisation resistance.

The administration of antimicrobial agents interferes with the individual microbial ecology.

First-generation β-lactams, aminoglycosides and polymyxins are antibiotics with little or no impact on the normal flora

humans harbor a characteristic collection of bacterial strains. The administration of antibiotics causes perturbations and transitions in these populations that can be detected by molecular analysis of the intestinal microflora. Regarding enterococcal species, a limited number of these is of importance for the gastrointestinal ecology and the food microflora, including *E. faecalis, E. faecium, E. durans/hirae, E. gallinarum* and *E. casseliflavus*. In the human gastrointestinal tract *E. faecium* is the most common species whereas in most animal species *E. faecalis* is at least present in the same amount [88, 89]. Especially in foods of animal origin such as cheese, pork meat, beef, poultry *E. faecalis* is very frequent. This is of special interest as glycopeptide resistance is most often found in human clinical *E. faecium* strains as well as in *E. faecium* from the environment or animal samples and less frequent in *E. faecalis* strains [88]. The understanding of gut microflora composition and of processes such as intestinal adherence, colonization, translocation, and immunomodulation will allow the definition of the interactions of "functional food"-borne beneficial bacteria with the gut. Intestinal microflora analysis should enable the development of a detailed knowledge of the microbial ecology of the human colon [89]. This knowledge is essential to derive scientifically valid probiotics [90].

The administration of antibiotics can modify the intestinal microflora resulting clinically in diarrhea and fungal infections that usually cease after treatment. Diseases associated with a deficient or compromised intestinal microflora include gastrointestinal tract infections, pseudomembranous colitis, inflammatory bowel disease including Crohn's disease and ulcerative colitis, irritable bowel syndrome, constipation, food allergies, cardiovascular disease, and certain cancers. Pseudomembranous colitis is an example of the deleterious effect of antimicrobial therapy that disturbs the normal ecologic balance of the bowel flora leading to an abnormal proliferation of *C. difficile* that releases a necrolytic toxin causing colitis [88, 89].

The effects of antibiotics on oropharyngeal, skin, and vaginal microflora may be important as well. Antibiotic therapy may cause alterations in the skin microbial flora with a decline in the number of bacteria regarding especially anaerobic bacteria (mostly *Peptostreptococcus spp.* and *Propionibacterium acnes*), aerobic streptococci, and *S. epidermidis*. On the other hand, antibiotic therapy increases significantly the number of *Candida albicans* isolates from the skin [91].

These effects of antibiotic therapy on the individual bacterial ecology depend on the absorption, route of elimination, and possible enzymatic inactivation and binding to fecal material of the agents. The exposure to antibiotics can interfere with the whole life of ecosystems by altering the quantitative and/or qualitative balance within different microbial populations [92].

Moreover, the exposure to antibiotics often results in antibiotic-resistant organisms that can transfer antibiotic resistance to other micro-organisms. This problem is particularly important because multiple-resistant organisms are often involved in severe nosocomial infections. By using antimicrobial agents that do not disturb colonization resistance, the risk of emergence and spread of resistant strains is reduced (Chapter 28).

In critically ill patients an impairment of host defenses can result in infections due to potential pathogens and antibiotics, that disturb the balance between aerobes and anaerobes and can increase the risk of superinfections following disregard for the patient's gut ecology.

Respect for the individual's ecology should be a prerequisite for every antibiotic policy and the use of antibiotics with little or no impact on the normal flora should always be encouraged. Antibiotics which are not active against the indigenous bacteria in the mouth and intestine and which - in case of activity - are not excreted to a significant degree via the intestine, saliva or skin are therefore preferred. First generation β-lactams, aminoglycosides and polymyxins are favorable from an ecological point of view [Chapter 12].

From a *global perspective* the ecological effects of antibiotic drugs are very important because the overuse of antibiotics has important consequences in public and environmental health [93] (Table 13).

The indiscriminate use of antibiotics has led to water contamination, selection and dissemination of antibiotic-resistant organisms, interfering with the fragile ecology of the microbial ecosystems. Damages caused by the overuse of antibiotics without the purpose of medical treatment include waterborne and foodborne infections by resistant bacteria, enteropathy, biosphere alteration, human and animal growth promotion [94] and the destruction of fragile interspecific competition in microbial ecosystems [93].

The veterinary use of antibiotics as growth promoters increases antibiotic resistance in animal bacteria and can result in antibiotic resistance in human pathogens. Transfer of antibiotic-resistant bacteria from animals to humans may occur via occupational exposure and via the food chain [94]. Resistance genes may transfer from bacteria of animals to human pathogens

Table 13. Respect for global microbial ecology

Requires antibiotics not to be used without the purpose of medical treatment

Prevents the dissemination of antibiotic-resistance

Reduces water contamination

Preserves the long-term efficacy of existing antibiotics

in the intestinal flora of humans. Appropriate use of antibiotics for food animals will preserve the long-term efficacy of existing antibiotics, support animal health and welfare, and limit the risk of transfer of antibiotic resistance to humans [94].

In addition to the transfer of microorganisms from animals to man, there is also evidence of resistance genes moving from humans into the animal population. This is important because of the amplification that can occur in animal populations.

Moreover, the use of antimicrobials is not restricted to animal husbandry but also occurs in horticulture (aminoglycosides in apple growing) and in some other industrial processes such as oil production [95].

In conclusion, commensals in ecosystems have a pronounced capacity for acquisition of resistance genes. *E. faecium* and *E. coli* in the gut flora or *Pseudomonas* species in aquatic environments are important examples. The transfer of antibiotic resistance can occur also via other routes including water and food plants (vegetables), in fact the transfer of resistance genes in aquatic environments has been demonstrated [95, 96].

Protein Binding

Serum protein binding of antimicrobial drugs may have important consequences on their action. In particular, high serum protein binding can reduce antimicrobial activity, tissue distribution, and the elimination of antibiotics. Binding percentages of 80 per cent or more have the potential to significantly reduce free drug levels and affect therapeutic efficacy. However, binding-induced alterations in drug elimination and differences in intrinsic antibacterial activity can often compensate for the inhibitory effect of high serum protein binding. The extent of protein binding is a major factor determining the concentration of active drug in serum and most extravascular fluids. As a general rule, agents with minimal protein binding penetrate into the tissues better than those that are highly protein bound, although they might be excreted much faster [97–99].

Therefore, agents that are highly protein bound may differ markedly from those that are minimally bound in terms of tissue penetration and half-life if they are excreted mainly by glomerular filtration. Among drugs that are less than 80-85% protein bound, differences appear to be of slight clinical importance [97].

Drugs may bind to different plasma proteins, including albumin. If the

roquinolones. Some ESBL producing micro-organisms have also acquired an AmpC-type β-lactamase. ESBL are often present in *E. coli* or *K. pneumoniae* but can be transferred to *P. mirabilis, Citrobacter, Serratia* and other AGNB. Detection of these enzymes is difficult. Micro-organisms may appear sensitive to certain antibiotics, like-third generation cephalosporins, at standard innoculum but have significantly elevated MIC at higher inocula. Every *E. coli* and *K. pneumoniae* with reduced susceptibility to these drugs or to aztreonam should be considered at risk of possessing these enzymes. All ESBL-producing organisms should be considered resistant to all penicillins, cephalosporins and aztreonam. If the organism is sensitive to β-lactam/β-lactamase inhibitor combinations the micro-organism should be considered susceptible although the use of these combinations is not ideal.

The treatment of infections caused by ESBL-producing strains is difficult because of the high risk of concomitant resistance to aminoglycosides, trimethoprim-sulfamethoxazole and fluoroquinolones. The susceptibility to third- and fourth- generation cephalosporins seen *in vitro* at higher inocula is associated with clinically significant reductions in efficacy *in vivo*. The carbapenems are the agents of choice against ESBL-producing bacteria because they are highly stable against β-lactamase hydrolysis although emergence of carbapenemase-producing organisms is a potential threat.

Different micro-organisms produce distinct β-lactamases, although most bacteria produce only one form of the enzyme. Regarding Gram-positive bacteria, they produce a large amount of β-lactamase, which is secreted extracellularly. These enzymes are usually inducible by substrates and encoded in a plasmid that may be transferred by bacteriophage to other bacteria. Regarding AGNB, they have small amounts of β-lactamases, however they are located in the periplasmic space between the inner and outer cell membranes. This location confers maximal protection, since the enzymes of cell-wall synthesis are on the outer surface of the inner membrane. β-lactamases of AGNB are encoded in chromosomes or plasmids, and they may be constitutive or inducible. The plasmids can be transferred between bacteria by conjugation [109].

β-lactamases may hydrolyze penicillins, cephalosporins, or both. However, the substrate of some of these enzymes is rather specific, so these often are described as either penicillinases or cephalosporinases [109].

Regarding cephalosporins, inactivation by hydrolysis of the β-lactam ring is their most prevalent mechanism of resistance. Cephalosporins show variable susceptibility to β-lactamases. Among the first-generation agents, cefazolin is more susceptible to hydrolysis than cephalothin. Cefoxitin, cefuroxime, and the third-generation cephalosporins are more resistant to hydrolysis due to β-lactamases produced by AGNB than first-generation cephalosporins.

Third-generation cephalosporins are susceptible to hydrolysis by inducible, chromosomally encoded (group 1) beta-lactamases. Induction of these β-lactamases can result from the treatment of infections due to AGNB with second- or third-generation cephalosporins and imipenem. Fourth generation cephalosporins, such as cefepime, are poor inducers of group 1 β-lactamases and are less susceptible to hydrolysis than are third-generation agents [109].

The inactivation of β-lactams antibiotics by β-lactamases can be inhibited by several drugs including sulbactam, clavulanic acid and tazobactam. These molecules can bind to β-lactamases and inactivate them. β-lactamase inhibitors are active against plasmid encoded β-lactamases but are inactive against the group 1 inducible chromosomal β-lactamases [1, 2, 109].

Although inactivaction of β-lactam antibiotics is an important and well described mechanism of resistance, the correlation between the susceptibility of an antibiotic to inactivation by β-lactamase and the ability of that antibiotic to kill the micro-organism is inconsistent. Penicillins hydrolyzed by β-lactamase are often effective against certain strains of β-lactamase-producing AGBN [1, 2, 109].

Regarding aminoglycosides, the mechanisms of bacterial resistance include: failure to penetrate by the antibiotic, low affinity of the drug for the bacterial ribosome, and inactivation of the drug by microbial enzymes. Inactivation of aminoglycosides is by far the most important mechanism of acquired microbial resistance in clinical practice [2, 110].

In the periplasmic space the aminoglycoside may become the substrate of several microbial enzymes that may phosphorylate, adenylate, or acetylate specific hydroxyl or amino groups respectively. Phosphorylation is the main mechanism of inactivation for aminoglycosides, it is determined by either Gram-positive or AGNB strains and it results in the complete inactivation of aminoglycosides. Aminoglycoside kinases include many enzymes like APH (3') I, II and III, APH (2"), APH (3"), APH (5") and APH (6), these enzymes require ATP and Mg. Some aminoglycosides are resistant to phosphorylation because of the presence of side chains, like amikacin, or because of the absence of specific hydroxyl groups, like tobramycin and gentamicin. Other enzymes like AAD (3"), AAD (2"), AAD (4') and AAD (6), adenilate aminoglycosides: AAD (4') is active especially agains tobramycin. Acetyltransferases are other bacterial enzymes able to inactivate aminoglycosides, they include AAC (3)-I, II, III and IV, AAC (2') and AAC (6')-1, 2, 3, and 4. They use ATP and acetyl-CoA to attach an acetyl group to an amino group [2]. Aminoglycosides inactivating enzymes are often encoded in plasmids and resistance transfer factors that may spread the genetic information by conjugation and transfer of DNA. Plasmids encoding aminoglycosides inactivating enzymes are common especially in hospital environments, and they have decreased the effectiveness of kanamycin, gentamicin and tobramycin [110]. Amikacin is less vulnerable to these inactivating enzymes because of protective molecular side chains, however, AAC(6')-I type enzymes (a group of 6'-N-acetyltransferases) can utilize amikacin as substrate and confer resistance to this antibiotic in addition to other aminoglycosides. Aminoglycosides inactivating enzymes are often bifunctional and they are able to modify different compounds (i.e. gentamicin, tobramycin, amikacin, kanamycin, and netilmicin). Therefore these aminoglycosides usually lose effectiveness together. Some gentamicin-resistant enterococci may be susceptible to streptomycin, because gentamicin and streptomycin are inactivated by different enzymes [2, 110].

Pharmacological strategies to inhibit aminoglycosides inactivating enzymes are under evaluation. Aminoglycoside kinases, enzymes that phosphorylate aminoglycosides have been shown to be related to eukaryotic protein kinases [111]. Several compounds target the antibiotic binding region of this enzyme and can result in its inhibition. Moreover, protein kinase inhibitors may interfere with the ATP-binding site of aminoglycoside-modifying enzymes [111]. Bifunctional aminoglycoside dimers could bind to the target site on the bacterial ribosome, while serving as poor substrates for modifying enzymes.

Endotoxin Neutralizing Antibiotics

Bacterial endotoxins are thought to play a fundamental role in the pathogenesis of sepsis and septic shock. Endotoxins are macromolecular constituents of the cell wall of AGNB included in their outermost layer where they take part in several functions including the maintenance of cell shape, the protection from bactericidal mechanisms, and the immune recognition of the host. Endotoxins are lipopolysaccharides composed by a carbohydrate chain of a variable size linked to another highly conserved chemical structure called lipid A composed of a bisphosphorylated diglucosamine backbone bearing up to seven acyl chains in ester and amide linkages [112]. The anionic and amphipathic nature of lipid A enables the interaction of a wide variety of cationic amphiphiles with the toxin. Bacterial growth and death is associated with the release of variable amount of endotoxins outside the bacteria. Inflammation and antibiotic therapy may increase the release of endotoxins. They trigger the septic response binding to specific receptors upon mononuclear phagocytes, endothelial cells and polymorphonuclear leucocytes. Therapies attenuating the mediator network triggered by endotoxins are double-edge swords impairing also the immuno-defence of the host. On the other side, the neutralization of endotoxins acting at the beginning of the septic cascade may be a more effective therapy. Because antibiotic therapy may increase the release of endotoxins, the use of endotoxin-neutralizing antibiotics may control the bacterial growth and, at the same time, may inhibit the effects of endotoxin, resulting in an immuno-modulating effect [112, 113] (Table 18).

Table 18. Antibiotics with endotoxin-neutralizing properties

Polymyxins

Magainins

Teicoplanin

Aminoglycosides

Antibiotics with endotoxin-neutralizing properties are polycationic molecules that can link the polianionic moieties of the lipopolysaccharides including polymyxins, teicoplanin and aminoglycosides [113, 114].

Polymyxins B and E and gramicidin S are bacterium-derived cationic antimicrobial peptides with endotoxin-neutralizing properties. Polymyxin B has been demonstrated to bind endotoxin in many biochemical studies. The biologic effects of this binding have also been the object of many animal studies in which polymyxin B has resulted in the reduction of endotoxin shock, pyrogenicity, Shwartzman reaction and endotoxin lethality. The parenteral use of polymyxin may be associated with side effects including nephrotoxicity [115-117]. Polymyxins have been widely used for selective decontamination of the digestive tract [Chapter 14].

Magainins are polycationic antibiotics with broad-spectrum activity, they have high affinity for lipopolysaccharides and lipid A [118].

Teicoplanin shows an endotoxin-neutralizing property that result in reduced level of TNF-α and IL-1 after stimulation with endotoxin. This property seems to depend on the primary amino group of the amino acid 1 and the alkyl moiety of the N-acyl-β-D-glucosaminyl group of the amino acid 4. Carboxamides derivatives of teicoplanin maintain the endotoxin-neutralizing property of the parent compound [119].

Aminoglycosides have endotoxin-neutralizing properties even if in this regard variable effects have been observed for different compounds of this class of antibiotics: tobramycin seems to be the most effective in regarding of endotoxin-neutralization. For the interaction between aminoglycosides and endotoxin to occur, the molecule of these antibiotics need at least four primary amino-groups, in fact netilmicin that has only three primary amino-groups lacks substantial endotoxin-neutralizing activity [120, 121].

Other nonpeptide antibiotics like pentamidine and some amino-quinolones seem to bind lipid A, probably the basic molecular structure supporting this property is a dicationic moiety.

The granules of neutrophils contain many cationic antimicrobial peptides with endotoxin-neutralizing activity including bactericidal/permeability-increasing protein (BPI), defensins, lactoferrin, antibacterial 15-kDa proteins (p15s), cathepsins, cathelicidins including cationic antimicrobial protein of 18 and 7 kDa (CAP 18 and CAP 7) and indolicidin [122, 123].

BPI binds lipopolysaccharides inhibiting the cytokine release associated with endotoxin stimulation, its amino-terminal fragment weighing 23 kDa seems to maintain the endotoxin-neutralizing proterty of BPI.

CAP 18 has many cationic amino acids concentrated in its C-terminal fragment weighing 7 kDa and corresponding to CAP 7. CAP 18 has antibacterial activity against Gram positive and AGNB. It binds endotoxin neutralizing it and inhibits the tissue factor production stimulated by endotoxin. The antimicrobial activity seems to be due to the interaction between cationic moieties of CAP 18 and CAP 7 and lipopolysaccharides in AGNB and lipoteichoic acids in Gram positives. Micetes and *Mycobacterium* spp. are resistant to the antimicrobial activity of CAP 18 and CAP 7. The use of γ globulin enriched in anti-endotoxin activities may prevent the binding of these toxins to receptors upon macrophage and the generation of inflammatory cytokines. The C-terminal domain of cathelicidin CAP18 has been coupled to immunoglobulin (Ig) G, this combination is thought to bind and neutralize LPS and to kill AGNB [122].

Recently, naturally processed hemoglobin fragments exhibited antimicrobial activity in humans. C-terminal fragments of γ-hemoglobin and β-hemoglobin seem to inhibit the growth of Gram-positive bacteria, AGNB and yeasts in micromolar concentrations. Moreover, they bind lipopolysaccharides reducing the biological activity of endotoxins [124].

The derivation of a pharmacophore for LPS recognition recently has led to the identification of novel and non-toxic molecules, the lipopolyamines. They bind and neutralize LPS both *in vitro* and in animal experiments.

A novel field of research focuses on intracellular endotoxin-binding molecules. Histones seem to bind lipoplysaccharides with affinities higher than that of polymyxin B. Histones seem to reduce the binding of LPS to the macrophage, and the endotoxin-induced production of TNF-α and nitric oxide by these cells. Histones may thus represent a new class of intracellular and extracellular LPS sensors [125, 126].

Toxicity of Glycopeptides: Teicoplanin vs Vancomycin

Vancomycin is widely used for severe Gram-positive bacterial infections, especially those caused by MRSA and CNS. Vancomycin has been associated with adverse effects including the red man syndrome, chest pain, hypotension, muscle spasm, ototoxicity, neutropenia, drug eruptions, fever, nephrotoxicity, thrombocytopenia and rarely pancytopenia and Stevens-Johnson syndrome [127].

The red man syndrome is an acute hypersensitivity reaction to vancomycin associated with flushing, pruritus and, occasionally, hypotension. It has an onset of few minutes and resolves over several hours after the infusion of the drug. The pathogenetic mechanism is a direct release of histamine from mast cells by non-immunological processes [127].

Vancomycin can also produce immunologically mediated adverse reactions like interstitial nephritis, lacrimation, linear IgA bullous dermatosis, exfoliative erythroderma, necrotizing cutaneous vasculitis and toxic epidermal necrolysis.

Neutropenia, thrombocytopenia, agranulocytosis and Stevens-Johnson syndrome have also been reported in association with vancomycin treatment. Vancomycin-associated neutropenia has an incidence of 2% and an onset of 9-30 days after the beginning of vancomycin treatment. Once the drug is discontinued, there is a rapid and complete recovery of the white blood cell count. The pathogenetic mechanism may be a peripheral destructive effect of vancomycin on neutrophils or an immunologically mediated mechanism. Therefore, the white cell count should be monitored in patients receiving vancomycin that should be discontinued in case of hematological abnormality [127].

Stevens-Johnson syndrome is an acute mucocutaneous disease with severe exfoliative dermatitis and mucosal involvement of the gastrointestinal tract and conjunctiva. The pathogenetic mechanism is an immunological cell-mediated toxicity. Stevens-Johnson syndrome may be associated with nephritis, lymphoadenopathy and hepatitis. The treatment includes discontinuation of vancomycin, antihistamines and steroids [127].

Given the number of clinically significant problems associated with vancomycin, the monitoring of serum concentrations is required.

In case of serious adverse reactions the replacement of vancomycin with teicoplanin may be successful [128, 129]. Adverse events have been demonstrated to be significantly less likely with teicoplanin than with vancomycin. This is particularly significant regarding nephrotoxicity that has a lower incidence with teicoplanin than with vancomycin [129, 130]. Red man syndrome is very rare following teicoplanin administration [130, 131]. A higher incidence of thrombocytopenia has been reported with teicoplanin, but at larger doses than those now recommended [130, 131]. Teicoplanin may rarely cause hypersensitivity reactions, such as itching and drug fever and anaphylactoid reactions like the red man syndrome. Many trials in immunocompromised patients have clearly demonstrated that teicoplanin is as effective as vancomycin, while it is associated with fewer adverse effects [129–132]. Moreover teicoplanin has the advantage of once daily administration that results in predictable serum levels not requiring the monitoring of serum concentrations [128].

New Perspectives against Gram-Positive Bacteria: the Lipopeptides

Daptomycin is the first of a new class of antibiotics called lipopeptides. It has activity against a wide range of Gram-positive bacteria [133, 134].

Mechanism of action. Daptomycin exerts its bactericidal activity by disrupting the function of plasma membrane without penetrating into the cytoplasm. The inhibition of the production of protein, DNA and RNA in the cells of bacteria has also been reported. Spontaneous acquisition of resistance *in vitro* seems to be rare [135].

Spectrum of antimicrobial action and clinical use. In *vitro*, daptomycin is active against *S. aureus*, *S. pyogenes*, *S. agalactiae*, group C and G β-hemolytic streptococci and vancomycin-susceptible *E. faecalis*. The drug may be very useful against multidrug-resistant, Gram-positive bacteria such as MRSA, VRE, and glycopeptide intermediate or resistant *S. aureus*. In September 2003, after almost 15 years of development, the Food and Drug Administration approved daptomycin for the treatment of complicated skin and soft tissue infections. Its efficacy in the treatment of more serious infections such as staphylococcal bacteremia is under investigation [136].

Pharmacologic properties. Daptomycin is eliminated primarily by glomerular filtration. In animal studies daptomycin exhibited linear pharmacokinetics, with a half-life of 0.9 to 1.4 h. The level of protein binding is 90%. Daptomycin demonstrates concentration-dependent killing and produces *in vivo* PAEs of 4.8 to 10.8 h [137]. The peak concentration/MIC (peak/MIC) ratio and 24-h AUC/MIC ratio are the pharmacologic parameters that best correlate with *in vivo* efficacy. The long PAE and potent bactericidal activity are the main advantages of daptomycin. Under conditions of high inoculum daptomycin is highly effective. The intravenous dose tested in pharmacokinetic studies has been a 0.5-hour intravenous infusion of 4 mg/Kg once a day [133, 134, 137].

Adverse reactions. Daptomycin seems to be safe and well tolerated. No adverse events related to the infusion have been reported. The most common adverse reactions include gastrointestinal disorders, injection site reactions, fever, headache, insomnia, dizziness, and rash. People receiving daptomycin should be monitored for the development of muscle pain or weakness, and blood tests measuring creatine phosphokinase levels should be monitored weekly [133, 134, 138].

References

1. Hardman JG, Limbird LE, Gilman AG (eds) (2001) Goodman & Gilman's. The pharmacological basis of therapeutics, 10th ed. Mc Graw-Hill Health Professions Division, New York
2. Giotti A, Genazzani E, Pepeu G, Periti P, Fantozzi R, Mugelli A, Mazzei T, Corradetti R. (1994) Farmacologia clinica e chemioterapia, 3rd ed. UTET, Torino
3. Rolinson GN (1986) Beta-lactam antibiotics. J Antimicrob Chemother 17:5–36
4. Allan JD, Eliopoulos GM, Moellering RC Jr (1986) The expanding spectrum of beta-lactam antibiotics. Adv Intern Med 31:119–146
5. Neu HC (1986) β-Lactam antibiotics: structural relationships affecting in vitro activity and pharmacologic properties. Rev Infect Dis 8[Suppl 3]:S237-S259
6. Malouin F, Bryan LE (1986) Modification of penicillin-binding proteins as mechanisms of beta-lactam resistance. Antimicrob Agents Chemother 30:1–5
7. Pauluzzi S (1986) Cephalosporins. Ann Ital Med Int 1:247–254
8. Park SY, Parker RH (1986) Review of imipenem. Infect Control 7:333–337
9. Pastel DA (1986) Imipenem-cilastatin sodium, a broad-spectrum carbapenem antibiotic combination. Clin Pharm 5:719–736
10. Brogden RN, Heel RC (1986) Aztreonam. A review of its antibacterial activity, pharmacokinetic properties and therapeutic use. Drugs 31:96–130
11. Goosen H (2003) Susceptibility of multi-drug-resistant *Pseudomonas aeruginosa* in intensive care units: results from the European MYSTIC study group. Clin Microbiol Infect 9:980–983
12. Nordbring F (1980) Clinical review of the aminoglycosides. Scand J Infect Dis. Suppl 23:S15–S19
13. Tok JB, Bi L (2003) Aminoglycoside and its derivatives as ligands to target the ribosome. Curr Top Med Chem 3:1001–1019
14. Smith CA, Baker EN (2002) Aminoglycoside antibiotic resistance by enzymatic deactivation. Curr Drug Targets Infect Disord 2:143–160
15. Bates DE (2003) Aminoglycoside ototoxicity. Drugs Today (Barc) 39:277–285
16. Tod M, Padoin C, Petitjean O (2000) Clinical pharmacokinetics and pharmacodynamics of isepamicin. Clin Pharmacokinet 38:205–223

17. Blondeau JM (2004) Fluoroquinolones: mechanism of action, classification, and development of resistance. Surv Ophthalmol 49 [Suppl 2]:S73–S78
18. Viale P, Pea F (2003) What is the role of fluoroquinolones in intensive care? J Chemother 15 [Suppl 3]:5–10
19. Hooper DC (2000) Mechanism of action and resistance of older and newer fluoroquinolones. Clin Infect Dis 31 [Suppl 2]:S24–S28
20. Hooper DC, Wolfson JS (1985) The fluoroquinolones: pharmacology, clinical uses, and toxicities in humans. Antimicrob Agents Chemother 28:716–721
21. Ackermann G, Rodloff AC (2003) Drugs of the 21st century: telithromycin (HMR 3647)—the first ketolide. J Antimicrob Chemother 51:497–511
22. Mazzei T, Mini E, Novelli A, Periti P (1993) Chemistry and mode of action of macrolides. J Antimicrob Chemother 31, Suppl C:1–9
23. Labro MT (2004) Macrolide antibiotics: current and future uses. Expert Opin Pharmacother 5:541–550
24. Feldman C (2004) Clinical relevance of antimicrobial resistance in the management of pneumococcal community-acquired pneumonia. J Lab Clin Med 143:269–283
25. Novelli A, Mini E, Mazzei T (2004) Pharmacological interactions between antibiotics and other drugs in the treatment of lower respiratory tract infections. Eur Respir Mon 28:1–26
26. Baldwin DR, Wise R, Andrews JM et al (1990) Azithromycin concentrations at the sites of pulmonary infection. Eur Resp J 3:886–890
27. Esposito S, Noviello S (2003) What is the role of glycopeptides in intensive care? J Chemother 15 [Suppl 3]:11–6
28. Malabarba A, Ciabatti R (2001) Glycopeptide derivatives. Curr Med Chem 8:1759–1773
29. Paradisi F, Corti G, Messeri D (2001) Antistaphylococcal (MSSA, MRSA, MSSE, MRSE) antibiotics. Med Clin North Am 85:1–17
30. Parenti F, Schito GC, Courvalin P (2000) Teicoplanin chemistry and microbiology. J Chemother 12 [Suppl 5]:5–14
31. Harding I, Sorgel F (2000) Comparative pharmacokinetics of teicoplanin and vancomycin. J Chemother 12 [Suppl 5]:15–20
32. Levin AS, Barone AA, Penco J, Santos MV, Marinho IS, Arruda EA, Manrique EI, Costa SF (1999) Intravenous colistin as therapy for nosocomial infections caused by multidrug-resistant *Pseudomonas aeruginosa* and *Acinetobacter baumannii*. Clin Infect Dis 28:1008–1011
33. Beringer P (2001) The clinical use of colistin in patients with cystic fibrosis. Curr Opin Pulm Med 7:434–440
34. Diekema DJ, Jones RN (2001) Oxazolidinone antibiotics. Lancet 358:1975–1982
35. Lundstrom TS, Sobel JD (2000) Antibiotics for gram-positive bacterial infections. Vancomycin, teicoplanin, quinupristin/dalfopristin, and linezolid. Infect Dis Clin North Am 14:463–474
36. De Gaudio AR, Di Filippo A (2003) What is the role of streptogramins in intensive care? J Chemother 15 [Suppl 3]:17–21
37. Hershberger E, Donabedian S, Konstantinou K, Zervos MJ (2004) Quinupristin-dalfopristin resistance in gram-positive bacteria: mechanism of resistance and epidemiology. Clin Infect Dis 38:92–98
38. Eliopoulos GM (2003) Quinupristin-dalfopristin and linezolid: evidence and opinion. Clin Infect Dis 36:473–481
39. Blondeau JM, Sanche SE (2002) Quinupristin/dalfopristin. Expert Opin Pharmacother 3:1341–1364

40. Gunderson BW, Ross GH, Ibrahim KH, Rotschafer JC (2001) What do we really know about antibiotic pharmacodynamics? Pharmacotherapy 21:302s–318s
40a. Mehrota R, De Gaudio R, Palazzo M (2004) Antibiotic pharmacokinetic and pharmacodynamic considerations in critical illness. Int Care Med 30:2145–2156
41. White CA, Toothaker RD, Smith AL, Slattery JT (1989) In vitro evaluation of the determinants of bactericidal activity of ampicillin dosing regimens against *Escherichia coli.* Antimicrob Agents Chemother 33:1046–1051
42. Thomson KS, Moland ES (2001) Cefepime, piperacillin-tazobactam and the inoculum effect in test with extended-spectrum beta-lactamase-producing *Enterobacteriaceae.* Antimicrob Agents Chemother 45:3548–3554
43. Hanberger H, Nilsson LE, Maller R, Nilsson M (1990) Pharmacodynamics of ß-lactam antibiotics on gram-negative bacteria: initial killing, morphology and postantibiotic effect. Scand J Infect Dis Suppl 74:118–123
44. Turnidge JD (1998) The pharmacodynamics of ß-lactams. Clin Infect Dis 27:10–22
45. Craig W, Rikardsdottir S, Watanabe Y (1992) In vivo and in vitro postantibiotic effects (PAEs) of azithromycin [abstr]. In: Program and abstracts of the 32nd Interscience Conference on Antimicrobial Agents and Chemotherapy. American Society for Microbiology, Washington DC p 45
46. MacArthur RD, Lolans V, Zar FA, Jackson GG (1984) Biphasic, concentration-dependent and rate-limited, concentration-independent bacterial killing by an aminoglycoside antibiotic. J Infect Dis 150:778–779
47. Ishida K, Kaku M, Irifune K, Mizukane R, Takemura H, Yoshida R, Tanaka H, Usui T, Suyama N, Tomono K (1994) In vitro and in vivo activities of macrolides against *Mycoplasma pneumoniae.* Antimicrob Agents Chemother 38:790–798
48. Novelli A, Fallani S, Cassetta MI, Arrigucci S, Mazzei T (2002) In vivo pharmacodynamic evaluation of clarithromycin in comparison to erythromycin. J Chemother 14:584–590
49. Den Hollander JG, Knudsen JD, Mouton JW, Fuursted K, Frimodt-Moller N, Verbrugh HA, Espersen F (1998) Comparison of pharmacodynamics of azithromycin and erythromycin in vitro and in vivo. Antimicrob Agents Chemother 42:377–782
50. Tessier PR, Kim MK, Zhou W, Xuan D, Li C, Ye M, Nightingale CH, Nicolau DP (2002) Pharmacodynamic assessment of clarithromycin in a murine model of pneumococcal pneumonia. Antimicrob Agents Chemother 46:1425–1434
51. Roosendaal R, Bakker-Woudenberg IA, van den Berghe-van Raffe M, Michel MF (1986) Continuous versus intermittent administration of ceftazidime in experimental *Klebsiella pneumoniae* pneumonia in normal and leukopenic rats. Antimicrob Agents Chemother 30:403–408
52. Nishida M, Murakawa T, Kamimura T, Okada N (1978) Bactericidal activity of cephalosporins in an in vitro model simulating serum levels. Antimicrob Agents Chemother 14:6–12
53. Craig WA (1995) Interrelationship between pharmacokinetics and pharmacodynamics in determining dosage regimens for broad-spectrum cephalosporins. Diag Microbiol Infect Dis 22:89–96
54. Vogelman B, Gudmundsson S, Leggett J, Turnidge J, Ebert S, Craig WA (1988) Correlation of antimicrobial pharmacokinetic parameters with therapeutic efficacy in an animal model. J Infect Dis 158:831–847
55. MacGowan AP, Bowker KE (1998) Continuous infusion of ß-lactam antibiotics. Clin Pharmacokinet 35:391–402
56. Cars O (1997) Efficacy of beta-lactam antibiotics: integration of pharmacokinetics

and pharmacodynamics. Diag Microbiol Infect Dis 27:29–33

57. Larsson AJ, Walker KJ, Raddatz JK, Rotschafer JC (1996) The concentration-independent effect of monoexponential and biexponential decay in vancomycin concentrations on the killing of *Staphylococcus aureus* under aerobic and anaerobic conditions. J Antimicrob Chemother 38:589–597

58. Knudsen JD, Fuursted K, Raber S, Espersen F, Frimodt-Moller N (2000) Pharmacodynamics of glycopeptides in the mouse peritonitis model of *Streptococcus pneumoniae* or *Staphylococcus aureus* infection. Antimicrob Agents Chemother 44:1247–1254

59. Ackerman BH, Vannier AM, Eudy EB (1992) Analysis of vancomycin time-kill studies with *Staphylococcus* species by using a curve stripping program to describe relationship between concentration and pharmacodynamic response. Antimicrob Agents Chemother 36:1766–1769

60. Rybak MJ, Houlihan HH, Mercier RC, Kaatz GW (1997) Pharmacodynamics of RP 59500 (quinupristin-dalfopristin) administered by intermittent versus continuous infusion against *Staphylococcus aureus*-infected fibrin-platelet clots in an in vitro infection model. Antimicrob Agents Chemother 41:1359–1363

61. Boswell FJ, Sunderland J, Andrews JM, Wise R (1997) Time-kill kinetics of quinupristin/dalfopristin on *Staphylococcus* with and without a raised MBC evaluated by two methods. J Antimicrob Chemother 39:29–32

62. Craig WA (1997) Postantibiotic effects and the dosing of macrolides, azalides and streptogramins. In: Zinner SH, Young LS, Acar JF, Neu HC (eds) Expanding indications for the new macrolides, azalides, and streptogramins. Marcel Dekker, New York pp 27–38

63. Rapp RP (1998) Pharmacokinetics and pharmacodynamics of intravenous and oral azithromycin: enhanced tissue activity and minimal drug interactions. Ann Pharmacother 32:785–793

64. Nightingale CH (1997) Pharmacokinetics and pharmacodynamics of newer macrolides. Pediatr Infect Dis J 16:438-443

65. Moore RD, Lietman PS, Smith CR (1987) Clinical response to aminoglycoside therapy: importance of the ratio of peak concentration to minimal inhibitory concentration. J Infect Dis 155:93–99

66. Kapusnik JE, Hackbarth CJ, Chambers HF, Carpenter T, Sande MA (1988) Single, large, daily dosing versus intermittent dosing of tobramycin for treating experimental pseudomonas pneumonia. J Infect Dis 158:7–12

67. Daikos GL, Jackson GG, Lolans VT, Livermore DM (1990) Adaptive resistance to aminoglycoside antibiotics from first-exposure down-regulation. J Infect Dis 162:414–420

68. Deziel-Evans LM, Murphy JE, Job ML (1986) Correlation of pharmacokinetic indices with therapeutic outcome in patients receiving aminoglycosides. Clin Pharm 5:319–324

69. Nicolau DP, Freeman CD, Belliveau PP, Nightingale CH, Ross JW, Quintiliani R (1995) Experience with a once-daily aminoglycoside program administered to 2,184 adult patients. Antimicrob Agents Chemother 39:650–655

70. Rotschafer JC, Rybak MJ (1994) Single daily dosing of aminoglycosides: a commentary. Ann Pharmacother 28:797–801

71. Gilbert DN (1991) Once-daily aminoglycoside therapy. Antimicrob Agents Chemother 35:399–405

72. Dudley MN, Blaser J, Gilbert D, Mayer KH, Zinner SH (1991) Combination therapy with ciprofloxacin plus azlocillin against *Pseudomonas aeruginosa*: effect of simulta-

neous versus staggered administration in an in vitro model of infection. J Infect Dis 164:499–506

73. Hyatt JM, Nix DE, Schentag JJ (1994) Pharmacokinetic and pharmacodynamic activities of ciprofloxacin against strains of *Streptococcus pneumoniae, Staphylococcus aureus*, and *Pseudomonas aeruginosa* for which MICs are similar. Antimicrob Agents Chemother 38:2730–2737

74. Thomas JK, Forrest A, Bhavnani SM et al (1998) Pharmaco-dynamic evaluation of factors associated with the development of bacterial resistance in acutely ill patients during therapy. Antimicrob Agents Chemother 42:521–527

75. Preston SL, Drusano GL, Berman AL et al (1998) Pharmaco-dynamics of levofloxacin: a new paradigm for early clinical trials. JAMA 279:125–129

76. Peterson ML, Hovde LB, Wright DH et al (1999) Fluoroquinolone resistance in *Bacteroides fragilis* following sparfloxacin exposure. Antimicrob Agents Chemother 43:2251–2255

77. Schentag JJ (1999) Antimicrobial action and pharmacokinetics/ pharmacodynamics: the use of AUIC to improve efficacy and avoid resistance. J Chemother 11:426–439

78. Azoulay-Dupuis E, Vallee E, Bedos JP, Muffat-Joly M, Pocidalo JJ (1991) Prophylactic and therapeutic activities of azithromycin in a mouse model of pneumococcal pneumonia. Antimicrob Agents Chemother 35:1024–1028

79. McNulty CA, Kane A, Foy CJ, Sykes J, Saunders P, Cartwright KA (2000) Primary care workshops can reduce and rationalize antibiotic prescribing. J Antimicrob Chemother 46:493–499

80. Carrie AG, Zhanel GG (1999) Antibacterial use in community practice: assessing quantity, indications and appropriateness, and relationship to the development of antibacterial resistance. Drugs 57:871–881

81. Vlahovic-Palcevski V, Morovic M, Palcevski G, Betica-Radic L (2001) Antimicrobial utilization and bacterial resistance at three different hospitals. Eur J Epidemiol 17:375–383

82. Fluckiger U, Zimmerli W, Sax H, Frei R, Widmer AF (2000) Clinical impact of an infectious disease service on the management of bloodstream infection. Eur J Clin Microbiol Infect Dis 19:493–500

83. Kollef MH (2001) Optimizing antibiotic therapy in the intensive care unit setting. Crit Care 5:189–195

84. Antonelli M, Mercurio G, Di Nunno S, Recchioni G, Deangelis G (2001) De-escalation antimicrobial chemotherapy in critically III patients: pros and cons. J Chemother 1:218–223

85. Gyssens IC (1999) Preventing postoperative infections: current treatment recommendations. Drugs 57:175–185

86. Meloni GA, Schito GC (1991) Microbial ecosystems as targets of antibiotic actions. Chemother 3 [Suppl 1]:179–181

87. Sullivan A, Edlund C, Nord CE (2001) Effect of antimicrobial agents on the ecological balance of human microflora. Lancet Infect Dis 1:101–114

88. Klein G (2003) Taxonomy, ecology and antibiotic resistance of enterococci from food and the gastro-intestinal tract. Int J Food Microbiol 88:123–131

89. Tannock GW (2001) Molecular assessment of intestinal microflora. Am J Clin Nutr 73 [Suppl 2]:410S–414S

90. Dunne C (2001) Adaptation of bacteria to the intestinal niche: probiotics and gut disorder. Inflamm Bowel Dis 7:136–145

91. Brook I (2000) The effects of amoxicillin therapy on skin flora in infants. Pediatr

Dermatol 17:360–363

92. Hoiby N (2000) Ecological antibiotic policy. J Antimicrob Chemother 46 [Suppl 1]:59–62 (discussion 63-5)
93. Zdziarski P, Simon K, Majda J (2003) Overuse of high stability antibiotics and its consequences in public and environmental health. Acta Microbiol Pol 52:5–13
94. Gaskins HR, Collier CT, Anderson DB (2002) Antibiotics as growth promotants: mode of action. Anim Biotechnol 13:29–42
95. Lathers CM (2002) Clinical pharmacology of antimicrobial use in humans and animals. J Clin Pharmacol 42:587–600
96. Teale CJ (2002) Antimicrobial resistance and the food chain. J Appl Microbiol 92 [Suppl]:85S–89S
97. Bergan T, Engeset A, Olszewski W (1987) Does serum protein binding inhibit tissue penetration of antibiotics? Rev Infect Dis 9:713–718
98. Muhle SA, Tam JP (2001) Design of Gram-negative selective antimicrobial peptides. Biochemestry 40:5777–5785
99. Nau R, Sorgel F, Prange HW (1998) Pharmacokinetic optimisation of the treatment of bacterial central nervous system infections. Clin Pharmacokinet 35:223–246
100. Wise R, Gillett AP, Cadge B, Durham SR, Baker S (1980) The influence of protein binding upon tissue fluid levels of six beta-lactam antibiotics. J Infect Dis 142:77–82
101. Bergan T, Engeset A, Olszewski W, Ostby N, Solberg R (1986) Extravascular penetration of highly protein-bound flucloxacillin. Antimicrob Agents Chemother 30:729-732
102. Roder BL, Frimodt-Moller N, Espersen F, Rasmussen SN (1995) Dicloxacillin and flucloxacillin: pharmacokinetics, protein binding and serum bactericidal titers in healthy subjects after oral administration. Infection 23:107–112
103. Singhvi SM, Heald AF, Schreiber EC (1978) Pharmacokinetics of cephalosporin antibiotics: protein-binding considerations. Chemotherapy 24:121–133
104. Hoffstedt B, Walder M (1981) Influence of serum protein binding and mode of administration on penetration of five cephalosporins into subcutaneous tissue fluid in humans. Antimicrob Agents Chemother 20:783–786
105. Nightingale CH, Klimek JJ, Quintiliani R (1980) Effect of protein binding on the penetration of nonmetabolized cephalosporins into atrial appendage and pericardial fluids in open-heart surgical patients. Antimicrob Agents Chemother 17:595–598
106. Kunst MW, Mattie H (1978) Cefazolin and cephradine: relationship between serum concentrations and tissue contents in mice. Infection 6:166–170
107. Singhvi SM, Heald AF, Gadebusch HH, Resnick ME, Difazio LT, Leitz MA (1977) Human serum protein binding of cephalosporin antibiotics in vitro. J Lab Clin Med 89:414–420
108. Bergan T (1990) Pharmacokinetic parameters and characteristics relevant to antimicrobial surgical prophylaxis. Scand J Infect Dis Suppl 70:31–35
109. Majiduddin FK, Materon IC, Palzkill TG (2002) Molecular analysis of beta-lactamase structure and function. Int J Med Microbiol 292:127–137
110. Tolmasky ME (2000) Bacterial resistance to aminoglycosides and beta-lactams: the Tn1331 transposon paradigm. Front Biosci 5:D20–D29
111. Burk DL, Berghuis AM (2002) Protein kinase inhibitors and antibiotic resistance. Pharmacol Ther 93:283–292
112. Lynn WA, Golenbock DT (1992) Lipopolysaccharide antagonists. Immunol Today 13:271–276
113. Focà A, Matera G, Berlingheri MC (1993) Inhibition of endotoxin activity by antibiotics. J Antimicrob Chemother 31:799

114. Zhang L, Dhillon P, Yan H, Farmer S (2000) Hancock RE. Interactions of bacterial cationic peptide antibiotics with outer and cytoplasmic membranes of *Pseudomonas aeruginosa*. Antimicrob Agents Chemother 44:3317–3321

115. Tsuzuki H, Tani T, Ueyama H, Kodama M (2001) Lipopolysaccharide: neutralization by polymyxin B shuts down the signaling pathway of nuclear factor kappaB in peripheral blood mononuclear cells, even during activation. J Surg Res 100:127–134

116. Tsubery H, Ofek I, Cohen S, Eisenstein M, Fridkin M (2002) Modulation of the hydrophobic domain of polymyxin B nonapeptide: effect on outer-membrane permeabilization and lipopolysaccharide neutralization. Mol Pharmacol 62:1036–1042

117. Bucklin SE, Lake P, Logdberg L, Morrison DC (1995) Therapeutic efficacy of a polymyxin B-dextran conjugate in experimental model of endotoxemia. Antimicrob Agents Chemother 39:1462–1466

118. Berkowitz BA, Bevins CL, Zasloff MA (1990) Magainins: a new family of membrane-active host defence peptides. Biochem Pharmacol 39:625-629

119. Focà A, Matera G, Berlinghieri MC (1993) Inhibition of endotoxin-induced interleukin 8 release by teicoplanin in human whole blood. Eur J Clin Microbiol Infect Dis 12:940–944

120. Focà A, Matera G, Iannello D et al (1991) Aminoglycosides modify the in vitro metachromatic reaction and murine generalized Shwartzman phenomenon induced by *Salmonella minnesota* R595 lipopolysaccharide. Antimicrob Agents Chemother 35:2161-2164

121. Artenstein AW, Cross AS (1989) Inhibition of endotoxin reactivity by aminoglycosides. J Antimicrob Chemother 24:826

122. Warren HS, Matyal R, Allaire JE, Yarmush D, Loiselle P, Hellman J, Paton BG, Fink MP (2003) Protective efficacy of CAP18106-138-immunoglobulin G in sepsis. J Infect Dis 188:1382–1393

123. Devine DA (2003) Antimicrobial peptides in defence of the oral and respiratory tracts. Mol Immunol 40:431–443

124. Liepke C, Baxmann S, Heine C, Breithaupt N, Standker L, Forssmann WG (2003) Human hemoglobin-derived peptides exhibit antimicrobial activity: a class of host defense peptides. J Chromatogr B Analyt Technol Biomed Life Sci 791:345-356

125. Augusto LA, Decottignies P, Synguelakis M, Nicaise M, Le Marechal P, Chaby R (2003) Histones: a novel class of lipopolysaccharide-binding molecules. Biochemistry 42:3929–3938

126. Nagaoka I, Hirota S, Niyonsaba F, Hirata M, Adachi Y, Tamura H, Heumann D (2001) Cathelicidin family of antibacterial peptides CAP18 and CAP11 inhibit the expression of TNF-alpha by blocking the binding of LPS to CD14(+) cells. J Immunol 167:3329–3338

127. Rocha JL, Kondo W, Baptista MI, Da Cunha CA, Martins LT (2002) Uncommon vancomycin-induced side effects. Braz J Infect Dis 6196–200

128. Menichetti F, Martino P, Bucaneve G, Gentile G, D'Antonio D, Liso V, Ricci P, Nosari AM, Buelli M, Carotenuto M, et al (1994) Effects of teicoplanin and those of vancomycin in initial empirical antibiotic regimen for febrile, neutropenic patients with hematologic malignancies. Gimema Infection Program. Antimicrob Agents Chemother 38:2041–2046

129. Janknegt R (1991) Teicoplanin in perspective. A critical comparison with vancomycin Pharm Weekbl Sci 13:153–160

130. Wood MJ (2000) Comparative safety of teicoplanin and vancomycin. J Chemother 12 [Suppl 5]:21–25

131. de Lalla F, Tramarin A (1995) A risk-benefit assessment of teicoplanin in the treatment of infections. Drug Saf 13:317–328
132. De Pauw BE, Novakova IR, Donnelly JP (1990) Options and limitations of teicoplanin in febrile granulocytopenic patients. Br J Haematol 76 [Suppl 2]:1–5
133. Fenton C, Keating GM, Curran MP (2004) Daptomycin. Drugs 64:445–455
134. Tedesco KL, Rybak MJ (2004) Daptomycin. Pharmacotherapy 24:41–57
135. Safdar N, Andes D, Craig WA (2004) In vivo pharmacodynamic activity of daptomycin. Antimicrob Agents Chemother 48:63–68
136. Cha R, Brown WJ, Rybak MJ (2003) Bactericidal activities of daptomycin, quinupristin-dalfopristin, and linezolid against vancomycin-resistant *Staphylococcus aureus* in an in vitro pharmacodynamic model with simulated endocardial vegetations. Antimicrob Agents Chemother 47:3960–3963
137. Pankuch GA, Jacobs MR, Appelbaum PC (2003) Postantibiotic effects of daptomycin against 14 staphylococcal and pneumococcal clinical isolates. Antimicrob Agents Chemother 47:3012–3014
138. Dvorchik B, Damphousse D (2004) Single-dose pharmacokinetics of daptomycin in young and geriatric volunteers. J Clin Pharmacol 44:612–620

Chapter 8

Systemic Antifungals

F. J. COOKE, T. ROGERS

Introduction

There is now widespread recognition of the importance of fungi as causes of life-threatening infections in critically ill patients. This increased awareness, which has developed especially over the past decade, is founded on studies that have been reported by the National Nosocomial Infection Surveillance Program in the United States [1, 2]. More recently, studies of secular trends and antifungal drug susceptibility of hospital-acquired candidemia conducted by the Centers for Disease Control Atlanta [3] and the SENTRY Antimicrobial Surveillance Program [4] respectively have also highlighted the growing significance of fungal infections.

Candida spp. are acknowledged to be the most frequent nosocomial fungal pathogens on intensive care units (ICU), whether the units are general or specialized in terms of their patient populations. On leukemia and hematopoietic stem cell transplant units, and to a lesser extent solid organ transplant services, mould infections, especially with Aspergillus spp., are increasing in incidence and have even higher mortality rates. Candida spp. have been reported by some North American centers to be their fourth most common cause of bloodstream infections (BSI) in ICU patients [5] and mortality rates due to candidemia have been reported to be as high as 60%. This experience has prompted studies that have investigated risk factors associated with this infection such as the National Epidemiology of Mycosis Survey (NEMIS), which was undertaken in six geographically separated academic centers in the United States [6]. By multivariate analysis the authors found that the factors independently associated with an increased risk of Candida BSI in adult patients were prior surgery, acute renal failure, receipt of parenteral nutrition, and the presence of a triple-lumen catheter in surgical patients. Interestingly, patients who underwent a surgical procedure or had a central vascular catheter in situ had an 11-fold increased risk of developing *Candida* BSI. The overall mortality rate of patients with *Candida* BSI was 41% compared with 8% in those without *Candida* BSI (*P* value <0.001). It is noteworthy that the incidence of *Candida* BSI varied widely between the participating institutions and that a high APACHE II score was not associated with a significantly increased risk of developing *Candida* BSI. The NEMIS group have also investigated candidemia among neonatal ICU patients [7]. Very low birth weight appeared to be the principal risk factor and the mortality was greater among candidemia patients compared with those neonates not infected (23% versus 4.7%).

The detection of *Candida* colonization at several body sites has been considered to be a risk factor for progression to an invasive infection. As a consequence, some authors recommend surveillance cultures; the finding of colonization at two or more sites, including candiduria, could be used to target patients at increased risk of invasive infection in whom pre-emptive therapy would be initiated. While this approach has been found clinically useful by some investigators, the NEMIS study [6] failed to show predictive value of either candiduria or rectal colonization.

There has been a changing epidemiology of *Candida* BSI over the past few years. Whereas *Candida albicans* formerly caused more than 80% of episodes, recent data from the SENTRY surveillance program reveal that the proportions of candidemia due to *C. albicans* in the United States, Latin America, Canada, and Europe were 55%, 45%, 60%, and 58%, respectively [8]. Overall, the most commonly represented species were *C. albicans* (55%), *C. glabrata* (15%), *C. parapsilosis* (15%), and *C. tropicalis* (9%). This changing picture has clinical relevance because *Candida* species other than *C. albicans* have less predictable susceptibility to fluconazole, an antifungal that has been widely used to treat candidemia and other *Candida* infections in ICU patients.

This chapter will review the systemically administered antifungal agents in current use, including recently licensed drugs, and also some new antifungals in development. Their role in managing invasive fungal infections in critical care patients will also be considered.

Antifungal Agents in Current Use

Polyenes

Amphotericin B and Lipid Formulations

Amphotericin B (Fungizone) has been extensively used to treat invasive fungal infections throughout the past 40 years [9] .Until recently it was regarded as the 'gold standard' therapeutic antifungal agent, particularly for infections with non-*albicans* species of *Candida* and *Aspergillus* spp.

Mechanism of action. By binding to ergosterol in fungal cell membranes, amphotericin B causes an increase in membrane permeability and thus loss of cell constituents. It is therefore a fungicidal drug in that it causes cell death. Theoretically amphotericin B shows selective toxicity to fungal cell membranes compared with human cell membranes. However, there are well-recognized problems with infusion-related reactions including chills, fevers, headache, nausea, and vomiting, and also nephrotoxicity in humans. Therefore lipid formulations of amphotericin B have been developed [10].

Spectrum of activity. Amphotericin B is the drug of choice for many deep fungal infections, as it has the broadest spectrum of activity of any licensed antifungal agent. Not only is it active against most *Candida* and *Aspergillus* spp., but also against *Cryptococcus neoformans* and the dimorphic fungi such as *Histoplasma capsulatum*. Notable exceptions include *Scedosporium spp., Fusarium spp., Candida lusitaniae, Aspergillus terreus,* and *Sporothrix schenckii.* Of note there are published data suggesting that lipid-based formulations may be more effective against zygomycetes and *Fusarium* species [11].

Reports of acquired resistance to amphotericin B are rare. There are, however, some published cases of relapsing cryptococcal disease in AIDS patients, where development of resistance to amphotericin B has been reported.

Pharmacological properties. Amphotericin B is normally administered intravenously together with a carrier such as desoxycholate, because it has very low oral bioavailability. The drug is highly protein bound (90%–95%) and penetration into the cerebrospinal fluid (CSF) is poor. It is widely distributed in body tissues, with a volume of distribution of 4 l/kg. It seems that hepatic dysfunction, renal impairment, and dialysis have little effect on serum levels. The usual intravenous dose is 0.7–1 mg/kg per day. In addition, oral and topical preparations are available in some countries for treating mucosal candidiasis or to suppress *Candida* overgrowth in the bowel.

A recent trial demonstrated that administration of conventional amphotericin B as a 24-h continuous infusion was better tolerated than traditional dosing [12]. The majority of patients were neutropenic and they were randomized to receive either amphotericin B at a dose of 0.95 mg/kg daily, infused over 4 h, or at a dose of 0.97 mg/kg as 24-h continuous infusions. There was a significant reduction in infusion-related reactions and better creatinine clearance in the continuous infusion arm. The authors advocated this approach for reducing the toxicity of amphotericin B. Together with the optimal use of pre-medications, this approach warrants further research.

Lipid formulations have been developed to overcome the problems associated with the nephrotoxicity of conventional amphotericin B. There are currently three widely licensed lipid formulations of amphotericin B, which are all given intravenously.

1. Liposomal amphotericin (Ambisome) is encapsulated in phospholipid-containing liposomes
2. Amphotericin B colloidal dispersion (ABCD, Amphocil, Amphotec) is complexed with cholesterol sulfate to form small lipid discs
3. Amphotericin B lipid complex (ABLC, Abelcet) is complexed with phospholipids to form ribbon-like structures.

The considerable expense associated with lipid preparations restricts their use in many healthcare settings. However, these are better tolerated than amphotericin B in terms of their nephrotoxicity, and all three formulations appear to be at least as therapeutically efficacious as amphotericin B. There are data suggesting that Ambisome results in fewer infusion-related reactions compared with Abelcet, which in turn causes fewer infusion-related side effects than Amphocil [13]. Further trials in high-risk patients would help to clarify the precise indications and usefulness of each formulation.

The lipid formulations can be given in higher doses (3–5 mg/kg per day) than the conventional drug, which is a clear advantage. Although their pharmacokinetics and pharmacodynamics are different, they are all distributed predominantly to the reticuloendothelial system, and so are particularly useful for treatment of fungal infections involving the liver, spleen, lung, and kidneys.

Clinical use of the lipid formulations has mainly been in treating suspected or proven invasive fungal infections complicating treatment of hematological malignancy. There are fewer clinical trial data from treating critical care patients; however, they are widely used in patients at risk of developing nephrotoxicity who do not tolerate amphotericin B. Dupont [10] concluded that further dose and cost-effectiveness studies are needed before these formulations can replace conventional amphotericin B.

Azoles

The azoles are grouped into the imidazoles [clotrimazole, miconazole (Daktarin) and ketoconazole (Nizoral)] and the triazoles [fluconazole (Diflucan), itraconazole (Sporanox), and voriconazole (VFend)] [14]. Over the last few years several as yet unlicensed triazoles have been developed, of which the most promising seem to be posaconazole and ravuconazole. These are still undergoing evaluation.

The triazoles are more often used in the ICU setting, and will be discussed below, focussing particularly on the newly licensed agent voriconazole. The imidazoles will not be considered further here.

Mechanism of action. The main sterol that makes up the fungal cell membrane is ergosterol and the azoles act on its synthetic pathway. They demonstrate selective toxicity because the predominant sterol in human cell membranes is cholesterol. Azoles bind to the heme of the enzyme cytochrome P-450 and then interfere with demethylation of the 14-methyl sterol intermediates, and thus inhibit synthesis of fungal cell membranes.

Spectrum of activity. The spectrum of activity of the triazoles is broad and includes *C. albicans, Cryptococcus neoformans, Coccidioides immitis, Blastomyces dermatitidis, Paracoccidioides brasiliensis, Histoplasma capsulatum,* and *Sporothrix schenckii.* However, fluconazole is less reliable against germ-tube negative yeasts, such as *Candida krusei* and *Candida glabrata, Fusarium* spp., and the zygomycetes. Resistance to fluconazole is increasingly recognized, particularly in AIDS patients, but this does not predict class resistance. Therefore comprehensive laboratory sensitivity testing and evaluation of minimum inhibitory concentrations is recommended for isolates cultured from sterile sites or invasive infections [15].

The other triazoles, itraconazole and voriconazole, have activity against *Aspergillus* spp. and better coverage of non-*albicans Candida* spp. Posaconazole may be clinically useful against some zygomycetes.

Pharmacological properties. Fluconazole can be administered orally and intravenously and these routes have identical pharmacokinetics. The adult dose ranges from 100 to 400 mg/day depending on the type of infection. For the treatment of systemic infection, the minimum daily dose is 400 mg. Absorption is not affected by gastric pH or food, and oral bioavailability is over 80%. Fluconazole is water soluble and weakly protein bound, so it penetrates well into the CSF (CSF concentrations may reach 60%–80% of serum levels). It is excreted by the kidney and although dose reduction may be required in renal impairment, therapeutic drug monitoring is rarely recommended. Overall, fluconazole is well tolerated, and can be given once daily because of the relatively long half-life of 7–10 h.

Itraconazole

Itraconazole was originally only administered orally at a dose of 3–5 mg/kg per day, as capsules or syrup. The oral bioavailability varies: acid conditions are required for absorption and the drug should ideally be taken with food. More recently an intravenous formulation has become available [16]. CSF penetration of itraconazole is poor because the plasma protein binding is very high. The drug is metabolized by the liver, so should not be prescribed for patients with liver disease. Dose adjustments are not required in renal impairment, but caution is needed for patients with cardiac failure. The intravenous cyclodextrin-based formulation provides more rapid and reliable drug serum concentrations [17].

Most in-patient clinical experience with itraconazole has been in prophylaxis or therapy of invasive fungal infections in patients with hematological malignancy. Prophylaxis studies with the oral formulations have given conflicting results but in a recent randomized trial of intravenous/oral itraconazole versus oral fluconazole, patients receiving itraconazole had significantly fewer proven invasive infections (9% versus 25%) in the first 180 days post allogeneic stem cell transplant [18]. Although there was no difference in overall mortality rates, death due to fungal infection was less frequent in itraconazole recipients (9% versus, 18%, 95% confidence interval -20.6 to 1.8, P=0.13). Itraconazole has been shown to be as effective as amphotericin B for the treatment of antibiotic-resistant febrile neutropenia in cancer patients [17] and produced a complete or partial response in 15 of 31 (48%) patients with invasive pulmonary aspergillosis [19].

Voriconazole

Voriconazole is derived from fluconazole. It has a broad spectrum of activity against *Candida* species (including *C. glabrata* and *C. krusei*), *Cryptococcus neoformans*, *Aspergillus spp.*, *Fusarium spp.*, *Scedosporium spp.*, and some other moulds [20, 21]. However, it is not active in vitro against the zygomycetes. It is available orally, with good bioavailability (96%) in healty volounteers and also intravenously as the cyclodextrin formulation. There is extensive tissue distribution, including the central nervous system. For intravenous therapy a loading dose of 6 mg/kg 12-hourly for the first 24 h is required, usually followed by 4 mg/kg twice daily. Orally, an initial loading dose of 400 mg every 12 h is given for 24 h followed by 200 mg twice daily. Dose adjustments are required for patients weighing less than 40 kg and children, according to the manufacturer's recommendations. The clinical pharmacology is complex and interactions with the different cytochrome enzyme systems may differ between ethnic groups. Therapeutic drug monitoring is not routinely recommended.

Voriconazole is more toxic than fluconazole, with the most common adverse effect reported in clinical trials being visual disturbance [22]. This has been reported in over 30% of patients, but all events to date have been transient. They include blurred vision, altered visual and/or colour perception, and photophobia, and commonly occur about 30 min post dose. They usually last for about 30 min and are more common early in the course of treatment. Mild hepatic abnormalities have also been reported in 10% of patients, but more severe hepatic toxicity can occur. Up to 20% of non-Indian Asians are at increased risk of hepatotoxicity, because of reduced metabolism of the drug by cytochrome P-450 enzymes. Rashes of mild severity, including photosensitivity, occur commonly but there are also reports of Stevens-Johnson syndrome and toxic epidermal necrolysis. Nausea and vomiting occur in 2% of cases.

Voriconazole has several important drug interactions [21]. For example it causes increased serum levels of co-administered ciclosporin or tacrolimus, but its levels are reduced if co-administered with rifampicin or phenytoin. Adverse interactions are likely when voriconazole is given with other drugs that are metabolized by the cytochrome P-450 enzyme system and the manufacturer's information sheet should be referred to prior to starting therapy.

There is extensive experience with voriconazole in clinical trials, including patients with invasive pulmonary aspergillosis, candidemia, rare mould and resistant yeast infections, and also as empirical therapy in febrile neutropenic patients. Its efficacy in treating invasive aspergillosis has been investigated in two studies. Denning et al. [23] treated 50 patients with voriconazole and compared them with 92 historical controls. Of those receiving voriconazole, 52% had a satisfactory response compared with 25% of controls. Voriconazole was better for treatment of pulmonary and disseminated disease than for disease of the central nervous system and other sites.

In a prospective randomized study voriconazole was compared with amphotericin B for primary treatment of invasive aspergillosis [22] followed by another licensed therapy if needed. In total 277 patients with probable or definite invasive aspergillosis were evaluated for a satisfactory response at week 12. There was a successful outcome in 52.8% in the voriconazole group compared with 31.6% in the amphotericin B group, i.e., a difference of 21.2% (95% confidence interval 10.4–32.9). Survival at 12 weeks was significantly better for those who received voriconazole (70.8% versus 57.9%, $P=0.02$). There were significantly fewer side effects with voriconazole.

In a multicenter randomized trial voriconazole was compared with liposomal amphotericin B as empirical therapy in 837 febrile neutropenic patients [24]. The overall responses were 26% and 30.6%, respectively, and although voriconazole failed a non-inferiority statistical evaluation it produced fewer breakthrough fungal infections (8 versus 21, $P=0.02$) had fewer infusion-related side effects and caused less renal toxicity.

In a double-blind randomized controlled trial [25] for treatment of esophageal candidiasis in 391 patients, most of whom had AIDS, oral voriconazole produced a similar overall response rate compared with oral fluconazole, with a slightly increased frequency of side effects, necessitating discontinuation of therapy.

Posaconazole

Posaconazole is an orally active triazole [26] with a broad spectrum of activity against yeasts and moulds, notably against *Rhizopus* [27]. It is only available orally, and bioavailability is variable although kinetics show linear absorption up to 800 mg. It is relatively well tolerated, without the visual disturbances reported with voriconazole. Phase 2 and 3 studies are in progress for therapy of invasive mycoses and for antifungal prophylaxis in high-risk hematological patients. An open non-comparative trial of 800 mg/day posaconazole to treat invasive fungal infections refractory to or intolerant of standard therapy showed complete or partial response at 1 month of 80% in candidiasis (n=10), 50% in aspergillosis (n=22), 80% in fusariosis (n=5), 58% in cryptococcosis (n=12), and 74% in other fungal infections (n=19) [28]. In this study the rate of adverse events was reported as 6%–12% (RY Hachem, personal communication).

Ravuconazole

Ravuconazole has a broad spectrum of activity, including *Candida* spp., *Aspergillus* spp., and other moulds. In an animal model of invasive aspergillosis it showed excellent activity [29]. The oral formulation has good bioavailability and has a very long half-life of 5-8 days. The further clinical development of this antifungal is unclear.

Flucytosine

Mechanism of action. Flucytosine is a fluorinated pyrimidine. It is converted by a fungal enzyme cytosine deaminase to 5-fluorouracil, which then inhibits the synthesis of RNA and DNA.

Spectrum of activity. The spectrum of activity of flucytosine is rather narrow and clinical use is largely restricted to the treatment of infections due to *Candida* spp. and *C. neoformans*. Drug resistance is likely to emerge if flucytosine is used as monotherapy so it is generally combined with other antifungal agents, such as amphotericin B. These two drugs demonstrate synergy in vitro and in vivo. Its main indications are for the treatment of severe life-threatening systemic infections, including cryptococcal meningitis, *Candida* meningitis, and endophthalmitis, and refractory candidemias [30].

Pharmacological properties. The oral formulation of flucytosine is not readily available in all countries, although it is well absorbed when given by this route. It can also be given intravenously, and the usual dose is 100 mg/kg/day, in divided doses. In patients with normal renal function the half-life is about 3 h. Protein binding is low (4%) so flucytosine penetrates organs, body fluids, and CSF extremely well. Doses should be modified in renal impairment as the drug is excreted by the kidney. In addition to monitoring renal function, serum drug concentrations of flucytosine and full blood counts should be monitored because flucytosine can cause myelosuppression and hepatotoxicity.

Echinocandins and Pneumocandins

The echinocandins and pneumocandins represent a new class of antifungals [31], which includes caspofungin, micafungin, and anidulafungin. They are cyclic hexapeptides, and have a novel mechanism of action. As a class they have good activity against *Candida* and *Aspergillus* spp., but they appear not to be active against *C. neoformans*, *Trichosporon*, *Fusarium*, or *Rhizopus*. There is currently no oral formulation so administration is by intravenous infusion.

Mechanism of action. The echinocandins and pneumocandins have a novel selective inhibitory effect on the fungal cell wall through inhibition of β 1, 3-D-glucan synthesis. This selective toxicity results in a favorable safety profile. There is also the added benefit of there being no cross-resistance with either the polyenes or azoles, which act on fungal cell membranes.

Caspofungin (Cancidas)

Caspofungin (Cancidas) is the first member of this group to be licensed for clinical use [32] for the treatment of patients with invasive *Aspergillus* infections refractory to other therapy. It is also effective in treatment of invasive candidiasis.

Spectrum of activity. Caspofungin is active against *Candida* and *Aspergillus spp.* [33], and is also active in vitro against dimorphic fungal pathogens and *Pneumocystis jiroveci*. However, it is not active against *C. neoformans* or some of the emerging moulds, notably *Fusarium* spp., and the zygomycetes. It is rapidly fungicidal for yeasts, but the activity against moulds is more complex.

Pharmacological properties. Caspofungin is only available as an intravenous formulation [34]. It has a convenient once-daily dosing regimen, and is usually given as an initial loading dose of 70 mg, then 50 mg once a day. The dose should be adjusted for patients with moderate hepatic insufficiency. No dose reduction is required in renal impairment and caspofungin is not removed by hemodialysis. The drug is relatively well tolerated, with only minimal renal toxicity. It is highly protein bound. Early studies indicated a clinically significant interaction between caspofungin and ciclosporin causing increased serum levels of caspofungin when the two drugs were co-administered. Elevation of liver enzymes has also been documented, such that when the two drugs are prescribed together, ciclosporin serum levels and hepatic function should be closely monitored. Co-administration with rifampicin may reduce caspofungin levels. Tacrolimus serum levels may also be reduced by caspofungin.

Clinical experience. Caspofungin has been evaluated in clinical trials for the treatment of oropharyngeal and esophageal candidiasis [35], invasive candidiasis [36], and aspergillosis [37], and also for empirical therapy of febrile neutropenia [38]. It was initially licensed for aspergillosis following the outcome of therapy in a series of adults with suspected or proven invasive aspergillosis who were all refractory to or intolerant of other antifungals. Most were being treated for hematological malignancy or were solid organ transplant recipients. There was a favorable response in 45% of recipients, which increased to 56% in patients who received more than 7 days of treatment. The response rates were poorer in allogeneic stem cell transplant recipients, in those with prolonged neutropenia, or patients with disseminated infection. In a randomized comparison with amphotericin B for treatment of invasive candidiasis involving 239 patients, caspofungin was as effective in producing a favorable response (71.7% versus 62.8%, 95% confidence interval -4.5 to 24.5) [36]. Most of the study patients were non-neutropenic, but had other underlying risk factors for candidiasis, and had documented candidemia. Caspofungin had significantly fewer drug-associated side effects than amphotericin B; 64% of the documented instances of candidemia in the caspofungin arm were due to species other than *C. albicans* and there was no difference in response rates relating to individual species. The conclusion from this study is that caspofungin is as effective as amphotericin B for treating invasive candidiasis but with far fewer and less significant side effects.

Micafungin

Micafungin was synthesized by chemical modification of an environmental mould *Coleophoma empedri*. It has been shown to have good activity against *Candida* and *Aspergillus* spp. in both in vitro [39] and animal models. Clinical experience has been limited to date.

Anidulafungin

Anidulafungin is also a semi-synthetic cyclic lipopeptide. It is not metabolized in the body but slowly chemically degraded and excreted into the intestine in an inactive form. No dose adjustment is required in either hepatic or renal failure. There are no serious known drug interactions to date. Overall it has a good safety profile. With similarly good activity against *Candida* and *Aspergillus* this drug is being developed for clinical use in esophageal candidiasis, candidemia, and invasive aspergillosis.

In a three-arm dose ranging study of the treatment of candidemia, 120 adults were randomized to one of three dosing regimens between 50 and 100 mg/day of anidulafungin [40]. Efficacy was evaluated at the end of therapy and at 2 weeks of follow-up. The mean APACHE II score ranged from13.7 to 15.3. Bloodstream isolates were identified as *C. albicans* in 52% and *C. glabrata* in

30% of cases. At the end of therapy a successful response was achieved in 82%–93% of patients; and at 2 weeks of follow-up the corresponding figures were 72%–86%. It was concluded that anidulafungin was effective across the dose range. It is now being evaluated in phase 3 trials.

Other Antifungal Drugs in Development

Development of a new antifungal agent might include the following requirements:
1. inhibition of fungal cell wall synthesis (and therefore fungicidal activity)
2. highly selective mode of action, and thus minimal adverse effects
3. high potency
4. convenient dosing and administration.

New formulations of current agents are continually being explored, for example the development of liposomal nystatin. In addition to new agents in pre-existing classes, the main advance is the discovery of new classes of antifungals with novel mechanisms of action [41]. The following new classes that act in different ways are therefore unlikely to show cross-resistance with pre-existing agents. This is a major advance, as one of the main challenges we currently face is the emergence of resistant isolates [42].

Pradimicins and benanomicins bind to cell wall mannoproteins, which results in osmotic lysis and leakage of the intracellular contents. They are therefore fungicidal. Nikkomycins are competitive inhibitors of the enzymes concerned with the synthesis of chitin. Sordarins target elongation factor 2 and cause inhibition of protein synthesis. They are active in vitro against *Candida*, filamentous fungi, and *Pneumocystis jiroveci*.

Further areas of research include laboratory methods of antifungal sensitivity testing and its correlation with in vivo activity, and work on the mechanisms of drug resistance [43]. The benefits of using antifungal combination therapy (such as the effects of blocking sequential steps in pathways) [44], and combination of antifungal agents with cytokines or antibodies [45], is also receiving much attention. Some antibacterial agents have been shown to have additive or synergistic activity with current antifungals, including rifampicin, fluoroquinolones, and azithromycin.

Clinical Uses of Systemic Antifungals

In recognition of the increased importance of invasive fungal infection in critical care patients there has been much interest in the use of antifungal agents for prophylaxis. This practice is well established, and of proven benefit, in severely immunocompromised neutropenic patients. However, the heterogeneity of most ICU patient populations has made evaluation of prophylaxis more challenging. In a review-based assessment of the findings of five studies in critically ill non-neutropenic patients [46] it was concluded that antifungal prophylaxis is only of value for selected patients. These include cases of liver transplantation or persistent intestinal perforation. This is also the conclusion of the Infectious Diseases Society of America practice guidelines on management of candidiasis [47]. Recent studies suggest that antifungal prophylaxis of very premature babies is efficacious [48] but again extension of this to all premature neonates is not recommended. Pre-emptive antifungal therapy is initiation of antifungals based on the patient having increased risk factors, either clinical or mycological, for invasive fungal infection. An example would be a patient with a fever and heavy *Candida* colonization at several body sites. Although it would appear this approach is being increasingly practised, it has not yet been validated in clinical trials and so cannot be recommended.

The most common use of systemic antifungal therapy is in a patient with documented fungemia or focal infection, e.g., peritonitis. Early randomized clinical trials comparing amphotericin B with fluconazole showed that either agent was equally effective in producing both clinical and mycological cure [47]. More recently Rex et al [46] evaluated these drugs as combination therapy compared with fluconazole alone but using a higher dose (800 mg/day) than in their earlier study [49]. While the combination reduced the duration of persistent candidemia there was no overall difference in mortality and the patients in the amphotericin B arm experienced more toxic side effects. It has been clearly shown that early exchange of central vascular catheters improves the response to antifungal therapy and this practice is strongly recommended [47]. Because of the increased incidence of *C. glabrata* infections, there are concerns about using fluconazole in cases of candidiasis where the species has yet to be identified. The trials that evaluated fluconazole therapy did not show that it was necessarily inferior to amphotericin B, but a consensus view is that the latter agent is preferred when this species has been identified as the pathogen. Caspofungin is an alternative treatment option for invasive candida infections and should soon be widely approved by regulatory authorities for this indication. It is more expensive than these other agents but this is the only obvious limiting factor to its more widespread use. Voriconazole has recently been compared with amphotericin B for this indication, but the results of the study are yet to be published.

Up to 10% of solid organ transplant recipients have an increased risk of developing either invasive candidiasis or aspergillosis, which is highest in heart or heart-lung transplant recipients and lowest in renal transplantation, but rates vary according to the transplant center. Various studies have been performed evaluating both the prophylactic and therapeutic use of antifungal agents [50].

In hematological malignancy patients, and especially allogeneic stem cell transplant recipients, the principal opportunistic mycosis is invasive aspergillosis. Antifungal prophylaxis is widely practised. Fluconazole has been shown to be effective for the prevention of both mucosal and invasive *Candida* infections in this setting [49]; however it has no useful clinical activity against *Aspergillus* spp. For this reason itraconazole is the preferred choice even though the protective efficacy of this azole has not always been clearly demonstrated. There are ongoing prospective studies evaluating voriconazole in this role for which it is currently not licensed in the United Kingdom.

For treatment of probable or proven invasive aspergillosis there are data that support the use of lipid amphotericin B formulations [13]. A recent prospective comparative trial showed voriconazole was superior to conventional amphotericin B and significantly reduced mortality at 12 weeks post start of therapy [22]. Either a lipid amphotericin or voriconazole would be acceptable therapy for aspergillosis. Voriconazole has an advantage in being also available as an oral formulation that can be used once patients are stable after a week or 10 days of intravenous therapy. Caspofungin has only been evaluated to date in an open non-comparative study, but looks to be a promising alternative to these other agents with a low incidence of side effects [37].

There is a less clear picture on which antifungal agents are the best choice for the so-called emerging mycoses, including invasive mould infections due to *Fusarium*, *Scedosporium* spp., and zygomycetes [11]; however, newer agents such as voriconazole appear to have a useful role in some of these relatively rare infections [51].

While combination therapy with amphotericin B and flucytosine may be indicated for the treatment of cryptococcosis or selected cases of invasive candidiasis, there are only limited clinical data to support combinations for other invasive mycoses either with established agents [44] or with the addition of one of the new antifungals [52]. These regimens are expensive, potentially more toxic, and so need to be tested in prospective trials.

References

1. Beck-Sague CM, Jarvis WR, and the National Nosocomial Infections Surveillance System (1993) Secular trends in the epidemiology of nosocomial fungal infections in the United States 1980-1990. J Infect Dis 167:1247-1251
2. Richards MJ, Edwards JR, Culver DH, Gaynes RP (1999) Nosocomial infections in medical intensive care units in the United States. National Nosocomial Infections Surveillance System. Crit Care Med 27:887-892

3. Trick WE, Fridkin SK, Edwards JR et al (2002) Secular trend of hospital-acquired candidemia among intensive care unit patients in the United States during 1989–1999. Clin Infect Dis 35:627–630

4. Pfaller MA, Diekema DJ (2002) Role of sentinel surveillance of candidemia: trends in species distribution and antifungal susceptibility. J Clin Microbiol 40:3551–3557

5. Edmond MB, Wallace SE, McClish DK et al (1999) Nosocomial bloodstream infections in United States hospitals: a three-year analysis. Clin Infect Dis 29:239–244

6. Blumberg HM, Jarvis WR, Soucie JM et al (2001) Risk factors for *Candida* bloodstream infections in surgical intensive care unit patients: the NEMIS prospective multicenter study. Clin Infect Dis 33:177–186

7. Saiman L, Ludington E, Pfaller M (2000) Risk factors for candidemia in neonatal intensive care unit patients. Pediatr Infect Dis J 19:319–324

8. Pfaller MA, Diekema DJ, Jones RN et al (2001) International surveillance of bloodstream infections due to *Candida* species: frequency of occurrence and in vitro susceptibilities to fluconazole, ravuconazole, and voriconazole of isolates collected from 1997 through 1999 in the SENTRY Antimicrobial Surveillance Program. J Clin Microbiol 39:3254–3259

9. Ellis D (2002) Amphotericin B: spectrum and resistance. J Antimicrob Chemother 49 [Suppl 1]:7–10

10. Dupont B (2002) Overview of the lipid formulations of amphotericin B. J Antimicrob Chemother 49 [Suppl 1]:31–36

11. Steinbach WJ, Perfect JR (2003) Newer antifungal therapy for emerging fungal pathogens. Int J Infect Dis 7:5–20

12. Eriiksson U, Seifert B, Schaffner A (2001) Comparison of effects of amphotericin B deoxycholate infused over 4 or 24 hours: randomised controlled trial. BMJ 322:579–582

13. Wingard JR (2002) Lipid formulations of amphotericins: are you a lumper or a splitter? Clin Infect Dis 35:891–895

14. Richardson MD, Warnock DW (2003) Fungal infection: diagnosis and management. Antifungal drugs. Blackwell, Massachusetts, pp 29–79

15. Rogers TR (2001) Optimal use of existing and new antifungal drugs. Curr Opin Crit Care 7:238–241

16. Boogaerts M, Winston DJ, Bow EJ et al (2001) Intravenous and oral itraconazole versus intravenous amphotericin B deoxycholate as empirical antifungal therapy for persistent fever in neutropenic patients with cancer who are receiving broad spectrum antibacterial therapy. Ann Intern Med 135:412–422

17. Slain D, Rogers DP, Cleary JD, Chapman SW (2001) Intravenous itraconazole. Ann Pharmacother 35:720–729

18. Winston DJ, Maziarz RT, Pranatharthi H et al (2003) Intravenous and oral itraconazole versus intravenous and oral fluconazole for long-term antifungal prophylaxis in allogeneic hematopoietic stem-cell transplant recipients. Ann Intern Med 138:705–713

19. Caillot D, Bassaris H, McGeer A (2001) Intravenous itraconazole by oral itraconazole in the treatment of invasive pulmonary aspergillosis in patients with hematologic malignancies, chronic granulomatous disease, or AIDS. Clin Infect Dis 33:e83–90

20 Johnson LB, Kaufmann CA (2003) Voriconazole: a new triazole antifungal agent. Clin Infect Dis 36:630–637

21. Gothard P, Rogers TR (2004). Voriconazole for serious fungal infections. Int J Clin Pract 54:74–80

22. Herbrecht R, Denning DW, Patterson TF et al (2002) Voriconazole versus amphotericin B for primary therapy of invasive aspergillosis. N Engl J Med 347:408–415

23. Denning DW, Ribaud P, Milpied N et al (2002) Efficacy and safety of voriconazole in the treatment of acute invasive aspergillosis. Clin Infect Dis 34:563–571
24. Walsh TJ, Pappas P, Winston DJ et al (2002) Voriconazole compared with liposomal amphotericin B for empirical antifungal therapy in patients with neutropenia and persistent fever. N Engl J Med 346:225–234
25. Ally R, Scharmann D, Kreisel W et al (2001) A randomized, double blind, double dummy, multicenter trial of voriconazole and fluconazole in the treatment of esophageal candidiasis in immunocompromised patients. Clin Infect Dis 33:1447–1454
26. Adis International Ltd (2003) Posaconazole:SCH56592. Drugs: 258–263
27. Pfaller MA, Messer SA, Hollis RJ et al (2002) Antifungal activities of posaconazole, ravuconazole, and voriconazole compared to those of itraconazole and amphotericin B against 239 clinical isolates of *Aspergillus* spp and other filamentous fungi: report from SENTRY Antimicrobial Surveillance Program, 2000. Antimicrob Agents Chemother 46:1032–1037
28. Hachem RY, Raad II, Afif CM et al (2000) An open, non-comparative multicenter study to evaluate efficacy and safety of posaconazole (SCH 56592) in the treatment of invasive fungal infections (IFI) refractory(R) to or intolerant(I) to standard therapy(ST). Abstracts of the 40th Interscience Conference on Antimicrobial Agents and Chemotherapy, p 372, abs no. 1109
29. Kirkpatrick WR, Perea S, Coco BJ, Patterson TF (2002) Efficacy of ravuconazole (BMS-207147) in a guinea pig model of disseminated aspergillosis. J Antimicrob Chemother 49:353–357
30. Francis P, Walsh TJ (1992) Evolving role of flucytosine in immunocompromised patients: new insights into safety, pharmacokinetics, and antifungal therapy. Clin Infect Dis 15:1003–1018
31. Denning DW (2002) Echinocandins: a new class of antifungal. J Antimicrob Chemother 49:889–893
32. Anonymous (2004) Caspofungin and voriconazole for fungal infections. Drugs Ther Bull 42:5–8
33. Deresinski SC, Stevens DA (2003) Caspofungin. Clin Infect Dis 36:1445–1457
34. Keating GM, Jarvis B (2001) Caspofungin. Drugs 61:1121–1129
35. Villanueva A, Arathoon EG, Gotuzzo E et al (2001) A randomized double-blind study of caspofungin versus amphotericin for the treatment of candidal esophagitis. Clin Infect Dis 33:1529–1535
36. Mora-Duarte J, Betts R, Rotstein C et al (2002) Comparison of caspofungin and amphotericin B for invasive candidiasis. N Engl J Med 347:2020–2029
37. Maertens et al (2002) Update of the multicenter, noncomparative study of caspofungin in adults with invasive aspergillosis refractory or intolerant to other antifungal agents: an analysis of 90 patients. Proceedings of the Interscience Conference on Antimicrobial Agents and Chemotherapy California September 27-30.
38. Walsh TJ, Teppler H, Donowitz GR et al (2004) Caspofungin versus liposomal amphotericin B for empirical antifungal therapy in patients with persistent fever and neutropenia. N Engl J Med 351:1391-1402
39. Ostrosky-Zeichner L, Rex JH, Pappas PG et al (2003) Antifungal susceptibility survey of 2,000 bloodstream *Candida* isolates in the United States. Antimicrob Agents Chemother 47:3149–3154
40. Krause DS, Reinhardt J, Vazquez JA et al (2004) Phase 2, randomised, dose-ranging study evaluating the safety and efficacy of anidulafungin in invasive candidiasis and candidemia. Antimicrob Agents Chemother 48:2021–2024
41. Odds FC, Brown AJ, Gow NA (2003) Antifungal agents: mechanisms of action. Trends

Microbiol 11:272–279

42. Rogers TR (2002) Antifungal drug resistance: does it matter? Int J Infect Dis 6 [Suppl 1]:S47–S53

43. Ghannoum MA, Rice LB (1999) Antifungal agents: mode of action, mechanisms of resistance, and correlation of these mechanisms with bacterial resistance. Clin Microbiol Rev 12:501–517

44. Kontoyiannis DP, Lewis RE (2004) Toward more effective antifungal therapy: the prospects of combination therapy. Br J Haematol 126:165–175

45. Matthews RC, Burnie JP (2004) Recombinant antibodies: a natural partner in combinatorial antifungal therapy. Vaccine 22:865–871

46. Rex JH, Sobel JD (2001) Prophylactic antifungal therapy in the intensive care unit. Clin Infect Dis 32:1191–1200

47. Rex JH, Walsh TJ, Sobel JD et al (2000) Practice guidelines for the treatment of candidiasis. Clin Infect Dis 30:662–678

48. Neely MN, Schreiber JR (2001) Fluconazole prophylaxis in the very low birth weight infant: not ready for prime time. Pediatrics 107:404–405

49. Rex JH, Pappas PG, Karchmen AW et al (2003) A randomized and blinded multicenter trial of high-dose fluconazole plus placebo versus fluconazole plus amphotericin B as therapy for candidemia and its consequences in non-neutropenic subjects. Clin Infect Dis 36:1221-1228

50. Gottfredsson M, Perfect JR (1999) Use of antifungal agents in the intensive care unit. Curr Opin Crit Care 5:381–390

51. Perfect JR, Marr KA, Walsh TJ et al (2003) Voriconazole treatment for less-common, emerging, or refractory fungal infections. Clin Infect Dis 36:1122–1131

52. Steinbach WJ, Stevens DA (2003) Review of newer antifungal and immunomodulatory strategies for invasive aspergillosis. Clin Infect Dis 37 [Suppl 3]:S157–S187

Chapter 9

Enteral Antimicrobials

M. Sanchez, B.P. Pizer, S.R. Alcock

Introduction

Individuals who are in reasonably good health may carry one or more of the six "normal" potentially pathogenic micro-organisms (PPM). They are *Streptococcus pneumoniae, Haemophilus influenzae, Moraxella catarrhalis, Escherichia coli, Staphylococcus aureus*, and *Candida albicans*. Carriage of the "opportunistic" or "abnormal" aerobic Gram-negative bacilli (AGNB), including *Klebsiella, Enterobacter, Proteus, Morganella, Citrobacter, Serratia, Acinetobacter*, and *Pseudomonas* species, and of methicillin-resistant *Staphylococcus aureus* (MRSA) in the oropharynx and gastrointestinal tract of healthy individuals is uncommon (Chapter 2). These nine "abnormal" bacteria are carried by patients with an underlying condition, either chronic or acute. Severity of illness is the most important factor in the conversion of the "normal" into the "abnormal" carrier state. Carriage of "abnormal" flora invariably leads to high concentrations, i.e., overgrowth of "abnormal" bacteria in the throat and gut of the critically ill [1]. Overgrowth is defined as $\geq 10^5$ of abnormal flora per milliliter of saliva and/or gram of feces [2]. Intestinal overgrowth with AGNB causes systemic immunosuppression [3]. Alimentary canal overgrowth has been shown to be an independent risk factor for endogenous infection, endotoxemia, emergence of resistance, transmission via hands of carers, and outbreaks (Chapter 2).

Eradication and Control of Carriage and Overgrowth of Abnormal Flora

The aim of enteral antimicrobials is the prevention and, if already present, the eradication of carriage and overgrowth of abnormal bacteria, including AGNB and

MRSA. Critically ill patients are unable to clear these "opportunistic" PPM due to their underlying disease (Chapter 2). Only the recovery from their underlying condition guarantees the return to the normal carrier state [4]. During the period of critical illness, antimicrobials are required to assist the intensive care unit (ICU) patient in the battle against gut overgrowth of abnormal flora.

Parenteral Antimicrobials

The most commonly used parenteral antimicrobials have been shown to clear the three oropharyngeal micro-organisms *S. pneumoniae*, *H. influenzae*, and *M. catarrhalis*. For example, cefotaxime is excreted into saliva in concentrations high enough to eradicate oropharyngeal carriage of these three "community" respiratory PPM [5]. The failure rate in clearing *E. coli* from the gut is substantially due to the non-lethal fecal concentrations following excretion via bile and mucus [5, 6]. Eradication of yeast carriage is almost impossible using systemic anti-fungals. A recent randomized controlled trial (RCT) evaluated the impact of fluconazole on throat and gut carriage of yeasts and reported that there was no significant difference between the group of critically ill patients who received fluconazole and the control group [7]. In the United Kingdom flucloxacillin is widely regarded as the anti-staphylococcal agent of choice, although there are no accurate data on the clearance of methicillin-sensitive *S. aureus* (MSSA) [8]. Effective eradication of MSSA from throat and gut has, however, been reported for cephradine [9].

Two grams of vancomycin produces vancomycin concentrations of between 6 and 11 µg/g of feces following intravenous administration, but enteral administration results in fecal levels between 3,000 and 24,000 µg/g of feces [10, 11]. These pharmacokinetic data may explain why systemic vancomycin has never been shown to clear MRSA. The same concept that salivary, fecal, and mucus concentrations are in general non-lethal for the AGNB carried in throat and gut applies to the commonly used systemic antimicrobials, including β-lactams, aminoglycosides, and fluoroquinolones [12–14]. Even the newer and more-potent carbapenems, and the combination of β-lactams and β-lactamase inhibitors, fail to clear AGNB, including *Pseudomonas* and *Acinetobacter* species [15, 16]. This highlights the importance of measuring drug levels at all relevant sites, in addition to blood levels.

Enteral Antimicrobials

The administration of enteral non-absorbable antimicrobials is based on the experience that critically ill patients given only parenteral antibiotics have harmful gut overgrowth with abnormal flora [17]. Selective decontamination of the digestive tract (SDD) is a maneuver designed to convert the "abnormal" carrier state into the "normal" carrier state. The purpose of SDD is to prevent or eradicate, if initially present, carriage and overgrowth of abnormal AGNB and MRSA. In addition, SDD also intends to eradicate MSSA and yeasts that are carried by varying percentages of healthy people. The overall aim of SDD using enteral antimicrobials is a reduction in mortality and morbidity following the recovery of the systemic immunity [18] and control of endogenous infection, a reduction in endotoxemia, and control of resistance and outbreaks. A combination of non-absorbable antimicrobials is given enterally to selectively decontaminate the digestive tract, i.e., to eradicate overgrowth of abnormal flora, leaving the indigenous flora, which are thought to play a role in the defence against carriage of abnormal bacteria, predominantly undisturbed. [19]. There are four criteria that antimicrobials should fulfil to qualify for the selective elimination of abnormal flora. (1) The antimicrobials should have a *narrow spectrum*. The antimicrobial spectrum should cover AGNB, MRSA, MSSA, and yeasts. The spectrum should not include the indigenous mostly anaerobic flora, in order that decontamination of abnormal flora is as selective as possible [20]. (2) They should be *non-absorbable* to achieve constant high intra-luminal antibiotic levels, which are lowered by absorption [21]. (3) They should show *minimal inactivation* by salivary, fecal, and food compounds, and no degradation by fecal enzymes produced by the indigenous anaerobic flora [22]. The interactions between feces, bacteria, and decontaminating antimicrobials determining the microbiologically active fecal concentrations are of great importance in the ultimate outcome of SDD. (4) The antimicrobials should be *bactericidal*. They should have low minimal bactericidal concentrations (MBC) for AGNB, MRSA, MSSA, and yeasts because there are no leukocytes in the human alimentary canal to assist decontaminating antimicrobials [23].

The most commonly used protocol is a combination of polymyxin and tobramycin to clear AGNB and MSSA, amphotericin or nystatin to eradicate yeasts, and enteral vancomycin in the case of MRSA [24].

Polymyxins are non-absorbable and cover AGNB, including *P. aeruginosa* and *Acinetobacter* species. However, polymyxins are not active against *Proteus*, *Morganella*, and *Serratia* species. Polymyxins are selective in that they are not active against the indigenous mainly anaerobic flora [25]. The mode of action is disruption of the bacterial cell wall, making the bacterial cell permeable and leading to cell death. This mechanism is independent of enzymatic systems [26]. Acquired resistance against polymyxins is extremely uncommon. Polymyxins are inactivated to a moderate extent by proteins, fiber, food, cell debris, and salivary and fecal compounds, and should therefore be given at a relatively high daily dose of 400 mg of polymyxin E (300 mg of polymyxin B) [25]. Polymyxins should be combined with an aminoglycoside due to the gap in activity against *Proteus*, *Morganella*, and *Serratia* species. The aminoglycoside should be active against *P. aeruginosa* because the polymyxins lose activity against this common ICU bacterium in the presence of feces. Polymyxins neutralize endotoxin [27].

Aminoglycosides have several attractive features for enteral use. They are active against a wide range of AGNB including *P. aeruginosa*, have a potent bactericidal activity similar to polymyxins, and there is also synergistic activity with polymyxins. Anti-pseudomonal aminoglycosides include gentamicin, tobramycin, and amikacin. They are non-absorbable and bactericidal by inhibiting protein synthesis. Tobramycin is the least inactivated by feces, followed by amikacin and gentamicin [28–30]. Tobramycin is considered to be selective in terms of leaving the indigenous flora undisturbed at doses lower than 500 mg/day [31]. Blood levels of tobramycin and gentamicin have been monitored during SDD [32–34]. Aminoglycoside levels were undetectable in most of the patients. Low concentrations of less than 1 mg/l were measured in ICU patients, particularly with renal impairment. Although the three anti-pseudomonal aminoglycosides and the polymyxins have a similar bactericidal activity, the total daily dose recommended for tobramycin is 320 mg, lower than the 400 mg for the polymyxins, which are inactivated to a moderate extent by fecal material. Aminoglycosides require the addition of polymyxins as the emergence of aminoglycoside neutralizing enzymes is not uncommon [35]. Polymyxins are thought to protect tobramycin from being inactivated by fecal enzymes. Tobramycin reduces endotoxin release [36].

Polyenes. The two polyenes used as decontaminating agents are amphotericin B and nystatin. They are bactericidal and highly selective, as fungi are the only PPM covered by polyenes. They bind to a sterol of the plasma membrane, alter the membrane permeability of the fungal cell leading to the leakage of essential metabolites, and finally fungal cell lysis occurs. Absorption of polyenes is minimal [33, 34] and emergence of resistance amongst yeasts and fungi against polyenes is very uncommon [37]. Fecal inactivation of polyenes is high, explaining the high daily dose of 2 g of amphotericin B and of 8×10^6 U of nystatin required for decontamination purposes [38, 39] (Table 1).

Glycopeptides. Of the two glycopeptides vancomycin and teicoplanin, most experience as decontaminating agent has been gathered for enteral vancomycin [10, 11]. Vancomycin is active against MRSA, but cannot be considered as a "selective" decontaminating agent as it covers the vast majority of the anaerobic *Clostridium* species. Thus, SDD protocols do not routinely include enteral vancomycin because of its negative impact on the gut ecology. Enteral vancomycin is only recommended for eradication of MRSA carriage and overgrowth, and should always be given in combination with polymyxin/

Table 1. Enteral antimicrobials for eradication of carriage of potential pathogens (*AGNB* aerobic Gram-negative bacilli, yeasts, *MRSA* methicillin-resistant *Staphylococcus aureus*)

Selective digestive decontamination		Total daily dose (4 daily)		
Target micro-organisms		<5 years	5–12 years	>12 years
Oropharynx				
AGNB	Polymyxin E with tobramycin	2 g of 2% paste or gel		
Yeasts	Amphotericin B or nystatin	2 g of 2% paste or gel		
MRSA	Vancomycin	2 g of 4% paste or gel		
Gut				
AGNB	Polymyxin E (mg)	100	200	400
	with tobramycin (mg)	80	160	320
Yeasts	Amphotericin B (mg)	500	1,000	2,000
	or nystatin (units)	2×10^6	4×10^6	8×10^6
MRSA	Vancomycin (mg)	20–40/kg	20–40/kg	500-2,000

tobramycin/amphotericin B (PTA) to offset the potential for AGNB and yeast overgrowth as a consequence of the use of a non-selective decontaminating agent [40]. The mode of action is bactericidal, as vancomycin is bound rapidly and irreversibly to the cell walls of sensitive bacteria, thereby inhibiting cell wall synthesis. Vancomycin absorption is rare [34]. Inactivation by proteins, fiber, food, and feces is substantial, hence the high daily dose of 2 g (Table 1).

Efficacy of Enteral Polymyxin/Tobramycin, Polyenes, and Vancomycin in the Eradication of Carriage and Over-growth of AGNB, Yeasts, and MRSA

Fifty-four RCTs evaluating SDD have been conducted in a total of 8,715 patients between 1987 and 2004 (Chapter 14). Polymyxin/tobramycin and polymyxin/gentamicin was used in 32 and 14 RCTs, respectively. A total of 38 RCTs show a significant reduction in infection, and 4 individual trials demonstrated a reduction in mortality. There are nine meta-analyses of RCTs on SDD and all invariably show a significant reduction in infection, five meta-analyses report a reduction in mortality.

Surveillance cultures of throat and rectum are an integral part of enteral antimicrobial protocols [19]. Monitoring the carrier state in the critically ill receiving enteral antimicrobials is essential, as only surveillance cultures allow monitoring of the compliance and efficacy of enteral antimicrobials. SDD is considered to be effective only if surveillance samples show the eradication of AGNB, MRSA, MSSA, and yeasts. Surveillance samples were taken in 47 of the 54 RCTs (87%). Throat and/or rectal swabs were evaluated in 83% of the trials, whilst gastric fluid was cultured in 46% of the SDD trials.

Aerobic Gram-Negative Bacilli

Most RCTs report an effective clearance of AGNB carriage following the administration of polymyxin/tobramycin. Abnormal carriage in the throat is eradicated within 3 days, whilst it takes 7 days for abnormal rectal carriage to be eradicated, depending on the return of peristalsis. A meta-analysis of the effect of SDD on AGNB carriage is underway (A. Aranguren, personal communication).

Yeasts

Data on yeast carriage were available in 27 RCTs. The enteral polyenes significantly reduced the odds ratio for carriage to 0.31 (0.18–0.54) [41].

Methicillin-Resistant *S. aureus*

Six RCTs included enteral vancomycin, but none of them analyzed the impact of enteral vancomycin on MRSA carriage and infections [34, 42–46]. A recent RCT evaluated the effect of a 4% vancomycin gel applied to the lower cheeks on oropharyngeal carriage of MRSA [47]. The oral vancomycin significantly reduced the odds ratio for oropharyngeal carriage to 0.25 (0.09–0.69).

Seven studies report fecal levels of one or more of the decontaminating agents polymyxin, tobramycin, gentamicin, amphotericin B, nystatin, and vancomycin [11, 31, 38, 39, 48–50]. Compared to polymyxin, tobramycin is less inactivated by fecal material. In one study fecal specimens contained tobramycin levels of at least 100 µg/g of feces following the daily intake of 300 mg of tobramycin [31]. In another study, individuals taking 600 mg of tobramycin daily showed >500 µg/g of fecal sample [48]. Polymyxin is moderately inactivated by mucosal cells, fiber, and feces, and hence the variation in fecal drug levels. Polymyxin was not detected in one-third of individuals who took 600 mg of polymyxin daily [49]. One-third had fecal levels exceeding 1,000 µg/g of feces, whereas the remaining individuals showed polymyxin levels of between 16 and 1,000 µg/g of feces. Tobramycin at a daily dose of 320 mg, added to 400 mg of polymyxin, is the most commonly used combination for the eradication of AGNB carriage and overgrowth, due to synergism and relatively less fecal inactivation [51]. The inactivation of vancomycin by fecal material is high. In one study, oral vancomycin was given at doses of 2 g daily for 7 days and the mean concentration of vancomycin in 25 stools obtained during treatment was 3,100±400 µg/g, with a range of 905–8,760 µg/g [17]. Fecal concentrations of the decontaminating agents polymyxin E and gentamicin were measured in 38 stool samples obtained from 15 patients [50]. The levels of both decontaminating antimicrobials were less than 20 µg/ml of feces in 10 stools. The remaining 28 samples showed fecal polymyxin E levels of 94±174 µg/ml (median 42 µg/ml, range 0–1,055 µg/ml) and gentamicin levels of 466±545 µg/ml (median 196 µg/ml, range 0–2,098 µg/ml). The inactivation of polyenes, including amphotericin B and nystatin, by fecal material, is high. Daily doses of 2,000 mg of amphotericin B or 8×10^6 U of nystatin were associated with fecal levels of 60 µg/g and 20 µg/g of feces, respectively [38, 39].

Most parenterally administered antimicrobials do not act upon gut flora. However, fluoroquinolones, including ciprofloxacin, have been shown to possess the pharmacokinetic characteristic of trans-intestinal secretion [52]. A substantial amount of intravenously administered ciprofloxacin is excreted via mucus rather than via bile (15% vs. 1%) leading to high fecal ciprofloxacin concentrations. The mean fecal level of ciprofloxacin was 108.7 µg/g of feces following the parenteral administration of a daily dose of 400 mg of ciprofloxacin [52]. The antifungal 5-flucytosine is a small molecule that also possess the pharmacokinetic property of trans-intestinal secretion, i.e., 10% of systematically administered 5-flucytosine is excreted via mucus into the gut [53]. The good penetration of flucytosine into most body tissues and fluids has been ascribed to its high water solubility, low molecular weight, and low protein binding. This feature of ciprofloxacin and 5-flucytosine can be useful in critically ill patients in whom rectal swabs remain positive for AGNB and yeasts following 1 week of polymyxin/tobramycin/amphotericin B. This failure of the classical PTA protocol may be due to AGNB and yeasts already translocated into the gut-associated lymphoid tissue on admission, and hence escaping the intra-luminal lethal activity of the non-absorbable PTA. Three days of high doses of intravenous ciprofloxacin or 5 flucytosine has been shown to assist effective SDD as measured by surveillance samples negative for AGNB and yeasts in patients with inflamed gut.

Apart from monitoring efficacy and compliance of enteral antimicrobials surveillance samples, in particular rectal swabs, provide the unique method of detecting antimicrobial resistance at an early stage, allowing prompt adjustment. In three RCTs [44, 54, 55] throat and rectal swabs were also cultured on agar plates containing 2 mg/l of polymyxin, 4 mg/l of tobramycin, and 6 mg/l of vancomycin. For example, *Proteus* and *Serratia* species intrinsically resistant to polymyxin may become resistant to tobramycin. There are reports that describe the enteral use of amikacin [56] and paramomycin [21] replacing tobramycin to establish eradication of tobramycin-resistant *Proteus* and *Serratia*, respectively.

Impact of Eradication of Abnormal Flora Using Enteral Antimicrobials on Clinical and Epidemiological Endpoints

Infectious Morbidity and Attributable Mortality

Infection control policies that include SDD have four fundamental features [19]. (1) The enteral antimicrobials aim to decontaminate the gastrointestinal tract; the enteral antimicrobials are combined with an oropharyngeal decontamination using a paste or gel containing 2% PTA. The aim of the oropharyngeal and intestinal non-absorbable antimicrobials is the prevention of secondary endogenous infections. (2) Parenteral antibiotics are given immediately on admission to control primary endogenous infections. (3) Hygiene is implemented to control exogenous infections. (4) Surveillance samples are collected to monitor the SDD protocol. The most complete meta-analysis demonstrated that enteral polymyxin with tobramycin or gentamicin significantly reduce AGNB infections [57]. Of the 54 RCTs, 42 evaluated the efficacy of the antifungal polyenes as part of SDD on yeast infections [41]. Enteral polyenes significantly reduced both patients with yeast infections and episodes of yeast infections. Lower airway infections due to MRSA were significantly reduced in the RCT using 4% vancomycin gel [47]. The most compelling evidence that infection is responsible for increased mortality derives from RCTs of SDD. Of the 54 RCTs, 2 trials of large sample size [14, 44] documented a significant absolute reduction of mortality of 8% in patients receiving the prophylactic regimen, combined with a significantly reduced relative risk for developing pneumonia of 0.20 (0.07–0.58) and bloodstream infections of 0.38 (0.17–0.83). While it is possible that these clinical benefits of SDD arise from reasons other than the prevention of both "early" primary endogenous and "late" secondary endogenous infections, e.g., reduced absorption of gut endotoxin, the most plausible interpretation of these recent data is that infection is responsible for a relative increase in risk of ICU mortality of 20%–40%. The most recent trial found a lower mortality risk in both medical and surgical patients and in all severity groups [14].

Endotoxemia

AGNB present in overgrowth in the gut are the major source of endotoxin in the human body. Up to 10 mg of fecal endotoxin per gram of feces has been measured in critically ill patients with gut overgrowth of AGNB [58]. For example, gut ischemia at the time of cardiac surgery and liver transplantation promotes transmural migration or translocation of AGNB present in concentrations of $\geq 10^5$ AGNB per gram of feces [59]. Most translocating AGNB are killed by the macrophages of the gut-associated lymphoid tissue, including the liver, with the aim of maintaining sterility of the bloodstream. However, the subsequent release of endotoxin may spill over into the bloodstream and lead to fluctuating levels of endotoxin in blood, i.e., endotoxemia [60]. The enteral combination of polymyxin/tobramycin has been shown to significantly reduce the fecal endotoxin load by a factor of 10^4 [61]. There are five RCTs evaluating the impact of SDD on endotoxemia, three during cardiopulmonary bypass [62–64] and two in liver transplant patients [65, 66]. Two trials report a significant reduction following SDD [62, 63], three trials failed to show a difference [64–66]. The cardiac patients received enteral polymyxin/tobramycin 3 days pre-operatively in the two positive studies. In the negative cardiac study, tobramycin was replaced by neomycin, a poor anti-endotoxin agent [67, 68]. In the two liver transplant studies, polymyxin/tobramycin was started 12 h pre-operatively and post-operatively only [69].

Antimicrobial Resistance

Perhaps the most intriguing aspect of the 17 years of clinical research into SDD is the experience that the addition of enteral antibiotics to parenteral antimicrobials may prolong the effectiveness of the antimicrobial agents [17]. The most rigorous and extensive meta-analyses demonstrate the virtual absence of any reported resistance, with all assessed RCTs being free of this problem and of subsequent super-infections and/or epidemics of multiresistant strains [56, 57]. This accords with data from four SDD studies in which the endpoint of resistance was evaluated over periods of 2, 2.5, 6, and 7 years [56, 70–72]. While two studies evaluating the emergence of resistant micro-organisms following the discontinuation of SDD failed to show any negative effect [72, 73]. The two recent trials with a significant reduction of mortality confirmed the absence of resistance [14, 44]. Indeed, the latest trial comparing patients on an SDD unit with patients receiving the parenteral antibiotic-only approach on a different ICU had significantly fewer carriers of multiresistant AGNB and *P. aeruginosa* in the SDD unit than on the control unit [14]. The extensive use of only parenteral antimicrobials had invariably led to antimicrobial resistance. Mechanisms contributing to an increase in the number of patients who carry resistant micro-organisms include (1) introduction of patients already carriers of resistant micro-organisms on admission to the unit; (2) selection and induction or mutation of resistant micro-organisms following antibiotic pressure; and (3) transmission of resistant micro-organisms whilst on the unit. Effective control of carriage/overgrowth using enteral antimicrobials guarantees control of import of resistance, control of induction or mutation at gut level, and significantly reduced transmission following the reduced number of carriers combined with a lower level of carriage of resistant micro-organisms (Chapter 13). MRSA, by design, is not covered by the SDD antimicrobials. Inevitably, SDD exerts selective pressure on this PPM, and hence six RCTs conducted in ICUs where MRSA was endemic at the time of the study showed a trend towards higher MRSA infection rates in patients receiving SDD [74–79]. Proponents of SDD have always accepted this possibility and proposed a strategy consisting of surveillance cultures to detect MRSA overgrowth in carriers combined with enteral vancomycin to control MRSA overgrowth [80, 81]. When there is a serious clinical MRSA problem occurring at least once a week, this approach can be used as a prophylactic policy in all high-risk groups. These patients should receive PTA combined with enteral vancomycin on admission after taking throat and rectal swabs throughout treatment on the ICU. With a less frequent incidence of less than one event per week, SDD that includes enteral vancomycin can be commenced as treatment after the swabs have been shown to be positive [82].

Transmission of Abnormal Flora via Hands of Carers

The high density of *S. aureus*, both methicillin sensitive and resistant, in the oropharynx and gut promotes skin carriage, hand and environmental contamination. Quantitative studies from the early 1950s demonstrated that overgrowth of *S. aureus* in the nasal cavity leads to skin carriage of *S. aureus* in 44% of individuals, but only in 16% if the level of contamination of nasal secretions was less than 10^5 *S. aureus* [83]. Airborne dissemination was also a function of the number of micro-organisms present in the nose. However, similar research from the late 1950s demonstrated that the "weight" of micro-organisms released to the environment by fecal carrier greatly exceeded that of the organisms released by nasal carrier [84, 85]. Twenty years later, the importance of fecal carriage of MRSA in children was shown from the air contamination studies during nappy changing when patients who were fecal carriers yielded the same type from the air [86]. More recently, gut overgrowth of MRSA was shown to be associated with a significant amount of MRSA dispersed from the perianal site into clothing and bedding, and hence into the environment [87]. Long-stay patients invariably have overgrowth in their throat and gut of $>10^9$ potential pathogens/ml of saliva or gram of feces [1]. Washing a patient or changing a nappy may lead to contamination of the hands of the health care workers to levels of $>10^6$ PPM/cm^2 of finger surface [88]. For hand hygiene to be effective, a disinfecting agent such as 0.5% chlorhexidine in 70% alcohol is required, and the procedure must take at least 2 min. Under these circumstances, the contamination levels are reduced at most by 10^4 micro-organisms, still leaving up to 10^2/cm^2 of finger surface [89]. These quantitative data show that the intervention of hand disinfecting in a busy ICU with a few long-stay patients can only ever hope to reduce transmission, but never abolish it [90]. From an SDD perspective, even under the hypothetical circumstances of completely clearing hand contamination, hand hygiene could never exert an influence on the major infection problem of primary endogenous infection with a magnitude of between 60% and 85% of all infections (Chapter 5). The intervention of hand disinfection also fails to clear oropharyngeal and gastrointestinal carriage and/or overgrowth of PPM present on arrival. However, high standards of hygiene, including hand disinfecting, are part of the SDD infection control protocol. This protocol aims to reduce the level of contamination below which transmission occurs. It is possible to achieve these low levels as the enteral antimicrobials eradicate throat and gut carriage of PPM and substantially reduce the overall density of PPM on the patient's skin. In this way, hand washing becomes more effective in controlling transmission of PPM and subsequent endogenous and exogenous infections.

Outbreaks

Observations on the characteristics of outbreaks of infection show that once approximately half the ICU population carries the outbreak strain in overgrowth concentrations of minimally 3+ on the semi-quantitative culturing scale [91], spread via the hands of carers is impossible to prevent, and an outbreak is difficult to avoid. Dissemination of AGNB invariably occurs whether there is oropharyngeal or intestinal overgrowth [92, 93]. In ICUs with ongoing endemicity of multiresistant *Klebsiella* [93, 94], *Candida parapsilosis* [95], and MRSA [40, 81], reinforcement of conventional hygiene measures including hand disinfecting invariably failed to stop the outbreaks. The introduction of enteral antimicrobials was reported to be successful in controlling AGNB, yeast, and MRSA outbreaks in five reports [40, 81, 93–95]. In a French study the patients were randomized and given either enteral antimicrobials or no enteral antimicrobials [93]. Fecal carriage of the extended-spectrum β-lactamase producing *Klebsiella* strain was cleared in 50% of the patients and the outbreak was under control within 8 weeks. In the Manchester ICU all patients received SDD and the *Klebsiella* outbreak was stopped within 3 weeks [94]. Similarly, gut carriage/overgrowth is the main source of *Candida* and MRSA, which are then transmitted via the hands of health care workers [40, 81, 95]. On the Liverpool neonatal ICU, enteral nystatin was given as a treatment to neonates who were identified to carry the outbreak strain of *Candida parapsilosis* and the outbreak was controlled within 14 weeks [95]. Enteral vancomycin was found to be an effective outbreak control measure in Italian [40] and Spanish ICUs [81] with MRSA endemicity. In the Spanish study, enteral vancomycin as part of SDD subsequently given as prophylaxis to all patients at high risk was more effective in controlling endemicity than enteral vancomycin administered to confirmed carriers only. The main concern about the use of enteral vancomycin is the selection of the vancomycin-resistant enterococci (VRE) [96]. Vancomycin resistance amongst low-level pathogens such as enterococci is an endemic problem in ICUs in the United States.

SDD, including enteral vancomycin, has been evaluated in four European studies in mechanically ventilated patients [40, 47, 81, 97]. None of the studies reported an increased infection rate due to VRE. They evaluated SDD including vancomycin in ICUs without VRE history, and in one study VRE was imported into the unit but no change in policy was required as rapid and extensive spread did not occur [81]. Recent literature shows that parenteral antibiotics that do not respect the patient's gut ecology, rather than high doses of enteral vancomycin, promote the emergence of VRE in the gut [98, 99].

Conclusions

SDD using enteral antimicrobials is now an evidence-based protocol. It is the best-ever evaluated intervention in intensive care medicine that reduces infectious morbidity and mortality. It is a cheap maneuver without side effects in terms of emergence of resistance. In ICUs using enteral antimicrobials, gut carriage of potential pathogens, both sensitive and resistant, is significantly reduced. However, hand disinfecting as a general hygiene procedure is still valuable and can be expected to be more effective in ICUs where all long-stay patients are successfully decontaminated, free from overgrowth of AGNB, yeasts, and *S. aureus*, thus subsequently reducing hand contamination and, consequently, the chance of transmission. SDD is the gold standard with which new maneuvers of infection control should be compared.

References

1. van Saene HKF, Taylor N, Donnell SC et al (2003) Gut overgrowth with abnormal flora: the missing link in parenteral nutrition-related sepsis in surgical neonates. Eur J Clin Nutr 57:548–553
2. Husebye H (1995) Gastrointestinal motility disorders and bacterial overgrowth. J Intern Med 237:419–427
3. Marshall JC, Christou NV, Meakins JL (1988) Small bowel overgrowth and systemic immuno-suppression in experimental peritonitis. Surgery 104:404–411
4. Ketai LH, Rypka G (1993) The course of nosocomial oropharyngeal colonisation in patients recovering from acute respiratory failure. Chest 103:1837–1841
5. Alcock SR (1990) Short-term parenteral antibiotics used as supplement to SDD regimens. Infection 18 [Suppl 1]:514–518
6. Sompolinsky D, Yaron V, Alkan WJ (1967) Microbiological changes in the human faecal flora following the administration of tetracyclines and chloramphericol. Am J Proctol 18:471–478
7. Garbino T, Lew DP, Romand JA et al (2002) Prevention of severe *Candida* infections in non-neutropenic, high risk, critically ill patients: a randomised, double-blind, place-

bo-controlled trial in patients treated by selective digestive decontamination. Intensive Care Med 28:1708–1717

8. Chang FY, Peacock JE, Musher MM et al (2003) *Staphylococcus aureus* bacteremia. Recurrence and the impact of antibiotic treatment in a prospective multicentre study. Medicine (Baltimore) 82:333–339

9. van Saene R, Fairclough S, Petros A (1998) Broad and narrow spectrum antibiotics: a different approach. Clin Microbiol Infect 4:56–57

10. Geraci JE, Heilman FR, Nicols DR et al (1956) Some laboratory and clinical experience with a new antibiotic, vancomycin. Proc Staff Meet Mayo Clin 31:564–582

11. Tedesco F, Markham R, Gurwith M et al (1978) Oral vancomycin for antibiotic-associated pseudomembranous colitis. Lancet II:226–228

12. D'Agata EMC, Venkataraman L, De Girolami P et al (1999) Colonisation with broad-spectrum cephalosporin-resistant Gram-negative bacilli in intensive care units during a non-outbreak period: prevalence, risk factors and rate of infection. Crit Care Med 27:1090–1095

13. Petros AJ, O'Connell M, Roberts C et al (2001) Systemic antibiotics fail to clear multi drug-resistant Klebsiella from a paediatric ICU. Chest 119:862–866

14. Jonge EJ de, Schultz M, Spanjaard L et al (2003) Effects of selective decontamination of the digestive tract on mortality and acquisition of resistant bacteria in intensive care: a randomised, controlled trial. Lancet 362:1011–1016

15. Corbella X, Montero A, Pujol M et al (2000) Emergence and rapid spread of carbapenem resistance during a large and sustained hospital outbreak of multi-resistant Acinetobacter baumannii. J Clin Microbiol 38:4086–4095

16. Toltzis PH, Yamashita T, Vilt L et al (1998) Antibiotic restriction does not alter endemic colonization with resistant Gram-negative rods on a paediatric intensive care unit. Crit Care Med 26:1893–1899

17. van Saene HKF, Petros AJ, Ramsay G, Baxby D (2003) All great truths are iconoclastic: selective decontamination of the digestive tract moves from heresy to level 1 truth. Intensive Care Med 29:677–690

18. Yao YM, Lu LR, Yu Y et al (1997) Influence of selective decontamination of the digestive tract on cell-mediated immune function and bacteria/endotoxin translocation in thermally injured rats. J Trauma 42:1073–1079

19. Baxby D, van Saene HKF, Stoutenbeek CP, Zandstra DF (1996) Selective decontamination of the digestive tract: 13 years on, what it is and what it is not. Intensive Care Med 22:699–706

20. van der Waaij D (1992) History of recognition and measurement of colonisation resistance of the digestive tract as an introduction to selective gastro-intestinal decontamination. Epidemiol Infect 109:315–326

21. Bodey GP (1981) Antibiotic prophylaxis in cancer patients: regimens of oral, non-absorbable antibiotics for prevention of infection during induction of remission. Rev Infect Dis 3:S259–S268

22. van Saene HKF, Stoutenbeek CP (1987) Selective decontamination. J Antimicrob Chemother 20:462–465

23. Harris JC, Dupont HL, Hornick RB (1972) Faecal leucocytes in diarrheal illness. Ann Intern Med 76:697–703

24. Stoutenbeek CP (1989) Topical antibiotic regimen. In: van Saene HKF, Stoutenbeek CP, Lawin P, Ledingham IM (eds) Infection control by selective decontamination. Springer Verlag, Berlin Heidelberg New York, pp 95–101

25. van Saene JJM, van Saene HKF, Tarko-Smith NJ, Beukeveld GJ (1988) *Enterobacteriaceae* suppression by three different oral doses of polymyxin E in human

volunteers. Epidemiol Infect 100:407–417
26.   Sogaard H (1982) The pharmacodynamics of polymyxin antibiotics with special reference to drug resistance liability. J Vet Pharmacol Ther 5:219–281
27.   Danner RL, Joiner KA, Rubin MR et al (1989) Purification, toxicity and anti-endotoxin activity of polymyxin B nonapeptide. Antimicrob Agents Chemother 33:1428–1432
28.   Veringa EM, van der Waaij D (1984) Biological inactivation by faeces of anti-microbial drugs applicable in selective decontamination of the digestive tract. J Antimicrob Chemother 14:605–612
29.   van Saene JJM, van Saene HKF, Stoutenbeek CP, Lerk CF (1985) Influence of faeces on the activity of anti-microbial agents used for decontamination of the alimentary canal. Scand J Infect Dis 17:295–300
30.   Hazenberg MP, Pennock-Schroder AM, van de Merwe JP (1985) Binding to and bacterial effect of aztreonam, temocillin, gentamicin and tobramycin on human faeces. J Hyg 95:255–263
31.   Mulder JG, Wiersma WE, Welling GW, van der Waaij D (1984) Low dose oral tobramycin treatment for selective decontamination of the digestive tract: a study in human volunteers. J Antimicrob Chemother 13:495–504
32.   Cavaliere F, Sciarra M, Crociani E et al (1988) Tobramycin serum levels during selective decontamination of the gastro-intestinal tract. Minerva Anestesiol 54:233–226
33.   Zobel G, Kuttnig M, Grubbauer HM et al (1991) Reduction of colonisation and infection rate during paediatric intensive care by selective decontamination of the digestive tract. Crit Care Med 19:1242–1246
34.   Gaussorgues P, Salord F, Sirodot M et al (1991) Nosocomial bacteremia in patients under mechanical ventilation and receiving beta-inotropic drugs; efficacy of digestive decontamination. Rean Soins Intens Med Urg 7:169–174
35.   Smith CA, Baker EN (2002) Aminoglycoside antibiotic resistance of enzymatic deactivation. Curr Drug Targets Infect Disord 2:143-160
36.   Sjolin T, Goscinski G, Lundholm M et al (2000) Endotoxin release from *Escherichia coli* after exposure to tobramycin: dose dependency and reduction in cefuroxime-induced endotoxin release. Clin Microbiol Infect 6:74–81
37.   Vandenbossche H, Dromer F, Improvisi I et al (1998) Antifungal drug resistance in pathogenic fungi. Med Mycol 36:119–128
38.   Hofstra W, deVries-Hospers HG, van der Waaij D (1979) Concentrations of nystatin in faeces after oral administration of various doses of nystatin. Infection 7:166–170
39.   Hofstra W, de Vries-Hospers HG, der Waaij D van (1982) Concentrations of amphotericin B in faeces and blood of healthy volunteers after oral administration of various doses. Infection 10:233–277
40.   Silvestri L, Milanese M, Oblach L et al (2002) Enteral vancomycin to control methicillin-resistant *Staphylococcus aureus* outbreak in mechanically ventilated patients. Am J Infect Control 30:391–399
41.   Silvestri L, Milanese M, Gregori D, van Saene HKF (2005) Impact of selective decontamination of the digestive tract on fungal carriage and infection: systematic review of randomised controlled trials. Intensive Care Med (in press)
42.   Bergmans DCJJ, Bonten MJM, Gaillard CA et al (2001) Prevention of ventilator-associated pneumonia by oral decontamination. Am J Respir Crit Care Med 164:382–388
43.   Korinek AM, Laisne MJ, Nicolas MH et al (1993) Selective decontamination of the digestive tract in neurosurgical intensive care unit patients: a double-blind, randomised, placebo-controlled study. Crit Care Med 21:1466–1473
44.   Krueger WA, Lenhart FP, Neeser G et al (2002) Influence of combined intravenous and topical antibiotic prophylaxis in the incidence of infections, organ dysfunctions and

mortality in critically ill surgical patients. Am J Respir Crit Care Med 166:1029–1037
45. Pugin J, Auckenthaler R, Lew DP, Suter PM (1991) Oropharyngeal decontamination decreases incidence of ventilator-associated pneumonia. JAMA 265:2704–2710
46. Schardey HM, Joosten U, Finke U et al (1997) The prevention of anastomotic leakage after total gastrectomy with local decontamination. Ann Surg 225:172–180
47. Silvestri L, van Saene HKF, Milanese M et al (2004) Prevention of MRSA pneumonia by oral vancomycin decontamination: a randomised trial. Eur Respir J 23:921–926
48. Bodey GP, Pan T (1980) Absorption of tobramycin after chronic oral administration. Curr Ther Res 28:394–401
49. Gotoff SP, Lepper MH (1965) Treatment of *Salmonella* carriers with colistin sulfate. Am J Med Sci 249:399–403
50. Misset B, Kitzis MD, Conscience G et al (1994) Mechanisms of failure to decontaminate the gut with polymyxin E, gentamicin and amphotericin B in patients in intensive care. Eur J Clin Microbiol Infect Dis 13:165–170
51. Stoutenbeek CP, van Saene HKF (1990) Infection prevention in intensive care by selective decontamination of the digestive tract. J Crit Care 5:137–156
52. Krueger WA, Ruckdeschel G, Unertl K (1999) Elimination of faecal *Enterobacteriaceae* by intravenous ciprofloxacin is not inhibited by concomitant sucralfate, a microbiological and pharmacokinetic study on patients. Infection 6:335–340
53. Daneshmend TK, Warnock DW (1983) Clinical pharmacokinetics of systemic antifungal drugs. Clin Pharmacokinet 8:17–42
54. Winter R, Humphreys H, Pick A et al (1992) A controlled trial of selective decontamination of the digestive tract in intensive care and its effect on nosocomial infection. J Antimicrob Chemother 30:73–87
55. Stoutenbeek CP, Saene HKF van, Zandstra DF (1987) The effect of oral non-absorbable antibiotics on the emergence of resistant bacteria in patients in an intensive care unit. J Antimicrob Chemother 19:513–520
56. D'Amico R, Pifferi S, Leonetti C et al (1998) Effectiveness of antibiotic prophylaxis in critically ill adult patients: systematic review of randomised controlled trials. BMJ 316:1275–1285
57. Liberati A, D'Amico R, Pifferi S et al (2004) Antibiotic prophylaxis to reduce respiratory tract infections and mortality in adults receiving intensive care [Cochrane Review]. In: The Cochrane Library, Issue 1, 2004. Chichester, UK: John Wiley & Sons, Ltd
58. van Saene HKF, Stoutenbeek CP, Faber-Nijholt R, van Saene JJM (1992) Selective decontamination of the digestive tract contributes to the control of disseminated intravascular coagulation in severe liver impairment. J Pediatr Gastroenterol Nutr 14:436–442
59. Fink MP, Mythen MG (1999) The role of gut-derived endotoxin in the pathogenesis of multiple organ dysfunction. In: Brade H, Opal SM, Vogel SN, Morrison DC (eds) Endotoxin in health and disease. Dekker, New York, pp 855–864
60. Cohen J (2000) The detection and interpretation of endotoxaemia. Intensive Care Med 26:S51–S56
61. van Saene JJM , Stoutenbeek CP, van Saene HKF et al (1996) Reduction of the intestinal endotoxin pool by three different SDD regimens in human volunteers. J Endotoxin Res 3:337–343
62. Martinez-Pellus AE, Merino P, Bru M et al (1993) Can selective digestive decontamination avoid the endotoxemia and cytokine activation promoted by cardiopulmonary bypass? Crit Care Med 21:1684–1689
63. Martinez-Pellus AE, Merino P, Bru M et al (1997) Endogenous endotoxemia of intestinal origin during cardiopulmonary bypass. Intensive Care Med 23:1251–1257

64. Bouter H, Schippers EF, Luelmo SAC et al (2002) No effect of pre-operative selective gut decontamination on endotoxemia and cytokine activation during cardio-pulmonary bypass: a randomised, placebo-controlled study. Crit Care Med 30:38–43
65. Bion JF, Badger I, Crosby HA et al (1994) Selective decontamination of the digestive tract reduces Gram-negative pulmonary colonisation but not systemic endotoxemia in patients undergoing elective liver transplantation. Crit Care Med 22:40–49
66. Maring JK, Zwaveling JH, Klompmaker IJ et al (2002) Selective bowel decontamination in elective liver transplantation: no improvement in endotoxaemia, initial graft function and post-operative morbidity. Transpl Int 15:329–334
67. Oudemans-van Straaten HM, vanSaene HKF, Zandstra DF (2003) Selective decontamination of the digestive tract: use of the correct antibiotics is crucial. Crit Care Med 31:334–335
68. Schippers EF, van Dissel JT (2003) Selective gut decontamination. Crit Care Med 31:2715–2716
69. van Saene HKF, Silvestri L, Bams JL et al (2003) Selective decontamination of the digestive tract: use in liver transplantation is evidence-based. Crit Care Med 31:1600–1601
70. Hammond JMJ, Potgieter PD (1995) Long term effects of selective decontamination on anti-microbial resistance. Crit Care Med 23:637–645
71. Leone M, Albanese J, Antonini F et al (2003) Long term (6-year) effect of selective digestive decontamination on anti-microbial resistance in intensive care, multiple-trauma patients. Crit Care Med 31:2090–2095
72. Tetteroo GWM, Wagenvoort JHT, Bruining HA (1994) Bacteriology of selective decontamination: efficacy and rebound colonisation. J Antimicrob Chemother 34:139–148
73. Saunders N, Hammond JMJ, Potgieter PD et al (1994) Mirobiological surveillance during selective decontamination of the digestive tract [SDD]. J Antimicrob Chemother 34:529–544
74. Gastinne H, Wolff M, Delatour F et al (1992) A controlled trial in intensive care units of selective decontamination of the digestive tract with non-absorbable antibiotics. The French study group on selective decontamination of the digestive tract. N Engl J Med 326:594–599
75. Hammond JMJ, Potgieter PD, Saunders GL et al (1992) Double-blind study of selective decontamination of the digestive tract in intensive care. Lancet 340:5–9
76. Ferrer M, Torres A, Gonzales J et al (1994) Utility of selective digestive decontamination in mechanically ventilated patients. Ann Intern Med 120:389–395
77. Wiener J, Itokazu G, Nathan C et al (1995) A randomised, double-blind, placebo-controlled trial of selective decontamination in a medical, surgical intensive care unit. Clin Infect Dis 20:861–867
78. Lingnau W, Berger J, Javorsky F et al (1997) Selective intestinal decontamination in multiple trauma patients: prospective, controlled trial. J Trauma 42:687–694
79. Verwaest C, Verhaegen J, Ferdinande P et al (1997) Randomised, controlled trial of selective decontamination in 600 mechanically ventilated patients in a multi-disciplinary intensive care unit. Crit Care Med 25:63–71
80. Sanchez Garcia M, Cambronero Galache JA, Lopez Diaz J et al (1998) Effectiveness and cost of selective decontamination of the digestive tract in critically ill intubated patients. Am J Respir Crit Care Med 158:908–916
81. de la Cal MA, Cerda E, van Saene HKF et al (2004) Effectiveness and safety of enteral vancomycin to control endemicity of methicillin-resistant *Staphylococcus aureus* in a medical/surgical intensive care unit. J Hosp Infect 56:175-183
82. van Saene HKF, Weir WI, de la Cal MA et al (2004) MRSA-time for a more pragmatic approach? J Hosp Infect 56:170-174

83. White A (1961) Relation between quantitative nasal cultures and dissemination of staphylococci. J Lab Clin Med 58:273–277
84. Brodie J, Kerr MR, Sommerville T (1956) The hospital staphylococcus. A comparison of nasal and faecal carrier states. Lancet I:19–20
85. Greendyke RM, Constantine HP, Magruder GB et al (1958) Staphylococci on a medical ward, with special reference to faecal carriers. Am J Clin Pathol 30:318–322
86. Hone R, Keane CT, Fitzpatrick S (1974) Faecal carriage of *Staphylococcus aureus* in infantile enteritis due to enteropathic *Escherichia coli*. Scand J Infect Dis 6:329–332
87. Brady LM, Thomson M, Palmer MA et al (1990) Successful control of endemic MRSA in a cardiothoracic surgical unit. Med J Aust 152:240–245
88. Salzman TC, Clark JJ, Klemm L (1967) Hand contamination of personnel as a mechanism of cross-infection in nosocomial infections with antibiotic-resistant Escherichia coli and *Klebsiella Aerobacter*. Antimicrob Agents Chemother 7:97–100
89. Nystrom B (1983) Optimal design/personnel for control of intensive care unit infection. Infect Control 4:388–390
90. Crossley K, Landesmann B, Zaske D (1979) An outbreak of infections caused by strains of *Staphylococcus aureus* resistant to methicillin and aminoglycosides. II. Epidemiology studies. J Infect Dis 139:280–287
91. Viviani M, van Saene HKF, Dezzoni R et al (2005) Control of imported and acquired methicillin-resistant *Staphylococcus aureus* [MRSA] in mechanically ventilated patients: a dose-response study of oral vancomycin to reduce absolute carriage and infection. Anaesth Intensive Care (in press)
92. Bonten MJM, Gaillard CA, Johanson WG et al (1994) Colonization in patients receiving and not receiving topical antimicrobial prophylaxis. Am J Respir Crit Care Med 150:1332–1340
93. Brun-Buisson C, Legrand P, Rauss A et al (1989) Intestinal decontamination for control of nosocomial multi-resistant Gram-negative bacilli: study of an outbreak in an intensive care unit. Ann Intern Med 110:873–881
94. Taylor ME, Oppenheim BA (1991) Selective decontamination of the gastro-intestinal tract as an infection control measure. J Hosp Infect 17:271–278
95. Damjanovic V, Connolly CM, van Saene HKF et al (1993) Selective decontamination with nystatin for control of a *Candida* outbreak in a neonatal intensive care unit. J Hosp Infect 24:245–259
96. Rice LB (2001) Emergence of vancomycin-resistant enterococci. Emerg Infect Dis 7:183-187
97. Sanchez M, Mir N, Canton R et al (1997) The effect of topical vancomycin on acquisition, carriage and infection with methicillin-resistant *Staphyloccocus aureus* in critically ill patients. A double-blind, randomized, placebo-controlled study (abstract). Abstracts of the 37th ICAAC, Toronto Canada, p 310
98. Stiefel U, Paterson DL, Pultz NJ et al (2004) Effect of increasing use of piperacillin/tazobactam on the incidence of vancomycin-resistant enterococci in four academic medical centres. Infect Control Hosp Epidemiol 25:380–383
99. Salgado CD, Giannetta ET, Farr BM (2004) Failure to develop vancomycin-resisteant *Enterococcus* with oral treatment of *Clostridium difficile*. Infect Control Hosp Epidemiol 25:413–417

Chapter 10

Evidence-Based Infection Control in the Intensive Care Unit

J. Hughes, N. Taylor, E. Cerda, M.A. de la Cal

Introduction

Nosocomial infection rates in the intensive care unit (ICU) are higher than in the general hospital population, the main reason being the severity of illness of ICU patients and hence the increased susceptibility to acquiring micro-organisms related to the ICU [1]. The unique environment of the ICU makes it more likely to encourage the emergence of infections due to multi-resistant potentially pathogenic microorganisms (PPMs) [2]. The ICU is the area in the hospital where the most severely ill patients are brought together. Practically all ICU patients, who require mechanical ventilation for >3 days receive antimicrobials. They are also cared for by larger numbers and a wider variety of healthcare workers (HCWs), which increases the risk of transmission of PPMs. Additionally, the often-urgent nature of critical care interventions can lead to sub-optimal practice of infection control [3]. This can lead to increased morbidity and mortality, become a drain on existing resources, and increase pressure on beds. However, it is also a quality and clinical governance issue [4, 5].

The three main clinical endpoints [6] for controlling infection in the ICU are to: (1) reduce high infection rates, (2) maintain low infection rates, and (3) control antibiotic resistance. Nosocomial infections are caused by micro-organisms acquired on the ICU following transmission via the hands of carers. Hence, the target of infection control is the control of transmission of often multi-resistant micro-organisms following breaches of hygiene.

Universally agreed infection control measures are basic hygiene standards, including hand hygiene, patient isolation, appropriate glove and gown usage, care of equipment, and standards for environmental cleanliness [7–9]. The role of device and antibiotic policies will be discussed in the following two Chapters 11 and 12. Although there are a number of studies on the benefits of such measures, in general, compliance with some or all of the practices is known to be sub-optimal and the evidence base is often poor or absent [10, 11]. Attempts to address some of the issues and to formulate national evidence-based guidelines for healthcare-associated infections have been addressed by the evidence-based practice in infection control (EPIC) project 2001 [11], Agency for Healthcare Research and Quality [10], and the Center for Disease Control and Prevention (CDC) [12, 13].

Why Do We Need Evidence-Based Practice in ICU?

Evidence-based practice (EBP) is defined as the "integration of best research evidence with clinical expertise and patient values" [14]. EBP is now recognized as a means of providing more effective health care by questioning the basis of many interventions and analyzing the available original clinical research in order to substantiate current practices and to form guidelines based on expert opinion where no other evidence currently exists [15]. EBP enables healthcare professionals to be confident that their interventions are informed by a current and appropriate knowledge base. It also helps ensure that practices and guidelines can be audited and measured against agreed standards. This is essential in the current healthcare climate and is high on many political agendas, particularly in relation to clinical governance directives [5]. The concept of EBP and its application is a key feature of clinical governance.

Although many infection control policies and recommendations have been attempted based on the available evidence, there is often a paucity of studies to support practices in infection control, with some procedures still based on ritual [16, 17]. Controlled clinical trials are difficult to undertake due to the large numbers of subjects required and the multiplicity of factors involved in infection control. In some cases, the difficulties of basing infection control practice on the best available evidence is often a problem due to the ethical considerations of conducting a randomized clinical trial. In addition, there are some areas of practice, such as hand decontamination, where there is some evidence to show it can help reduce infection, but compliance is often poor [18].

The National Health Service Executive in the United Kingdom [19] stated that all clinical guidelines should be classified according to: randomized controlled trials, other robust experimental or observational studies, or more limited evidence usually based on expert opinion and endorsed by respected authorities.

The CDC guidelines [12, 13] based their evidence on:

Category IA. Strongly recommended for implementation and supported by well-designed, experimental, clinical, or epidemiological studies

Category IB. Strongly recommended for implementation and supported by certain experimental, clinical, or epidemiological studies and a strong theoretical rationale

Category II. Suggested for implementation and supported by suggestive clinical or epidemiological studies or a theoretical rationale

No recommendation. Unresolved issue. Practices for which insufficient evidence or no consensus regarding efficacy exist

This classification has been used in Tables 1 and 2.

Table 1. Recommendations for hand hygiene (*HCWs* healthcare workers)a

Recommendation	Level of evidence
When hands are visibly dirty or contaminated with proteinaceous material or are visibly soiled with blood or other body fluids, wash hands with either a non-antimicrobial soap and water or an antimicrobial soap and water	IA
If hands are not visibly soiled, use an alcohol-based hand rub for routinely decontaminating hands in all other clinical situations described in items	IC
Decontaminate hands after contact with a patient's intact skin (e.g., when taking a pulse or blood pressure, and lifting a patient)	IB
Decontaminate hands after contact with body fluids or excretions, mucous membranes, non-intact skin, and wound dressings if hands are not visibly soiled	IA
Decontaminate hands after removing gloves	IB
Before eating and after using a restroom, wash hands with a non-antimicrobial soap and water or with an antimicrobial soap and water	IB
No recommendation can be made regarding the routine use of non-alcohol-based hand rubs for hand hygiene in healthcare settings	Unresolved issue
When decontaminating hands with an alcohol-based hand rub, apply product to palm of one hand and rub hands together, covering all surfaces of hands and fingers, until hands are dry	IB
When washing hands with soap and water, wet hands first with water, apply an amount of product recommended by the manufacturer to hands, and rub hands together vigorously for at least 15 seconds, covering all surfaces of the hands and fingers. Rinse hands with water and dry thoroughly with a disposable towel. Use towel to turn off the faucet	IB
Provide personnel with efficacious hand-hygiene products that have low irritancy potential, particularly when these products are used many times per shift. This recommendation applies to products used for hand antisepsis before and after patient care in clinical areas and to products used for surgical hand antisepsis by surgical personnel	IB

→ *Cont.*

→ **Table 1** *Cont.*

Recommendation	Level of evidence
Do not add soap to a partially empty soap dispenser. This practice of "topping up' dispensers can lead to bacterial contamination of soap	IA
Provide HCWs with hand lotions or creams to minimize the occurrence of irritant contact dermatitis associated with hand antisepsis or handwashing	IA
As part of a multidisciplinary program to improve hand hygiene adherence, provide HCWs with a readily accessible alcohol-based hand-rub product	IA
To improve hand hygiene adherence among personnel who work in areas in which high workloads and high intensity of patient care are anticipated, make an alcohol-based hand rub available at the entrance to the patients' room or at the bedside, in other convenient locations, and in individual pocket-sized containers to be carried by HCWs	IA

For a more detailed description see [10, 11, 13]

Table 2. Recommendations for protective clothing and care of equipment and environment[a]

Recommendation	Level of evidence
Select protective equipment on the basis of an assessment of the risk of transmission of micro-organisms	II
Gloves Wear gloves (clean, non-sterile gloves are adequate) when touching blood, body fluids, secretions, excretions, and contaminated items. Put on clean gloves just before touching mucous membranes and non-intact skin. Change gloves between tasks and procedures on the same patient after contact with material that may contain a high concentration of micro-organisms. Remove gloves promptly after use, before touching non-contaminated items and environmental surfaces, and before going to another patient, and wash hands immediately to avoid transfer of micro-organisms to other patients or environments	IB
Mask and eye protection Wear a mask or a face shield to protect mucous membranes of the eyes, nose, and mouth during procedures and patient-care activities that are likely to generate splashes or sprays of blood, body fluids, secretions, and excretions	IB
Gown Wear a gown (a clean, non-sterile gown is adequate) to protect skin and to prevent soiling of clothing during procedures and patient-care activities that are likely to generate splashes or sprays of blood, body fluids, secretions, or excretions. Select a gown that is appropriate for the activity and amount of fluid likely to be encountered. Remove a soiled gown as promptly as possible, and wash hands to avoid transfer of micro-organisms to other patients or environments	IB

→ *Cont.*

→ **Table 2.** *cont.*

Isolation Place a patient who contaminates the environment or who does not (or cannot be expected to) assist in maintaining appropriate hygiene or environmental control in a private room. If a private room is not available, consult with infection control professionals regarding patient placement or other alternatives	IB
Patient-care equipment Handle used equipment soiled with blood, body fluids, secretions, and excretions in a manner that prevents skin and mucous membrane exposures, contamination of clothing, and transfer of micro-organisms to other patients and environments. Ensure that reusable equipment is not used for the care of another patient until it has been cleaned and reprocessed appropriately. Ensure that single-use items are discarded properly	IB
Environmental control Ensure that the hospital has adequate procedures for the routine care, cleaning, and disinfecting of environmental surfaces, beds, bedrails, bedside equipment, and other frequently touched surfaces, and ensure that these procedures are being followed	IB
Handle, transport, and process used linen soiled with blood, body fluids, secretions, and excretions in a manner that prevents skin and mucous membrane exposures and contamination of clothing, and that avoids transfer of micro-organisms to other patients and environments	IB

For a more detailed description see [10–12]

The Five Main Infection Control Maneuvers to Control Transmission

Hand Hygiene

Hand washing is often referred to as the single most important means of preventing the transmission of healthcare-associated infections (Table 1) [13, 20]. Several studies have shown that the transmission of PPMs from one patient to another via the hands of healthcare workers can result in adverse patient outcomes [21, 22]. The EPIC guidelines based on a systematic review of the available literature suggest that effective hand decontamination can significantly reduce infection rates in high-risk areas such as the ICU. Although there is no level one evidence, i.e., randomized controlled trials, and the ethical approval for such a study would be non-existent, the evidence is based on expert consensus opinion and several observational epidemiological studies [9, 23, 24]. Therefore, hands must be decontaminated and dried thoroughly immediately before each direct patient contact/care episode and after any activity or contact that can result in hands becoming contaminated.

There are various studies that look at differing products for hand decontamination. Some studies suggest that soap and water is as effective as handwashing products containing antimicrobial agents for decontaminating hands and removing transient micro-organisms [24]. Antimicrobial liquid soap preparations will reduce transient micro-organisms and resident flora and result in hand asepsis. Alcohol-based hand rubs alone are not effective in removing physical dirt or soiling, but will result in substantial reductions in transient micro-organisms. A recent prospective, randomized clinical trial with crossover design, paired data, and blind evaluation in a Spanish ICU demonstrated that alcoholic solutions alone were effective in reducing the number of colony forming units (CFU) on hands after hand washing by 88.2% compared with 49.6% after soap and water [25].

Overall the EPIC project review failed to find compelling evidence for the general use of antimicrobial agents over soap or one antimicrobial agent over another. From the available evidence, based on a review of expert opinion, the authors suggest that acceptability of agents and hand hygiene techniques are the most essential factors for the selection of the best products and compliance with handwashing.

Hand decontamination is, however, often poorly performed and several studies demonstrate that compliance is sub-optimal [26, 27]. The various reasons suggested for this include availability of hand decontamination facilities and harsh hand care products causing skin damage. ICUs should therefore have enough sinks with easy access to wash hands. The increased availability of alcohol gel hand rubs, which contain emollients, has also been found to increase compliance [28]. Regular hand decontamination training sessions/audits with compliance could also help increase awareness [29, 30].

However, it must also be appreciated that the saliva or feces of critically ill patients contain high concentrations of PPMs (>10^8 CFU/g of feces), and after contact with such a patient hand contamination can often exceed 10^5 cfu/cm^2 of finger surface area. Hand decontamination with 0.5% chlorhexidine in 70% alcohol effectively clears micro-organisms from the hands, but only if the contamination is <10^4 CFU [31]. Therefore, hand decontamination can only be expected to reduce transmission and not eradicate it completely.

Gloves, Gowns and Aprons (Personal Protective Equipment)

Some healthcare-associated infections may easily be transferable between patients by direct transmission via hands of HCW [32] or via inanimate objects such as equipment. The most common PPMs are vancomycin-resistant enterococci (VRE), methicillin-resistant *Staphylococcus aureus* (MRSA), *Clostridium difficile*, and (often resistant) aerobic Gram-negative bacilli (AGNB). The ICU may often not know the carrier state of a patient on admission and it is imperative that standard (formerly referred to as universal infection control blood and body fluid) precautions are practised by all HCW. Personal protective equipment should be easily accessible to all HCW in the ICU to ensure compliance with standard precautions [33] and to comply with Health and Safety regulations such as the Personal Protective Equipment Regulations (1994), which are compulsory in some countries, e.g., United Kingdom [34].

Gloves and aprons should be used routinely when handling blood and/or body fluids from all patients to protect the HCW and prevent transmission to other susceptible individuals. These measures ensure all patients are treated equally without breaching confidentiality.

Latex gloves are one of the most effective barriers against micro-organisms [32], although several studies have shown poor compliance [26, 27], with gloves not always being worn when required, or conversely being worn for prolonged periods and hands not being washed following removal, leading to potential hand contamination. Gloves can also cause adverse reactions and skin sensitivity in both the HCW and patients [32] and their use should not be indiscriminate. Risk assessments should be undertaken to establish when to use gloves and which particular type of glove to use [32]. Sterile gloves should be worn for all invasive procedures, contact with sterile sites, and non-intact skin. Non-sterile gloves are suitable for all procedures, which involve contact with mucous membranes, and where a risk assessment has indicated exposure to blood or body fluids, secretions, and excretions. Gloves should also be single-use items and discarded after each activity as clinical waste, followed by hand decontamination.

Disposable plastic aprons are just as effective as gowns in protecting the clothing of HCW. Many studies advocate gown usage to prevent the transmission of PPMs, in particular C. difficile and VRE [26, 35, 36]. However, although many of the studies demonstrated a reduction in the incidence of infection due to the above PPMs, it was difficult to differentiate between individual factors, including severity of illness, type of underlying disease, and the use of antibiotics. Antibiotics that respect the patient's normal flora, i.e., ecology, have been shown to control VRE and C. difficile, [37, 38]. Furthermore, a systematic review undertaken by the EPIC project authors identified two randomized controlled trials where gown usage in special care baby units failed to reduce infection rates [39, 40]. However, where there is a possibility of contamination of the clothing of HCW with blood or body fluids, it is recommended that disposable plastic aprons be worn. Gowns are only required where there is a risk of gross contamination or splashing, such as in major burn patients or severe trauma, and in this event the gowns should be made of a fluid-repellent material.

In the ICU or emergency department the HCW should also have access to facial or eye protection. Although facemasks have not been found to be beneficial, personal respiratory protection is required for patients with tuberculosis

The Minimum Infection Database

The traditional infection surveillance systems are based on the recommendations of the CDC [71, 72]. The aim of this approach is to provide a simple and efficient tool:

1) to define the rates of the most relevant ICU-acquired infections, i.e., pneumonia related to mechanical ventilation, bloodstream infections related to intravascular devices, and urinary tract infections related to bladder catheters
2) to monitor the trend of these rates in the ICU
3) to assess the impact of any preventive measure (Fig. 2).

The infection indicators recommended by the CDC are based on the relative weight of the following criteria: (1) clear case definition; (2) ease of surveillance system, importance of the event; (3) potential of intervention to reduce rates; (4) availability of denominator device-days; (5) ease of collection of the denominator device-days [73].

The selected indicators include:

Ventilator-associated pneumonia rate=number of ventilator-associated pneumonia/number of ventilator-days

Central line associated bloodstream infection rate=central line-associated bloodstream infections/number of central line-days

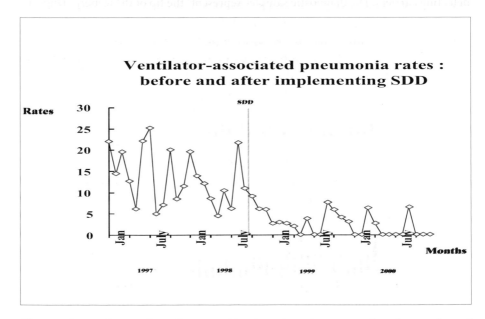

Fig. 2. The incidence of ventilator-associated pneumonia expressed as the number of pneumonias divided by 1,000 ventilation-days significantly decreased following implementation of selective digestive decontamination (SDD) form 12.4 to 3.6 ($P<0.001$) [80]

Urinary catheter-associated urinary tract infection rate=number of urinary catheter-associated urinary tract infection/number of urinary catheter-days.

This minimum data set has been proposed for use in the ICU, even in those with limited resources, because of the low workload for data acquisition and the relevance of the information retrieved [74–76].

Nevertheless the use of diagnostic samples may only underestimate the level of transmission of PPMs because diagnostic samples are generally taken on clinical indication for microbiological confirmation. Moreover, diagnostic samples do not detect transmission [62, 68].

The strengths and the weaknesses of both infection surveillance systems, based on surveillance samples and diagnostic samples, are summarized in Table 3.

Table 3. Strengths and weaknesses of both surveillance methods of infection only and of infection combined with carriage

Strengths	Weaknesses
Surveillance of infection (solely diagnostic samples)	Surveillance of infection (solely diagnostic samples)
• Already routine • Easy to fulfil • Number of infections per 1,000 device-days: useful to know the trends in infection rates in one unit	• Substantial delay between the detection of a problem and the implementation of the appropriate measures to control it, because of the extra work required to identify the pathogenesis of the problem • Cost-effectiveness: has to be tested • Time cut-off of 48 h: not accurate for the estimation of infection due to ICU micro-organisms • Value of method for interhospital comparison: limited • Detection of resistance, transmission and outbreaks: late
Surveillance of infection/carriage (diagnostic samples combined with surveillance samples)	Surveillance of infection/carriage (diagnostic samples combined with surveillance samples)
• More accurate estimation of infections due to ICU-acquired micro-organisms • Early implementation of the appropriate preventive measures according to the pathogenesis of the infections • Detection of resistance at an early stage • Detection of transmission at an early stage • Indispensable in control of an outbreak • Monitoring the efficacy of selective digestive decontamination	• Workload for laboratory is higher • Cost-effectiveness: has to be tested • Value of method for interhospital comparison: has to be tested • Surveillance cultures: unpopular amongst traditional microbiologists

How to Implement an Infection Control Program

Implementing an effective evidence-based infection control program in the ICU not only relies on establishing and reviewing the best available evidence, but it is essential that the evidence is practical and easy to utilize in order to achieve compliance with the recommended guidelines and policies.

1. The intensivist together with an ICU nurse interested in infection control, in general, take the initiative to design an infection control program. They invite the infection control team of the hospital, the clinical microbiologist, and pharmacist to join the ICU infection control team. In some cases the hospital infection control team approaches ICU staff to develop the program.

2. The resultant ICU infection control team defines the content of the infection control program that should initially include:

   (a) How to implement the five infection control maneuvers (hand hygiene, protective clothing, isolation, care of the equipment, and care of the environment) in order to control the transmission of PPMs

   (b) The definition of the population who may benefit from SDD and how to implement it [77, 78]

   (c) The minimum data set to evaluate the quality of infection control (Fig. 2)

   (d) The surveillance cultures (throat and rectum) targeting carriage of resistant PPMs, i.e., MRSA, *P. aeruginosa*, *Acinetobacter spp.* (Fig. 1)

   (e) How to report the results of the database and liaize with HCW.

   Regular meetings of the ICU infection control team are indispensable to discuss current patient-related problems and relevant infection control issues.

3. Regular surveillance samples to monitor carriage of patients who receive SDD in order:

   (a) To identify the preventative measure to be implemented

   (b) To monitor the efficacy of SDD in eradicating the abnormal carrier state (Fig. 3)

4. The antibiotic policy and surveillance of antimicrobial usage are discussed in Chapters 12 and 28.

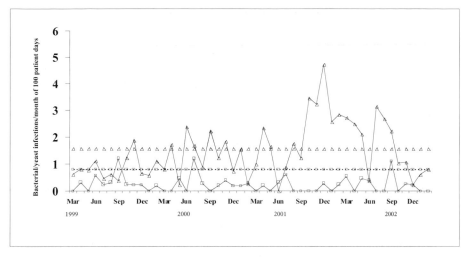

Fig. 3. The incidence density of secondary endogenous (□) and exogenous infections (Δ) due to newly acquired micro-organisms that were not present in the admission flora. Micro-organisms causing exogenous infections were not cultured from the surveillance samples of throat and rectum. Secondary endogenous infections were due to micro-organisms that had been through a digestive tract phase. The micro-organisms were acquired on the pediatric intensive care unit in both types of infection. Two thresholds were used for exogenous and secondary endogenous infections, respectively. The thresholds were calculated at the 95 % confidence interval from the first 24 months of data, assuming the infection rate data conforms to the Poisson distribution. Exogenous infections rose above the threshold on twenty occasions whereas secondary endogenous infections were above the threshold three times (from Sarginson RE, Taylor N, Reilly N, Baines PB, Van Saene HKF (2004) Infection in prolonged pediatric critical illness: A prospective four-year study based on knowledge of the carrier state. Crit Care Med 32:839-847, with permission) [59]

References

1. Waterer GW, Wunderink RG (2001) Increasing threat of Gram-negative bacteria. Crit Care Med 4 [Suppl]:N75–N81
2. Warren DK, Fraser VJ (2001) Infection control measures to limit antimicrobial resistance. Crit Care Med 29:N128–N134
3. Fridkin SK (2001) Increasing prevalence of antimicrobial resistance in intensive care units. Crit Care Med 4 [Suppl]:N64–N68
4. Masterton RG, Teare EL (2001) Clinical governance and infection control in the United Kingdom. J Hosp Infect 47:25–31
5. NHS Executive (1999) Health Service Circular 1999/132 Governance in the New NHS 21 May. Department of Health, London
6. Condon RE, Haley RW, Lee JT et al (1988) Does infection control control infection? Arch Surg 123:250–256
7. Wenzel RP (ed) (1993) Prevention and control of nosocomial infections, 2nd edn. Williams and Wilkins, Baltimore, USA

double-lumen central venous catheters were evaluated in patients after cardiac surgery ($n=77$) and did not significantly reduce bacterial catheter contamination compared with the control catheters [26]. However, in another study, silver impregnation of the internal and external surfaces of a central venous catheter was investigated for antimicrobial activity. Catheter-associated infections were diagnosed in the silver group in 5.26/1,000 catheter days and 18.34/1,000 catheter days in the control group, indicating a reduction rate of 71.3% ($p<0.05$). The silver-coated catheter appeared to be effective if the internal surface was also impregnated [27].

The results of clinical trials of antiseptic-coated central venous catheters are controversial. Maki et al. [28] studied 403 catheters in 158 adults scheduled to receive a central venous catheter in a medical-surgical ICU of a 450-bed university hospital. Participants received either a standard triple-lumen polyurethane catheter or a catheter impregnated with chlorhexidine and silver sulfadiazine. In this study the clorhexidine-silver sulfadiazine catheter was well tolerated and reduced the incidence of catheter-related infection. It also extended the time that non-cuffed central venous catheters could be safely left in place for the short term, which should allow cost savings [28].

George et al. [29] observed that using an antiseptic- (chlorhexidine and silver sulfadiazine) impregnated catheter in a group of patients with thoracic organ transplantation, the contamination rate was reduced from 25 of 35 standard catheters to 10 of 44 study catheters ($p<0.002$, 68% reduction). Similarly, the incidence of concomitant infection by the same organism at another site of infection was reduced from 10 of 35 standard catheters to 4 of 44 study catheters ($p<0.03$), a 63% reduction [29].

Different results were obtained in a tertiary care medical center on 282 patients who required central venous catheter placement. Despite a marked decrease in catheter site colonization and catheter-related infection rates, the central venous catheter coated with silver sulfadiazine and chlorhexidine did not significantly reduce the incidence of catheter-related septicemia [30].

The incidence of local catheter infection and catheter-related bacteremia was evaluated in 308 surgical critically ill patients with triple-lumen central venous catheters coated with a combination of chlorhexidine and silver sulfadiazine. The use of chlorhexidine and silver sulfadiazine reduced the incidence of significant bacterial growth on both the tip and intradermal segments of coated triple-lumen catheters, but had no effect on the incidence of catheter-related bacteremia [31].

However, in a series of 105 patients with central venous catheters placed while they were in the emergency room (neurotrauma, medical/surgical critically ill patients), there was a reduction in catheter contamination and in frequency of catheter removal when the patients received a chlorhexidine- and silver sulfadiazine–impregnated catheter [32].

In another study similar results on colonization were observed in 351 catheters inserted in 228 ICU patients. However, the reduction in catheter-related sepsis [8 infections (4.7%), versus 3 infections (1.7%)] was not statistically significant [33]. Similar results on colonization were observed in a total of 204 critically ill patients with 235 central venous catheters. These patients received either a standard triple-lumen polyurethane catheter or an antiseptic catheter impregnated with chlorhexidine and silver sulfadiazine. The study showed that central venous catheters with antiseptic coating were safe and had less risk of being contaminated by bacteria and fungi than standard catheters [34].

Furthermore, the use of benzalkonium chloride-impregnated central venous catheters failed to decrease the incidence of catheter-related contamination and bacteremia in patients treated with intensive chemotherapy for acute leukemia, lymphoma, or solid tumors [35].

Hence, the antiseptic-coated catheter appears to reduce catheter contamination, but the ability to prevent catheter-related infection has to be demonstrated in further studies.

A multicenter randomized clinical trial of antiseptic-coated catheters was performed in 281 hospitalized patients who required 298 triple-lumen, polyurethane venous catheters. Contamination occurred in 36 (26%) uncoated catheters and 11 (8%) coated catheters ($p<0.001$). CRBI developed in 7 patients (5%) with uncoated catheters and no patients with coated catheters ($p<0.01$). Multivariate logistic regression analysis showed that coating catheters with minocycline and rifampin was an independent protective factor against catheter-related contamination ($p<0.05$) [36].

Recently, Darouiche et al. [37] compared the rates of catheter contamination and CRBI associated with two different antibiotic-impregnated triple-lumen catheters (minocycline and rifampin covering the luminal and external surfaces versus chlorhexidine and silver sulfadiazine covering only the external surface). These catheters were inserted in high-risk adult patients and were expected to remain in place for 3 days or more. Catheters impregnated with minocycline and rifampin were a third more likely to be contaminated than catheters impregnated with chlorhexidine and silver sulfadiazine [28 of 356 catheters (7.9%) versus 87 of 382 (22.8%), $p<0.001$]. CRBI was one-twelfth more likely in catheters impregnated with minocycline and rifampin [1 of 356 (0.3%) versus 13 of 382 (3.4%) for those impregnated with chlorhexidine and silver sulfadiazine ($p<0.002$)] [37]. However, this study suggested that the growth of microorganisms cultured from the tip of a catheter could be reduced by the residual antimicrobial activity of the bound antibiotic [38].

In pediatric patients a prospective double-blind randomized controlled study was performed to determine whether heparin bonding (HB) reduces the incidence of catheter-related thrombosis and infection in critically ill children. The study was performed in 209 patients, admitted to the ICU and needing a central venous line (CVL). The study shows a significant reduction in the incidence of infection and thrombosis associated with the use of a HB CVL [39]. We would like to recommend the use of this HB catheter, but more studies are necessary to evaluate the use of antibiotic and antiseptic-coated central venous catheters in pediatric patients.

Two randomized controlled trials have been published in the last few years on the insertion site (femoral versus subclavian). The subclavian site is useful. However, in a randomized clinical trial of 336 patients with femoral tunnelled catheters, there was a reduction of patients who developed systemic catheter-related sepsis [relative risk 0.25 (CI 0.09–0.72), $p=0.005$] and of positive quantitative culture on the catheter tip [relative risk 0.48 (CI 0.23–0.99), $p=0.045$] [40].

Another randomized controlled clinical trial was conducted on 289 critically ill adult patients receiving a first central venous catheter. Patients were randomly assigned to undergo central venous catheterization at the femoral site ($n=145$) or the subclavian site ($n=144$). Femoral catheterization was associated with a higher incidence rate of overall infectious complications (19.8% versus 4.5%, $p<0.001$, incidence density of 20 versus 3.7 per 1,000 catheter-days) and of major infectious complications (clinical sepsis with or without bloodstream infection, 4.4% versus 1.5%, $p=0.07$, incidence density of 4.5 versus 1.2 per 1,000 catheter-days) [41].

Pulmonary Artery Catheters

Pulmonary artery catheters are widely used for the hemodynamic management of critically ill patients. The frequency of pulmonary artery CRBI may have decreased in recent years for several reasons: (1) insertion through an introducer on teflon which is more resistant to microbial adherence than the formerly used polyvinyl chloride; (2) shorter duration of use of pulmonary catheters compared with other central venous catheters; (3) widespread use of HB pulmonary catheter in which the heparin is associated with benzalkonium chloride, a compound with some antimicrobial activity; (4) the use of a sheath during the insertion. Generally the optimal time to maintain the pulmonary catheter on site seems to be no more than 4 days [42].

In conclusion, intravascular device policies can be summarized as follows: (1) educate the staff and apply a surveillance program with a restrictive antibiotic policy; (2) hand washing needs adequate attention, (3) always use barrier precautions during the insertion; (4) consider a cutaneous antisepsis and the use of dressing (a sterile gauze is adequate and less expensive); (5) the routine change of central catheters is not necessary and expensive; (6) a decreased manipulation of administration sets, with a more careful technique and less-frequent set replacement may reduce the risk of infection; (7) the literature does not offer clear indications on the prophylactic use of antimicrobial agents before or during the insertion of an intravascular device.

The effects of some proposed device management methods on CRBI infection are summarized in Table 1.

Table 1. Proposed device management based on guidelines of 1996 and on randomized controlled trials of the last 5 years for prevention of catheter-related bloodstream infection (CRBI) (*ICU* intensive care unit)

Device management	Effect on CRBI prevention	References
Use a restrictive antibiotic control program	Positive	[4]
Perform an infection surveillance system	Positive	[5]
Stress nurse/physician hand hygiene in the ICU	Positive	[3, 6-10]
Use 0.5% tincture of chlorhexidine instead of 10% povidone–iodine	Uncertain	[11, 12]
Use a transparent dressing instead of standard dressing	Uncertain or negative	[13, 14]
Remove any intravascular device only when clinically indicated	Positive	[15, 16]
Replace administration sets no more than every 72 h	Positive	[3]
Decrease manipulation of administration sets	Positive	[3]
Teicoplanin given at the time of insertion	Negative	[19]
Use midline catheters	Positive	[21]
Rotate peripheral venous sites every 48–72 h	Positive	[3]
Remove peripheral venous catheters at the signs of phlebitis	Positive	[3]
Apply topical antimicrobial ointment	Negative	[3]
Define an IV therapy dedicated team	Positive	[22]
Replace arterial catheters no more frequently than every 4 days	Positive	[3, 23]
Use multilumen central venous catheters instead of single lumen	Positive	[24]
Use silver-coated central venous catheters	Uncertain	[26]
Use silver impregnation of the internal and external surfaces of the catheter	Positive but uncertain on infection	[36-38]
Use antiseptic-impregnated catheters	Positive on contamination but uncertain on infection	[28-35]
Use antibiotic-coated catheters	Positive on contamination but uncertain on infection	[36-38]
In pediatric patients use a heparin bonding catheter	Positive	[39]
Prefer subclavian instead of non-tunnelled femoral site	Positive	[40, 41]
Maintain the arterial pulmonary catheter on site no more than 4 days	Positive	[42]

Device Policies to Prevent VAP

VAP typically refers to nosocomial pneumonia developing more than 48 h following endotracheal intubation and mechanical ventilation. VAP is associated with approximately a 4-day increase in length of ICU stay and an attributable mortality of approximately 20%–30% [43].

Fixed VAP risk factors include underlying cardiorespiratory disease, neurological injury, and trauma. Modifiable VAP risk factors (Table 2) include some aspects of general ICU management and ventilator and airway management [43].

There is a great deal of controversy about the methods for the prevention of this infection. Prevention of VAP relies on basic infection control practices and on many specific strategies interfering with colonization routes, e.g., selective decontamination of the digestive tract (Chapter 14).

Infection control for VAP should also consider practices based on staff education and infection surveillance programs. It seems to be useful to educate healthcare workers about the risks of bacterial pneumonia and the procedures that patients need. For example, 16 intensive care nurses were trained to improve the practice of endotracheal suctioning. This showed significant improvements in both knowledge and practice [44]. It also seems necessary to conduct a surveillance program for bacterial pneumonia in ICU patients at high risk for nosocomial pneumonia to determine trends and identify potential problems, including data regarding the causative micro-organisms and their antimicrobial susceptibility patterns. Data should be presented as rates (e.g., number of infected patients or infections per 100 ICU days or per 1,000 ventilator-days) to facilitate intra-hospital comparisons [45, 46].

In order to avoid person-to-person transmission of bacteria we should respect some general recommendations regarding hand washing, barrier precautions, and the suction of respiratory tract secretions. The use of a multi-use closed-system suction catheter instead of the single-use open-system catheter for prevention of pneumonia seems to reduce the incidence rate of VAP without demonstrating any adverse effects [47].

To avoid the transmission of micro-organisms we should consider the sterilization or disinfection and maintenance of equipment and devices following these procedures: sterilize or use high-level disinfection for semi-critical equipment or devices, for example items that come into direct or indirect contact with the lower respiratory tract. Do not routinely sterilize or disinfect the internal machinery of mechanical ventilators and do not change the breathing circuit more frequently than every 48 h including tubing and exhalation valve. The elimination of routine ventilator circuit changes can reduce medical care costs without increasing the incidence of nosocomial pneumonia in patients who require prolonged mechanical ventilation [48]. At present, there are no rec-

Table 2. Risk factors for ventilator-associated pneumonia (from reference [43]) (*COPD* chronic obstructive pulmonary disease, *ARDS* acute respiratory distress syndrome, *OSF*, organ system failure)

Related to population	Age
	Cardiorespiratory disease
	COPD
	ARDS
	Coma
	Neurosurgery
	Head trauma, polytrauma
	Burns
	OSF
Ventilatory and airway management	Mechanical ventilation
	Intracuff pressure < 20 cmH$_2$O
	Reintubation
	24-h circuit changes
	Tracheostomy
	Failed subglottic aspiration
General ICU management	Enteral nutrition
	Supine positioning
	Aspiration
	H2-receptor antagonists
	Paralytic agents
	Antibiotics
	Transport out of the ICU

ommendations for the maximum length of time after which the breathing circuit and the attached bubbling or humidifier of a ventilator should be changed. Sterilize reusable breathing circuits and bubbling or humidifiers, or subject them to high-level disinfection between their use on different patients. Periodically drain and discard any condensation that collects in the tubing of a mechanical ventilator, taking precautions not to allow condensation to drain towards the patient. Wash hands after performing the procedure or handling the fluid. It does not seem necessary to place a filter at the distal end of the expiratory-phase tubing of the breathing circuit to collect condensation. Do not place bacterial filters between the humidifier reservoir and the inspiratory-phase tubing of the breathing circuit of a mechanical ventilator. Always use sterile water to fill the humidifier [49].

An unresolved issue is the use of a hygroscopic condenser/humidifier or a heat and moisture exchanger (HME) rather than a heated humidifier. In 1997, Rathgeber et al. [50] demonstrated that a HME with electric filters prevents

47. Combes P, Fauvage B, Oleyer C (2000) Nosocomial pneumonia in mechanically venti-
     lated patients, a prospective randomised evaluation of the Stericath closed suctioning
     system. Intensive Care Med 26:878–882
48. Kollef MH, Shapiro SD, Fraser VJ et al (1995) Mechanical ventilation with or without
     7-day circuit changes. A randomized controlled trial. Ann Intern Med 123:168–174
49. Favero MS (1989) Principles of sterilization and disinfection. Anesth Clin N Am
     7:941–949
50. Rathgeber J, Kietzmann D, Mergeryan H et al (1997) Prevention of patient bacterial
     contamination of anaesthesia-circle-systems: a clinical study of the contamination
     risk and performance of different heat and moisture exchangers with electret filter
     (HMEF). Eur J Anaesthesiol 14:368–373
51. Boots RJ, Howe S, George N et al (1997) Clinical utility of hygroscopic heat and moi-
     sture exchangers in intensive care patients. Crit Care Med 25:1707–1701
52. Memish ZA, Oni GA, Djazmati W et al (2001) A randomized clinical trial to compare
     the effects of a heat and moisture exchanger with a heated humidifying system on the
     occurrence rate of ventilator-associated pneumonia. Am J Infect Control 29:301–305
53. Kirton OC, DeHaven B, Morgan J et al (1997) A prospective, randomized comparison
     of an in-line heat moisture exchange filter and heated wire humidifiers: rates of ven-
     tilator-associated early-onset (community-acquired) or late-onset (hospital-acquired)
     pneumonia and incidence of endotracheal tube occlusion. Chest 112:1055–1059
54. Davis K Jr, Evans SL, Campbell RS et al (2000) Prolonged use of heat and moisture
     exchangers does not affect device efficiency or frequency rate of nosocomial pneu-
     monia. Crit Care Med 28:1412–1418
55. Blunt MC, Young PJ, Patil A, Haddock A (2001) Gel lubrication of the tracheal tube cuff
     reduces pulmonary aspiration. Anesthesiology 95:377–381
56. Holdgaard HO, Pedersen J, Jensen RH et al (1998) Percutaneous dilatational tracheo-
     stomy versus conventional surgical tracheostomy. A clinical randomised study. Acta
     Anaesthesiol Scand 42:545–550
57. Garibaldi RA (1993) Hospital acquired UTI. In: Wenzel RP (ed) Prevention and con-
     trol: nosocomial infections, 2nd edn. Williams and Wilkins, Baltimore, pp 600-610
58. Wilson C, Sandhu SS, Kaisary AV (1997) A prospective randomized study comparing
     a catheter-valve with a standard drainage system. Br J Urol 80:915–917
59. Karchmer TB, Giannetta ET, Muto CA et al (2000) A randomized crossover study of sil-
     ver-coated urinary catheters in hospitalized patients. Arch Intern Med 160:3294–3298
60. Darouiche RO, Smith JA Jr, Hanna H et al (1999) Efficacy of antimicrobial-impregna-
     ted bladder catheters in reducing catheter-associated bacteriuria: a prospective, ran-
     domized, multicenter clinical trial. Urology 54:976–981

Chapter 12

Antibiotic Policies in the Intensive Care Unit

H.K.F. VAN SAENE, N.J. REILLY, A. DE SILVESTRE, G. NARDI

Why Does an Intensivist Need an Antibiotic Policy?

Every intensive care unit (ICU) should have well-structured guidelines on the use of antimicrobial agents to guarantee that patients requiring intensive care receive appropriate antimicrobials for a relevant period to prevent and treat infections. These guidelines should meet the therapeutic needs of the consultants and allow the intensivist, clinical microbiologist, and pharmacist to monitor efficacy, toxicity, including allergy and diarrhea, and side-effects, such as the emergence of resistant strains and subsequent outbreaks of superinfections. Calculation of infection rates is only feasible following the implementation of an antibiotic policy. Apart from audit and research, antimicrobial guidelines aid educational programs and enable the clinical pharmacist to control drug expenditure.

Main Feature of Antibiotic Guidelines

The main feature of an antibiotic policy in the ICU is the use of a minimum of well-established antimicrobial agents that are associated with a minimum of side-effects, but also allow the control of the three patterns of ICU infections due to the 15 potentially pathogenic micro-organisms (PPM) (Chapters 4 and 5).

Antimicrobials Chosen on the Basis of Three Characteristics

Preservation of Indigenous Flora

Control of the abnormal flora, including (potentially resistant) aerobic gram-negative bacilli (AGNB) and methicillin-resistant *Staphylococcus aureus*

(MRSA), by normal indigenous mainly anaerobic flora is termed "microbial ecology" [1]. The normal flora has been shown to provide resistance to acquisition and subsequent carriage of PPM, and constitutes the microbial component of the carriage defense (Chapter 2). Antimicrobial agents that are active against the indigenous anaerobic flora, and that are excreted into throat and gut via saliva, bile, and mucus in lethal concentrations, may suppress the indigenous flora. Diarrhea and candidiasis are well known side-effects of commonly used antibiotics. The use of antimicrobial agents that disregard ecology leads to an impaired microbial factor of the carriage defense and promotes overgrowth of abnormal AGNB [2] and MRSA [3], as well as *Clostridium difficile* [4] and vancomycin-resistant enterococci (VRE) [5]. Narrow-spectrum antimicrobials can be defined as antimicrobials that only cover the 15 aerobic PPM, leaving the indigenous normal flora more or less intact [6]. Broad-spectrum antimicrobials are not only active against the 15 disease-causing PPM but also affect the normal indigenous anaerobic flora that contributes to physiology rather than infection. From an ecological perspective, ampicillin, amoxycillin, and flucloxacillin are antimicrobials with a spectrum that is broader than that of cephradine and cefotaxime [7–11]. The most recent ever more potent antimicrobials generally belong to the group of ecology disregarding antimicrobials that predispose to, e.g., AGNB, MRSA, and yeast overgrowth and subsequent superinfection [3, 12–15] (Table 1).

Table 1. Classification of parenteral antimicrobials based on respect for ecology

Indigenous flora friendly	Indigenous flora suppressing
Challenge studies in volunteers	
cephradine	ampicillin
cefotaxime	amoxicillin
Comparative studies in patients	
cephradine	amoxicillin
penicillin	ampicillin
Observational studies in patients	
gentamicin	flucloxacillin
tobramycin	amoxicillin + clavulanic acid
amikacin	piperacillin + tazobactam
polymyxins	ciprofloxacin
polyenes	carbapenems
metronidazole	macrolides

Limitation of the Emergence of Resistant Microbes by Using Antimicrobials with the Lowest Resistance Potential

If resistance occurs during drug development or clinical trials, or within 2 years of general use, the antibiotic has a high resistance potential [16]. Ceftazidime-resistant, ciprofloxacin-resistant, and imipenem-resistant *Pseudomonas aeruginosa* were reported during clinical trials and early after were introduced for general use [17–19]. Antimicrobials with little or no resistance potential include cephradine, piperacillin, cefotaxime, amikacin, and meropenem (Table 2) [19–22]. Three observations have emerged from this historical experience: (1) each antibiotic class has one or more antimicrobials capable of causing antibiotic resistance, but this is not a class phenomenon; antibiotic resistance is agent specific; (2) resistance is not related to duration of use; and (3) resistance is not related to volume of use.

Table 2. Classification of parenteral antimicrobials based on the potential for resistance

Low resistance	High resistance
piperacillin	ampicillin
cephradine	ceftazidime
cefotaxime	gentamicin
cefepime	ciprofloxacin
amikacin	imipenem
levofloxacin	
meropenem	

The underlying mechanisms explaining the difference between antibiotics with a high and a low resistance potential are not fully understood, but are thought to be based on specific antibiotic resistance mechanisms. For example, among the aminoglycosides, only gentamicin has been associated with widespread *P. aeruginosa* resistance, but amikacin continues to be effective against most gentamicin-resistant *P. aeruginosa*. Gentamicin is an aminoglycoside that is highly susceptible to inactivation by a variety of enzymes at six different loci on the gentamicin molecule, but amikacin has only one such vulnerable point that is subject to enzyme inactivation [23]. It was postulated that the substitution of amikacin for gentamicin would decrease *P. aeruginosa* susceptibilities to gentamicin. The substitution of amikacin for gentamicin decreased gentamicin-resistant *P. aeruginosa* when amikacin was used in the same volume as gentamicin, and no subsequent resistance problems developed. Some institutions with renewed gentamicin susceptibility to *P. aeruginosa* returned to using gentamicin as the major hospital aminoglycoside (i.e., rotating formularies) [24]. Predictably, gentamicin-resistant *P. aeruginosa* isolates returned to previous levels and were perpetuated as long as gentamicin was the primary aminoglycoside used in the hospital and ICU. Some people believe that these aminoglycoside lessons of the past should be applied to the problems of *P. aeruginosa* resistant to ceftazidime, ciprofloxacin, and imipenem. The substitution of cefepime, levofloxacin, and meropenem for ceftazidime, ciprofloxacin, and imipenem may decrease or even eliminate resistant *P. aeruginosa* from the ICU environment [25–27]. According to the concept of low and high resistance potential of antimicrobial agents, the key to controlling antibiotic resistance is agent related, and is not class, duration, or volume associated.

Control of Inflammation by Using Antimicrobials with Anti-endotoxin/Inflammation Properties

Lipopolysaccharide (LPS) or endotoxin is the major component of the outer membrane of AGNB, and is thought to be a key molecule in the induction of generalized inflammation. LPS causes the production and release from host effector cells of various pro-inflammatory cytokines and other mediators of inflammation, such as nitric oxide and prostaglandins. The degree to which these mediators are released depends, in part, on the amount of LPS that is presented to CD14-bearing effector cells such as monocytes, macrophages, and polymorphonuclear leukocytes. Therefore, it is possible that factors that affect the amount of LPS that is released in vivo may modulate the inflammatory response associated with AGNB infection. Several in vitro and animal studies show that antimicrobial agents may differentially release LPS from AGNB [28, 29]. They also demonstrated that antibiotics associated with substantial release of endotoxin result in the generation of higher levels of pro-inflammatory cytokines, and suggested that the use of antimicrobials associated with the release of lower amounts of LPS leads to lower levels of cytokinemia and better outcome. Carbapenems such as imipenem and meropenem have been shown to release a small amount of endotoxin, whilst third-generation cephalosporins such as ceftazidime and cefotaxime are associated with far greater release of endotoxin [30]. Three clinical trials failed to support this hypothesis that differential antibiotic-induced endotoxin release is of clinical significance, as there were no significant differences in clinical parameters (temperature, blood pressure, or heart rate) or plasma endotoxin and cytokine levels [31–33].

Fluoroquinolones such as ciprofloxacin release substantial amounts of endotoxin compared with the aminoglycosides gentamicin and tobramycin and with the polymyxins both E (colistin) and B [34, 35]. Although not active against AGNB, glycopeptides, including teicoplanin [36] and vancomycin [37], and polyenes, such as amphotericin B [38], have been shown to downregulate the LPS-induced cytokine release (Table 3).

Table 3. Classification of antimicrobials based on their anti-inflammation propensities

Inflammation controlling	Inflammation promoting
aminoglycosides	β-lactams
glycopeptides	cefotaxime ceftazidime
polymyxins	
polyenes	fluoroquinolones ciprofloxacin
carbapenems	

The classification of antimicrobials using these three criteria of flora friendliness, low resistance potential, and anti-inflammation propensity is not evidence based, i.e., not evaluated in randomized trials. However, despite the lack of level 1 evidence, we found the available data compelling and difficult to ignore in selecting antimicrobials for our antibiotic policy.

The use of a limited number of antimicrobial agents allows the control of the 15 potential pathogens implicated in the three types of ICU infections. The main groups are: (1) the β-lactams, i.e., antibiotics with a β-lactam ring in their structure such as penicillins and cephalosporins, (2) the aminoglycosides, e.g., tobramycin, (3) the polymyxins, e.g., polymyxin E or colistin, (4) the glycopeptides, e.g., vancomycin, and (5) polyenes such as amphotericin B.

All these antimicrobial agents are lethal to micro-organisms. The polymyxins, glycopeptides, and polyenes have a rapid action on the microbial cell membrane. The β-lactams interfere with the cell wall synthesis, a slower mechanism of action. The aminoglycosides inhibit the synthesis of protein, but still kill microbes in the rest phase. These differences in mechanism of action may explain why aminoglycosides and polyenes are more toxic to the ICU patient than β-lactams when parenterally administered. Table 4 shows the spectrum of activity of the five main antimicrobial groups according to the minimal bactericidal concentration (MBC) for the 15 PPMs. The MBC of an antimicrobial agent is defined as the amount of the antimicrobial (mg/l) required to establish irreversible inhibition in the test tube, without the support of the killing activity of the leukocytes of the ICU patient. Leukocytes of the critically ill are thought to be less effective in killing PPM than those of a healthy population [39]. Antimicrobial agents with an MBC of ≤1 mg/l for PPM are in general suitable for clinical use. Non-toxic antibiotics such as the β-lactams are ideal for systemic administration, and high doses (50-100 mg/kg per day) can be given. The more toxic agents, such as the polymyxins and the polyenes, can be safely applied enterally and topically in high doses. Polyenes given parenterally are toxic and the daily doses are in the order of milligrams (1.5 mg/kg per day for amphotericin B). Aminoglycosides and glycopeptides, although toxic, are administered systemically in lower doses (5–25 mg/kg per day).

Antimicrobial Use for Both Prophylaxis and Therapy Falls into Three Categories

Parenteral Antimicrobials

Parenteral antimicrobials aim to prevent and, if already present, to eradicate colonization/infection of the internal organs, including blood, lungs, and bladder. Systemic prophylaxis is generally accepted in surgery [40]. The aim is to achieve a tissue concentration at the time of the surgical trauma in order to prevent wound infections. Patients who require intensive care due to an acute trauma or worsening of the underlying disease invariably receive invasive devices, including ventilation tube, urinary catheter, and intravascular lines. These interventions are well known risk factors for lower airway, bladder, and bloodstream infections in the ICU patient whose immunoparalysis is at its nadir during the 1st week of admission. This is the time period during which primary endogenous infections occur. Only the immediate administration of parenteral antimicrobials enables the prevention of this type of infection and the early therapy of an already incubating primary endogenous infection. If the primary endogenous infection is the indication for admission to the ICU, parenteral antimicrobials are required to treat the established infection. The philosophy that prevention of infection is always better than cure dictates the immediate administration of systemic antibiotics to a critically ill patient requiring mechanical ventilation. Hence, systemic cefotaxime is an integral part of the concept of the prophylactic protocol of selective decontamination of the digestive tract (SDD) [41].

The criteria for parenteral antibiotics include flora friendliness and low resistance potential (after excretion into throat and gut via saliva, bile, and mucus) and anti-inflammation propensity. In addition, the pharmacokinetic properties should include a high excretion in the target organs and in particular in the bronchial secretions. The ratio of the antimicrobial level in the target organ and the MBC (Table 4) determine the efficacy against a particular micro-

Table 4. Spectrum of activity of the commonly used antimicrobial agents for the 15 potential pathogens expressed by the minimal bactericidal concentration (MBC) (mg/l)

PPM	Penicillin G	Cephradine	Cefotaxime	Ceftazidime	Aminoglycosides e.g. tobramycin	Polymyxins e.g. polymyxin E	Glycopeptides e.g. vancomycin	Polyenes e.g. amphotericin B
"Normal"								
S. pneumoniae	0.1		0.2	(2)				
H. influenzae			0.06	0.2	1			
M. catarrhalis			1	1	1			
E. coli			0.02	0.2	0.2	0.1		
S. aureus		1	1	(8.0)	0.2		0.05	
Candida spp								0.05
"Abnormal"								
Klebsiella			0.1	0.1	0.1	0.1		
Proteus			0.1	0.1	0.2			
Morganella			0.1	0.1	0.2			
Citrobacter			0.3	0.3	0.1	0.1		
Enterobacter			0.2	0.2	0.1	0.1		
Serratia			1	1	0.2			
Acinetobacter			(8)	(8)	0.1	0.1		
Pseudomonas			-	0.1	0.1	0.5		
MRSA							1.0	

PPM, potentially pathogenic micro-organisms; *MRSA*, methicillin-resistant *Staphylococcus aureus*

organism (Chapter 7). Protein binding should be minimal. The parenteral antimicrobial requires a good safety profile in terms of allergy, nephro- and ototoxicity, and influence on hemostasis. Finally, the target PPM is a criterion of paramount importance for the choice of a parenteral antimicrobial. Primary endogenous infections are caused by both "normal", e.g., *Streptococcus pneumoniae*, *Haemophilus influenzae*, and *S. aureus*, and "abnormal" potential pathogens, including AGNB and MRSA. General health before admission to the ICU influences the carrier state (Chapter 2). Previously healthy individuals such as trauma, burn, acute liver, and pancreatitis patients only carry normal potential pathogens, whilst patients with chronic underlying diseases, including chronic obstructive pulmonary disease, diabetes, and alcoholism, may carry AGNB and MRSA. It is obvious that patients referred to the ICU from other hospitals or wards are highly likely to be carriers of abnormal potential pathogens. Taking these criteria into consideration there are only a few antimicrobials suitable for prophylaxis. The first- and second-generation β-lactams cover the normal potential pathogens, but are less effective against the abnormal AGNB. Cefotaxime, a third-generation cephalosporin, has an adequate spectrum towards both normal and abnormal AGNB, with the exception of *P. aeruginosa* and *Acinetobacter* species. Ceftazidime adequately covers AGNB, but at the expense of *S. aureus*. Cefepime may be a suitable alternative for ceftazidime. Three randomized SDD trials used the fluoroquinolones ciprofloxacin and ofloxacin as systemic prophylaxis despite the inadequate cover of *S. pneumoniae* [42–44]. Most SDD studies employed cefotaxime as parenteral antimicrobial. Many patients admitted to a medical/surgical ICU receive peri-operative prophylaxis. This surgical prophylaxis may be replaced by cefotaxime as soon as SDD is started. In patients in whom prosthetic material has been implanted, an appropriate endocarditis prophylaxis should also be given. It is not uncommon that patients with a generalized inflammation state on admission to the ICU receive an aminoglycoside to control inflammation, in addition to cefotaxime.

Colonization of the lower airways, in particular with *S. aureus*, MRSA, *P. aeruginosa*, and *Aspergillus fumigatus*, may persist despite adequate systemic therapy. Cephradine, vancomycin, polymyxin E, cefotaxime, ceftazidime, gentamicin, tobramycin, and amphotericin B can be nebulized to achieve higher antibiotic concentrations in the lower airways. The ventilation tube is often contaminated and has to be changed and replaced by a new tube following nebulization. Surveillance swabs of the oropharynx are required to monitor the efficacy of the therapy. Chapter 23 discusses in detail the fundamental features of infection therapy: (1) sterilization of the infected internal organ using parenteral antibiotic(s); (2) source elimination with enteral antibiotics; (3) removal or change of the foreign device; and (4) evaluation of efficacy of therapy using surveillance samples.

Enteral Non-Absorbable Antimicrobials

Enteral non-absorbable antimicrobials aim to prevent and, if already present, to eradicate carriage and overgrowth of abnormal flora from throat and gut. The abnormal carrier state always precedes secondary endogenous infections. Whilst parenteral antimicrobials are required to control primary endogenous infections, enteral non-absorbable antibiotics aim to prevent secondary endogenous infections [45]. The commonly used decontaminating agents include polymyxin E, tobramycin, amphotericine B, or nystatin and vancomycin. They all fulfil the three requirements of narrow spectrum or ecology friendliness, low resistance potential, and anti-inflammation properties. Additionally, they are non-absorbable in order to achieve high salivary and fecal concentrations, and as all antimicrobials they are inactivated by fiber, cells, and fecal material to varying extents. Tobramycin and polymyxin are minimally and moderately inactivated, respectively. The polyenes and vancomycin require high oral doses due to a high inactivation rate (Chapter 9). For decontaminating agents to be effective, a minimal contact time between antimicrobial and abnormal potential pathogen of 15 min is required. This contact time is no problem in the stomach and gut due to ileus, and is guaranteed by the application of a paste or a gel in the oropharynx. High failure rates of oral sprays and rinses of antimicrobials have been reported (Chapter 27). Apart from nystatin, all antimicrobials used for SDD are administered parenterally in spite of their toxicity. Toxicity is a lesser problem following enteral administration, even in high doses. Chapter 9 discusses the significant reductions in carriage of AGNB, yeasts, and MRSA following the enteral use of polymyxin/tobramycin, polyenes, and vancomycin. Interestingly, amongst the 15 target PPMs, three micro-organisms *P. aeruginosa*, *Candida* species, and MRSA are less easy to completely clear from the throat and/or gut. It is not uncommon that the surveillance swabs yield very low concentrations of yeasts, MRSA, and *P. aeruginosa* even during long-term SDD use. Apparently, reducing overgrowth to very low growth densities is sufficient to control infection, resistance, and transmission [46, 47].

Topical Antimicrobials

Topical antimicrobials aim to prevent and, if already present, to eradicate colonization/infection of abnormal flora from wounds in which plastic devices may be present such as tracheostoma and gastrostoma. Wounds, in particular burn wounds, are prone to acquisition and subsequent exogenous colonization/infection with potential pathogens such as *P. aeruginosa* and MRSA, without previous carriage in the digestive tract. Gels including aquaform and intrasite are very suitable for the application of antimicrobials to burn wounds [48]. The concentration of for example polymyxin E or vancomycin is in general 2%. Each application has to be preceded by debridement of the wound and cleaning with a disinfecting agent such as 2% tauroline, to remove necrotic tissue that may inactivate polymyxin E or vancomycin. The transparent gels allow careful inspection of wound healing and granulating tissue. Tracheostoma and gastrostoma are artificially created long-term wounds kept open by plastic devices. Potential pathogens such as *P. aeruginosa* and non-*aeruginosa*, *Acinetobacter baumannii*, and *S. aureus*, both methicillin sensitive and resistant, have an intrinsic affinity for plastic. Colonization/infection of exogenous origin is not uncommon in patients with tracheostoma and/or gastrostoma. As it is virtually impossible to sterilize plastic using parenteral agents, the devices have to be removed and the wounds to be cleaned with taurolin. A thin layer of a paste containing 2% of polymyxin E and/or vancomycin is applied to the stoma before a new device is put in. Obviously prevention of colonization/infection of tracheostoma and gastrostoma using the paste twice daily throughout ICU treatment is preferred to therapy of colonization/infection [49].

Efficacy in Relation to Duration of Antimicrobial Therapy

Parenteral Antimicrobials

The prevention of primary endogenous infection is the main reason for the use of parenteral antimicrobials, being one of the crucial components of the SDD protocol. Supplementary prophylaxis is the second reason for its use [50]: cover during establishment of SDD on mucosal surfaces, cover for procedurally released micro-organisms, and elimination from mucosal surfaces of PPM resistant to the enteral antimicrobials, e.g., *S. pneumoniae* is resistant to polymyxins, aminoglycosides, and polyenes.

The duration of parenteral prophylaxis as an integral part of SDD depends on the type of carrier state, i.e., normal versus abnormal. The maximum period of parenteral prophylaxis is 5 days for patients with abnormal flora. The oropharynx and gut (not rectal cavity) are expected to be free from abnormal AGNB and MRSA within 3 days of enteral antimicrobials. In patients who were previously healthy, a shorter period of 3 or even 2 days has been shown to be effective [51].

According to the guidelines of the American Thoracic Society, lower airway infections due to normal potential pathogens, including *H. influenzae* and *S. aureus*, should be treated for 7–10 days, whereas episodes caused by *P. aeruginosa* and *Acinetobacter species* should be treated for at least 14–21 days [52]. The guidelines are based on 'expert' opinion. There is only one randomised controlled trial evaluating whether a short course of intravenous antimicrobial therapy of 1 week is as effective as a prolonged treatment of equal or more than

2 weeks [53]. These investigators showed that there is no evidence to support an antibiotic course exceeding one week. A third approach for determining the duration of antibiotic therapy is the use of inflammation markers including C-reactive protein. Five prospective studies show that a course of appropriate antimicrobials of <1 week results in significant improvements of clinical, radiographic, and microbiological parameters [54-58].T here is no evidence to support the superiority of a 2-week course of intravenous antibiotics over a 1-week course, which prompted us to implement a parenteral antibiotic policy of 5 days, followed by a careful evaluation of the patients' clinical, radiographic, and microbiological parameters [59, 60].

Enteral Antimicrobials

The administration of enteral antimicrobials using a paste or gel and a suspension into the throat and gut, respectively, is indicated so long as the patient is immunoparalyzed, i.e., at high risk of acquiring abnormal flora and subsequently of developing an infection. SDD is generally given throughout the ICU treatment or, in practice, until extubation.

There is general consensus that long-term use of enteral polymyxin E/tobramycin/amphotericin B in the correct concentrations in throat and gut abolishes oropharyngeal and gastric carriage of the target PPM within a few days. Eradication of rectal carriage appears to depend on the presence of peristalsis and may vary until the patient produces faeces [61].

Topical Antimicrobials

Three days of topical application of polymyxin E/tobramycin/amphotericin B and/or vancomycin into wounds or tracheostoma or gastrostoma has been shown to eradicate the potential pathogens using daily sampling [48, 49]. Prevention of colonization/infection of wounds and stomas obviously requires the application of the topical antibiotics throughout the ICU treatment [49].

Endpoints of Antimicrobial Policies

A new antimicrobial agent launched by the pharmaceutical industry or a new antibiotic policy implemented in the ICU should be assessed using four main endpoints including morbidity, mortality, antimicrobial resistance, and costs (Table 5). The pharmaceutical industry is not often able to provide that information. If the superinfection rate associated with a particular antimicrobial is known, that figure is often diluted by the number of all patients enrolled in all

Table 5. Endpoints of antimicrobial policies

(i) Efficacy: clinical endpoints

- reduction in infectious morbidity (superinfection)
- reduction in mortality following the immediate administration of empirical antimicrobial

(ii) Safety: microbiological endpoints [using surveillance samples]

- impact on ecology: yeasts, *Clostridium* difficile (diarrhea)
- antimicrobial resistance: supercarriage of aerobic Gram-negative bacilli, methicillin-resistant *Staphylococcus aureus*, vancomycin-resistant enterococci

(iii) Costs

- duration: an antimicrobial course of <1 week is as good as that of ≥ 2 weeks
- is the newer more expensive antimicrobial superior than the older cheaper one in terms of efficacy and safety

studies, whether community, hospital-, or ICU-based, as denominator. Superinfection rates are invariably higher in the critically ill patients requiring intensive care, including mechanical ventilation, compared with patients staying on hospital wards. The more severely ill the patient population studied, the higher the superinfection rate. The mortality should be assessed following the immediate administration of the antimicrobial(s), as the delay of adequate therapy is associated with increased mortality [62, 63]. Immediate administration of an antimicrobial agent always implies an empirical decision in the absence of any knowledge of the causative micro-organism, although of course reasonable assumptions can be made depending upon the presentation of the disease [60]. It is highly likely that the patient carries "normal" potential pathogens in their admission flora if the patient was previously healthy (trauma, burn, acute liver failure, and pancreatitis patients). Patients with chronic underlying diseases, including alcoholism, chronic obstructive pulmonary disease, and diabetes, often import "abnormal" potential pathogens in their flora on admission. Patients referred from other hospitals or from the wards are generally ill and may bring abnormal bacteria associated with the hospital ecology into the ICU. Surveillance samples of throat and rectum taken at the time of admission may help in identifying the normal versus abnormal carrier state. These samples are also required to assess the impact of an antibiotic on the patient's ecology, and to monitor secondary or supercarriage of resistant bacteria. This information is invariably missing for most new antibiotics or antibiotic policies. New antibiotics are also recommended for 10 or more days and are always more expensive than the older antimicrobials that are often out of patent and inexpensive.

Our antimicrobial policy using the above criteria is shown in Chapter 18. A prospective, observational cohort study was performed over four years (1999–2003) to assess the efficacy, side-effects, and costs of this antibiotic policy. Only critically ill children requiring 4 or more days of intensive care were included in the epidemiological descriptive study [64]. This study group represents the sicker patients with longer pediatric ICU stays. Approximately two-thirds of pediatric ICU admissions did not meet the 4-day stay entry criterion for the study, and are not included in the denominator for infection rates. Short-stay patients have a low risk of developing secondary endogenous and exogenous infection, and we believe they should not be reported in the denominator of pediatric ICU infection rates. A total of 1,241 children were included in the study. There were 520 children with infections, an overall infection rate of 41.9%, viral infections accounted for 14.5% and bacterial/yeast infections for 33.0%. The incidence of blood stream infection and lower airway infection was 21.0 and 9.1 episodes per 1,000 patient-days; 13.3% of the children were infected with a micro-organism acquired on the pediatricICU; 4.0% of admitted patients developed infections due to resistant micro-organisms. The mortality in the study group was 9.6%.

References

1. Vollaard EJ, Clasener HAL (1994) Colonisation resistance. Antimicrob Agents Chemother 335:409–414
2. Vlaspolder F, Zeeuw G de, Rozenberg-Arska M et al (1987) The influence of flucloxacillin and amoxicillin with clavulanic acid on the aerobic flora of the alimentary tract. Infection 15:241–244
3. Harbarth S, Liassine N, Dharan S et al (2000) Risk factors for persistent carriage of methicillin-resistant *Staphylococcus aureus*. Clin Infect Dis 31:1380–1385
4. Shek FW, Stacey BSF, Rendell J et al (2000) The rise of *Clostridium difficile*: the effect of length of stay, patient age and antibiotic use. J Hosp Infect 45:235–237
5. Donskey CJ, Chowdry TK, Hecker MT et al (2000) Effect of antibiotic therapy on the density of vancomycin-resistant enterococci in the stool of colonised patients. N Engl J Med 343:1925–1932
6. van Saene R , Fairclough S, Petros A (1998) Broad- and narrow-spectrum antibiotics: a different approach. Clin Microbiol Infect 4:56–57
7. Buck AC, Cooke EM (1969) The fate of ingested *Pseudomonas aeruginosa* in normal persons. J Med Microbiol 2:521–525
8. van Saene HKF, Stoutenbeek CP, Geitz JN et al (1988) Effect of amoxycillin on colonisation resistance in human volunteers. Microb Ecol Health Dis 1:169–177
9. Vollaard EJ, Clasener HAL, Janssen AJHM et al (1990) Influence of amoxicillin on microbial colonisation resistance in healthy volunteers. A methodological study. J Antimicrob Chemother 25:861–871
10. Vollaard EJ, Clasener HAL, Janssen AJHM et al (1990) Influence of cefotaxime on microbial colonisation resistance in healthy volunteers. J Antimicrob Chemother

49. Morar P, Makura Z, Jones A et al (2000) Topical antibiotics on tracheostoma prevents exogenous colonisation and infection of lower airways in children. Chest 117:513–518
50. Alcock SR (1990) Short-term parenteral antibiotics used as a supplement to SDD regimens. Infection 13 [Suppl 1]:S14–S18
51. Sirvent JM, Torres A, El-Ebiary M et al (1997) Protective effect of intravenously administered cefuroxime against nosocomial pneumonia in patients with structural coma. Am J Respir Crit Care Med 155:1729–1734
52. Hospital-acquired pneumonia in adults: diagnosis, assessment of severity, initial antimicrobial therapy, and preventative strategies (1995). A consensus statement. Am J Respir Crit Care Med 153:1711–1725
53. Chastre J, Wolff M, Fagon JY et al (2003) Comparison of 8 vs 15 days of antibiotic therapy for ventilator-associated pneumonia in adults. A randomised trial. JAMA 290: 2588-2598
54. A'Court CHD, Garrard CS, Crook D et al (1993) Microbiological lung surveillance in mechanically ventilated patients, using non-directed bronchial lavage and quantitative culture. Q J Med 86:635–648
55. Montravers P, Fagon JY, Chastre J et al (1993) Follow-up protected specimen brushes to assess treatment in nosocomial pneumonia. Am Rev Respir Dis 147:38–44
56. Singh N, Rogers P, Atwood CW et al (2000) Short-course empiric antibiotic therapy for patients with pulmonary infiltrates in the intensive care unit. Am J Respir Crit Care Med 162:505–511
57. Dennesen PJW, van derVen AJAM, Kessels AGH et al (2001) Resolution of infectious parameters after antimicrobial therapy in patients with VAP. Am J Respir Crit Care Med 163:1371–1375
58. Ibrahim EH, Ward S, Sherman G et al (2001) Experience with a clinical guideline for the treatment of ventilator-associated pneumonia. Crit Care Med 29:1109–1115
59. Condon RE (2002) Bacterial resistance to antibiotics. Arch Surg 137:1417–1418
60. Torres A, Ewig S (2004) Diagnosing ventilator-associated pneumonia. N Engl J Med 350:433-435.
61. Ledingham I McA, Alcock SR, Eastaway AT et al (1988) Triple regimen of selective decontamination of the digestive tract, systemic cefotaxime, and microbiological surveillance for prevention of acquired infection in intensive care. Lancet I:785-790
62. Luna CM, Vujacich P, Niederman MS et al (1997) Impact of BAL data on the therapy and outcome of ventilator-associated pneumonia. Chest 111:676–685
63. Alvarez-Lerma F and the ICU-acquired Pneumonia Study Group (1996) Modification of empiric antibiotic treatment in patients with pneumonia acquired in the intensive care unit. Intensive Care Med 22:387–394
64. Sarginson RE, Taylor N, Reilly N et al (2004) Infection in prolonged pediatric critical illness: a prospective four year study based on knowledge of the carrier state. Crit Care Med 32: 839-847

Outbreaks of Infection in Intensive Care Units-Usefulness of Molecular Techniques for Outbreak Analysis

V. Damjanovic, X. Corbella, J.I. van der Spoel, H.K.F. van Saene

Introduction

In the first edition of the book *Infection Control in ICU* (1998) we described our experience with four outbreaks of infection on a neonatal intensive care unit (NICU) [1]. Subsequently we analyzed ten outbreaks of infection due *Pseudomonas aeruginosa* on NICU. For that exercise, we designed a framework for the description and analysis of an outbreak of infection based on 13 pieces of information [2]. This particular framework serves as the basis of this chapter.

This chapter describes the analysis of a total of 57 outbreaks [3–59] occurring on not only NICU [3–27] but also on pediatric (PICU) [28–37] and adult intensive care units (AICU) [38–59]. These 57 outbreaks were selected for their employment of molecular techniques in the analysis of the micro-organisms involved in the outbreaks. Traditionally, all isolates obtained during the outbreak were required to be identical to be the cause of the outbreak. Several techniques, including serotyping, biotyping, and antibiogram, were applied, but were not found to be reliable. The recent advent of molecular techniques has greatly improved the determination of outbreak isolates. These techniques are currently accepted as the gold standard. The three objectives of this analysis of 57 outbreaks are: (1) to assess whether outbreaks are invariably due to one clone of an outbreak strain; (2) to evaluate the impact of molecular techniques on the analysis of all key data relevant to the outbreak; (3) to clarify the contribution of molecular techniques to the management of an outbreak.

Methods of Analysis of Outbreaks

Search Strategy

We searched for outbreak reports published between 1 January 1990 and 30 June 2002. Studies were identified through Medline. The MeSH keywords used were 'intensive care unit', 'adult ICU', 'pediatric ICU' and 'neonatal ICU', and 'outbreaks'. All studies that tested the strains involved using molecular biological techniques were selected.

Definitions

Definitions were given for the key data (Table 1) that were not readily available in the outbreak reports: morbidity, carriage rate, information on the type of outbreak, i.e., endogenous versus exogenous development and clonality.

For the calculation of *morbidity* the following definition was used. Morbidity was defined in this study as the number of patients who developed an infection due to the outbreak strain divided by the total number of patients who were carriers of the outbreak strain in nose, throat, and/or gut, i.e., *endogenous* pathogenesis [1, 2]. In case of an *exogenous* infection, morbidity was defined as the number of patients who developed an exogenous infection divided by the number of patients who acquired the outbreak strain in normally sterile sites such as blood, lower airways, bladder, and wounds.

In many studies the term colonization was used to refer to persistence of the outbreak strain in the patient. In this analysis carriage was used (Table 1). With regard to the type of the outbreak, the terms *endogenous* and *exogenous* were only used following interpretation of the evidence from the cited report.

An outbreak was considered to be *monoclonal*, if one clone amongst the others investigated was the cause of the outbreak. *Polyclonal* outbreaks were due to more than one clone. Those with one predominant strain were distinguished from those without one predominant strain.

Framework of the Analysis

The original framework was comprised of 13 key data [2]. Two key data were added to the present analysis: (1) clonality results (monoclonal/polyclonal) were added to the endogenous or exogenous type of outbreak and (2) risk factor analysis (case-control studies). All 57 outbreaks were screened for 15 different key data related to the three elements crucial in the development of an outbreak of infection: source/organism, transmission, and susceptible host.

Table Presentation (Table 1)

In total, 57 outbreaks, 25 on the NICU [3–27], 10 on the PICU [28–37], and 22 on the AICU [38–59], were retrieved from the literature. The causative micro-organisms were presented in the following order: in alphabetical order aerobic Gram-negative bacilli (AGNB), yeasts, methicillin-sensitive (MSSA) and resist-ant *Staphylococcus aureus* (MRSA), coagulase-negative staphylococci, *Bacillus cereus*, and *Enterococcus faecium*. Within the same outbreak strain, outbreaks were presented chronologically, and in cases of the same year, the outbreaks were tabled using the first author in alphabetical order. There were two out-breaks of carriage, not infection, due to *Klebsiella oxytoca* [15] and *P. aerugi-nosa* [33] and one pseudo-outbreak caused by *Staphylococcus epidermidis* [26].

Results

Table 1 shows the 15 key data for the three different types of intensive care: NICU, PICU, and AICU.

Neonatal Intensive Care Unit

There were 13 outbreaks that were retrieved from the first half of the 1990s; the other 12 originated from the second part of the decade. Half of the outbreaks (13) were reported from Europe, 8 from North America (7 from USA), and 2 each from Australia and Africa. Six outbreaks that lasted for less than 2 months were retrieved. There were 11 studies describing outbreaks with duration vary-ing between 2 months and 1 year. Only 3 studied outbreaks lasting between 1 and 2 years and 4 prospective outbreaks of longer than 2 years were found in the literature search. One study did not report the duration of the outbreak.

Of the reported outbreaks, 60% were caused by *Klebsiella* (5), *Enterobacter* (4), *Acinetobacter* (3), and *Pseudomonas* (3). Application of molecular tech-niques was a criterion for inclusion in the analysis. Three studies from the early 1990s used plasmid profile analysis. All other studies employed analysis of chromosomal DNA, the majority of which were pulsed-field gel electrophoresis (PFGE) (7), arbitrary primed polymerase chain reaction (PCR) (4), and several other PCR variations (4). Different clones were labeled with different capital let-ters, e.g., A, B, C, etc. In the case of minor genetic variation, the capital letters were followed by an apostrophe, e.g., A', B', C', etc. Unique and different clones were denoted by X. Generally, more than 10 isolates were tested (19/25 out-breaks, 76%) in each of the outbreaks.

Table 1. Main characteristics (key data) of outbreak infection in intensive care units (ICU)

Location year duration	Organism		Source		Mode of transmission
	Species and strain clonality no. identical/ no. tested	Sensitivity to antibiotics used as 1st line	Inanimate	Animate	
[3] Nijmegen (Netherlands) 1998, 1999 2-year Prospective study	*Acinetobacter* (genomospecies 3 predominant) 29A,3B,3C/38; 3X	Not stated Resistant to amoxicillin cefuroxime	Not found	Not found	Hands of staff presumed
[4] Ghent (Belgium) 1993 1st outbreak 1 month 2nd outbreak 2 months	1st outbreak *Acinetobacter junii* 4/4	Not stated S not mentioned	Not found	Not found	Not identified
	2nd outbreak *Acinetobacter baumannii* 6/6	Not stated Decreased S to ampicillin, cefuroxime, colistin + SXT	Not found	Not found	Not identified
[5] Leiden (Netherlands) 1995 2 weeks	*Acinetobacter junii* 12A, 4B/18 2X	Not stated R to β-lactams	Not found	Not found	Not identified

RDS, respiratory distress syndrome; *S*, sensitive; *R*, resistant; *SXT*, cotrimoxazole; *RTI*, respiratory tract infection; *UTI*, urinary tract infection. Letter A, B = different clones; A', B' = minor genetic variation; X, unique, different from each other and from separate clones; *Surveillance cultures include throat and/or rectum (others)

Neonates				Surveillance cultures*		Type of outbreak Endogenous or exogenous: monoclonal or polyclonal	Outbreak control measures
Susceptibility		No. of infected neonates	% Morbidity	% carriage rate			
Average, or range birth weight (g)	Predominant underlying condition	Predominant infection	% Mortality	Before outbreak	During outbreak		
590-3, 310	Prematurity and RDS	18, Septicemia, pneumonia	? Not reported	-- --	-- (Env.) --	Secondary endogenous polyoclonal (one predominant)	Strict hygiene, carbapenem treatment 'disinfection' of wounds
Not stated Not stated	Prematurity Prematurity	4, 3 colonized 1 RTI 6 5 colonized 1 RTI	? 3 died due to other causes ? 0	-- -- -- --	-- -- -- --	? Monoclonal ? Monoclonal	Not reported Not reported
Not stated	Not mentioned	6 Septicemia	 0	+ 0	+ 25	? Polyclonal (2 infants infected with 2 strains)	Not reported

cont. →

Table 1. *cont.* →

Location year duration	Organism		Source		Mode of transmission
	Species and strain clonality no. identical/ no. tested	Sensitivity to antibio- tics used as 1st line	Inanimate	Animate	
[6] South Miami (USA) 1984-1988 4 years	*Citrobacter diversus* NICU infants: 7A,5B/16; 3X (2 from 1 infant) Other than NICU infants (community): 4A,3A', 3B,3B'/16; 3X	Not stated R to kanamycin, streptomy- cin, mezlocillin	Authors: Parallel strain groups in NICU infants and outside of NICU supports a theory of multiple source introduction of different C. diversus strains into the NICU rather than repeated intra-NICU spread of a few strains Source not found		
[7] Non-USA hospital ? USA hospital ?	*Enterobacter sakazakii* 26/27 (3 patients, 24 formula)	Not stated R to cephalo- sporins	Contami- nated dried infant formula	--	Direct from the source
	5/5 (3 patients, 1 formula, 1 blender)	Not stated R to cephalo- sporins	Contami- nated dried infant formula	--	Direct from the source
[8] London (UK) 1992-1993 3 months	*Enterobacter cloacae* 8/8	Not stated R to penicillins + cephalo- sporins	Blood gas analyzer	--	Hands of staff presumed

NEC, necrotising enterocolitis; *CHD*, congenital heart disease; *CRF*, chronic renal failure;

Neonates				Surveillance cultures*		Type of outbreak Endogenous or exogenous: monoclonal or polyclonal	Outbreak control measures
		No. of infected neonates	% Morbidity	% carriage rate			
Susceptibility							
Average, or range birth weight (g)	Predo-minant underlying condition	Predo-minant infection	% Mortality	Before outbreak	During outbreak		
Not stated	Not mentioned	18 (includes colonized) UTI Septicemia, meningitis	? Not reported	+ ?	+ ?	Primary endogenous polyclonal	Nurse-patient cohorting, no efficacy was evident
Not stated	Not mentioned	3 Meningitis	100 33	-- --	-- --	Exogenous monoclonal	Not stated but presumably by destro-ying the external source (dried Formula)
Not stated	Not mentioned	3 Septicemia	? 0	-- --	-- --	Exogenous monoclonal	
Not stated	Prematurity	5 Septicemia	? 0	-- --	+ (axilla, groin, tracheal secre-tion, environ-ment) ?	? Monoclonal	Gloves when using the machine. Disinfection of the sampling port of the machine

cont. →

Table 1. *cont.* →

Location year duration	Organism		Source		Mode of transmission
	Species and strain clonality no. identical/ no. tested	Sensitivity to antibiotics used as 1st line	Inanimate	Animate	
[9] Nijmegen (Netherlands) 1993 3 months	*Enterobacter cloacae* 24A,5B,4C,2D/38; 3X	Not stated R to cephalosporins	--	One neonate	'cross contamination' according to authors
[10] Gauteng (South Africa) 1996 2 months	*Enterobacter cloacae* 10/13; 3X; Identical: 3 patients, 6 environment, 1 hands of staff	Not stated R to penicillins + cephalosporins	Amino acid cocktail solution (not sealed bottles)	--	Administration of amino acid cocktail
[11] Durban (South Africa) 1989 3 weeks	*Klebsiella pneumoniae* Serotype X17, all identical plasmid profiles	Not stated R to many including amikacin and cephalosporins	--	Neonates	Hands of staff
[12] London (UK) 1992 4 months	*Klebsiella pneumoniae* All identical (number not stated)	Not stated R to cephalosporins, β-lactam + β-lactamase inhibitor combinations	--	Neonates (gut carriage)	Hands of staff presumed

Neonates				Surveillance cultures*		Type of outbreak Endogenous or exogenous: monoclonal or polyclonal	Outbreak control measures
Susceptibility		No. of infected neonates	% Morbidity	% carriage rate			
Average, or range birth weight (g)	Predo-minant underlying condition	Predo-minant infection	% Mortality	Before outbreak	During outbreak		
Not stated	Prematurity	6 colonized or infected	? Not reported	-- --	-- --	Secondary endogenous polyclonal (one predomi-nant)	Barrier isolation, aseptic techniques, hand washing
Not stated	NEC	9 Septicemia	? 100 (?NEC)	-- --	-- (Environ-ment) --	Exogenous monoclonal	Retrieving all suspected solutions; emphasis on hand washing
1400	Prematurity RDS	3 Septicemia (2) Pneumonia (1)	33 0	--	-- (Nasal, umbili-cal, environ-ment)	Secondary endogenous monoclonal	Isolation; hand disinfec-tion; disinfection of ventilator tubing
16 days to 8 months	CHD CRF	14 Wound, septicemia	? 21.4	-- --	-- --	? Monoclonal	Restricting admission; isolation of infected and colonized patients; strict hand washing

cont. →

Table 1. *cont.* →

Location year duration	Organism		Source		Mode of transmission
	Species and strain clonality no. identical/ no. tested	Sensitivity to antibio- tics used as 1st line			
			Inanimate	Animate	
[13] Parramatta (Australia) 1995-1996 8 months	*Klebsiella pneumoniae* 4/5; 1X	R to vancomycin and gentamicin	--	Neonates	Hands of staff presumed
[14] Amsterdam (Netherlands) 1997 4 mohths	*Klebsiella pneumoniae* 8/9; 1X	Not stated R to gentamicin and β-lactams	--	Neonates	Hands of staff presumed
CCS, low birth weight, shorter gestational age and length of stay were risk factors;					
[15] Saint Etienne (France) 1996-1997 6 months	*Klebsiella oxytoca* NICU = 1 clone PBU = different clone (figures not given)	Not stated R to amoxicillin, ticarcillin, piperacillin; S to amino- glycosides, fluoro- quinolones	--	Neonates	Enteral feeding procedure
[16] Freiburg (Germany) 1991-1992 5 months	*Pseudomonas aeruginosa* Patients: 2A, 1B/3 Tap water (8 faucets): 17A,5B,6C,3D/38	Not stated S not mentioned	Tap water from faucets on the ward	--	Directly from tap water with which neonates were bathed

CCS, case-control study; *PBU,* premature baby unit

Neonates				Surveillance cultures*		Type of outbreak Endogenous or exogenous: monoclonal or polyclonal	Outbreak control measures
		No. of infected neonates	% Morbidity	% carriage rate			
Susceptibility							
Average, or range birth weight (g)	Predo-minant underlying condition	Predo-minant infection	% Mortality	Before outbreak	During outbreak		
600-3700	Gastro-intestinal surgery, NEC	7 Septicemia	? 28.6	-- --	-- --	? Monoclonal	Altering empiric antibiotic treatment to imipenem and van-comycin, hand-washing
627-1720	Prematurity	3 Pneumonia (2) Septicemia (1)	23.1 30	-- --	+ (Environ-ment) ?	Secondary endogenous monoclonal	Replacing gentamicin with amikacin, hand disinfection
'Low birth weight'	Prematurity	PBU: 30 carriers NICU: numbers not given	? Not reported	+ ?	+ ?	Outbreak of 'carriage', independent monoclonal in each of the two units	Hand wash-ing, isolation, cohorting, using gloves during feeding conlrolled the outbreak
Not stated	Prematurity	3 Septicemia (1) Meningitis (1) Pneumonia (1)	? 0	-- --	-- --	Exogenous monoclonal (faucets car-rying the infec-ting strain in proximity to the infected patients)	Faucets aera-tors changed twice weekly and autocla-ved (coloni-zation redu-ced but *Pseu-domonas* still present in tap water)

cont. →

Table 1. *cont.* →

Location year duration	Organism		Source		Mode of transmission
	Species and strain clonality no. identical/ no. tested	Sensitivity to antibiotics used as 1st line			
			Inanimate	Animate	
[17] Melborne (Australia) ? 10 months	*Pseudomonas aeruginosa* 16A,2B,1C/I9	Not stated R to ticarcillin, ticarcillin + clavulanic acid	Blood gas analyzer	Patients	Hands of staff presumed
[18] Oklaoma City (USA) 1997-1998 1 year 3 months	*Pseudomonas aeruginosa* Neonates: 15A,3B/20 Staff: 2A,1B/3	Not stated S not mentioned	--	Neonates	Staff fingers/nails
CCS, exposure to two nurses both with long finger nails (one natural and one artificial) were risk factors for acquiring colonization/infection with P. *aeruginosa*					
[19] Mexico City (Mexico) 1995 5 months	*Serratia marcescens* 24A,4B/33	Not stated R to ampicillin, aminoglycosides, aztreonam, SXT	--	Index case from another hospital	
			Cross-transmission between patients		
[20] Ghent (Belgium) 1991-1993 1 year 10 months	*Sphingomonas paucimobilis* Neonates (temp probes): 26/31 Environmental contacts: 5X	Not stated R to piperacillin, aztreonam, temocillin, polymyxin B	The ventilator temperature for probes	--	Contaminated droplets from the temperature probe flowing back to the endotracheal tube

Neonates				Surveillance cultures*		Type of outbreak Endogenous or exogenous: monoclonal or polyclonal	Outbreak control measures
Susceptibility		No. of infected neonates	% Morbidity	% carriage rate			
Average, or range birth weight (g)	Predo-minant underlying condition	Predo-minant infection	% Mortality	Before outbreak	During outbreak		
1760	Prematurity	16 Septicemia, pneumonia	? 3	-- --	+ (nose) ?	? Polyclonal (one predomi-nant)	Vigilant hand washing
500->2500	Prematurity	34 Septicemia, endotracheal colonization	33 50	-- --	-- (Environ-ment) --	? Polyclonal (oligoclonal)	Improved hand was-hing; restriction of use of long finger nails
Not stated	Not mentioned	23 Septicemia	? Not reported	-- --	-- --	? Polyclonal (one predomi-nant)	Strict hand was-hing, cohor-ting, wearing gloves during catheter manipula-tion
Not stated	Not mentioned	85 with tracheal coloniza-tion (no infection)	0 0	-- --	-- --	Exogenous monoclonal	Hand disin-fection (did not control the oubreak), steam sterili-zation of the ventilator temperature probes did

cont. →

Table 1. *cont.* →

Location year duration	Organism		Source		Mode of transmission
	Species and strain clonality no. identical/ no. tested	Sensitivity to antibiotics used as 1st line			
			Inanimate	Animate	
[21] Winston-Salem (USA) 1990 5 weeks	*Candida albicans* 3A/5; 2X	Intrinsically R to all antibiotics	Retrograde syringes in TPN	--	Retrograde medication administration
[22] Liverpool (UK) 1990 4.5 months	*Candida parapsilosis* 19A,11B/30	Intrinsically R to all antibiotics	--	Neonates (gut carriage)	Hands of staff presumed
[23] New York (USA) 1989 3 months	MRSA 8A,2B/1O	Not stated R to methicillin	'the spread of more than a single strain of MRSA among hospitalized patients or from health care worker's suggested by the authors Source not found		

HMD, hyaline membrane disease; *IVH* intraventricular hemorrhage; *CLD,* chronic lung disease; *SDD,* selective decontamination of the digestive tract

Neonates				Surveillance cultures*		Type of outbreak Endogenous or exogenous: monoclonal or polyclonal	Outbreak control measures
Susceptibility		No. of infected neonates	% Morbidity	% carriage rate			
Average, or range birth weight (g)	Predo-minant underlying condition	Predo-minant infection	% Mortality	Before outbreak	During outbreak		
1400	Patent ductus arteriosus, 4 had surgical repair	5 Candidemia	100	--	--	Exogenous	Cohorting infected and exposed in-fants, use of gloves for all infant contact, chlorhexidine for hand washing. Us-ing syringes only once and IV tubing changes every 24 h terminat-ed the outbreak
			40	--	--	monoclonal	
1002	Prematurity, HMD, IVH, CLD	6 Candidemia	20	+	+	Secondary endogenous	Cohorting carriers, enhanced level of hygiene, SDD with nystatin
				10%	40% at peak; 10% to-wards end	polyclonal (one predomi-nant)	
			33				
550-3487	Prematurity	10 Septicemia, meningitis, osteomye-litis	?	--	-- (nose + groin)	? Polyclonal (one predomi-nant)	Cohorting of infected and colonized infants. Hexachloro-phene hand washing
			30	--	20		

cont. →

Table 1. *cont.* →

Location year duration	Organism		Source		Mode of transmission
	Species and strain clonality no. identical/ no. tested	Sensitivity to antibiotics used as 1st line	Inanimate	Animate	
[24] Dallas (USA) 1988-1991 3 years	MRSA 35/36	Not stated R to methicillin	--	Neonates	Hands of staff presumed
[25] Leeds (UK) 1992-1996 5 years	*Staphylococcus aureus* MSSA 38/40	Not stated R to penicillin		Staff nasal carriers	Hands of staff
[26] New York (USA) ? 3 months	*Staphylococcus epidermidis* 2A,2B,2C/15; 9X	Not stated R to oxacillin, erythromycin, cefuroxime + gentamicin	--	Not found	Not identified
[27] Amsterdam (Netherlands) 1998 3 months	*Bacillus cereus* 35/35 (infected + colonized neonates, balloons + nurses)	Not stated S not mentioned	Balloons used in manual ventilation	Neonates	Blowing the organism into the respiratory tract; hands of staff

CCS, lower gestational age and birth weight and longer total length of stay were risk factors,

ICN, infection control nurse

Neonates				Surveillance cultures*		Type of outbreak Endogenous or exogenous: monoclonal or polyclonal	Outbreak control measures
Susceptibility		No. of infected neonates	% Morbidity	% carriage rate			
Average, or range birth weight (g)	Predominant underlying condition	Predominant infection	% Mortality	Before outbreak	During outbreak		
Not stated	Not mentioned	43 (including colonized) Septicemia, meningitis, osteomyelitis	? Not reported	-- --	+ (Anterior nares, axillae) 40	? Monoclonal	Dedication of an ICN to tighten infection control practices. Triple dye application to umbilical stumps of all infants on admission to NICU
<1500 (175 neonates)	Prematurity	202 (including colonization) Conjunctivitis, RTI, septicemia	? Not reported	-- --	-- (Staff nasal environment)	? Monoclonal	Hand hygiene
675-1588	Immaturity	12 Septicemia NEC	? Not reported	-- --	-- --	? 'pseudo-outbreak' no single endemic strain	Prevention of intravascular catheter colonization
825-2780	RDS(2) Perinatal asphyxia (1) Prematurity	3 Septicemia (35 respiratory tract colonization)	7.9 33.3	-- --	+ (umbilicus, armpits) ?	Secondary endogenous monoclonal	Sterilization of the balloons

cont. →

Table 1. *cont.* →

Location year duration	Organism		Source		Mode of transmission
	Species and strain clonality no. identical/ no. tested	Sensitivity to antibiotics used as 1st line			
			Inanimate	Animate	
[28] Paris (France) Pediatric Burns Unit 1996 2 months	*Alcaligenes xylosoxidans* 12/12	Not stated Antibiotics not used, poor sensitivity to chlorhexidine	Diluted solution- of chlorhexidine	--	Treatment with contaminated spray
[29] Taipei (Taiwan) 1987 1 month 1988-1989 2 months	*Enterobacter cloacae* Cluster 1: 4A/4 Cluster 2: 9B/9 4 isolates blood, 5 distilled water	Not stated 1st outbreak S to cephalosporins + aminoglycosides 2nd outbreak R to β-lactams + aminoglycosides	Cluster 1? Cluster 2: distilled water, respiratory humidifier	--	Contaminated distilled water
[30] Madrid (Spain) 1997-1998 8 months *CCS,* age<12 weeks and prior treatment with 3 rd generation cephalosporins and aminoglycosides were risk factors for colonization/infection with multiresistant *K. pneumoniae*	*Klebsiella pneumoniae* 10/10	Not stated R to 3rd generation cephalosporins, aminoglycosides commonly used (gentamicin + tobramycinin)	--	Index case (16-day-old neonate)	Not identified

Pediatrics				Surveillance cultures*		Type of outbreak Endogenous or exogenous: monoclonal or polyclonal	Outbreak control measures
Susceptibility		No. of infected children	% Morbidity	% carriage rate			
Average, and/or range age	Predominant underlying condition	Predominant infection	% Mortality	Before outbreak	During outbreak		
6.9 years 9 months to 15 years	Burns	6 Wounds	100 0	-- --	-- --	Exogenous monoclonal	Decontamination of the atomizers, chlorhexidine dilution under aseptic conditions
?	? All 8 children required ventilation	Cluster 1: 4 septicemias Cluster 2: 4 septicemias	? Not reported ? Not reported	-- -- --	-- -- --	1 Exogenous monoclonal 2 Exogenous monoclonal	Changing distilled water container
1 day to 5 years	Surgery for congenital heart abnormalities	4 (6 colonized) Bacteremia	? 25	+ ?	+ ?	? Monoclonal	Patient isolation, gloves, gowns etc during procedures, cleaning + disinfection of environmental equipment. Restricted use of 3rd generation cephalosporins + aminoglycosides

cont. →

Table 1. *cont.* →

Location year duration	Organism		Source		Mode of transmission
	Species and strain clonality no. identical/ no. tested	Sensitivity to antibio- tics used as 1st line			
			Inanimate	Animate	
[31] Omaha (USA) 1997-1999 21 months	*Klebsiella pneumoniae* 14/23; 9X	Not stated R to exten- ded spectrum β-lactams	Not found	Not found	Not identified
[32] Taoyman (Taiwan) 1997 5 months 1998 1 month	*Klebsiella pneumoniae* 21A/39; 15X A = 8 patients, 1 rectal swab from carrier, 10 sink swabs, 2 hands of staff	Not stated R to β-lactams and genta- micin	Hand- washing sinks	--	Hands of staff
[33] Paris (France) 1989 2 months	*Pseudomonas aeruginosa* 11/13; 2X 5 patients with identical strain	R to tobramycin, S to colistin used in total digestive decontam- ination	--	Patients with fecal carriage	Hands of staff suggested by authors
[34] Johannesburg (South Afiica) Pediatric oncology unit 3 months	*Pseudomonas pickettii* 3A,2B/6; 1 X	R to β-lactams, S to amino- glycosides	'sterile' distilled water	--	Flushing the patients indwelling Hickman lines with contamina- ted water

Pediatrics				Surveillance cultures*		Type of outbreak Endogenous or exogenous: monoclonal or polyclonal	Outbreak control measures
Susceptibility		No. of infected children	% Morbidity	% carriage rate			
Average, and/or range age	Predominant underlying condition	Predominant infection	% Mortality	Before outbreak	During outbreak		
2.0 years (0.4-11.6)	Liver + intestinal transplants	23 UTI, bacteremia, RTI	56 20	-- --	-- --	? Polyclonal (one predominant)	Not mentioned
5-70 days	Prematurity	8 Bacteremia	? 0	-- --	-- (Environ-ment) ?	? Secondary endogenous monoclonal	Reinforcing hand-washing, cohorting infected patients, disinfecting sinks with bleach, reducing the splatter
3 months - 6 years	Immuno-deficiency	6 with gut carriage including 4 undergoing total digesti-ve deconta-mination (vancomycin, tobramycin, colistin)	? Not reported	+ ?	+ ?	? Monoclonal 'Outbreak of carriage'	Not mentioned
19 months - 9 years	Nephro-blastoma, neuro-blastoma	7 Septicemia	100 0	-- --	-- --	Exogenous polyclonal (one predominant)	The use of contamina-ted water disconti-nued

cont. →

Table 1. *cont.* →

Location year duration	Organism		Source		Mode of transmission
	Species and strain clonality no. identical/ no. tested	Sensitivity to antibio- tics used as 1st line			
			Inanimate	Animate	
[35] Mexico City (Mexico) 1997 2 months P1CU	*Pseudomonas aeruginosa* 14A, 2B,7x/23	Not stated R to β-lactams + amino- glycosides	Not found	Not found	Cross- contam- ination suggested by authors
[36] Vancouver (Canada) 1991-1992 ? 8 months	*Serratia marcescens* 5A,4B,2C,1D/12	Not stated 3/12 R to cephalo- sporins	Not found	Not found	'Respiratory care suction involved'
[37] Philadelphia (USA) 1995 8 months	*Serratia marcescens* 'Heterogenicity of strains demonstrated' (data not given)	Not stated Sensitivity not mentioned	Not found	Not found	Hands of staff suggested by authors

CCS, surgery >3 h and exposure to one particular person were risk factors

Pediatrics				Surveillance cultures*		Type of outbreak Endogenous or exogenous: monoclonal or polyclonal	Outbreak control measures
Susceptibility		No. of infected children	% Morbidity	% carriage rate			
Average, and/or range age	Predo-minant underlying condition	Predo-minant infection	% Mortality	Before outbreak	During outbreak		
6 years	Congenital heart, neurologi-cal, lung and neo-plastic diseases	11 Septicemia Not reported	?	-- --	+ (Environ-ment) ?	? Polyclonal (one predomi-nant)	Strict hand was-hing, gloves during any catheter manipula-tion, super-vision of antibiotic use
1 month - 5 years	Post open heart, post neuro-surgery	12 (or coloni-zed) Bacteremia (6)	? Not reported	-- --	-- --	? Polyclonal	Change in disinfectant for respira-tory com-ponent to 1% final concentra-tion of gluteral-dehyde
0-545 days	Cardiac disease or surgical procedure	8 (+ 6 coloni-zed) Bacteremia, UTI	? Not reported	-- --	-- --	? Polyclonal	Contact isolation precautions, hand washing, environ-mental cleaning

cont. →

Table 1. *cont.* →

Location year duration	Organism		Source		Mode of transmission
	Species and strain clonality no. identical/ no. tested	Sensitivity to antibio- tics used as 1st line			
			Inanimate	Animate	
[38] Nottingham (UK) 1992-93 6 months	*Acinetobacter* spp. 9/10	Not stated R to β-lactams + amino- glycosides	Not found	Not found	Not identified
[39] Houston (USA) 1992 10 weeks	*Acinetobacter baumannii* 16/16 (also 9/9 from two other Houston hospitals but S to ciprofloxacin)	R to β-lactams + amino- glycosides (only S to imipenem/ cilastin)	--	Index patient with acute pneumo- nia	Not identified

CCS, therapy with 3rd generation cephalosporins, placement of central venous catheters and total parenteral nutrition were risk factors

[40] Cork (Ireland) 1993 2 x 3 months	*Acinetobacter baumannii* 6A, 6B/29 17X	Not stated S not mentioned	Not found	Not found	Not identified

Adults				Surveillance cultures*		Type of outbreak Endogenous or exogenous: monoclonal or polyclonal	Outbreak control measures
Susceptibility		No. of infected patients	% Morbidity	% carriage rate			
Average, and/or range age	Predominant underlying condition	Predominant infection	% Mortality	Before outbreak	During outbreak		
40.4 17-73	Multiple trauma, head injury/ neuro-surgery, post operative support	11 26 colonized Pneumonia (8), bacteremia (3), wounds	? 36	-- --	-- (Environ-ment) --	? Monoclonal	Isolation, cohort nursing, disposable aprons + gloves, hand washing with chlorhexidine, closure of the unit
55	? 24/25 (96%) used mechanical ventilation	9 (+ 16 colonized) Pneumonia (5) bacteremia (6)	36 52	-- --	-- --	? Monoclonal (The concurrent isolation of a single clone in several hospitals due to circulation of staff and patients amongst hospitals)	Contact isolation. A cohort of nurses for A. baumannii +ve patients, hand washing, equipment not shared outside the cases, proper control of antibiotics
?	?	28 Wounds	? Not reported	-- --	-- --	? Polyclonal	Rigidity enforced

cont. →

Table 1. *cont.* →

Location year duration	Organism		Source		Mode of transmission
	Species and strain clonality no. identical/ no. tested	Sensitivity to antibiotics used as 1st line			
			Inanimate	Animate	
[41] Nedlands (Australia) 1993-1994 2 years	*Acinetobacter baumannii* 41A, 5B/46	Not stated R to β-lactams + aminoglycosides clone B also resistant to ciprofloxacin	--	Hand carriage	Hands of staff
[42] Nashville (USA) SICU 1998 5 months (2 without intervention, when attack rate rose from 3 to 16/100 patient/month)	*Acinetobacter baumannii* 18/18	Not stated Multi-drug R, S only to imipenem + amikacin	Not found	Not found	Not identified
CCS, surgery >3 h and exposure to one particular person were risk factors					
[43] Barcelona (Spain) 1997-1998 18 months prospective study	*Acinetobacter baumannii* Authors example: 1A,2B,1C,6D,2E/12 6m before intervention: 25D,4E/29 6m after intervention: 4D,12E/16	R to carbapenem (in 62% of patients) also R to other β-lactams, aminoglycosides, ciprofloxacin	Environment (secondary to contamination)	Patients	'Horizontal'
Risk factors: previous carriage, carbapenems, admission to unit with a high density of patients with the outbreak strain					

Adults				Surveillance cultures*		Type of outbreak Endogenous or exogenous: monoclonal or polyclonal	Outbreak control measures
Susceptibility		No. of infected patients	% Morbidity	% carriage rate			
Average, and/or range age	Predominant underlying condition	Predominant infection	% Mortality	Before outbreak	During outbreak		
51 16-79	Multiple trauma, head injury, cardiac surgery	27 (+18 colonized) Pneumonia	60	--	--	Secondary endogenous	Hand washing, protective clothing, decontamination of equipment, use of gentamincin + cephalosporins restricted
			0	--	--	polyclonal (one predominant)	
41	Traumas	18 Pneumonia, bacteremia, wound	Daily point prevalence determined	--	+ (Environment)	?	Strict infection control measures
			Not reported	--	?	Monoclonal	
48.7 with CR 57.3 with CS	Polytrauma, major digestive surgery, cardio-pulmonary surgery	189 (+124 colonized) RTI, bacteremia, wounds	1	--	+	Not elucidated Polyclonal- one predominant before intervention, the other during intervention	Sequential closure for decontamination; redesign of the units; education + hand washing; restriction of carbapenem use
			20 (with CR) 21 (with CS)	--	?		

CR, carbapenem resistant strains; CS, carbapenem sensitive strains

cont. →

Table 1. *cont.* →

Location year duration	Organism		Source		Mode of transmission
	Species and strain clonality no. identical/ no. tested	Sensitivity to antibio- tics used as 1st line			
			Inanimate	Animate	
[44] Marseille (France) 1994-1995 7 months	*Enterobacter cloacae* 21/21	Highly R to fluoro- quinolones after treatment	Not found	Not found	Not identified
			'Nosocomially acquired' –sample ≥ 48 h after admission		
[45] Brussels (Belgium) 1994-1995 9 months	*Enterobacter aerogenes* 24/24	Not stated, Multi-drug R, including the emergence of imipenem resistance	--	Index case patient	Hands of staff
CCS, no risk factors identified					
[46] Athens (Greece) 1994-1995 3 months	*Klebsiella pneumoniae* 6/6	Not stated R to β-lactams	Not found	Not found	Not identified
[47] Sao Paolo (Brazil) 1991 3 months	*Pseudomonas aeruginosa* 7/14	Not stated R to aminogly- cosides, extended spectrun β-lactams, fluoro- quinolones	Not found	Not found	Not identified

Adults				Surveillance cultures*		Type of outbreak Endogenous or exogenous: monoclonal or polyclonal	Outbreak control measures
Susceptibility		No. of infected patients	% Morbidity	% carriage rate			
Average, and/or range age	Predominant underlying condition	Predominant infection	% Mortality	Before outbreak	During outbreak		
?	Acute renal and respiratory failure	15 RTI UTI	? / Not reported	-- / --	-- / --	? / Monoclonal	Reducing the prescription of fluoro-quinolones
56.5	Multiple traumas, respiratory failure, cardiac surgery	15 Pneumonia, UTI, Bacteremia (19 colonized)	44 / 38	-- / --	+ (Hands of ICU workers) / ?	Secondary exogenous / monoclonal	Isolation, hand disinfection, tube sterilisation of mechanical ventilators every 48h, cohort nursing of colonized patients (gut carriers)
?	?	6 Bacteremia	? Not reported	-- / --	-- / --	? / Monoclonal	?
?	?	14 RTI, surgical wounds	? Not reported	-- / --	+ / ?	? / Monoclonal	? After the ICU reconstruction 'the control measures reemphasized'

cont. →

Table 1. *cont.* →

Location year duration	Organism		Source		Mode of transmission
	Species and strain clonality no. identical/ no. tested	Sensitivity to antibiotics used as 1st line			
			Inanimate	Animate	
[48] Iowa (USA) 1990 1 month	*Pseudomonas aeruginosa* Patents: 3A/4 Nurse: 1A/1	Not stated S not mentioned	Not found	Not found	Hands of a nurse
[49] Freiburg (Germany) 1992 2 months	*Pseudomonas aeruginosa* 3A, 2B/5	Not stated R to β-lactams	--	Index patient	Not identified
[50] Maastricht (Netherlands) 1994-1995 10 months	*Pseudomonas aeruginosa* 5A, 3B/50, 42X	R to Amoxicillin/ clavulanic acid S to gentamicin	--	Carriers on admission	Not identified
[51] Pau (France) 1995-1998 3 years	*Pseudomonas aeruginosa* 15/15	R to ceftazidime S to amikacin	--	Index patient with pneumonia	Not identified
[52] Varese (Italy) 1998-1999 10 months	*Pseudomonas aeruginosa* 4A,4A'/8	Not stated R to aminoglycosides, β-lactams + ciprofloxacin	--	Index patient	Not identified

Adults				Surveillance cultures*		Type of outbreak Endogenous or exogenous: monoclonal or polyclonal	Outbreak control measures
Susceptibility		No. of infected patients	% Morbidity	% carriage rate			
Average, and/or range age	Predo-minant underlying condition	Predo-minant infection	% Mortality	Before outbreak	During outbreak		
31-87	Motor vehicle accidents	9 RTI, surgical wounds	30%	--	+ (Hand, of staff)	?	Careful hand washing between
			Not reported	--	?	Monoclonal	contact with different patients
? 19-71	Heart, lung + bowel disease	5 SWI (1) VAP (5)	?	--	--	Secondary endogenous polyclonal	?
			0	--	--		
58 17-93	Medical surgical trauma	? many carriers VAP	?	+	+	Primary endogenous polyclonal	?
			Not reported	The main daily prevalence 34%			
57.5	Brain + lung disease	64 RTI in mechani-cally ventilated	?	--	--	Secondary endogenous	Treatment with cefepime, amikacin
			31	--	--	monoclonal	combina-tion and hygiene measures
?	?	18 Sepsis UTI	? Not reported	--	--	Secondary endogenous	Strict hygie-ne, carbape-nem treat-
				--	--	monoclonal	ment 'disin-fection' of wounds

SWI, surgical wound infection; *VAP*, ventilator associated pneumonia

cont. →

Table 1. *cont.* →

Location year duration	Organism		Source		Mode of transmission
	Species and strain clonality no. identical/ no. tested	Sensitivity to antibio- tics used as 1st line			
			Inanimate	Animate	
[53] Kaysen (Turkey) ICUS 2000 3 months	*Serratia marcescens* (in 15 patients) misc AGNB in 5 patients *S. marcescens* 9/9	Not stated R to many, S to amikacin, cipro- floxacin, imipenem	Not found	Not found	Conta- minated theater linen
[54] Richmond (USA) 1998-1999 10 months	*Serratia marcescens* (and *Enterobacter cloacae* in 25% of pa- tients) *S. marcescens* 24/25 *E. cloacae* 7/7	Not stated S not mentioned	Parenteral narcotic (fentanyl) contami- nated by a therapist	--	Infusion of contamina- ted narcotic
CCS, length of stay, fentanyl administration and exposure to two particular respiratory therapists were risk factors					
[55] Albany, NY (USA) 1991 2 months	MRSA 5/7 (4 from patients, 1 from a nurse identical)	Not stated R to methi- cillin, eryth- romycin, ciprofloxacin	--	Patients	Using a common bathtub
[56] New York (USA) 1988-1991 3 years	MRSA Cluster I: Labour + delivery, Summer 1988 - 12 (4 patients, 4 staff; 4 environment) /12 Cluster 2: MICU, Spring 1990 - 6A, 2B/10, 2X (all patients) Cluster 3: OHU, Fall 1990 5A/6, X (3 patients, 2 environment) SICU: 4B,2C/6, 1X	Not stated R to methicillin Not stated R to methicillin	Not found Not found	Not found Not found Index patient Not found	Not identified Not identified Not identified Not identified

MICU, medical ICU; *SICU*, surgical ICU; *OHU*, open heart unit

Adults				Surveillance cultures*		Type of outbreak Endogenous or exogenous: monoclonal or polyclonal	Outbreak control measures
Susceptibility		No. of infected patients	% Morbidity	% carriage rate			
Average, and/or range age	Predominant underlying condition	Predominant infection	% Mortality	Before outbreak	During outbreak		
Not stated	AVR MVR Bypass	17 Bacteremia, mediastinitis	7 30	-- --	-- --	Exogenous monoclonal	Review of the central sterilisation unit with strict control measures for effective sterilization
7	Surgery for trauma	26 Septicemia 31% (8 patients had polymicrobial septicemia)	100 12	-- --	-- (Environ -ment) -- --	Exogenous monoclonal	Termination of employment of the implicated health care wolker
?	Psoriasis, skin ulcers, AIDS	7 Bacteremia	21.2 0	-- --	-- --	? Monoclonal	The use of the bathtub discontinued
? ? ? ?	? ? ?	7 neonates, 8 mothers (1 mother infected, others colonized) 7 (2 bacteremia, 5 colonized) 5 wounds 3 wounds	6.7 0 28.6 0 ? 0 ? 0	-- -- -- -- -- -- -- --	-- -- -- -- -- -- -- --	? Monoclonal (unrelated to other clones) Polyclonal (one predominant) Monoclonal Polyclonal (one predominant)	All clusters: patient isolation, screening of staff, topical bacitracin to carriers of MRSA, educating staff

AVR, arterial valve replacement; *MVR*, mitral valve replacement

cont. →

What Is SDD?

SDD is a maneuver designed to convert the "abnormal" carrier state (see Chapter 2) into the "normal" carrier state using non-absorbable antimicrobials. The practice of SDD has four fundamental features termed the classical Stoutenbeek's tetralogy [3, 4] (Fig. 1, Table 2).

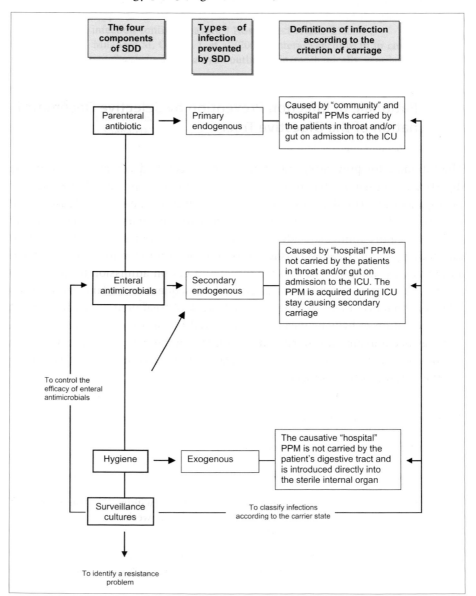

Fig. 1. The Stoutenbeek's tetralogy of selective decontamination of the digestive tract (SDD) and the type of infection prevented/controlled by each component. (*PPM* potentially pathogenic microorganism, *ICU* intensive care unit) (from Silvestri L, Lenhart FP, Fox MA (2001) Prevention of intensive care unit infections. Curr Anaesth Crit Care 12:35-40, with permission)

Table 2. Full four component protocol of SDD

Target PPM and antimicrobials	Total daily dose (4x daily)		
	<5 years	5–12 years	>12 years
1. enteral antimicrobials			
A. oropharynx			
AGNB: polymyxin E with tobramycin		2 g of 2% paste/gel	
Yeasts: amphotericin B, or nystatin		2 g of 2% paste/gel	
MRSA: vancomycin		2 g of 4% paste/gel	
B. Gut			
AGNB: polymyxin E (mg)	100	200	400
with tobramycin (mg)	80	160	320
Yeasts: amphotericin B (mg),	500	1,000	2,000
or nystatin (units)	2×10^6	4×10^6	8×10^6
MRSA: vancomycin (mg)	20-40/Kg	20-40/Kg	500/2,000
2. parenteral antimicrobials			
cefotaxime (mg)	150/Kg	200/Kg	4,000
3. hygiene			
4. surveillance cultures of throat and rectum on admission, Monday, Thursday			

PPM, potentially pathogenic micro-oganism; *AGNB,* aerobic Gram-negative bacilli; *MRSA,* methicillin-resistant *Staphyloccoccus aureus*

1. enteral antimicrobials given throughout the treatment on ICU, in combination with
2. parenteral antibiotics given immediately on admission for 4 days
3. hand hygiene throughout the treatment on ICU
4. surveillance cultures of throat and rectum on admission and twice weekly thereafter

This strategy selectively targets the 15 PPMs and the high-level pathogens, such as *Streptococcus pyogenes*, which contribute to mortality. By design, SDD does not target low-level pathogens, including anaerobes, viridans streptococci, enterococci, and coagulase-negative staphylococci as, in general, they only cause morbidity. The most-important feature of SDD is the enteral administration of non-absorbable polymyxin E/tobramycin to eradicate the abnormal aerobic Gram-negative bacilli (AGNB). This results in decontamination of the digestive tract. Critically ill patients are unable to clear these pathogens due to their underlying disease. Intestinal overgrowth with AGNB causes systemic immunoparalysis [4]. Enteral polymyxin E/tobramycin promotes recovery of systemic immunity [4] and prevention or eradication of abnormal AGNB in the throat and gut, and effectively controls aspiration and translocation of these micro-organisms into the lower airways and blood, respectively. Enteral antimicrobials are effective in the control of secondary endogenous infections. However, the use of enteral antibiotics does not affect primary endogenous and exogenous infections. The second component is the immediate administration of an adequate parenteral antimicrobial to control primary endogenous pneumonia and septicemia. Cefotaxime has been used in most randomized trials to cover both "community" and "hospital" pathogens. In adding enteral to parenteral antibiotics, the original pre 1980s antibiotics remain useful, without the development of antimicrobial resistance (Chapter 28). Thirdly, high standards of hygiene are indispensable for reducing hand contamination and subsequent transmission from external sources. Finally, surveillance samples of the throat and rectum are taken on admission and twice weekly thereafter. These are an integral component of the SDD protocol. Knowledge of the carrier state allows the compliance with and efficacy of this prophylactic protocol to be monitored.

Effectiveness of SDD

In total, 54 randomized controlled trials (RCTs) have been undertaken over 20 years of clinical research (Table 3) [5–58]. SDD was actively researched during the 1990s and after a short interval there has been a revival in new randomized

Table 3. General characteristics of the 54 randomized trials (*A*, amphotericin B; *Ami*, amikacin; *Cipro*, ciprofloxacin; *G*, gentamicin; *I*, intestine; *Nali*, nalixidic; *Neo*, neomycin; *Net*, netilmicin; *Nor*, norfloxacin; *Ny*, nystatin; *O*, oropharynx; *Oflox*, ofloxacin; *P*, polymyxin; *Pip*, piperacillin; *T*, tobramycin; *Van*, vancomycin)

Author	Patients	Parenteral	AGNB	Enteral Yeasts	S. aureus	Site
Abele-Horn et al. [5]	Trauma	Cefotaxime	PT	A		O, -
Aerdts et al. [6]	Mixed	Cefotaxime	P Nor	A		O, I
Arnow et al. [7]	Liver transplantation	Cefotaxime/ ampicillin (2 arms)	PG	Ny		O, I
Barret et al. [8]	Pediatric, burns	Pip/ami/ van (2 arms)	PT	A		-, I
Bergmans et al. [9]	Mixed	Antibiotics (40%) (2 arms)	PG	--	Van	O, -
Bion et al. [10]	Liver transplantation	Cefotaxime/ ampicillin (2 arms)	PT	A (2 arms)		O, I
Blair et al. [11]	Mixed	Cefotaxime	PT	A		O, I
Boland et al. [12]	Trauma	Cefotaxime	PT	Ny		O, I

→ Cont.

→ Table 3. Cont.

Author	Patients	Parenteral	AGNB	Enteral Yeasts	S. aureus	Site
Bouter et al. [13]	Cardiac	Flucloxacillin (2 arms)	P Neo	--		-, I
Brun-Buisson et al. [14]	Mixed	--	P Neo Nali	--		-, I
de la Cal et al. [17]	Burns	Cefotaxime	PT	A		O, I
Cerra et al. [15]	Mixed	--	Nor	Ny		-, I
Cockerill et al. [18]	Mixed	Cefotaxime	PG	Ny		O, I
Ferrer et al. [19]	Respiratory	Cefotaxime (2 arms)	PT	A		O, I
Finch et al. [20]	Mixed	Cefotaxime	PG	A		O, I
Flaherty et al. [21]	Cardiac	Cefazolin (2 arms)	PG	Ny		O, I
Gastinne et al. [22]	Mixed	Antibiotics (65%)(2 arms)	PT	A		O, I
Gaussorges et al. [23]	Mixed	Antibiotics (2 arms)	PG	A	Van	-, I
Georges et al. [24]	Trauma	Amoxycillin +clav (2 arms)	P Net	A		O, I
Hammond et al. [25]	Respiratory	Cefotaxime (2 arms)	PT	A		O, I
Hellinger et al. [26]	Liver transplantation	Ceftizoxime (2 arms)	PG	Ny (2 arms)		O, I
Jacobs et al. [27]	Neurosurgical	Cefotaxime	PT	A		O, I
de Jonge et al. [16]	Mixed	Cefotaxime	PT	A		O, I
Kerver et al. [28]	Mixed	Cefotaxime	PT	A		O, I
Korinek et al. [29]	Neurosurgical	--	PT	A	Van	O, I
Krueger et al. [30]	Surgical, trauma	Ciprofloxacin	PG	--	Van	O, I
Laggner et al. [31]	Mixed	Amoxycillin+clav (70%) (2 arms)	G	A (2 arms)		O, -

→ Cont.

→ **Table 3. cont.**

Author	Patients	Parenteral	AGNB	Enteral Yeasts	S. aureus	Site
Lingnau et al. [32]	Trauma	Ciprofloxacin (3 arms)	PT P Cipro	A A		O, I O, I
Luiten et al. [33]	Pancreatitis	Cefotaxime	P Nor	A		O, I
Martinez-Pellus et al. [34]	Cardiac	--	PT	A		-, I
Martinez-Pellus et al. [35]	Cardiac	--	PT	A		-, I
Palomar et al. [36]	Mixed	Cefotaxime	PT	A		O, I
Pneumatikos et al. [37]	Trauma	--	PT	A		O, -
Pugin et al. [38]	Surgical, trauma	--	P Neo	--	Van	O, -
Quinio et al. [39]	Trauma	Cefazolin (38%) (2 arms)	PG	A		O, I
Rayes et al. [40]	Liver transplant	Ceftriaxone/ metronidazole (2 arms)	PT	A		-, I
Rocha et al. [41]	Medical, trauma	Cefotaxime	PT	A		O, I
Rodriguez-Roldan et al. [42]	Mixed	--	PT/Net	A		O, -
Rolando et al. [43]	Liver failure	Cefuroxime	PT	A		O, I
Rolando et al. [44]	Liver failure	Ceftazidime/ flucloxacillin (2 arms)	PT	A (2 arms)		O, I
Ruza et al. [45]	Pediatric	--	PT	Ny		-, I
Sanchez-Garcia et al. [46]	Mixed	Ceftriaxone	PG	A		O, I
Schardey et al. [47]	Gastrectomy	Cefotaxime (2 arms)	PT	A	Van	-, I

→ Cont.

→ Table 3. cont.

Author	Patients	Parenteral	AGNB	Enteral Yeasts	S. aureus	Site
Smith et al. [48]	Pediatric, liver transplant	Cefotaxime/ ampicillin (2 arms)	PT	A		O, I
Stoutenbeek et al. [49]	Trauma	Cefotaxime (2 arms)	PT	A		O, I
Stoutenbeek et al. [50]	Trauma	Cefotaxime	PT	A		O, I
Tetteroo et al. [51]	Esophagectomy	Cefotaxime	PT	A		O, I
Ulrich et al. [52]	Mixed	Trimethoprim	P Nor	A		O, I
Unertl et al. [53]	Neurosurgical	--	PG	A		O, I
Verwaest et al. [54]	Mixed	Cefotaxime Ofloxacin	PT Oflox	A A		O, I
Wiener et al. [55]	Mixed	--	PG	Ny		O, I
Winter et al. [56]	Mixed	Ceftazidime	PT	A		O, I
Zobel et al. [57]	Pediatric, Cardiac	Cefotaxime	PG	A		O, I
Zwaveling et al. [58]	Liver transplantation	Cefotaxime/ tobramycin (2 arms)	PT	A		O, I

SDD trials (Fig. 2). The randomized trials not only differ in combining enteral and/or parenteral antimicrobials, they also show large variations in the antimicrobials used. The classical Stoutenbeek's tetralogy has been evaluated in 17 RCTs [11, 16, 17, 19, 25, 27, 28, 36, 41, 43, 48-51, 54, 56, 58]. Infection was significantly reduced in all but 12 studies. In those 12 negative studies the reduction was not significant [8, 14, 19, 22, 25, 26, 31, 32, 44, 54, 55, 58]. Only 2 studies showed a significant reduction in mortality following an intention-to-treat basis [16, 30]. The first study included 527 patients, and the reduction in mortality was significant with a relative risk of 0.69 [95% confidence interval (CI) 0.51–0.95]. The second study included 924 patients; both ICU [odds ratio (OR) 0.60, 95% CI 0.42–0.82] and hospital (OR 0.71, 95% CI 0.53–0.94) mortality were significantly reduced. In order to quantify the impact of SDD on infection and mortality meta-analysis is required.

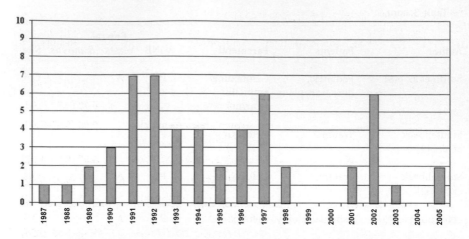

Fig. 2. Fifty-four randomized trials of SDD from 1987 to 2005

Meta-Analyses of Randomized Trials of SDD

Nine meta-analyses have been performed on RCTs only (Table 4) [59–67]. The most rigorous meta-analysis [66] showed that SDD reduces the OR for lower airway infections to 0.35 (95% CI 0.29–0.41) and mortality to 0.78 (95% CI 0.68–0.89), with a 6% overall mortality reduction from 30% to 24%. In surgical patients the benefit is even higher, with the risk of lower airway infections reduced by 81% (OR 0.19, 95% CI 0.15–0.26), bloodstream infections reduced by 49% (OR 0.51, 95% CI 0.34–0.75), and mortality reduced by 30% (OR 0.70, 95% CI 0.52–0.93) [63]. The reason for this difference in improvement is that surgical patients are in general younger and do not suffer from chronic under-lying diseases, whereas medical patients are older and often have incurable conditions such as diabetes, chronic obstructive pulmonary disease, and heart failure. In the 53rd and latest SDD trial the randomization unit was the ICU and not the patient, as in all previous trials [16]. This Dutch study of 934 patients is the largest single study yet undertaken. The primary endpoint was mortality as opposed to infectious morbidity, and the risk of mortality was significantly reduced to 0.6 (95% CI 0.4–0.8) in the unit where SDD was administered to all patients. In contrast, the patient was the "randomization unit" in the previous 52 trials; therefore, half the population was not decontaminated. However, the likelihood is high that those control patients, albeit not receiving SDD, will still benefit from the intervention as concurrent patients were subjected to a lower risk of microbial acquisition and carriage, acquired infection, and infection-related mortality. This dilution risk due to the control group being present with decontaminated patients at the same time in the same unit is termed "contam-

Table 4. Nine meta-analyses of randomized trials of SDD

Author	Year	Studies (n)	Patients (n)	Endpoints	Results
SDD trialists' group [59]	1993	22	4,142		Odds ratio
				Mortality	0.90 (0.79–1.04)
				Parenteral and enteral antibiotics	0.80 (0.67–0.97)
				Only enteral antibiotics	1.07 (0.86–1.32)
				Pneumonia	0.37 (0.31–0.43)
				Parenteral and enteral antibiotics	0.33 (0.27–0.40)
				Only enteral antibiotics	0.43 (0.33–0.56)
Kollef [60]	1994	16	2,270		Difference in risk
				Mortality	0.019 (-0.016 to 0.054)
				Pneumonia	0.145 (0.016–0.174)
Heyland et al. [61]	1994	24	3,312		Relative risk
				Mortality	0.87 (0.79–0.97)
				Parenteral and enteral antibiotics	0.81 (0.71–0.95)
				Only enteral antibiotics	1.00 (0.83–1.19)
				Pneumonia	0.46 (0.39–0.56)
				Parenteral and enteral antibiotics	0.48 (0.39–0.60)
				Only enteral antibiotics	0.49 (0.32–0.59)
D'Amico et al. [62]	1998	33	5,727		Odds ratio
				Mortality	
				Parenteral and enteral antibiotics	0.80 (0.69–0.93)
				Only enteral antibiotics	1.01 (0.84–1.22)
				Pneumonia	
				Parenteral and enteral antibiotics	0.35 (0.29–0.41)
				Only enteral antibiotics	0.56 (0.46–0.68)

cont. →

→ **Table 4** *cont.*

Author	Year	Studies (*n*)	Patients (*n*)	Endpoints	Results
Nathens et al. [63]	1999	11	Not mentioned		Odds ratio
				Mortality	
				Surgical patients	0.70 (0.52–0.93)
				Parenteral and enteral antibiotics	0.60 (0.41–0.88)
				Only enteral antibiotics	0.86 (0.59–1.45)
				Non-surgical patients	0.91 (0.71–1.18)
				Parenteral and enteral antibiotics	0.75 (0.53–1.06)
				Only enteral antibiotics	1.14 (0.77–1.68)
				Pneumonia	
				Surgical patients	0.19 (0.15–0.26)
				Non-surgical patients	0.45 (0.33–0.62)
Redman et al. [64]	2001	Not mentioned	Not mentioned		Odds ratio
				Pneumonia	
				Parenteral and enteral antibiotics	0.31 (0.20–0.46)
				Only enteral antibiotics	0.40 (0.29–0.55)
Silvestri et al. [65]	2003	42	6,263		Odds Ratio
				Fungal carriage	0.32 (0.19-0.53)
				Fungal infections	0.31 (0.19-0.51)
				Fungemia	0.49 (0.13-1.95)
Liberati et al.[66]	2004	36	6,922		Odds ratio
				Mortality	
				Parenteral & enteral antibiotics	0.78 (0.68-0.89)
				Only enteral antibiotics	0.97 (0.81-1.16)
				Pneumonia	
				Parenteral & enteral antibiotics	0.35 (0.29-0.41)
				Only enteral antibiotics	0.52 (0.43-0.63)
Safdar et al.[67]	2004	4 (Liver transpl.)	259		Relative risk
				Infection	0.88 (0.73-1.09)
				Gram negative infection	0.16 (0.07-0.37)
				Mortality	0.82 (0.22-2.45)

ination bias". The design of the latest trial has avoided this type of bias and may explain the highest reported mortality reduction to date. Translating this information into pragmatic terms, only 5 ICU patients need to be treated with SDD to prevent 1 case of pneumonia, and 21 ICU patients need to be treated to prevent 1 death [66]. The number needed to be treated to prevent 1 death in the latest study of de Jonge et al. is 12 [16].

Conclusions and Future Research

SDD is the only evidence-based maneuver that prevents infection and mortality in the critically ill. The target micro-organisms of SDD include the "normal" PPMs including *Streptococcus pneumoniae* and methicillin-sensitive *Staphylococcus aureus* (MSSA) and the "abnormal" AGNB, including *Klebsiella*, *Acinetobacter*, and *Pseudomonas* species. Methicillin-resistant *S. aureus* (MRSA), by design, is not covered by the original protocol of SDD, and, hence, seven randomized trials conducted in ICU where MRSA was endemic at the time of the study, showed a trend towards higher MRSA infection rates in patients receiving SDD [17, 19, 22, 25, 32, 54, 55]. These observations suggest that the parenteral and enteral antimicrobials of the SDD protocol, i.e., cefotaxime, polymyxin, tobramycin, and amphotericin B, select and promote MRSA. Under these circumstances, SDD requires the addition of oropharyngeal and intestinal vancomycin. Two RCTs show that the addition of vancomycin to SDD is an effective and safe maneuver [68, 69].

The Cochrane Library meta-analysis [66] - the only one that includes the first ever RCT on antimicrobial resistance [16] - reports that SDD does not lead to resistance amongst AGNB but, even better, the addition of enteral polymyxin/tobramycin to the parenteral antimicrobials reduces resistance compared with the parenteral antibiotics only. This is in line with a previous RCT demonstrating that enteral antimicrobials control extended spectrum β-lactamase producing *Klebsiella* [14]. Reports claiming resistance are invariably of low level evidence including before-after studies [70]. SDD implemented in two American ICUs with endemic vancomycin resistant enterococci (VRE) did not lead to an increased number of VRE infections [7, 26]. VRE did not emerge in any of the RCTs using enteral vancomycin [9, 23, 29, 30, 38, 47]. Antimicrobial resistance, being a long-term issue, has been evaluated in eight SDD studies monitoring antimicrobial resistance between 2 and 7 years, and bacterial resistance with SDD has not been a clinical problem [71-78].

A proper analysis of cost-effectiveness has not been performed. A Spanish Working Party has undertaken a cost-effectiveness analysis of the 54 RCTs and the nine meta-analyses using the decision tree analytic model [79, 80].

References

1. Sirvent JM, Torres A, Vidaur L, Armengol J, de Battle J, Bonet A (2000) Tracheal colonisation within 24 h of intubation in patients with head trauma: risk factor for developing early-onset ventilator-associated pneumonia. Intensive Care Med 26:1369–1372
2. Sirvent JM, Torres A, El-Ebiary M, Castro P, de Battle J, Bonet A (1997) Protective effect of intravenously administered cefuroxime against nosocomial pneumonia in patients with structural coma. Am J Respir Crit Care Med 155:1729–1734
3. Stoutenbeek CP, van Saene HKF, Miranda DR, Zandstra DF (1984) The effect of selective decontamination of the digestive tract on colonization and infection rate in multiple trauma patients. Intensive Care Med 10:185–192
4. van Saene HKF, Petros AJ, Ramsay G, Baxby D (2003) All great truths are iconoclastic: selective decontamination of the digestive tract moves from heresy to level 1 truth. Intensive Care Med 29:677–690
5. Abele-Horn M, Dauber A, Bauernfeind A, Russwurm W, Seyfarth-Metzger I, Gleich P, Ruckdeschel G (1997) Decrease in nosocomial pneumonia in ventilated patients by selective oropharyngeal decontamination (SOD). Intensive Care Med 23:1878–1895
6. Aerdts SJA, van Dalen R, Clasener HAL, Festen J, van Lier HJJ, Vollaard EJ (1991) Antibiotic prophylaxis of respiratory tract infection in mechanically ventilated patients. A prospective, blinded, randomized trial of the effect of a novel regimen. Chest 100:783–791
7. Arnow PA, Caradang GC, Zabner R, Irwin ME (1996) Randomized controlled trial of selective decontamination for prevention of infections following liver transplantation. Clin Infect Dis 22:997–1003
8. Barret JP, Jeschke MG, Herndon DN (2001) Selective decontamination of the digestive tract on severely burned pediatric patients. Burns 27:439–445
9. Bergmans DCJJ, Bonten MJM, Gaillard CA et al (2001) Prevention of ventilator-associated pneumonia by oral decontamination. A prospective, randomized, double-blind, placebo-controlled study. Am J Respir Crit Care Med 164:382–388
10. Bion JF, Badger I, Crosby HA et al (1994) Selective decontamination of the digestive tract reduces Gram-negative pulmonary colonization but not systemic endotoxemia in patients undergoing elective liver transplantation. Crit Care Med 22:40–49
11. Blair P, Rowlands BJ, Lowry K, Webb H, Armstrong P, Smilie J (1991) Selective decontamination of the digestive tract: a stratified, randomized, prospective study in a mixed intensive care unit. Surgery 110:303–310
12. Boland JP, Sadler DL, Stewart W, Wood DJ, Zerick W, Snodgrass KR (1991) Reduction of nosocomial respiratory tract infections in the multiple trauma patients requiring mechanical ventilation by selective parenteral and enteral antisepsis regimen (SPEAR) in the intensive care (abstract). Abstracts of the 17th Congress of Chemotherapy, Berlin, nn. 0465
13. Bouter H, Schippers EF, Luelmo SAG, Versteegh MIM, Ros P, Guiot HFL, Frolich M, van Dissel JT (2002) No effect of preoperative selective gut decontamination on endotoxemia and cytokine activation during cardiopulmonary bypass: a randomized, placebo-controlled study. Crit Care Med 30:38–43
14. Brun-Buisson C, Legrand P, Rauss A et al (1989) Intestinal decontamination for control of nosocomial multiresistant gram-negative bacilli. Study of an outbreak in an intensive care unit. Ann Intern Med 110:873–881
15. Cerra FB, Maddaus MA, Dunn DL, Wells CL, Kostantinides NN, Lehman SL, Mann HJ (1992) Selective gut decontamination reduces nosocomial infections and length of stay but not mortality or organ failure in surgical intensive care unit patients. Arch

Surg 127:163–169

16. de Jonge E, Schultz M, Spanjaard L, Bossuyt PPM, Vroom B, Dankert J (2003) Effects of selective decontamination of the digestive tract on mortality and acquisition of resistant bacteria in intensive care: a randomised controlled trial. Lancet 362:1011–1016

17. Cal MA de la, Cerda E, Garcia-Hierro P et al (2002) Survival benefit in severely burned patients receiving selective decontamination of the digestive tract: a randomised, placebo controlled, double blind trial. Med Intens 26:152

18. Cockerill FR, Muller SR, Anhalt JP et al (1992) Prevention of infection in critically ill patients by selective decontamination of the digestive tract. Ann Intern Med 117:545–553

19. Ferrer M, Torres A, Gonzalez J et al (1994) Utility of selective decontamination in mechanically ventilated patients. Ann Intern Med 120:389–395

20. Finch RG, Tomlinson P, Holliday M, Sole K, Stack C, Rocker G (1991) Selective decontamination of the digestive tract (SDD) in the prevention of secondary sepsis in a medical/surgical intensive care unit (abstract). Abstracts of the 17th Congress of Chemotherapy, Berlin, no. 0471

21. Flaherty J, Nathan C, Kabins SA, Weinstein RA (1990) Pilot trial of selective decontamination for prevention of bacterial infection in an intensive care unit. J Infect Dis 162:1393–1397

22. Gastinne H, Wolff M, Delatour F, Faurisson F, Chevret S, for the French Study Group on selective decontamination of the digestive tract (1992) A controlled trial in intensive care units of selective decontamination of the digestive tract with nonabsorbable antibiotics. N Engl J Med 326:594–599

23. Gaussorges P, Salord F, Sirodot M, Tigaud S, Cagnin S, Gerard M, Robert D (1991) Efficacité de la décontamination digestive sur la survenue des bacteriemies nosocomiales chez les patients sous ventilation mécanique et recevant des betamimetiques. Rean Soins Intens Med Urg 7:169–174

24. Georges B, Mazerolles M, Decun J-F et al (1994) Decontamination digestive selective: resultats d'une etude chez le polytraumatise. Rean Urg 3:621–627

25. Hammond JMJ, Potgieter PD, Saunders GL, Forder AA (1992) Double-blind study of selective decontamination of the digestive tract in intensive care. Lancet 340:5–9

26. Hellinger WC, Yao JD, Alvarez S et al (2002) A randomized, prospective, double blinded evaluation of selective bowel decontamination in liver transplantation. Transplantation 73:1904–1909

27. Jacobs S, Foweraker JE, Roberts SE (1992) Effectiveness of selective decontamination of the digestive tract (SDD) in an ICU with a policy encouraging a low gastric pH. Clin Intensive Med 3:52–58

28. Kerver AJH, Rommes JH, Mevissen-Verhage EAE, Hulstaert PF, Vos A, Verhoef J, Wittebol P (1988) Prevention of colonization and infection in critically ill patients: a prospective randomized study. Crit Care Med 16:1087–1093

29. Korinek AM, Laisne MJ, Nicolas MH, Raskine L, Deroin V, Sanson-Lepors MJ (1993) Selective decontamination of the digestive tract in neurosurgical intensive care unit patients: a double-blind, randomized, placebo-controlled study. Crit Care Med 21:14661473

30. Krueger WA, Lenhart F-P, Neeser G et al (2002) Influence of combined intravenous and topical antibiotic prophylaxis on the incidence of infections, organ dysfunctions, and mortality in critically ill surgical patients. A prospective, stratified, randomized, double-blind, placebo-controlled clinical trial. Am J Respir Crit Care Med 166:1029–1037

31. Laggner AN, Tryba M, Georgopulos A et al (1994) Oropharyngeal decontamination with gentamicin for long-stay ventilated patients on stress ulcer prophylaxis with sucralfate? Wien Klin Wochenschr 106:15–19

tion and causative micro-organism [7]. In medical patients the attributable length of ICU stay is longer and the attributable mortality greater than in surgical patients. A matched cohort study suggests that VAP is not linked to mortality, at least in surgical patients [8]. There was no difference in attributable length of stay or mortality between trauma and non-trauma patients or between those with early (<7 days) or late-onset pneumonia [9].

Mortality in VAP is influenced by the pathogenicity of the micro-organism, host defense, and the adequacy of antibiotic treatment. The occurrence of late-onset VAP due to high-risk pathogens is the most-important predictor of hospital mortality among patients developing VAP. Risk stratification should be used to identify patients with resistant micro-organisms. Prior treatment with antibiotics during hospitalization, prolonged length of hospital stay, and the presence of invasive devices are well-recognized risk factors [10].

Pathogenesis

"Early Onset" VAP

Half of all VAP cases were diagnosed within 4 days of admission to the ICU in an Italian multi-center study [11]. A classification system was proposed to distinguish "early onset pneumonia" from "late-onset pneumonia" using a time cut-off of 4 days. Various time periods have been suggested, according to the causative micro-organisms. George et al. [5] used a time cut-off of 5 days of MV. *Streptococcus pneumoniae* and *Haemophilus influenzae* were predominant in the pneumonias occurring within 5 days, whilst aerobic Gram-negative bacilli (AGNB), in particular *Pseudomonas aeruginosa*, caused lower airway infections after 5 days. Episodes of VAP involving anaerobic bacteria (23%) occurred more often in the first 5 days [12]. The anaerobes were of oropharyngeal or dental origin. This emphasizes the fact that VAP might be caused by the aspiration of contaminated oropharyngeal secretions or leakage around the artificial airway. Early onset VAP was defined as a lower airway infection acquired within 7 days of MV in a French study [6]. In patients who had not received prior antimicrobial treatment, these cases of VAP were generally due to sensitive AGNB, *H. influenzae*, methicillin-sensitive *Staphylococcus aureus*, or *S. pneumoniae*. The late-onset VAP in patients receiving prior antibiotics was mainly caused by potentially resistant bacteria, including methicillin-resistant *S. aureus*, *P. aeruginosa*, *Acinetobacter baumannii*, and *Stenotrophomonas maltophilia*.

Rello et al. [13] showed that leakage of contaminated subglottic secretions around the cuff of the endotracheal tube is the most important risk factor for pneumonia within the first 8 days of intubation. The incidence of VAP in this period was apparently lower in patients receiving antibiotic treatment for previous or concomitant infection than in patients not receiving antimicrobial agents. The authors reported a trend towards a higher risk of pneumonia among patients with persistent intracuff pressures below 20 cmH_2O. Only 10% of the first episodes of VAP occurred before day 7 of MV in patients with ARDS, compared with 40% of the episodes in patients without ARDS [4].

VAP occurring within 48 h of intubation. Although these pneumonias do not strictly fulfil the definition of VAP [1], some authors include these infections into the category of "early onset pneumonia". Their pathogenesis differs from the "classical nosocomial pneumonia" for the following reasons. The aspiration of oropharyngeal (gastric) fluid, the acute retention of tracheobronchial secretions following an accident, or a disease of sudden onset, e.g., stroke, intoxication, may provoke a massive microbial inoculation of the lungs. This may occur before admission to the ICU or at the very time of endotracheal intubation. Rello et al. [14] studied 250 intubated patients during the first 48 h after intubation and found that 12.8% developed pneumonia. Multivariate analysis demonstrated cardiopulmonary resuscitation and continuous sedation as risk factors for VAP. Antibiotic treatment provided protection against this type of pneumonia. The authors concluded that risk factors for pneumonia in intubated patients change over time in the same patient.

"Late-Onset" VAP

Trouillet et al. [6] studied the risk for VAP due to potentially resistant bacteria such as MRSA, *P. aeruginosa*, *A. baumannii*, and *S. maltophilia*. The incidence of VAP for these micro-organisms was 57%. Three variables remained independently associated with these infections: duration of MV ≥7 days, prior antibiotic use, and previous use of broad-spectrum antibiotics, including third-generation cephalosporins, imipenem, and fluoroquinolones. Late-onset pneumonia in patients who had recently received antibiotic treatment was generally caused by potentially resistant pathogens. George et al. [5] confirmed that *Pseudomonas* spp. and MRSA were predominant in late-onset VAP (>5 days of MV).

ARDS patients are often treated with antibiotics early in the course of the syndrome. Hence the onset of VAP is frequently delayed beyond the 1st week of MV and is then caused mainly by MRSA and other multi-resistant micro-organisms [4]. In conclusion, the definition of early onset pneumonia varies considerably depending whether the time of hospital admission, admission to the ICU, or intubation is chosen as the reference point. If the time of ICU admission is chosen, patients may already have been extensively colonized during their previous hospital stay and, consequently, differences in micro-organisms causing early and late-onset pneumonia are no longer evident [15].

patients receiving MV if two or more of the following clinical features are present: temperature >38°C or <36°C; leukopenia or leukocytosis, purulent tracheal secretions, and decreased PaO_2. In the absence of such findings, no further investigations are required, and observation will suffice (grade B). If two or more of these abnormalities are present, a chest X-ray should be evaluated. If the findings are normal, other causes of the abnormal clinical features should be investigated (grade C). If the X-ray shows alveolar infiltrates or an air bronchogram sign, or if the findings have worsened, the panel recommends one of two management options.

The first option involves quantitative testing and the second empirical treatment and non-quantitative (qualitative) testing. Figure 1 shows the VAP diagnostic algorithm [22]. These two options are offered (grade D) because of insuf-

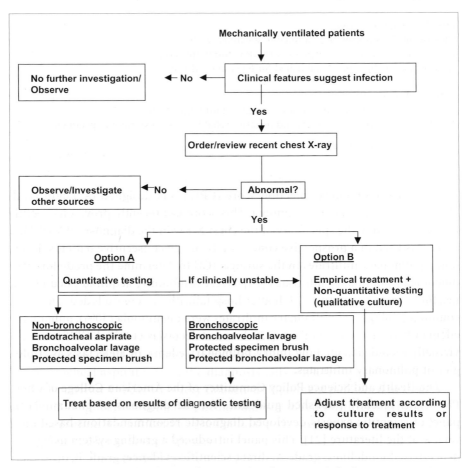

Fig. 1. Diagnostic algorithm for ventilator associated pneumonia [22]

ficient high-level evidence to indicate that quantitative testing produces better clinical outcomes than empirical treatment. While invasive tests may avoid the use of antibiotics for clinically insignificant organisms, no direct evidence or consensus indicates the superiority of one invasive test over another (grade B).

There Is no "Gold Standard" for the Diagnosis of VAP

All strategies for diagnosing VAP differ because of the lack of an irrefutable reference test ("gold standard") for the validation of diagnostic criteria and techniques. The use of histology as reference for VAP allows detection of all stages of pneumonia but cannot differentiate clinically symptomatic from asymptomatic, persistent, or resolving infection. The use of quantitative cultures of lung tissue as a reference for VAP reflects the total bacterial burden of the sample. However, colonization and infection can not be distinguished. A combination of both as reference for VAP is more likely to reflect clinically symptomatic infection but still may be vulnerable to potential biases arising from early stages of pneumonia, non-infectious lung injury, and concurrent antimicrobial treatment. In our experience, quantitative cultures of lung tissue did not reliably discriminate between the presence and absence of histological pneumonia [23].

Specific limitations of the post-mortem lung biopsy approach include the selection of a population not necessarily representative of all MV patients, the risk of overestimation of lung injuries in histological samples from severely ill patients, and sampling errors due to the multifocal nature of VAP. To minimize these potential pitfalls we used a combination of the histological presence of pneumonia with positive quantitative cultures of lung tissue samples as the reference test [24]. We thought that this approach would allow us to distinguish between foci of residual pneumonia and active and clinically symptomatic pneumonia. The results are shown in Table 2.

A high rate of false-positive results was obtained from the chest X-ray, probably due to alternative diagnoses that may cause pulmonary infiltrates mimicking VAP, such as alveolar hemorrhage, atelectasis, pulmonary infarction, and the fibroproliferative phase of ARDS. The technical limitations of portable chest radiography may hinder interpretation of radiographs. The combination of infiltrates on the chest X-ray with two of three clinical criteria had a reasonable diagnostic accuracy.

Negative microbiological results in the presence of clinically suspected VAP must not therefore be a reason for withholding antibiotics, unless an alternative diagnosis is clearly established.

We believe that the key point in clinical practice is to find a balance between the information provided by clinical judgement and the microbiology of the lower airways, and not to withhold antibiotics if VAP is clinically suspected.

Table 2. Association of clinical and microbiological diagnoses for VAP [24] (*TBA* tracheo-bronchial aspirates, *PSB* protected sample brushing, *BAL* bronchoalveolar lavage)[a,b]

Histology plus lung tissue culture	Clinical diagnosis (chest radiograph plus 2 of the 3 clinical criteria)	Non-invasive microbiological diagnosis (TBA)	Invasive microbiological diagnosis (PSB, BAL, protected BAL)	Both non-invasive and invasive microbiological diagnoses
Positive (pneumonia present)	False-negative 4/25 (16%)	Adequate 3/4 (75%)	Adequate 3/4 (75%)	Adequate 3/4 (75%)
Negative (pneumonia absent)	False-positive 3/25 (12%)	Adequate 3/3 (100%)	Adequate 1/3 (33%)	Adequate 2/3 (67%)
Positive (pneumonia present)	Correct positive 9/25 (36%)	Inadequate 3/9 (33%)	Inadequate 1/9 (11%)	Inadequate 1/9 (11%)
Negative (pneumonia absent)	Correct negative 9/25 (36%)	Inadequate 1/9 (11%)	Inadequate 4/9 (44%)	Inadequate 5/9 (55%)

[a]Cut-off points for sampling techniques: TBA specimens were considered positive in the presence of $\geq 10^5$ cfu/ml, PSB specimens $>10^3$ cfu/ml, and protected BAL and BAL specimens $>10^4$ cfu/ml

[b]Adequate=antibiotic treatment would have been administered or withheld adequately in the presence of a false or positive clinical diagnosis; inadequate=antibiotic treatment would have been administered or withheld inadequately in the presence of a correct positive or negative clinical diagnosis

Are Invasive Respiratory Sampling Techniques Better than Non-invasive? Could Immediately Direct examination (Gram Stain) of Respiratory Samples Be Helpful?

Some studies use blind or fiberoptic bronchoalveolar lavage (BAL) [25, 26] or plugged telescoping catheter (PTC) [27]. However, blind procedures are more widely available. Solé Violán et al. [26] compared management based on quantitative cultures obtained by protected sample brushing (PSB) and BAL via bronchoscopy or non-bronchoscopic BAL (PBAL) with management based on clinical judgement and non-quantitative cultures of tracheal aspirates. There were no differences in mortality and morbidity between the two strategies. Invasive diagnostic techniques showed a greater ability to narrow the initial empirical antibiotic regimen compared with the less invasive approach.

Two randomized trials have demonstrated that diagnosing pneumonia less frequently following invasive sampling is not associated with a reduction in mortality [17, 28]. A French randomized trial of 413 patients, in which 204 were managed invasively with PSB versus 209 patients managed non-invasively with tracheal aspirates, failed to show a survival benefit at 28 days (30.9% versus 38.8%, $p=0.10$) using restrictive antibiotic prescribing policies [17]. A Spanish randomized trial of 77 patients, comparing an invasive diagnostic approach ($n=39$) with a non-invasive tracheal aspirate method ($n=38$), found that the 30-day outcome of pneumonia was not influenced (38% versus 46%, $p=0.48$) by the techniques used for microbial investigation [28]. Additionally, both trials evaluated the emergence of antimicrobial resistance as a secondary endpoint. In the French trial the proportions of resistant isolates obtained from lower airway secretions were similar in both invasive (61.3%) and non-invasive (59.8%) groups, despite significantly less use of antibiotics in the invasive group. The Spanish trial reported identical high isolation rates of 58.3% of resistant bacteria (MRSA and *P. aeruginosa* in both groups).

Bonten et al. [29] demonstrated that antibiotic therapy could be stopped in patients with negative quantitative cultures with no adverse effect in terms of recurrence of VAP or mortality in a study with 138 patients evaluated using bronchoscopic specimens.

The design of the study of Timsit et al. [30] was based on the assumption that bronchoscopy with direct examination of BAL fluid generally leads to a rapid and appropriate treatment of nosocomial pneumonia in ventilated patients. This strategy led to effective treatment of 87% of VAP cases. Surprisingly, the appropriateness of the initial treatment was unrelated to patient outcome. The authors admit that these results cannot be extrapolated to other teams who are not familiar with distal sampling 24 h a day.

Nevertheless, many physicians continue to use EA and clinical features in diagnosing VAP. The sensitivity and specificity of quantitative tests of EA vary widely in their ability to diagnose VAP. Qualitative EA cultures usually identify organisms found by invasive tests. EA cultures have high sensitivity. However, qualitative EA cultures often recover multiple organisms, including non-pathogens. EA tests have a moderate positive predictive value. If a qualitative EA culture is negative, VAP is unlikely unless the patient has received antibiotic therapy. EA tests have a moderately high specificity [31].

A decision tree has been proposed for the early diagnosis and management of suspected VAP based on the Gram stain of lower airway samples obtained via blind or fiberoptic-guided PTC and of EA [27]. There are three scenarios. Firstly, if the Gram stain of EA is negative, VAP is very unlikely. No empirical antibiotic treatment for pneumonia is needed pending culture results. Secondly, if the Gram stain of PTC is positive, VAP is very likely. Early empirical antibiotic treatment is based on the Gram stain of the lower airway secretions and on epidemiological data. When culture results are obtained, the antibiotic treatment may be maintained, adapted, or stopped. Thirdly, if the EA Gram stain is

Semi-Recumbent Position (45°)

Although the oropharynx is generally considered to be the internal source of PPM causing pneumonia, some investigators believe that PPM carried in the stomach may contribute to the development of pneumonia. This concept of the gastro-pulmonary route implies that supine patient positioning increases the risk of gastric reflux, aspiration, and pneumonia. Semi-recumbent positioning, defined as elevation of the head of the bed to 45°, is hypothesized to decrease the risk for pneumonia during ventilation.

Two RCTs have evaluated the effect of the semi-recumbent positioning on the incidence of pneumonia. The first small RCT (n=86) found that ventilating patients in the semi-recumbent position significantly reduced pneumonia [41]. There was no difference in mortality. Patients were excluded if they had undergone abdominal or neurological surgery within 7 days, had shock refractory to vasoactive therapy, or had required readmission within 1 month. The second large multicenter RCT (n=221) failed to confirm the positive results of the first RCT [42].

Selective decontamination of the digestive tract using parenteral and enteral antimicrobials has been evaluated in 54 RCTs and in 9 meta-analyses, and showed an absolute mortality reduction of 8% [43] (Chapter 14).

Empirical Antibiotic Treatment

Regardless of the diagnostic method used, the American Thoracic Society (ATS) Consensus Group suggests an empirical initial therapy, based on the severity of the patient's disease and the stage of onset, using antibiotics to cover special pathogens in patients with specific risk factors [18]. According to these guidelines, VAP due to *H. influenzae* and methicillin-sensitive *S. aureus* should be treated for 7–10 days, whereas episodes caused by *P. aeruginosa* and *Acinetobacter* spp. should be treated for at least 14–21 days. However, a substantial failure rate in empirical antibiotic treatment for VAP has been reported. In patients receiving prior antibiotic treatment, episodes of late-onset VAP were mainly caused by potentially resistant bacteria [6]. Moreover, previous antibiotic treatment decreased the sensitivity of microbiological studies [23]. There is only one RCT on the duration of antibiotic treatment showing no difference in outcome in patients receiving 1 week of antibiotics compared with 2 weeks [44].

Do we need a decision rule to guide us in prescribing antibiotics? Singh et al. [45] used a modified CPIS (Table 4) to determine the "likelihood" of pneumonia [45]. CPIS ≤6 implied that the patient was unlikely to have bacterial pneumonia. CPIS was used, not as a diagnostic tool as originally proposed by Pugin et al. [19], but as a screen for decision-making regarding antibiotic ther-

Table 4. Calculation of clinical pulmonary infection score (adapted from Pugin et al. [19] by Singh et al. [45]) (*ARDS* adult respiratory distress syndrome)

Temperature (°C)

≥36.5 and ≤38.4=0 point
≥38.5 and ≤38.9=1 point
≥39 and ≤36=2 points

Blood leukocytes (/mm3)

≥4,000 and ≤11,000=0 point
≥4,000 or ≤11,000=1 point plus band forms ≥50%=add 1 point

Tracheal secretions

Absence of tracheal secretions=0 point
Presence of non-purulent tracheal secretions=1 point
Presence of purulent tracheal secretions=2 points

Oxygenation: PaO_2/FiO_2 (mmHg)

240 or ARDS (ARDS defined as PO_2/FiO_2, or equal to 200, pulmonary arterial wedge pressure ≤18 mmHg and acute bilateral infiltrates)=0 point
≤240 and no ARDS=2 points

Pulmonary radiography

No infiltrate=0 point
Diffuse (or patchy) infiltrate=1 point
Localized infiltrate=2 points

Progression of pulmonary infiltrate

No radiographic progression=0 point
Radiographic progression (after CHF and ARDS excluded)=2 points

Culture of tracheal aspirate

Pathogenic bacteria cultured in rare or light quantity or no growth=0 point
Pathogenic bacteria cultured in moderate or heavy quantity=1 point
Same pathogenic bacteria seen on Gram stain, add 1 point

(CPIS at baseline was assessed on the basis of the first five variables. CPIS at 72 h was calculated based on all seven variables taking into consideration the progression of the infiltrate an culture results of then tracheal aspirate. A score >6 at baseline or at 72 h was considered suggestive of pneumonia)

sical criteria followed by the immediate administration of adequate antibiotics after obtaining lower airway secretions [61].

References

1. Pingleton SK, Fagon JY, Leeper KV Jr (1992) Patient selection for clinical investigation of ventilator-associated pneumonia. Criteria for evaluating diagnostic techniques. Chest 102:553S–556S
2. Richards MJ, Edwards JR, Culver DH, Gaynes RP (1999) Nosocomial infections in medical intensive care units in the United States. National Nosocomial Infections Surveillance System. Crit Care Med 27:887–892
3. Alberti C, Brun-Buisson C, Burchardi H et al (2002) Epidemiology of sepsis and infection in ICU patients from an international multicentre cohort study. Intensive Care Med 28:108–121
4. Chastre J, Trouillet JL, Vuagnat A et al (1998) Nosocomial pneumonia in patients with acute respiratory distress syndrome. Am J Respir Crit Care Med 157:1165–1172
5. George DL, Falk PS, Wunderink RG et al (1998) Epidemiology of ventilator-acquired pneumonia based on protected bronchoscopic sampling. Am J Respir Crit Care Med 158:1839–1847
6. Trouillet JL, Chastre J, Vuagnat A et al (1998) Ventilator-associated pneumonia caused by potentially drug resistant bacteria. Am J Respir Crit Care Med 157:531–539
7. Hubmayr RD (2002) Statement of the 4th International Consensus Conference in Critical Care on ICU-Acquired Pneumonia—Chicago, Illinois, May 2002. Intensive Care Med 28:1521–1536
8. Papazian L, Bregeon F, Thirion X et al (1996) Effect of ventilator-associated pneumonia on mortality and morbidity. Am J Respir Crit Care Med 154:91–97
9. Heyland DK, Cook D, Griffith L et al for the Canadian Critical Care Trials Group (1999) The attributable morbidity and mortality of ventilator-associated pneumonia in the critically ill patient. Am J Respir Crit Care Med 159:1249–1256
10. Kollef MH (2001) Hospital-acquired pneumonia and de-escalation of antimicrobial treatment. Crit Care Med 29:1473–1475
11. Langer M, Cigada M, Mandelli M et al (1987) Early-onset pneumonia: a multicenter study in intensive care units. Intensive Care Med 140:342–346
12. Doré P, Robert R, Grollier G et al (1996) Incidence of anaerobes in ventilator-associated pneumonia with use of a protected specimen brush. Am J Respir Crit Care Med 153:1292–1298
13. Rello J, Soñora R, Jubert P et al (1996) Pneumonia in intubated patients: role of respiratory airway care. Am J Respir Crit Care Med 154:111–115
14. Rello J, Diaz E, Roque M et al (1999) Risk factors for developing pneumonia within 48 hours of intubation. Am J Respir Crit Care Med 159:1742–1746
15. Ibrahim EH, Ward S, Sherman G et al (2000) A comparative analysis of patients with early onset versus late onset nosocomial pneumonia in the ICU setting. Chest 117:1434–1442
16. A. Torres, J Carlet and European Task Force on Ventilator-Associated Pneumonia (2001) Ventilator-associated pneumonia. Eur Repir J 17:1034–1045
17. Fagon JY, Chastre J, Wolff M et al (2000) Invasive and noninvasive strategies for management of suspected ventilator-associated pneumonia. A randomized trial. Ann Intern Med 132:621–630

18. American Thoracic Society (1995) Hospital-acquired pneumonia in adults: diagnosis, assessment of severity, initial antimicrobial therapy, and preventive strategies. A consensus statement. Am J Respir Crit Care Med 153:1711–1725

19. Pugin J, Auckenthaler R, Mili N et al (1991) Diagnosis of ventilator-associated pneumonia by bacteriologic analysis of bronchoscopic and non bronchoscopic "blind" bronchoalveolar lavage fluid. Am Rev Respir Dis 143:1121–1129

20. Singh N, Falestiny MN, Reed MJ et al (1998) Pulmonary infiltrates in the surgical ICU. Prospective assessment of predictors of etiology and mortality. Chest 114:1129–1136

21. The American College of Chest Physicians (2000) Evidence based assessment of diagnostic tests for ventilator associated pneumonia. Chest 117:177S–218S

22. Grossman RF, Fein A (2000) Evidence-based assessment of diagnostic tests for ventilator-associated pneumonia. Executive summary. Chest 117:177S–181S

23. Torres A, Fàbregas N, Ewig S et al (2000) Sampling methods for ventilator-associated pneumonia: validation using different histologic and microbiological references. Crit Care Med 28:2799–2804

24. Fàbregas N, Ewig S, Torres A et al (1999) Clinical diagnosis of ventilator associated pneumonia revisited: comparative validation using immediate post-mortem lung biopsies. Thorax 54:867–873

25. Ibrahim EH, Ward S, Sherman G et al (2001) Experience with a clinical guideline for the treatment of ventilator-associated pneumonia. Crit Care Med 29:1109–1115

26. Solé Violán J, Arroyo Fernández J, Bordes Benítez A et al (2000) Impact of quantitative invasive diagnostic techniques in the management and outcome of mechanically ventilated patients with suspected pneumonia. Crit Care Med 28:2737–2741

27. Blot F, Raynard B, Chachaty E et al (2000) Value of Gram stain examination of lower respiratory tract secretions for early diagnosis of nosocomial pneumonia. Am J Respir Crit Care Med 162:1731–1737

28. Ruiz M, Torres A, Ewig S, Marcos MA et al (2000) Noninvasive versus invasive microbial investigation in ventilator-associated pneumonia. Evaluation of outcome. Am J Respir Crit Care Med 162:119–125

29. Bonten MJ, Bergmans DC, Stobberingh EE et al (1997) Implementation of bronchoscopic techniques in the diagnosis of ventilator-associated pneumonia to reduce antibiotic use. Am J Respir Crit Care Med 156:1820–1824

30. Timsit JF, Cheval C, Gachot B et al. (2001) Usefulness of a strategy based on bronchoscopy with direct examination of bronchoalveolar lavage fluid in the initial antibiotic therapy of suspected ventilator-associated pneumonia. Intensive Care Med 27:640–647

31. Cook D, Mandell L (2000). Endotracheal aspiration in the diagnosis of ventilator-associated pneumonia. Chest 117:195S–197S

32. Kollef MH (1999) The prevention of ventilator-associated pneumonia. N Engl J Med 340:627–634

33. Tablan OC, Anderson LJ, Arden NH et al (1994) Guideline for prevention of nosocomial pneumonia. The Hospital Infection Control Practices Advisory Committee, Centers for Disease Control and Prevention. Infect Control Hosp Epidemiol 15:588–625

34. Cook D, De Jonghe B, Brochard L et al (1998) Influence of airway management on ventilator-associated pneumonia. JAMA 279:781–787

35. Torres A, Gatell JM, Aznar E, El-Ebiary M et al (1995) Re-intubation increases the risk of nosocomial pneumonia in patients needing mechanical ventilation. Am J Respir Crit Care Med 152:137–141

36. Girou E, Schortgen F, Delclaux C et al (2000) Association of non invasive ventilation with nosocomial infections and survival in critically ill patients. JAMA 284:2376–2378

37. Mahul P, Auboyer C, Jospe R et al (1992) Prevention of nosocomial pneumonia in intubated patients: respective role of mechanical subglottic secretions drainage and stress ulcer prophylaxis. Intensive Care Med 18:20–25

38. Valles J, Artigas A, Rello J et al (1995) Continuous aspiration of subglottic secretions in preventing ventilator-associated pneumonia. Ann Intern Med 122:179–186

39. Kollef MH, Skubas NJ, Sundt TM (1999) A randomised clinical trial of continuous aspiration of subglottic secretions in cardiac surgery patients. Chest 116:1339–1346

40. Smulders K, van der Hoeven H, Weers-Pothoff I et al (2002) A randomised clinical trial of intermittent subglottic secretion drainage in patients receiving mechanical ventilation. Chest 121:858–862

41. Drakulovic MB, Torres A, Bauer TT et al (1999) Supine body position as a risk factor for nosocomial pneumonia in mechanically ventilated patients: a randomised trial. Lancet 354:1851–1858

42. van Nieuwenhoven CA, van Tiel FH, Vandenbroucke-Grauls C et al (2002) The effect of semi-recumbent position on development of ventilator-associated pneumonia (VAP) (abstract). Intensive Care Med 27 [Suppl 2]:S285

43. van Saene HKF, Petros AJ, Ramsay G, Baxby D (2003) All great truths are iconoclastic: selective decontamination of the digestive tract moves from heresy to level 1 truth. Intensive Care Med 29:677–690

44. Chastre J, Wolff M, Fagon JY et al (2003) Comparison of 8 vs 15 days of antibiotic therapy for ventilator-associated pneumonia in adults. JAMA 290:2588–2598

45. Singh N, Rogers P, Atwood CW et al (2000) Short-course empiric antibiotic therapy for patients with pulmonary infiltrates in the intensive care unit. A proposed solution for indiscriminate antibiotic prescription. Am J Respir Crit Care Med 162:505–51143

46. Rello J, Sa-Borges M, Correa H et al (1999) Variations in etiology of ventilator-associated pneumonia across four treatment sites. Implications for antimicrobial prescribing practices. Am J Respir Crit Care Med 160:608–613

47. Luna CM, Vujacich P, Niederman MS et al (1997) Impact of BAL data on the therapy and outcome of ventilator-associated pneumonia. Chest 111:676–685

48. Kollef MH (2000) Inadequate treatment of nosocomial infections is associated with certain empiric antibiotic choices. Crit Care Med 28:3456–3464

49. Dupont H, Mentec H, Sollet JP et al (2001) Impact of appropriateness of initial antibiotic therapy on the outcome of ventilator-associated pneumonia. Intensive Care Med 27:355–362

50. van Saene HKF, Damjanovic V, Murray AE et al (1996) How to classify infections in intensive care units–the carrier state, a criterion whose time has come? J Hosp Infect 33:1–12

51. Sarginson RE, Taylor N, Reilly N et al (2004) Infection in prolonged pediatric critical illness: a prospective four year study based on knowledge of the carrier state. Crit Care Med 32:839-847

52. de Latorre FJ, Pont T, Ferrer A et al (1995) Pattern of tracheal colonisation during mechanical ventilation. Am J Respir Crit Care Med 152:1028–1033

53. Cardenosa Cendrero JA, Sole-Violan J, Bordes Benitez A et al (1999) Role of different routes of tracheal colonisation in the development of pneumonia in patients receiving mechanical ventilation. Chest 116:462–470

54. Ewig S, Torres A, El-Ebiary M et al (1999) Bacterial colonization patterns in mechanically ventilated patients with traumatic and medical head injury. Incidence, risk factors, and association with ventilator-associated pneumonia. Am J Respir Crit Care Med 159:188–198

55. Bregeon F, Ciais V, Carret V et al (2001) Is ventilator-associated pneumonia an independent risk factor for death? Anesthesiology 94:551–553

56. Dennesen PJW, van der Ven AJAM, Kessels AGH et al (2001) Resolution of infectious parameter after antimicrobial therapy in patients with ventilator-associated pneumonia. Am J Respir Crit Care Med 163:1371–1375

57. Hayon J, Figliolini C, Combes A et al (2002) Role of serial routine microbiologic culture results in the initial management of ventilator-associated pneumonia. Am J Respir Crit Care Med 165:41–46

58. Montravers P, Veber B, Auboyer C et al (2002) Diagnostic and therapeutic management of nosocomial pneumonia in surgical patients: results of the Eole study. Crit Care Med 30:368–375

59. Flanagan PG (1999) Diagnosis of ventilator-associated pneumonia. J Hosp Infect 41:87–99

60. Rello J, Diaz E (2001) Optimal use of antibiotics for intubation-associated pneumonia. Intensive Care Med 27:337–339

61. Torres A, Ewig S (2004) Diagnosing ventilator-associated pneumonia. N Engl J Med 350:433–435

Chapter 16

Bloodstream Infections Including Endocarditis and Meningitis

J. VALLÉS, R. FERRER, P. FERNÁNDEZ-VILADRICH

Introduction

Patients in intensive care units (ICUs), representing 8%–15% of hospital admissions, suffer a disproportionately high percentage of nosocomial infections compared with patients in non-critical care areas [1–6]. The severity of the underlying disease, invasive diagnostic and therapeutic procedures, contaminated life-support equipment, and the prevalence of resistant micro-organisms are critical factors in the high rate of infection in the ICUs [7]. Ventilator-associated pneumonia and bacteremia are the most frequent nosocomial infections diagnosed in the ICU, and this distribution is related to the widespread use of mechanical ventilation and intravenous catheters. Recent data compiled through the National Nosocomial Infections Surveillance System (NNIS) of the Centers for Disease Control and Prevention between 1992 and 1997 in the United States revealed that bloodstream infections accounted for almost 20% of nosocomial infections in ICU patients, 87% of which were associated with a central line [8].

Bloodstream infection continues to be a severe, and often life-threatening, disease. Despite the availability of potent antimicrobial agents and sophisticated life-support facilities, bacteremia continues to be a serious infection, with high rates of morbidity and mortality. In the ICU, patients are exposed to many conditions that favor the development of bacteremia, and several studies have analyzed the epidemiology and prognosis of ICU-acquired bloodstream infections [5–7, 9, 10]. Donowitz et al. [4] reported that bloodstream infections are 7.4 times more likely to occur in ICU patients than in ward patients, with an infection rate in the ICU of 52 episodes per 1,000 admissions compared with 7 episodes per 1,000 admissions in a general ward ($p<0.001$). Trilla et al. [9], in a study of the risk factors for nosocomial bloodstream infection in a large Spanish university hospital, found that among other variables, the admission to an ICU was linked to a marked increase in the risk of nosocomial bloodstream infection (odds ratio=2.37, 95% confidence interval 1.67–3.38, $p=0.02$). Studies conducted in critically ill patients in recent years show that the incidence of nosocomial bloodstream infection in the ICU ranges from 27 to 67 episodes per 1,000 admissions [11–14] (Table 1), depending on the type of ICU (surgical, medical, or coronary care unit), the severity of illness, the use of invasive devices, and the length of ICU stay.

However, 40% of patients admitted to the ICU present infections acquired in the community, and 17% present bacteremia [15]. The incidence of patients with community acquired bacteremia admitted to a general ICU is about 9–10 episodes per 1,000 admissions [16, 17], representing 30%–40% of all episodes of bacteremia in the ICU (Fig. 1).

Table 1. Rates of nosocomial bloodstream infection in the intensive care unit (ICU)

Year	Type of ICU	Episodes of nosocomial bloodstream infection per 1,000 admissions	Reference
1994	Medical-surgical ICU	67.2	Rello et al. [11]
1994	Surgical ICU	26.7	Pittet et al. [13]
1996	Adult ICUs, multicenter study	41	Brun-Buisson et al. [14]
1997	Adult ICUs, multicenter study	36	Vallés et al. [12]

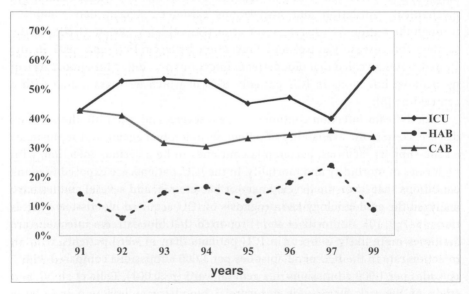

Fig. 1. Distribution of bacteremias in the medical-surgical ICU of Hospital Sabadell (Period 1991-1999) ICU: ICU-acquired bacteremia; HAB: Hospital-acquired bacteremia; CAB: Community acquired bacteremia

The aim of this chapter is to discuss the clinical importance of bloodstream infection in the ICU, including nosocomial and community episodes and specifically to emphasize the characteristics and prognosis of critically ill patients with endocarditis and meningitis admitted to the ICU.

Pathophysiology of Bloodstream Infection

Invasion of the blood by micro-organisms usually occurs via one of two mechanisms: drainage from the primary focus of infection via the lymphatic system to the vascular system, or direct entry from needles (e.g., in intravenous drug users) or other contaminated intravascular devices, such as catheters or graft material. The presence of bloodstream infection represents either the failure of an individual's defenses to localize an infection at its primary site or the failure of a physician to remove, drain, or otherwise sterilize that focus. Ordinarily, host defenses respond promptly to a sudden influx of micro-organisms, particularly by efficient phagocytosis by macrophages or the mononuclear phagocytic system that help clear the blood within minutes to hours. Clearance may be less efficient when micro-organisms are encapsulated, or it may be enhanced if the host has antibodies specific for the infecting organism. Clearance of the bloodstream is not always successful. Examples of this include bloodstream infections associated with intravascular foci and endovascular infections and episodes that occur in individuals whose host defense mechanisms either are too impaired to respond efficiently or are simply overwhelmed [10].

For that reason, the presence of living micro-organisms in blood is of substantial clinical importance; it is an indicator of disseminated infection and, as such, generally indicates a poorer prognosis than that associated with localized disease.

Definitions

Nosocomial bloodstream infection in the ICU is defined in a patient with a clinically significant blood culture positive for a bacterium or fungus that is obtained more than 72 h after admission to the ICU or if it is directly related to an invasive manipulation on admission to the ICU (e.g., urinary catheterization or insertion of an intravenous line). In contrast, a community acquired bacteremia is defined when the infection develops in a patient prior to hospital and ICU admission, or if this episode of bacteremia develops within the first 48 h of hospital and ICU admission, and is not associated with any procedure performed after hospital or ICU admission. When a culture is unexpectedly positive (in the absence of signs or symptoms) or when only one of several cultures is positive for a micro-organism, it can often be dismissed as a contaminant. Every positive blood culture, however, should be carefully evaluated before being dismissed as insignificant [18].

Bloodstream infections may be classified as primary or secondary according to the source of the infection [19]. Primary bloodstream infection occurs without any recognizable focus of infection with the same organism at another site at the time of positive blood culture, and secondary bloodstream infections develop subsequent to a documented infection with the same micro-organism at another site. Episodes secondary to intravenous or arterial lines have traditionally been classified as primary bacteremias. However, if local infection (defined as redness, tenderness, and pus) is present at the site of an intravascular line, and if the semiquantitative (yielding >15 colonies) or quantitative culture of a segment catheter is positive for the same strain as in the blood cultures, they may be classified as secondary bacteremias. According to this definition, in the absence of an identified source, primary bacteremias should be designated bacteremias of unknown origin [11, 12, 20].

According to clinical patterns of bacteremia, it may also be useful to categorize bloodstream infection as transient, intermittent, or continuous [10]. Transient bacteremia, lasting minutes to hours, is the most common, and occurs after manipulation of infected tissues (e.g., abscesses), during certain surgical procedures, when procedures are undertaken that involve contaminated or colonized mucosal surfaces (e.g., gastrointestinal endoscopy), and, predictably, at the onset of acute bacterial infections such as pneumonia, meningitis, and complicated urinary infections. Intermittent bacteremia is that which occurs, clears, and then recurs in the same patient due to the same micro-organism. Classically, this type of bacteremia is associated with undrained closed space infections, such as intra-abdominal abscesses. Continuous bacteremia is characteristic of infective endocarditis as well as other endovascular infections, such as arterial graft infections, and suppurative thrombophlebitis associated with intravenous line infections commonly seen in critically ill patients. Bacteremias may also be categorized as unimicrobial or polymicrobial depending on the number of microorganisms isolated during a single bacteremic episode.

Blood cultures that are found to be positive in the laboratory but do not truly reflect bloodstream infection in the patient have been termed contaminant bacteremias or, more recently, pseudobacteremias [18]. Several techniques are available to assist the clinician and microbiologist in interpreting the clinical importance of a positive blood culture. The categorical decision to consider the bloodstream infection as true infection or a contaminant should take into account the patient's clinical history, physical findings, body temperature at the time of the blood culture, leukocyte count and differential cell counts, the identity of the micro-organism isolated, and the result of cultures from other sites. The type of micro-organism isolated may have some predictive value: common blood isolates that always or nearly always (>90%) represent true infection include *Staphylococcus aureus*, *Escherichia coli*, and other members of the *Enterobacteriaceae*, *Pseudomonas aeruginosa*, *Streptococcus pneumoniae*, and *Candida albicans*. Other micro-oganisms such as *Corynebacterium* spp., *Bacillus* spp., and *Propionibacterium acnes* rarely (<5%) represent true bacteremia. More problematic are the viridans group streptococci, which represent true bloodstream infection in 28% of cases, enterococci in 78%, and coagulase-negative staphylococci (CNS) in 15% [21, 22].

The number of positive blood cultures of the total number performed is frequently used to determine the clinical significance of the isolate, but recent data suggest that this technique is flawed. Mirret et al. [23] examined the significance of CNS in blood cultures. For conventional two-bottle culture sets, 49% of those classified as significant infections and 68% classified as contaminants grew in one bottle, whereas 51% of pathogens and 68% of contaminants grew in both bottles. The degree of overlap is so great that it is difficult to predict the clinical significance based on the number of positive bottles. It is important to note that although CNS have frequently been considered as contaminants in the past, recent studies have shown that even a single blood culture positive for these micro-organisms is frequently associated with clinically relevant episodes of bacteremia [24–26].

Microbiology

Nosocomial Bloodstream Infection

The spectrum of micro-organisms that invade the bloodstream in patients with nosocomial infections during their stay in the ICU has been evaluated in several recent studies. Although almost any micro-organism can produce bloodstream infection, staphylococci and Gram-negative bacilli account for the vast majority of cases.

Currently, the leading pathogens among cases of nosocomial bloodstream infection in the ICU are Gram-positive micro-organisms, representing nearly half of the organisms isolated [11–13, 27] (Table 2). CNS, *S. aureus* and enterococci are the most frequent Gram-positive bacteria in all studies, and CNS is isolated in 20%–30% of all episodes of bloodstream infection. Gram-negative bacilli are responsible for 30%–40% of bloodstream infection episodes, and the remaining cases are mostly due to *Candida* spp. Polymicrobial episodes are relatively common, representing about 10%. Anaerobic bacteria are isolated in fewer than 5% of cases.

Table 2. Micro-organisms causing nosocomial bloodstream infection in adult ICUs (*CNS* coagulase-negative staphylococci)

Reference	Gram-positive micro-organisms	Gram-negative micro-organisms	Fungi	Polymicrobial episodes
Rello et al. [11]	44.1% CNS *S. aureus* Enterococci	40.5% *P. aeruginosa* *E. coli* *Enterobacter* spp.	5.4% *Candida* spp.	9.9%
Pittet et al. [13]	51.0% CNS *S. aureus* Enterococci	39.0% *Enterobacter* spp. *Klebsiella* spp. *S. marcescens*	4.8% *Candida* spp.	21%
Vallés et al. [12]	49.8% CNS *S. aureus* Enterococci	32.6% *P. aeruginosa* *A. baumannii* *K. pneumoniae*	4.4% *Candida* spp.	12.7%
Jamal et al. [27]	46.8% CNS *S. aureus* Enterococci	36.6% *Enterobacter* spp. *S. marcescens* *K. pneumoniae*	17.6% *Candida* spp.	9.8%

Among Gram-positive bloodstream infections, the incidence of the pathogens is similar in the different ICUs, CNS being the most frequently isolated organism and *S. aureus* the second commonest pathogen in all studies. Only the incidence of strains with antibiotic resistance, such as methicillin-resistant *S. aureus* (MRSA) or vancomycin-resistant enterococci (VRE), differs substantially according to the characteristics of individual institutions, and depending on whether they become established as endemic nosocomial pathogens in the ICU. In contrast, the Gram-negative species isolated from nosocomial bloodstream infections in the ICUs of different institutions show marked variability. The relative contribution of each Gram-negative species to the total number of isolates from blood varies from hospital to hospital and over time. The antibiotic policy of the institution may induce the appearance of highly resistant micro-organisms and the emergence of endemic nosocomial pathogens, in particular *Pseudomonas* spp., *Acinetobacter* spp., and *Enterobacteriaceae* with extended-spectrum β-lactamase (ESBL).

The incidence of polymicrobial and anaerobic bloodstream infections depends on the incidence of surgical patients in each ICU, because in two-thirds of these bacteremic episodes the origin is an intra-abdominal infection.

Community Acquired Bloodstream Infection

In the bacteremic episodes acquired in the community and admitted to the ICU, the incidence of Gram-positive and Gram-negative micro-organisms is similar and approximately 10% are polymicrobial episodes. *E. coli, S. pneumoniae,* and *S. aureus* are the leading pathogens, and the prevalence of these micro-organisms is related to the main sources of bacteremia found in these patients, such as urinary, pulmonary tract, and unknown origin [16, 17] (Table 3).

Table 3. Micro-organisms and sources of community acquired bacteremias admitted to the ICU (GNB: gram-negative bacilli; GPC: gram-positive cocci)

Reference	Sources		Microorganisms	
Forgacs et al. [16]	Pulmonary	38.5%	*S. pneumoniae*	32.3%
	Genitourinary	23.0%	*E. coli*	27.2%
	Endocarditis	8.0%	*S. aureus*	13.5%
	Biliary tract	5.9%	Other GNB	14.2%
	Other	11.1%	Other GPC	8.2%
	Unknown origin	20.0%	Other	14.2%
Vallés et al. [17]	Pulmonary	20.0%	*S. pneumoniae*	28.1%
	Abdominal	20.1%	*E. coli*	17.9%
	Genitourinary	19.8%	*S. aureus*	14.9%
	Other	10.3%	Other GNB	18.6%
	Unknown origin	29.2%	Other GPC	9.5%
			Other	11.07%

Sources

According to a more recent analysis, most (70%) nosocomial bloodstream infections in the ICU are secondary bacteremias, including the bloodstream infections related to an intravascular catheter infection. The remaining 30% are bacteremias of unknown origin. Table 4 summarizes the sources of nosocomial bacteremias in the ICU in several recent series [11–13, 28]. As shown, intravascular catheter-related infections and respiratory tract infections are the leading causes of secondary episodes.

The source of nosocomial bloodstream infections varies according to the micro-organism. CNS and *S. aureus* commonly complicate intravenous infections, whereas Gram-negative bacilli are the main etiology for secondary bloodstream infections following respiratory tract, intra-abdominal, and urinary tract infections. Most bacteremias of unknown origin are caused by

Table 4. Major sources of nosocomial bloodstream infection in the ICUs

Type of infection	Rello et al. [11] (%)	Pittet et al. [13] (%)	Vallés et al. [17] (%)	Edgeworth et al. [28] (%)
Intravenous catheter	35	18	37.1	62
Respiratory tract	10	28	17.5	3
Intra-abdominal infection	9	NA	6.1	6.9
Genitourinary tract	3.6	5.4	5.9	2.4
Surgical wound or soft tissue	8	8	2.4	3
Other	7	14.5	2.9	-
Unknown origin	27	20	28.1	22.4

Gram-positive micro-organisms, mainly CNS, and they may originate in device-related infections not diagnosed at the time of development of the bloodstream infection.

Among community acquired bloodstream infections, lower respiratory tract, intra-abdominal and genitourinary infections represent more than 80% of episodes of bacteremia admitted to the ICU. Approximately 30% of episodes are of unknown origin, including mainly meningococcal and staphylococcal infections [16, 17].

Systemic Response to Bloodstream Infection

Bloodstream infection and fungemia have been simply defined as the presence of bacteria or fungi in blood cultures. Four stages of systemic response of increasing severity have been described: the systemic inflammatory response syndrome (SIRS), which is identified by a combination of simple and readily available clinical signs and symptoms (i.e., fever or hypothermia, tachycardia, tachypnea, and changes in blood leukocyte count); sepsis, in patients in whom the SIRS is caused by documented infection; severe sepsis when patients have a dysfunction of the major organs; and septic shock, which describes patients with hypotension and organ dysfunction in addition to sepsis. As sepsis progresses to septic shock, the risk of death increases substantially. Early sepsis is usually reversible, whereas many patients with septic shock succumb despite aggressive therapy.

The presence of organisms in the blood is one of the most reliable criteria for characterizing a patient with sepsis or one of its more severe presentations, such as severe sepsis or septic shock.

In a recent multicenter study, Brun-Buisson et al. [14] analyzed the relationship between bloodstream infection and severe sepsis in adult ICUs and general wards in 24 hospitals in France. In this study, of the 842 episodes of clinically significant bloodstream infection recorded, 162 (19%) occurred in patients hospitalized in ICUs. Three hundred and seventy-seven episodes (45%) of bloodstream infection were nosocomial, and their incidence was 12 times greater in ICUs than in wards. The frequency of severe sepsis during bloodstream infection differed markedly between wards and ICUs (17% versus 65%, $p<0.001$). The nosocomial episodes acquired in the ICU represented an incidence of 41 episodes per 1,000 admissions and the incidence of severe sepsis among patients with nosocomial bloodstream infection in the ICU was 24 episodes per 1,000 admissions.

Another recent multicenter study reported by our group [12] analyzed exclusively nosocomial bloodstream infections acquired in adult ICUs of 30 hospitals in Spain, and classified their systemic response according to new definitions as sepsis, severe sepsis, and septic shock. Among 590 episodes of nosocomial bloodstream infection, the host reaction was classified as sepsis in 371 episodes (62.8%), severe sepsis in 109 episodes (18.5%), and septic shock in the remaining 110 (18.6%). The systemic response differed markedly according to the source of the bloodstream infection. Bloodstream infections associated with intravascular catheters showed the lowest rate of septic shock (12.8%), whereas those secondary to lower respiratory tract or intra-abdominal tract infections showed the highest incidence of severe sepsis and septic shock. In the study by Brun-Buisson et al. [14], in patients hospitalized in ICUs, intravascular catheter-related bloodstream infection was also associated with a lower risk of severe sepsis (odds ratio=0.2, 95% confidence interval 0.1–0.5, $p<0.01$).

The systemic response may differ according to the micro-organism causing the episode of bloodstream infection. Gram-negative organisms and *Candida* spp were associated with a higher incidence of severe sepsis and septic shock in our multicenter study [12], whereas CNS were responsible for the lowest incidence of septic shock. The multicenter study of Brun-Buisson et al. [14] analyzed ICU bloodstream infections separately and found the episodes caused by CNS to be also associated with a reduced risk of severe sepsis (odds ratio=0.2, $p=0.02$) relative to other organisms.

These results suggest that the source of infection and probably the type of micro-organism causing the episode of bloodstream infection, especially if a species other than CNS is involved, may be important in the development of severe sepsis and septic shock.

Among community acquired episodes, the incidence of severe sepsis and septic shock is higher than in nosocomial episodes, in part because the severity of the systemic response is the reason for ICU admission. In the multicenter French study, 74% of community acquired episodes presented severe sepsis or septic shock on admission to the ICU. In the multicenter Spanish study carried out in 30 ICUs in 1993 and in 1998, the incidence of severe sepsis and septic shock was also 75%. In this study, Gram-negative micro-organisms and the urinary and intra-abdominal infections were associated more frequently with septic shock [17].

Risk Factors for Nosocomial Bloodstream Infection in the ICU

The conditions that predispose an individual to bloodstream infection include not only underlying host conditions but also therapeutic, microbial, and environmental factors. The illnesses that have been associated with an increased risk of bloodstream infection include hematological and non-hematological malignancies, diabetes mellitus, renal failure requiring dialysis, chronic hepatic failure, immune deficiency syndromes, and conditions associated with the loss of normal skin barriers such as serious burns and decubitus ulcers. In the ICU, therapeutic maneuvers associated with an increased risk of nosocomial bloodstream infection include the placement of intravascular and urinary catheters, endoscopic procedures, and drainage of intra-abdominal infections.

Several risk factors have been associated with the acquisition of bloodstream infection by specific pathogens. CNS are mainly associated with central venous line infection and with the use of intravenous lipid emulsions. *Candida* spp. infections are related to the exposure to multiple antibiotics, hemodialysis, isolation of *Candida* from sites other than the blood, azotemia, and the use of indwelling catheters. In a recent analysis of risk factors for nosocomial candidemia in ICU patients with nosocomial bloodstream infections, we found that exposure to more than four antibiotics during the ICU stay (odds ratio 4.10), parenteral nutrition (odds ratio 3.37), previous surgery (odds ratio 2.60), and the presence of solid malignancy (odds ratio 1.57) were independently associated with the development of *Candida* spp. infection [29].

Prognosis

Nosocomial Bacteremia

In a recent study, Bueno-Cavanillas et al. [30] analyzed the impact of nosocomial infection on the mortality rate in an ICU. The overall crude relative risk of mortality was 2.48 (95% confidence interval=1.47–4.16) in patients with a nosocomial infection compared with non-infected patients. When the type of infection was evaluated, the risk of mortality for patients with bloodstream infection was 4.13 (95% confidence interval=2.11–8.11).

The risk of dying is influenced by the clinical condition of the patient and the rate at which complications develop. Analysis using prognostic stratification systems (such as the APACHE scoring system) indicates that factoring in the patients' age and certain physiological variables results in more accurate estimates of the risk of dying. Variables associated with the high care-fatality rates include acute respiratory distress syndrome (ARDS), disseminated intravascular coagulation (DIC), renal insufficiency, and multiple organ dysfunction (MOD). Microbial variables are less important, although high care-fatality rates have been observed for patients with bloodstream infection due to *P. aeruginosa*, *Candida* spp., and for patients with polymicrobial bloodstream infection.

The crude mortality from bloodstream infection is often 35%–60%, ranging from 12% to 80%. The attributable mortality defines the mortality directly associated with the episode of bloodstream infection, and excludes the mortality attributable to underlying conditions. It averages 26%, but varies according to the specific micro-organisms involved. CNS averaged 13.6%, enterococci, 31%, and *Candida* spp. 38% [24, 31].

Pittet et al. [13] in 1994 analyzed the attributable mortality, excess of length, and extra costs to nosocomial bloodstream infection in a surgical ICU. In this case-control study, the crude mortality rate was 50%, differing significantly from the matched controls (15%, $p<0.01$). In consequence, the attributable mortality associated with nosocomial bloodstream infection was 35%. Those authors also observed that the median length of hospital stay for cases was 14 days longer than for controls. Furthermore, nosocomial bloodstream infection was associated with a doubling of time of surgical ICU stays, and consequently with a significant economic burden.

In another study of nosocomial bloodstream infection in a medical-surgical ICU reported by Rello et al [11], the overall mortality was 31.5%, and 65.7% of all deaths were directly attributable to infection. Bloodstream infection of intra-abdominal, lower respiratory tract, or unknown origin was associated with a poor prognosis. A logistic regression analysis defined intra-abdominal origin ($p=0.01$, odds ratio 15.7) and the presence of shock ($p<0.004$, odds ratio 3.3) as independently influencing the risk of death.

A number of factors have been hypothesized as being associated with mortality in bloodstream infection. The most widely recognized prognostic factors are age, severity of the patient's underlying disease, and the appropriateness of antimicrobial therapy. Other factors potentially related to the outcome of bloodstream infection include a multiple source of infection, secondary infection, bloodstream infection caused by some difficult-to-treat organisms such as *Pseudomonas* and *Serratia* spp., polymicrobial bloodstream infection, and factors related to host response, such as the occurrence of hypotension, shock, or organ failure. In a French multicenter study of bloodstream infection and severe sepsis in ICUs and wards of 24 hospitals, Brun-Buisson et al. [14] reported that bloodstream infection due to *E. coli* or CNS was associated with a lower risk of severe sepsis and death, whereas *S. aureus* and Gram-positive organisms other than CNS were associated with an increased risk of death. The results of that study emphasize the impact of end-organ dysfunction (i.e., severe sepsis and septic shock) on the prognosis of bloodstream infection.

In the multicenter study of nosocomial bloodstream infection carried out by our group [12] in 30 Spanish ICUs, crude mortality was 41.6%, and 56% of all deaths were directly attributable to the bloodstream infection. The crude mortality was correlated with the severity of the systemic response; it was as high as 80% among patients with septic shock, compared with 26% among patients whose bacteremic episodes were manifested exclusively as sepsis.

Pittet et al. [32] recently conducted a large cohort study to determine prognostic factors of mortality in ICU patients with positive blood cultures. They analyzed 173 patients with bacteremia, of which 53.1% were nosocomially acquired. Among patients with bacteremic sepsis, 75 died (43%); in 81%, the cause of death was considered to be directly or indirectly related to the infection. In this study, the best two independent prognostic factors were the APACHE II score at the onset of sepsis (odds ratio 1.13, 95% confidence interval 1.08–1.17, $p<0.001$) and the number of organ dysfunctions developing thereafter (odds ratio 2.39, 95% confidence interval 2.02–2.82, $p<0.001$). This study suggests that in ICU patients with positive blood cultures outcome can be predicted by the severity of illness at onset of sepsis and the number of vital organ dysfunctions developing subsequently.

Community Acquired Bacteremia

Patients admitted to the ICU with community acquired bacteremia present a crude mortality of approximately 40%, compared with a mortality of 18% in bacteremic patients admitted to general wards [17, 33]. This elevated mortality is in part due to the severity of the systemic response in these patients that it is the cause of admission to the ICU [17]. In addition to the severity of the systemic response (severe sepsis and septic shock) and associated complications, the appropriateness of empiric antimicrobial treatment is the most important variable influencing the outcome of these patients [17]. The incidence of inappropriate antibiotic treatment of community acquired bacteremias admitted to the ICU in two recent studies ranged between 15% and 20% and the mortality among patients with empiric inappropriate antibiotic treatment is more than 70% [17, 34].

Conclusions

Nosocomial bloodstream infections occur two to seven times more often in critically ill patients than in ward patients. Recent studies have shown that the incidence rate ranges between 26 and 67 episodes per 1,000 ICU admissions, depending on the type of ICU.

Patients with nosocomial ICU bloodstream infection have a higher prevalence of intravenous lines and respiratory sources of infection than ward patients in whom urinary tract infection is the most prevalent source of bloodstream infection.

Gram-positive micro-organisms are the most prevalent cause of nosocomial bloodstream infection in ICU patients. This high incidence is related to the high prevalence of bloodstream infection associated with intravascular catheters in critically ill patients, and the multiple antibiotic therapy used for Gram-negative infections in ICU patients, which results in the selection of Gram-positive micro-organisms.

Currently, Gram-negative micro-oganisms cause between 30% and 40% of ICU-acquired bloodstream infections, and multiresistant organisms, such as *P. aeruginosa*, *Serratia* spp., or *A. baumannii*, are the most frequently isolated pathogens.

The attributable mortality from nosocomial bloodstream infections is high in critically ill patients, and the infection is associated with excessively long ICU and hospital stays, and a significant economic burden.

The incidence rate of community acquired bacteremia in adult ICUs is 10 episodes/1,000 admissions. *S. pneumoniae, S. aureus, and E. coli* represent more than 80% of micro-organisms causing community acquired bacteremia in the critically ill patients. Most episodes are associated with severe sepsis or septic shock, and they are associated with a high mortality, and in the majority of cases directly related to the infection. The severity of the systemic response and the appropriateness of empiric antibiotic treatment significantly influence the prognosis of these patients.

Infective Endocarditis

Magnitude of the Problem

Infective endocarditis (IE) usually refers to bacterial or fungal infection within the heart valves. Despite improvements in outcome due to advances in antimicrobial treatment and enhanced ability to diagnose and treat complications, substantial morbidity and mortality result from this infection. Currently IE represents the fourth leading cause of life-threatening infectious disease syndromes (after urosepsis, pneumonia, and intra-abdominal sepsis) [35]. Patients with prosthetic cardiac valves, users of illicit parenteral drugs, and patients with mitral valve prolapse, instead of rheumatic heart disease, account for the majority of cases of endocarditis.

Of persons with native valve IE who do not use parenteral drugs, 60%–80% have an identifiable predisposing cardiac lesion. Mitral valve prolapse is the underlying lesion in 30%–50% of cases, rheumatic heart disease in 30%, and congenital heart disease in 10%–20% of cases [36, 37]. IE on a native valve in a non-drug abuser remains predominantly a disease of men (male/female ratio 3:1) [38].

IE in intravenous drug abusers represents about 20%–50% of all cases of endocarditis, affecting mainly the tricuspid valve in men (male/female ratio 3:1) with a mean age of 30 years [39]. Prosthetic valve infection accounts for 20% of all causes of IE. The overall frequency of endocarditis in patients with prosthetic valves is 1%–4% [40]. By convention, prosthetic valve IE is termed early when symptoms appear within 60 days of valve insertion and late when they occur thereafter. Early prosthetic valve IE reflects contamination arising in the perioperative period. The rate is about 0.75% of all such patients. Late prosthetic valve IE occurs after valves have been endothelialized. The overall incidence has been estimated at 0.2%–0.5% per patient-year.

Pathophysiology of IE

Intracardiac pressure gradients that induce turbulent blood flow are detected clinically as heart murmurs, some of which are recognized risk factors for the development of IE. In the usual sequence of events, turbulent blood flow results in endothelial damage followed by platelet and fibrin deposition at the site of damage, forming a focus of non-bacterial thrombotic endocarditis. Transient bacteremia (or fungemia) with organisms that display tissue adhesion structures leads to microbial attachment and inclusion in the platelet/fibrin thrombus to form a vegetation. These vegetations may enlarge through the formation of successive layers of clot and micro-organisms. Colonies of bacteria and fungi within a vegetation are relatively resistant to antibiotic penetration. This unique microbial environment within the vegetation determines the need for prolonged therapy with high doses of microbicidal agents to achieve a microbiological cure in patients with IE.

Diagnostic Criteria

The diagnosis of bacterial endocarditis has long been based on a constellation of history, physical examination, laboratory data including blood cultures, and an assessment of the patient's risk factors and underlying diseases. Many patients complain only of fever and fatigue and are found to have a new cardiac murmur. The disease, however, presents in a myriad of ways. Friable vegetations may result in embolic features, such a stroke, meningitis, blindness, myocardial infarction, or arterial occlusion. Some patients will initially appear septic, some will present with autoimmune disease, and others with congestive heart failure secondary to rapid destruction of a heart valve. Embolic signs on physical examination, such as Osler's nodes, Janeway lesions, Roth's spots, and splinter hemorrhages are less often seen today because of the rapid institution of antibiotic therapy in most patients. Although positive results on blood cultures are very helpful in diagnosis, some patients with IE will have persistently negative cultures. Other patients with positive blood cultures may appear to have endocarditis but be found to have another focus of infection instead. For these reasons, standardized diagnostic criteria for endocarditis have long been sought.

In 1994 Durack et al. [41] from Duke University proposed a diagnostic strategy called the Duke criteria. These Duke criteria (Table 5) combine important diagnostic parameters (persistent bacteremia, new regurgitant murmurs, and vascular complications) with echocardiographic findings. The Duke criteria consider the diagnosis as definitive when two major criteria are present or when there are one major and three minor criteria or five minor criteria. The diagnosis is also definitive when there are micro-organisms in a vegetation demonstrated by culture or when histology confirms the presence of vegetations or intracardiac abscess showing active endocarditis. Several studies have demonstrated that the Duke criteria have a high sensitivity and specificity [42, 43]. Thus, on the basis of the weight of clinical evidence involving nearly 1,700 patients in the current literature, it would appear that patients suspected of having IE should be evaluated with the Duke criteria as a primary diagnostic framework [35].

Blood cultures are critical in the diagnosis of IE. However, some patients are found to have the disease despite negative cultures. The main reasons for culture-negative IE are prior antimicrobial treatment and the presence of some organisms that require special culture techniques [44]. The HACEK bacteria group are particularly difficult to grow by standard methods, requiring prolonged incubation and subculturing to chocolate agar. Nutritionally deficient streptococci cause about 5% of cases of IE and need supplements in the standard medium to grow. Fungal endocarditis also presents frequently with negative blood cultures and *Coxiella burnetti* can cause Q-fever endocarditis with negative blood cultures. In samples of resected heart valves from patients with culture-negative endocarditis made available at surgery, molecular techniques will be increasingly useful in determining the etiological agent [45].

Table 6. Microbiology of endocarditis [102]

		Predisposing conditions	Clinical course
Gram-positive cocci	S. viridans	Trauma, dental manipulations	Subacute (most-common cause), rarely acute
	Enterococcus: S. liquefaciens, S. zymogenes, E. faecalis, E. faecium	Source: urological or intestinal tracts, oral cavity	Acute or subacute
	S. bovis	Cancer of the colon, Crohn's disease, ulcerative colitis	Subacute, rarely acute
	Peptostreptococcus		Subacute, rarely acute
	S. pyogenes		Acute, may produce intracardiac complications
	S. pneumoniae	Other extracardiac foci of infection	Uncommon acute disease
	Other species of streptococci: S. mutans		
	S. aureus	Cardiac surgery, intravenous drug use, infections of the skin, osteomyelitis	Acute (most-common cause). High frequency of intracardiac complications. Disseminated extracardiac infections are common
	S. epidermidis	Most-common organism infecting prosthetic valves	Subacute or chronic
Gram-positive bacilli	Erysipelothrix insidiosa	Acquired from fish, birds, cats	Acute
	Lactobacillus	Dental procedures	
	Listeria monocytogenes	Involves natural and prosthetic valves	High incidence of systemic embolization
	Corynebacteria (Propionibacterium acnes and others), Corynebacterium diphtheriae, Bacillus cereus, Bacillus subtilis, Rothia dentocariosa	Uncommon causes	Subacute in general

cont. →

	Organism	Epidemiology/Source	Course
Gram-negative cocci	N. gonorrhoeae	Not always related to genital infection	Frequent intra- and extracardiac complications requiring surgery
	N. meningitidis	Always secondary to bacteremia	Acute
	Other Gram-negative cocci: N. flava, M. catarrhalis, N. pharyngis, N. mucosa, Megasphaera elsdenii	Uncommon causes	Subacute in general
Gram-negative bacilli	Escherichia coli, Enterobacter, Klebsiella pneumoniae, Proteus	Urological tract origin: manipulation, preceding infection	Subacute, rarely acute
	Pseudomonas aeruginosa	Drug addicts or superinfections during therapy of another infection	Acute emboli produce necrosis of walls of blood vessels
	Other species of Pseudomonas and Salmonella	Gastrointestinal tract is the source in 50%	Course often acute
	Haemophilus	Rare	High frequency of embolization
	Brucella	Rare	Occasionally acute. Bulky vegetations
	Pasteurella	Animal bite or scratch	
	Acinetobacter		Acute or subacute. Cardiac failure and embolization in >50% of cases
	Serratia	Drug addicts	Subacute course with large emboli
	Campylobacter	Dental manipulation	
	Streptobacillus moniliformis	Related to rat bite	
	Cardiobacterium hominis	Uncommon, pharyngeal orgin	Subacute
	Actinobacillus actinomycetemcomitans, Flavobacterium, Edwardsiella tarda, Citrobacter diversus	Uncommon	Subacute
			Course subacute
Yeast and fungi	Candida	One-third follow cardiac surgery, 20% related to superinfections	Course subacute. Emboli occlude large arteries
	Histoplasma capsulatum	Uncommon	

Table 6 *cont.*

	Predisposing conditions	Clinical course
Aspergillus	Immunocompromised patients. Prosthetic valves most commonly involved. Infection of mural endocardium common	Subacute course
Other yeasts and fungi: *Penicillium, Phialophora, Hormodendrum, Paecilomyces, Curvilacea.*	Uncommon	
Other organisms *Mycobacterium chelonei*	Porcine bioprostheses infected prior to insertion	Subacute course
Mycobacterium tuberculosis	Complication of disseminated tuberculosis	Subacute course
Coxiella burnetti	In the course of Q fever	Subacute course
Actinomyces israelii	Very rare	
Nocardia israelii	Very rare	
Bacteroides	Rare	Usually subacute
Fusobacterium	Rare	May be fulminant
Legionella sp.	Involves prosthetic valves	

Table 7. Suggested regimens for therapy of native valve endocarditis due to penicillin-susceptible viridans streptococci and *Streptococcus bovis* (*IV* intravenous, *IM* intramuscular)

Antibiotic	Dosage and route	Duration (weeks)
Penicillin G sodium	12-18 million U IV/24 h in 6 doses	4
Ceftriaxone sodium	2 g/24 h IM or IV	4
Penicillin G sodium plus	12-18 million U IV/24 h in 6 doses	2
Gentamicin sulfate	1 mg/kg IM or IV/8 h	2
Vancomycin hydrochloride	30 mg/kg IV/24 h in 2 doses	4

Vancomycin therapy is recommended for patients allergic to β-lactams

mg/ml of penicillin for inhibition, combination therapy with penicillin (4 weeks) and gentamicin (2 weeks) is indicated.

Vancomycin hydrochloride is an effective alternative and the drug of choice in patients with immediate-type hypersensitivity to penicillins and other β-lactam antibiotics.

S. pneumoniae, S. pyogenes, and B, C, and G streptococci. Endocarditis caused by these streptococci is relatively uncommon. No formal recommendations for optimal empirical treatment of *S. pneumoniae* IE can be made because an increasing number of penicillin-resistant pneumococci are now recognized. However, in accordance with the current recommendations for meningitis, it is prudent to initiate therapy with cefotaxime and a glycopeptide until the results of the susceptibility testing can be obtained.

Based on limited published data for the treatment of endocarditis caused by *S. pyogenes*, penicillin G potassium given intravenously is recommended and a first-generation cephalosporin is an acceptable alternative. In general, strains of group B, C, and G streptococci are more resistant to penicillin and some authorities recommend the addition of gentamicin to penicillin (or cephalosporin) therapy for at least the first 2 weeks of a 4- to 6-week course of antimicrobial therapy.

Enterococci (Table 8). Although according to standard taxonomy there are at least 12 species within the genus *Enterococcus, Enterococcus faecalis* and *Enterococcus faecium* are the major enterococci isolated from clinical sources.

Treatment of enterococcal endocarditis is complicated because the organisms are relatively resistant to penicillin, expanded-spectrum penicillins, or vancomycin. Furthermore, enterococci are uniformly resistant to cephalosporins and are generally resistant to standard therapeutic concentra-

with intravenous vancomycin. The role of supplemental gentamicin in native valve endocarditis due to methicillin-resistant staphylococci is similar to that described for methicillin-sensitive staphylococci. Although aminoglycosides have been added to the vancomycin regimen, there is evidence of synergistic nephrotoxic effects without clinical evidence of enhanced efficacy.

Treatment regimens for staphylococcal endocarditis that occurs on native cardiac valves differ from those required for treatment of staphylococcal endocarditis that occurs on prosthetic valves or on other prosthetic materials.

CNS causing prosthetic valve endocarditis are usually methicillin resistant, particularly when endocarditis develops within 1 year of surgery. Unless susceptibility to methicillin can be conclusively demonstrated, CNS causing prosthetic valve endocarditis should be assumed to be methicillin resistant, and treatment should be designed accordingly. Vancomycin and rifampin are administered for a minimum of 6 weeks, with gentamicin use limited to the initial 2 weeks of therapy. If the CNS are resistant to gentamicin, an aminoglycoside to they are is susceptible is substituted for gentamicin. If the organism is resistant to all available aminoglycosides, aminoglycoside treatment should be omitted.

Considering the high mortality rate associated with prosthetic valve endocarditis caused by coagulase-positive staphylococci, combination therapy with nafcillin or oxacillin, rifampin, and an aminoglycoside (first 2 weeks) seems prudent. When methicillin-resistant organisms are encountered, regimens containing vancomycin must be used.

HACEK micro-organisms. These micro-organisms grow slowly in standard blood culture media, and recovery may require prolonged incubation. Typically, only a fraction of the blood culture bottles from patients with HACEK endocarditis demonstrate growth. The microbiology laboratory should be asked to retain blood cultures for 2 weeks or longer in patients who have a clinical illness suggestive of endocarditis but whose blood cultures are initially negative. Conversely, bacteremia caused by HACEK micro-organisms in the absence of an obvious focus of infection is highly suggestive of endocarditis, even in the absence of typical physical findings.

The drugs of choice for the treatment of HACEK endocarditis are the third-generation cephalosporins cefotaxime sodium or ceftriaxone [58]. The duration of therapy for native valve infection should be 3–4 weeks, and the duration of therapy for prosthetic valve endocarditis should be 6 weeks. The HACEK group is susceptible in vitro to trimethoprim-sulfamethoxazole, fluoroquinolones, and aztreonam. Based on these susceptibility data, these antimicrobial agents could be considered as alternative regimens in patients unable to tolerate β-lactam therapy.

Surgical Treatment

The major indication for surgical intervention is progressive congestive failure due to valvular dysfunction. Other surgical indications include: fungal endocarditis, persistent sepsis despite antimicrobial therapy, rupture of aneurysm of sinus of Valsalva, and new onset of an auricular-ventricular conduction disturbance. Indications for cardiac surgery are presented in Table 10.

Table 10. Ratings of indications for surgery in acute infective endocarditis (IE) (*CHF* congestive heart failure)[103]

5+	4+	3+	2+	+
Severe CHF	Kissing infection of anterior leaflet of mitral valve and aortic valve	Compensated CHF on medical therapy	Subclinical CHF	Nonstreptococcal IE
Fungal endocarditis (except due to *Histoplasma*)		Recurrent emboli	Single embolic episode	Vegetation in echocardiography
Persistent sepsis (>72 h) despite antimicrobial treatment			Isolated IE of aortic valve or more than one valve	Isolated IE of mitral valve
Rupture of aneurysm of sinus of Valsalva			Small perivalvular dehiscence	
New onset of A-V conduction disturbances, myocardial abscess, significant perivalvular dehiscence, or observed tilting movement of valve				

A-V, auriculoventricular. Surgery is rarely indicated for right-sided endocarditis

Conclusion

Despite substantial improvements in the management and diagnosis of IE in recent years, important mortality and morbidity persists from this infection. Treatment of this infection requires a multidisciplinary approach among health care providers from a variety of backgrounds. Prompt recognition and management of the major complications of IE, such as heart failure, splenic abscess, or mycotic aneurysms, are also essential to successful patient outcome. It is essential to continue funding research on endocarditis in order to provide more information on the pathophysiology of the disease, as well as novel and better treatment and prophylactic strategies.

Acute Bacterial Meningitis

Bacterial meningitis is defined as the inflammation of both leptomeninges and the cerebrospinal fluid (CSF) that they contain, when caused by bacterial organisms. As a rule, the infectious process also affects the ependymus and ventricular CSF [59]. The most frequent bacterial meningitis are those due to pyogenic organisms that usually cause the typical clinical picture of acute meningitis with purulent CSF. Other non-pyogenic bacterial agents that can also cause meningitis that often runs a subacute or chronic course and presents with clear CSF showing a predominantly lymphocytic pleocytosis will not be considered in this chapter.

Epidemiology and Etiology

Acute bacterial meningitis is a common disease worldwide [59]. It mainly occurs in the community setting, although it has been frequent in the nosocomial setting [60], where it is mainly a complication of neurosurgical procedures. In this chapter, we will mainly focus on community acquired meningitis, which is more frequently a bacteremic illness. Its incidence varies widely, depending on factors such as age, geographic region, socioeconomic level, and, especially, the existence of a hyperendemic or epidemic situation of meningococcal disease, since only meningococcal meningitis may occur in an epidemic form. A recent estimate of the incidence of bacterial meningitis in the United States was between 2 and 3 per 100,000 people per year [61]. Because of the systematic vaccination of infants with the *H. influenzae* conjugated vaccine in industrialized countries, the incidence of meningitis caused by this organism has greatly declined [62, 63]. Consequently, today bacterial meningitis prevails in adults [61].

Currently, the most common pathogens causing community acquired bacterial meningitis at all ages (except in neonates) are *S. pneumoniae* and *Neisseria meningitidis*, followed by *Listeria monocytogenes*, which usually affects both the elderly and those patients with immunosuppressive illnesses or therapies. *H. influenzae, S. agalactiae, Enterococcus* spp., *S. aureus*, and Gram-negative bacilli also occasionally infect this immunosuppressed population [59–61].

Pathogenesis

Organisms can reach the central nervous system via several pathways [59]. Frequently, they arrive there via the bloodstream from a distant focus of infection. This mechanism is thought to occur in the majority of cases of meningococcal and listerial meningitis, as well as in many cases of pneumococcal meningitis and meningitis due to *H. influenzae*. Any bacteria can occasionally cause meningitis by this mechanism. Organisms can also reach the central nervous system from an infectious focus in the vicinity such as otitis media, sinusitis, pericranial CSF, cranial fistula, brain abscess, surgical wound, or through a catheter for ventricular drainage. Table 11 shows the relationships between the various foci of infection and the etiological agents.

Table 11. Relationship between foci of infection and etiological agents of community acquired bacterial meningitis in adults

Foci of infection	Most-frequent etiological agents
Acute pharyngitis (with or without purpuric lesions)	*Neisseria meningitidis*
Acute otitis media	*Streptococcus pneumoniae*
Cholesteatomatous otitis media*	*Proteus* spp., *Streptococcus* spp., *Bacteroides* spp.
Chronic sinusitis*	Anaerobic bacteria, *Streptococcus* spp.
Post-traumatic pericranial fistula	*Streptococcus pneumoniae*
Bacterial pneumonia	*Streptococcus pneumoniae*
Dental infection*	*Streptococcus milleri*
Chronic bronchial or lung infection*	Anaerobic bacteria, *Streptococcus* spp.
Abdominal or urinary infection	*Escherichia coli, Klebsiella pneumoniae*
Acute endocarditis	*Staphylococcus aureus, S. pneumoniae*
Subacute endocarditis*	*Enterococcus faecalis, Streptococcus viridans*
No apparent focus in teenagers	*Neisseria meningitidis*
No apparent focus in the elderly or immunosuppressed patients	*Listeria monocytogenes, Streptococcus pneumoniae, Streptococcus agalactiae*
Any focus in patients with	*Pseudomonas aeruginosa, Enterobacteriaceae,*
Neutropenia or cancer	*Listeria monocytogenes,* Gram-positive cocci

* A focal intracranial suppuration should be ruled out

Once organisms have reached the CSF, they quickly multiply. Several cytokines are released and create an inflammatory process that increases blood-brain barrier permeability and produces cytotoxic and vasogenic brain edema, intracranial hypertension, ischemic phenomena, and neuronal damage. This inflammatory process and its negative consequences may be greatly increased when cell wall fragments are massively released after bacteriolytic antibiotics are administered. However, bacterial growth in the meningeal spaces frequently leads to a secondary bacteremia that may contribute to morbidity. In particular, hemodynamic instability or shock, if not properly treated, will worsen the neurological process by lowering the cerebral perfusion pressure and increasing brain ischemia [64–66].

Clinical Manifestations

Clinical manifestations are due to the meningeal inflammation and its neurological consequences, the original source of infection, and possible concurrent primary or secondary septicemia.

The characteristic elements of the meningeal syndrome are fever, headache, nausea or vomiting, meningismus, and impairment of consciousness level. High fever is the most frequent sign, and is usually preceded by chills of variable intensity. However, fever may be absent in the elderly and in immunosuppressed patients, as well as in those who are in shock or have been given antipyretic drugs. Likewise, meningismus may also be absent during the first few hours of the meningeal process, in deep comatose patients, and also in the elderly or immunosuppressed. Moreover, there are several circumstances in which the clinician must be alerted to the possibility of concurrent bacterial meningitis: the confused or agitated patient with pneumonia, alcoholism, or liver cirrhosis in whom abnormal mental or behavioral signs could be attributed to hypoxemia, alcoholic deprivation, or hepatic encephalopathy, or those patients who present with fever and either seizures or an ischemic brain event.

Seizures are a frequent complication of bacterial meningitis. They have repeatedly been associated with higher mortality and neurological sequelae [60, 67–69]. In adults, they occur much more frequently in pneumococcal meningitis than in meningitis caused by other pathogens. Thus about 30% of adults with pneumococcal meningitis convulse [60, 70]. Moreover, the majority of these seizures occur precociously. In our experience, about 10% of adults with pneumococcal meningitis have already convulsed when first visited, and another 20% convulse after antibiotic treatment has been initiated, usually during the first 24 or 48 h of treatment. Some patients go on to status epilepticus. Additional impairment of the consciousness level and signs of brain herniation also often occur after the initiation of antibiotic treatment. Other neurological complications, such as brain infarcts due to cortical thrombophlebitis or arteritis, occur in about 15% of adults with bacterial meningitis [71]. Early death related to one of these complications occurring when CSF has already been sterilized by appropriate antibiotic therapy is a common experience when treating patients with pneumococcal meningitis (and occasionally other types of bacterial meningitis). This may be explained in part by the CSF inflammatory burst. That is why, with the intention of preventing these neurological complications, for more than a decade now, we have been administering very early adjunctive therapy to all adult patients with suspected pneumococcal meningitis and those with bacterial meningitis of any other etiology showing signs of high intracranial hypertension [72].

Of paramount importance are symptoms and signs due to a primary focus of infection, because they point to the etiological agent and orient the most-appropriate approach to treatment. Thus, when bacterial meningitis is preceded by *respiratory symptoms* a classical meningeal pathogen such as meningococcus, pneumococcus or *H. influenzae* is probably the cause [73]. Meningitis due to *L. monocytogenes* will not usually be preceded by respiratory symptoms. The existence of previous or concurrent *sore throat* occurs in about 40% of teenagers and adults with meningococcal disease [67]. Acute bacterial meningitis is the most frequent intracranial complication of acute otitis media at all ages. About 35% of adult pneumococcal meningitis cases are a complication of an attack of acute otitis media [70, 74]. A brain abscess is the most frequent intracranial complication of cholesteatomatous chronic otitis media, in which the classical meningeal pathogens are not usually implicated [75]. Thus, in patients with both meningeal signs and otitis, ascertaining the type of otitis has diagnostic and therapeutic consequences. A lumbar puncture should be performed without delay if the otitis media is acute, whereas a computed brain scan should first be performed if it is chronic, in order to rule out a suppurative intracranial collection that may have presented as bacterial meningitis. A pericranial fistula is likely to be present if the patient has suffered, even many years before, from a cranial or facial trauma, an operation involving either the ethmoid or sphenoid sinuses or the otic cavities, or if they have had CSF rhinorrhea or recurrent episodes of bacterial meningitis. *S. pneumoniae* is also the most frequent cause of bacterial meningitis in this setting, although other respiratory pathogens such as *H. influenzae, N. meningitidis,* or streptococci of the *viridans* group may also be the cause [74].

Septicemia may be both the cause and the consequence of the meningeal infection, and may cause distant infection, such as arthritis or endocarditis, or shock. A maculo-petechial or purpuric skin rash is characteristic of meningococcal septicemia, although it may also be due to other micro-organisms.

Diagnosis

When a diagnosis of bacterial meningitis is suspected, a lumbar puncture should be performed immediately, the CSF opening pressure must be recorded and its aspect observed. In cases with a non-acute clinical course, especially if a focal neurological deficit or papilledema is found, and in patients who present with a primary focus of infection that characteristically is complicated by a brain abscess, such as chronic cholesteatomatous otitis media, chronic sinusitis, and dental or anaerobic lung infection, a computed tomography (CT) brain scan should be performed prior to the lumbar puncture. Seizures are quite frequent in bacterial meningitis, so in themselves they do not constitute an indication for brain scanning prior to lumbar puncture if the illness runs an acute course.

CSF may appear either clear or only slightly cloudy during the first few hours of the illness, in some cases of severe meningococcal sepsis with meningitis, and in meningitis due to *L. monocytogenes*. In these cases, there may be either no CSF cells or only slight pleocytosis. However, white blood cell counts between 1,000 and 5,000/µl are common in fully established bacterial meningitis, with the percentage of polymorphonuclear cells between 90% and 100%. As an exception, a significant percentage of lymphocytic cells is frequently found in meningitis caused by *L. monocytogenes* [76]. CSF protein is usually elevated in bacterial meningitis, the most frequent range being from 1 to 5 g/l. Reduced CSF glucose occurs in about 50% of bacterial meningitis cases and CSF glucose is often almost undetectable. However, normal CSF glucose does not rule out a diagnosis of bacterial meningitis.

An urgent CSF Gram stain is especially advised in order to optimize empirical antibiotic therapy. Results are positive in less than 25% of cases of listerial meningitis, in about 50%–60% of meningococcal, staphylococcal, and Gram-negative bacillar meningitis, and in more than 80% of pneumococcal meningitis. CSF cultures are positive in about 70% of meningococcal meningitis and in 85%–90% of the other etiologies. CSF cultures are often sterile in patients who have received prior effective antibiotic therapy. Other diagnostic microbiological techniques such as latex agglutination, co-agglutination, or counter-immunoelectrophoresis have not proved informative, especially in adults, and therefore have not entered clinical practice. The polymerase chain reaction of the CSF is very useful in selected cases in which the etiological diagnosis has epidemiological implications, as may occur in meningococcal disease [77].

Blood cultures should always be performed in acute bacterial meningitis because if they are positive they will establish the etiological diagnosis [78]. On occasion, they are the only means of supporting the diagnosis, as sometimes occurs in patients who have suffered from severe cranial trauma and in whom it is not possible to obtain CSF. For instance, in the absence of a respiratory infection, positive blood cultures for *S. pneumoniae* or *H. influenzae* make the diagnosis of post-traumatic bacterial meningitis probable in such circum-stances and constitute an indication for urgent therapy. The frequency of posi-tive blood cultures in bacterial meningitis ranges from 40% in meningococcal meningitis to more than 85% in pneumococcal meningitis. Culture of pharyn-geal secretions in Tayer-Martin media is also recommended in suspected meningococcal disease. If positive, it supports the diagnosis if CSF and blood cultures are negative and it indicates appropriate prophylaxis to be given to intimate contacts. Gram stain and cultures of specimens from any possibly infected portal of entry should also be performed.

Polymorphonuclear leukocytosis is usually found in bacterial meningitis. However, the white cell blood count may be normal or even low. Leukopenia constitutes a bad prognostic sign that indicates severe sepsis, as does thrombo-cytopenia and impairment of the coagulation factors, as frequently occurs in meningococcal disease. A certain degree of hypokalemia may also be related to septicemia, and hyponatremia may be due to inappropriate secretion of antidi-uretic hormone, more often in children than in adults. A chest radiographic examination should always be performed. Other radiological tests such as CT of the paranasal sinuses, CT of the base of the skull, or magnetic resonance imag-ing of brain should be performed if necessary.

Differential Diagnosis

Several conditions, both infectious and non-infectious, may occasionally be confused with bacterial meningitis [59]. Among the most frequent are acute viral meningitis or meningoencephalitis and acute disseminated encephalomyelitis that may initially present with a predominance of polymor-phonuclear cells in CSF. Some cases of tuberculous meningitis of very acute onset may also show this CSF polymorphonuclear predominance. Chemical meningitis, such as that produced when radiological contrast media or certain anesthetics or materials from a dermoid or parasite cyst are introduced into the subarachnoid space, can also produce both a clinical syndrome and CSF cyto-chemical alterations similar to those seen in acute bacterial meningitis. Occasionally, a spontaneous or post-surgical subarachnoid hemorrhage with fever may suggest bacterial meningitis.

Therapy

Bacterial meningitis constitutes a medical emergency that must be rapidly treated in order to minimize both mortality and neurological sequelae. Mortality is still high and has not changed significantly over the antibiotic era, in spite of the very effective antibiotics available and the therapeutic develop-ments that are provided in ICUs [60, 79]. Of note is the fact that in developed countries, the overall mortality of pneumococcal meningitis in adults is 30% [60, 70, 71]. This mortality is mainly caused by the early neurological complications. All of these neurological complications may also occur in bacterial meningitis of other etiologies, although with a lesser frequency than in pneumococcal meningitis. For instance, these complications cause death in a low percentage of patients with meningococcal meningitis (about 2% overall), the majority of deaths in meningococcal disease being due to fulminant meningococcemia [67]. When these complications, especially brain herniation, do occur, brain damage is frequently irreversible, and measures to lower inflammation and cranial hypertension are usually late. Although a general rule for the treatment of bacterial meningitis is not to delay antibiotic treatment, since significant delays will certainly increase mortality and neurological sequelae, early antibiotic treatment may not only be insufficient to avoid neurological complications, especially those associated with pneumococcal meningitis, but may even favor their development through their bacteriolytic effect. Therefore, since in these cases the administration of appropriate adjunctive therapy may be even more urgent than that of the antibiotic itself, we will begin with that aspect of therapy.

Early adjunctive therapy. An initial perfusion of mannitol may occasionally be lifesaving by rapidly lowering cranial hypertension [80, 81]. In deeply comatose patients, consciousness level frequently improves rapidly after mannitol has been given. This improvement may be manifested by passing from coma to an agitated state. Moreover, improvement of the bradycardia and respiratory rhythm irregularities that these patients sometimes present may also be observed.

With regard to anti-inflammatory treatment, there is general agreement about the convenience of administering dexamethasone to children with bacterial meningitis [82]. Dexamethasone reduces neurological and audiological sequelae in children with meningitis due to *H. influenzae* type b [83]. This may also be true for pneumococcal meningitis, provided it is given before or at the same time as antibiotic therapy. Even in children with meningococcal meningitis a slight beneficial effect has been observed [84]. The administration of dexamethasone during the first 48 h of therapy has not been associated with significant adverse events [84]. Early dexamethasone therapy has also been associated with reduced mortality of adult patients with pneumococcal meningitis, but since the experience published to date is limited [85] and controlled studies are lacking, its indication for purulent meningitis continues to be controversial. However, there is a tendency to recommend the use of dexamethasone in at least some cases of bacterial meningitis in adults [86]. In our experience [72], and that of others [87], early adjunctive treatment consisting of a single bolus dose of mannitol (1 g/kg), dexamethasone during the first 2 days (after an initial loading dose of 8–12 mg) and sodium phenytoin (18 mg/kg for the first 24 h and then 2 mg/kg every 8 h for 10 days) to prevent seizures has significantly lowered the mortality of pneumococcal meningitis in adults to less than 15%. We therefore recommend such treatment in all cases of suspected pneumococcal meningitis, as well as in meningitis of other etiologies when the opening pressure of lumbar CSF is higher than 30 cm of water. We have already administered such treatment to many adult patients with bacterial meningitis without significant adverse events. If this therapy is conducted appropriately, many patients with severe neurological disease will improve rapidly and the need for more aggressive measures may be avoided. However, hospitalization in an ICU is obligatory for those patients who convulse in spite of adjunctive therapy in order to better control seizures, in those with other severe neurological complications that require mechanical support, hyperventilation, and monitoring of cranial hypertension, and, obviously, for those patients who have hemodynamic instability or shock [88].

Antibiotic treatment. In those patients with cutaneous lesions suggestive of meningococcal sepsis, antibiotic therapy must be immediately instituted. If not, antibiotic therapy may be delayed as much as 30 min in order to perform a CSF Gram stain and institute pre-antibiotic adjunctive therapy when indicated. Initial antibiotic treatment must be based on both the epidemiological and clinical data and the CSF Gram stain result (Table 12). Empirical antibiotic treatment can later be modified if the results of cultures yield the etiological agent.

Meningococcal meningitis must be treated with a broad-spectrum cephalosporin such as ceftriaxone, 50 mg/kg every 24 h, or cefotaxime 50 mg/kg every 6 or 8 h. This treatment is more convenient than penicillin if the susceptibility of the causal strain to penicillin is not known, since a variable percentage of meningococci is moderately resistant to this antibiotic (MIC between 0.1 and 1 mg/l) [89]. In penicillin-allergic patients, the elective alternative is chloramphenicol, 25 mg/kg every 6 h, with a maximum of 4 g/day. However, of great concern is the recent emergence, albeit anecdotal, of high-level chloramphenicol resistance in *N. meningitidis* isolates [90].

Aztreonam, 30 mg/kg every 6 h, may also be appropriate for these patients, but it shows reduced activity towards penicillin-resistant meningococci [91]. The recommended duration of treatment for meningococcal meningitis is 7 days, although shorter courses such as 4 days are equally safe and efficient [92, 93].

Appropriate antibiotic treatment of pneumococcal meningitis requires knowledge of the causal strain's susceptibility to penicillin and to broad-spectrum cephalosporins. By performing an E-test directly on initial culture plates it is possible to obtain preliminary information about the susceptibility of the causal strain in less than 24 h [94]. Until that susceptibility is known, the rec-

Table 12. Empiric antibiotic therapy of community acquired bacterial meningitis in adults based on foci of infection and cerebrospinal fluid Gram stain

Probable etiological agent	Elective therapy	Alternative therapies
Neisseria meningitidis	Cefotaxime, ceftriaxone	Chloramphenicol, aztreonam, meropenem*
Streptococcus pneumoniae	High-dose cefotaxime plus vancomycin	Vancomycin plus rifampin**
Haemophilus influenzae	Cefotaxime, ceftriaxone	Aztreonam
Listeria monocytogenes	Ampicillin plus gentamicin	Cotrimoxazole
Enterobacteriaceae	Cefotaxime, ceftriaxone	Aztreonam
Pseudomonas aeruginosa	Ceftazidime plus tobramycin	Aztreonam
Staphylococcus aureus	Cloxacillin or vancomycin	Vancomycin
Unknown	Ceftriaxone or high-dose cefotaxime plus vancomycin (plus ampicillin)***	Vancomycin plus aztreonam (plus co-trimoxazole)***

* Meropenem might also be a useful alternative therapy for the majority of etiological agents
** (See reference [104])
***Ampicillin or co-trimoxazole are added if *Listeria monocytogenes* is considered

ommended antibiotic therapy is the combination of a third-generation cephalosporin with vancomycin [86]. If dexamethasone is concurrently administered, vancomycin at the recommended dosage for adult patients (30 mg/kg per day) does not reach reliable CSF levels [95], and CSF cefotaxime levels may also be insufficient for some cephalosporin-resistant pneumococcal strains [96]. Moreover, it is not certain whether both antibiotics are synergistic against all pneumococcal strains. This is why we recommend that high-dose cefotaxime (300–400 mg/kg per day, with a maximum dose of 24 g/day) always be initially administered to adults with pneumococcal meningitis [97]. This is not necessary in children for whom the dosage of vancomycin is higher (60 mg/kg per day) and usually sufficient to cure the infection, even if dexamethasone is given concurrently [98]. After results of susceptibility tests are known, antibiotic therapy may be modified (Table 13).

If the causal strain shows penicillin and cephalosporin resistance, a second lumbar puncture must be performed at 36–48 h of treatment, in order to assess the evolution of CSF cultures and to test CSF antibiotic levels and/or bactericidal titers. The usual length of therapy for pneumococcal meningitis is 10 days.

Table 13. Antibiotic therapy for adult meningitis caused by *Streptococcus pneumoniae* (*MIC* minimal inhibitory concentration)

Organism susceptibility	Elective therapy	Alternative therapies
Penicillin-sensitive*	Penicillin G	Chloramphenicol**, Vancomycin plus rifampin
Penicillin-resistant and:		
Cefotaxime-sensitive^	Cefotaxime, Chloramphenicol**, Ceftriaxone	Vancomycin plus rifampin
Cefotaxime-resistant^^	High-dose cefotaxime, Chloramphenicol**, High-dose cefotaxime plus vancomycin	Vancomycin plus rifampin

*MIC of penicillin <0.12 mg/l
**If the causal strain is chloramphenicol sensitive
^MIC of cefotaxime <1 mg/l
^^MIC of cefotaxime ≥1 mg/l

If the patient has a CSF pericranial fistula, he must undergo prompt surgery in order to avoid new episodes of bacterial meningitis.

Meningitis due to *L. monocytogenes* is best initially treated with the combination of ampicillin (250 mg/kg per day) with gentamicin (5–6 mg/kg per day) [99]. If gentamicin is administered on a once a day schedule, higher CSF levels will be reached and higher bactericidal activity will possibly be achieved. However, in order to avoid its ototoxicity in this usually older population it can be discontinued after a few days of therapy. For penicillin-allergic patients, the elective antibiotic consists of a high dose of co-trimoxazole that may be administered orally if necessary. The length of therapy for listerial meningitis ranges from 3 to 6 weeks, depending on both the immunological status of the patient and the presence of listerial cerebritis. In order to rule out this latter process, we recommend that magnetic resonance imaging of the brain be performed on all patients with this disease.

H. influenzae meningitis must be treated with a third-generation cephalosporin. Ten days of therapy are usually sufficient. Community acquired meningitis caused by enterobacteriaceae (more often *E. coli* or *K. pneumoniae*) are rare, and may occur as a complication of bacteremia from urinary, intestinal, or pneumonic origin, usually in patients with diabetes mellitus, liver cirrhosis, or chronic alcoholism. A third-generation cephalosporin also constitutes the elective treatment, which must be extended to 3 or 4 weeks. Community acquired *S. aureus* meningitis usually occurs in the setting of endocarditis, septicemia, or spinal abscess. A high intravenous dose of methicillin or cloxacillin

diction of mortality from bacteremic sepsis. A dynamic analysis of ICU patients. Am J Respir Crit Care Med 153:684–693

33. Carton JA, García-Velasco G, Maradona JA, Perez F, Asensi V, Arribas JM (1988) Bacteriemia extrahospitalaria en adultos. Análisis prospectivo de 333 episodios. Med Clin (Barc) 90:525–530

34. Ibrahim EH, Sherman G, Ward S, Fraser VJ, Kollef MH (2000) The influence of inadequate antimicrobial treatment of bloodstream infections on patient outcomes in the ICU setting. Chest 118:146–155

35. Bayer AS, Bolger AF, Taubert KA, Wilson W, Steckelberg J, Karchmer AW et al (1998) Diagnosis and management of infective endocarditis and its complications. Circulation 98:2936–2948

36. Weinberger I, Rotenberg Z, Zacharovitch D, Fuchs J, Davidson E, Agmon J (1990) Native valve infective endocarditis in the 1970s versus the 1980s: underlying cardiac lesions and infecting organisms. Clin Cardiol 13:94–98

37. McKinsey DS, Ratts TE, Bisno AL (1987) Underlying cardiac lesions in adults with infective endocarditis. The changing spectrum. Am J Med 82:681–688

38. von Reyn CF, Levy BS, Arbeit RD, Friedland G, Crumpacker CS (1981) Infective endocarditis: an analysis based on strict case definitions. Ann Intern Med 94:505–518

39. Weisse AB, Heller DR, Schimenti RJ, Montgomery RL, Kapila R (1993) The febrile parenteral drug user: a prospective study in 121 patients. Am J Med 94:274–280

40. Heimberger TS, Duma RJ (1989) Infections of prosthetic heart valves and cardiac pacemakers. Infect Dis Clin North Am 3:221–245

41. Durack DT, Lukes AS, Bright DK (1994) New criteria for diagnosis of infective endocarditis: utilization of specific echocardiographic findings. Duke Endocarditis Service. Am J Med 96:200–209

42. Hoen B, Beguinot I, Rabaud C et al (1996) The Duke criteria for diagnosing infective endocarditis are specific: analysis of 100 patients with acute fever or fever of unknown origin. Clin Infect Dis 23:298–302

43. Sekeres MA, Abrutyn E, Berlin JA et al (1997) An assessment of the usefulness of the Duke criteria for diagnosing active infective endocarditis. Clin Infect Dis 24:1185–1190

44. Abraham AK, Neutze JM, MacCulloch D, Cornere B (1984) Culture negative infective endocarditis. Aust N Z J Med 14:223–226

45. Goldenberger D, Kunzli A, Vogt P, Zbinden R, Altwegg M (1997) Molecular diagnosis of bacterial endocarditis by broad-range PCR amplification and direct sequencing. J Clin Microbiol 35:2733–2739

46. Heiro M, Nikoskelainen J, Engblom E, Kotilainen E, Marttila R, Kotilainen P (2000) Neurologic manifestations of infective endocarditis: a 17-year experience in a teaching hospital in Finland. Arch Intern Med 160:2781–2787

47. Paschalis C, Pugsley W, John R, Harrison MJ (1990) Rate of cerebral embolic events in relation to antibiotic and anticoagulant therapy in patients with bacterial endocarditis. Eur Neurol 30:87–89

48. Wilson WR, Karchmer AW, Dajani AS et al (1995) Antibiotic treatment of adults with infective endocarditis due to streptococci, enterococci, staphylococci, and HACEK microorganisms. American Heart Association. JAMA 274:1706–1713

49. Karchmer AW, Moellering RC Jr, Maki DG, Swartz MN (1979) Single-antibiotic therapy for streptococcal endocarditis. JAMA 241:1801–1806

50. Francioli P, Etienne J, Hoigne R, Thys JP, Gerber A (1992) Treatment of streptococcal endocarditis with a single daily dose of ceftriaxone sodium for 4 weeks. Efficacy and outpatient treatment feasibility. JAMA 267:264–267

51. Stamboulian D, Bonvehi P, Arevalo C et al (1991) Antibiotic management of outpatients with endocarditis due to penicillin-susceptible streptococci. Rev Infect Dis 13 [Suppl 2]:S160–S163
52. Fantin B, Carbon C (1992) In vivo antibiotic synergism: contribution of animal models. Antimicrob Agents Chemother 36:907–912
53. Eliopoulos GM (1993) Aminoglycoside resistant enterococcal endocarditis. Infect Dis Clin North Am 7:117–133
54. Caputo GM, Archer GL, Calderwood SB, DiNubile MJ, Karchmer AW (1987) Native valve endocarditis due to coagulase-negative staphylococci. Clinical and microbiologic features. Am J Med 83:619–625
55. Karchmer AW, Archer GL, Dismukes WE (1983) *Staphylococcus epidermidis* causing prosthetic valve endocarditis: microbiologic and clinical observations as guides to therapy. Ann Intern Med 98:447–455
56. Chambers HF (1993) Short-course combination and oral therapies of *Staphylococcus aureus* endocarditis. Infect Dis Clin North Am 7:69–80
57. Torres-Tortosa M, de Cueto M, Vergara A et al (1994) Prospective evaluation of a two-week course of intravenous antibiotics in intravenous drug addicts with infective endocarditis. Grupo de Estudio de Enfermedades Infecciosas de la Provincia de Cadiz. Eur J Clin Microbiol Infect Dis 13:559–564
58. Francioli PB (1993) Ceftriaxone and outpatient treatment of infective endocarditis. Infect Dis Clin North Am 7:97–115
59. Tunkel AR, Scheld WM (1994) Acute meningitis. In: Mandell GL, Bennet JE, Dolin R (eds) Principles and practice of infectious diseases. Churchill Livingstone, New York, pp 831–865
60. Durand ML, Calderwood SB, Weber DJ et al (1993) Acute bacterial meningitis in adults. A review of 493 episodes. N Engl J Med 328:21–28
61. Schuchat A, Robinson K, Wenger JD et al (1997) Bacterial meningitis in the United States in 1995. Active Surveillance Team. N Engl J Med 337:970–976
62. Adams WG, Deaver KA, Cochi SL et al (1993) Decline of childhood *Haemophilus influenzae* type b (Hib) disease in the Hib vaccine era. JAMA 269:221–226
63. Liptak GS, McConnochie KM, Roghmann KJ, Panzer JA (1997) Decline of pediatric admissions with *Haemophilus influenzae* type b in New York State, 1982 through 1993: relation to immunizations. J Pediatr 130:923–930
64. Saez-Llorens X, Ramilo O, Mustafa MM, Mertsola J, McCracken GH Jr (1990) Molecular pathophysiology of bacterial meningitis: current concepts and therapeutic implications. J Pediatr 116:671–684
65. Quagliarello V, Scheld WM (1992) Bacterial meningitis: pathogenesis, pathophysiology, and progress. N Engl J Med 327:864–872
66. Pfister HW, Fontana A, Tauber MG, Tomasz A, Scheld WM (1994) Mechanisms of brain injury in bacterial meningitis: workshop summary. Clin Infect Dis 19:463–479
67. Viladrich PF (1993) Thesis: Enfermedad meningocócica en adolescentes y adultos (Hospital de Bellvitge, 1977-1990). Universitat de Barcelona, Spain
68. Casado FJ, Garcia Teresa MA, Cambra F et al (1997) Multicenter prospective study on severe bacterial meningitis in children. An Esp Pediatr 47:466–472
69. Lacroix J, Deal C, Gauthier M, Rousseau E, Farrell CA (1994) Admissions to a pediatric intensive care unit for status epilepticus: a 10-year experience. Crit Care Med 22:827–832
70. Viladrich PF, Buenaventura I, Gudiol F et al (1986) Meningitis neumocócica del adulto. Estudio de 141 episodios. Med Clin (Barc) 87:569–574
71. Pfister HW, Feiden W, Einhaupl KM (1993) Spectrum of complications during bacte-

tion of symptoms, and that treatment for 10 days is no more effective than treatment for 5 days.

Goals of management of secondary peritonitis are summarized in Table 2. Several studies have identified *E. coli* and *B. fragilis* as the main target organisms for antibiotic therapy [2, 15]. The current practice of early empirical administration of antibiotics targeted against these bacteria is well established. However, issues concerning the choice and timing of drugs, the need for surgical cultures, and the duration of postoperative administration are controversial.

Despite several published options, antibiotic therapy for secondary peritonitis is simple. The emerging concepts suggest that less, in terms of number of drugs and duration of treatment, is better [2]. Furthermore, recent studies suggest that monotherapy with a single broad-spectrum antibiotic that includes full activity against *E. coli* may be equal or superior to polytherapy with multiple drug combinations [15-19].

The surgical strategy depends on the source of the infection [20, 21], the degree of peritoneal contamination, the clinical condition of the patient, and

Table 2. Principles for the management of peritonitis and indications for staged abdominal repair

Supportive measures	To combat hypovolemia and shock and maintain adequate tissue oxygenation
	To treat bacteria not eliminated by surgery with antibiotics
	To support failing organ systems
	To provide adequate nutrition
Operative treatment	Repair and/or control the source of infection
	Evacuate bacterial inoculum, pus, and adjuvants
	Treat abdominal compartment syndrome
	Prevent or treat persistent and recurrent infection or verify both repair and purge
Staged abdominal repair	Critical patient condition, due to hemodynamic instability, precluding definitive repair
	Excessive peritoneal edema (abdominal compartment syndrome, pulmonary, cardiac, renal, or hepatic dysfunction, decreased visceral perfusion) preventing abdominal closure without under tension
	IA pressure > 15 mmHg
	Massive abdominal wall loss
	Impossible to eliminate or to control the source of infection
	Incomplete debridement of necrotic tissue
	Uncertainty of viability of remaining bowel
	Uncontrolled bleeding (the need for packing)

the concomitant disease. Moreover, early goal-directed therapy provides significant benefits with respect to outcome in patients with severe sepsis and MOF [22]. Ideally, a severe IA infection should be cured with a single surgical procedure; unfortunately, infection often persists or recurs. Traditionally, severe peritonitis has been treated by performing a midline laparotomy to identify and eliminate the source of infection. In certain instances, complete control of the infective focus is not feasible during the first operation [2]. While elimination of the focus and reduction of contamination are accepted as conditions of successful treatment, surgical procedures differ for the treatment of residual infection. The following major approaches have been developed: (1) continuous closed postoperative lavage; (2) planned relaparotomy; and (3) open treatment by laparostomy.

Continuous peritoneal lavage takes the whole concept of lavage to an extreme, the hypothesis being that continual IA irrigation will enhance the removal of bacteria and their products, and improve the time to resolution [23]. Various forms of peritoneal lavage are routinely used in management of patients with peritonitis. There is little evidence that supports this approach in either the clinical and scientific literature; moreover, it has been documented that lavage damages mesothelial cells, dilutes agents that are involved in peritoneal defense, and may spread previously contained infection.

The planned relaparotomy approach involves reoperations at fixed intervals, irrespective of the clinical condition of the patient, to prevent development of further septic fluid collections, so precluding their systemic effects. Adverse effects of planned relaparotomies are frequent and include damage to abdominal wall structures and IA viscera. Open management facilitates frequent re-exploration and, by treating the entire peritoneal cavity as one large infected collection, continuous exposure for maximal drainage. Furthermore, it serves to reduce the high IA pressure caused by peritoneal edema associated with fluid resuscitation and inflammation, thus obviating the deleterious systemic consequences of the abdominal compartment syndrome [24]. GIT fistulas and abdominal wall defects have plagued simple open management; these complications should be minimized by introduction of temporary abdominal closure devices, such as artificial mesh-zipper techniques.

Tertiary peritonitis develops late in the postoperative course, presents clinically as sepsis, and is associated with a sterile peritoneal cavity or particular microbiology. Further antimicrobial administration and surgical interventions may contribute to peritoneal superinfection with yeasts and other low level pathogens [2]. The low virulence of these organisms, which represent a marker of tertiary peritonitis and not its cause, reflects the global immunodepression of the affected patients.

Pathophysiology

The pathogenesis of AP remains poorly understood. A number of factors can initiate this process, including obstruction or overdistention of the pancreatic duct, exposure to ethanol and other toxins, hypertriglyceridemia, hypercalcemia, increased permeability of the pancreatic duct, and hyperstimulation of the gland. These diverse factors initiate an inappropriate activation of zymogens. Ischemia of the organ appears to transform mild edematous AP into severe hemorrhagic/necrotizing forms of the disease [30, 31]. The mechanisms of AP and resulting complications are reported in Fig. 2. The necrotic pancreas

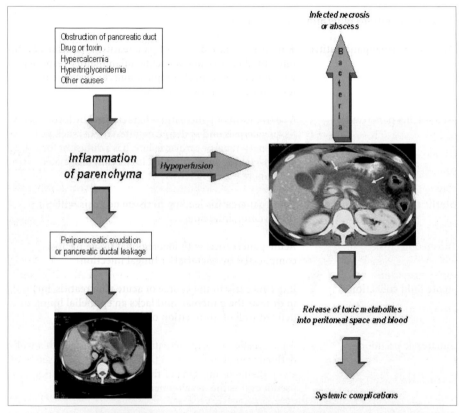

Fig. 2. Mechanisms of acute pancreatitis and resulting complications. Acute pancreatitis can be triggered by several events, resulting in inflammation of the parenchyma. Ischemia of the organ appears to transform mild edematous pancreatitis into severe necrotizing forms of the disease. Pseudocysts can develop if pancreatic juices and debris leak into the peripancreatic spaces. Necrotic parenchyma becomes secondarily infected in 40%–60% of cases, usually with aerobic Gram-negative bacilli translocated from the gastrointestinal tract. Alternatively, the necrotic pancreas may release toxic factors into the peripancreatic spaces, peritoneal cavity, or systemic circulation, leading to local or systemic complications. Computed tomography scans show a pancreatic pseudocyst, and lack of enhancement, representing necrosis, of the head, body and tail of the pancreas (*arrows*)

becomes secondarily infected in 40%–60% of cases, usually with aerobic Gram-negative bacilli translocated from the GIT [31, 32]. Enteric organisms predominate and polymicrobial infection is common. Fungal infection is recognized with increased frequency, and the presence of *Candida* spp. is associated with increased mortality [33].

Presentation and Classification

Severe AP is diagnosed if three or more of Ranson's criteria are present, if the APACHE II score is 8 or more, or if one or more of the following are present: shock, renal insufficiency, and pulmonary insufficiency. Pancreatic glandular necrosis is usually associated with necrosis of peripancreatic fat, and by definition, it represents a severe form of AP. The risk of infected necrosis increases with the amount of glandular necrosis and the time from the onset of AP, peaking at 3 weeks. The overall mortality in severe AP is approximately 30%. As long as necrotizing AP remains sterile, the mortality rate is approximately 10%, but at least triples if there is infected necrosis. In addition, patients with sterile necrosis and high severity-of-illness scores accompanied by MOF, shock, or renal insufficiency have significantly higher mortality. Deaths occur in two phases. Early deaths (1-2 weeks after AP onset) are due to MOF caused by the release of inflammatory mediators and cytokines. Late deaths result from systemic or local infection. Local infections, so-called secondary pancreatic infections, are represented by pancreatic abscess, infected pseudocyst, and infected necrosis. By definition, pancreatic abscess and infected pancreatic pseudocysts are associated with little or no necrosis. In contrast, patients with diffuse or focal areas of non-viable pancreatic parenchyma, often associated with peripancreatic fat necrosis, are categorized as having infected or non-infected pancreatic necrosis.

Recognition

Dynamic intravenous contrast-enhanced abdominal CT diagnoses pancreatic necrosis radiographically. Because the normal pancreatic microcirculation is disrupted during necrotizing AP, affected portions of the pancreas do not show normal contrast enhancement. The lack of normal contrast enhancement may be better detected several days after initial clinical presentation. Contrast-enhanced CT is the gold standard for the non-invasive diagnosis of pancreatic necrosis, with an accuracy of more than 90% when there is more than 30% glandular necrosis [34].

Sterile and infected necrosis can be difficult to distinguish clinically, since both may produce fever, leukocytosis, and severe abdominal pain. The distinction is important, because mortality among patients with infected necrosis

Table 6. Etiology of pleural effusions (PE) (ARDS acute respiratory distress syndrome)

PE characteristic	Diseases
Transudative	Congestive heart failure (most-common transudative PE), hepatic cirrhosis with and without ascites, nephrotic syndrome, peritoneal dialysis/continuous ambulatory peritoneal dialysis, hypoalbuminemia (e.g., severe starvation), glomerulonephritis, superior vena cava obstruction, urinothorax
Exudative	Malignant disorders (metastatic disease to the pleura or lungs, primary lung cancer, mesothelioma, Kaposi sarcoma, lymphoma, leukemia), infectious diseases (bacterial, fungal, parasitic, and viral infections, infection with atypical organisms such as *Mycoplasma*, *Rickettsiae*, *Chlamydia*, *Legionella*), GIT diseases (pancreatic disease, Whipple disease, IA abscess, esophageal perforation, abdominal surgery, diaphragmatic hernia, endoscopic variceal sclerotherapy), collagen vascular diseases (rheumatoid arthritis, systemic lupus erythematosus, drug-induced lupus syndrome, immunoblastic lymphadenopathy, Sjögren syndrome, familial Mediterranean fever, Churg-Strauss syndrome, Wegener granulomatosis), benign asbestos effusion, Meigs syndrome (benign solid ovarian neoplasm associated with ascites and pleural effusion), drug-induced primary pleural disease (nitrofurantoin, dantrolene, methysergide, bromocriptine, amiodarone, procarbazine, methotrexate, ergonovine, ergotamine, oxprenolol, maleate, practolol, minoxidil, bleomycin, interleukin-2, propylthiouracil, isotretinoin, metronidazole, mitomycin), injury after cardiac surgery (Dressler syndrome), uremic pleuritis, yellow nail syndrome, ruptured ectopic pregnancy, electrical burns
Exudative/transudative	Pulmonary embolism, hypothyroidism, pericardial disease (inflammatory or constrictive), atelectasis, trapped lung (usually a borderline exudate), sarcoidosis (usually an exudate), amyloidosis
Miscellaneous	Hemothorax, following coronary artery bypass graft surgery, after lung or liver transplant, milk of calcium PE, ARDS, systemic cholesterol emboli, iatrogenic misplacement of lines or tubes into the mediastinum or the pleural space, radiation pleuritis, necrotizing sarcoid granulomatosis, ovarian hyper stimulation syndrome, postpartum PE (immediate or delayed), rupture of a silicone bag mammary prosthesis, rupture of a benign germ cell tumor into the pleural space (e.g., benign mediastinal teratoma, syphilis, echinococcosis)

An empyema may occur by direct contamination of the pleural space through wounds of the chest, by hematological spread, by direct extension from lung parenchymal infections, by rupture of an intrapulmonary abscess or infected cavity, or by extension from the mediastinum. Most often, empyemas are the results of a primary infectious process in the lung.

Frequency and Mortality/Morbidity

In industrialized countries, the relative annual incidence of PE is estimated to be 320 per 100,000 people. The approximate PE annual incidences are based on major underlying disease processes, such as congestive heart failure, bacterial pneumonia, malignancy, pulmonary embolus, and cirrhosis with ascites, pancreatitis, collagen vascular disease, and tuberculosis. PE morbidity and mortality are directly related to cause, stage of disease at the time of presentation, and biochemical findings in the pleural fluid. Morbidity and mortality rates of patients with pneumonia and PE are higher than those of patients with pneumonia alone.

Symptoms and Physical Findings

The clinical manifestations of PE are variable and often are related to the underlying disease process. The most commonly associated symptoms are progressive dyspnea, cough (typically non-productive), and pleuritic chest pain. Dyspnea is the most common clinical symptom at presentation, and usually indicates a large effusion [82, 84].

Chest pain may be mild or severe. It is typically described as sharp or stabbing, is exacerbated with deep inspiration, and is pleuritic. Pain may be localized to the chest wall or referred to the ipsilateral shoulder or upper abdomen, usually because of diaphragmatic involvement. Other signs and symptoms occurring with pleural effusions are associated more closely with the underlying disease process. An acute febrile episode, purulent sputum production, and pleuritic chest pain may occur in patients with PE associated with aerobic bacterial pneumonia [85].

Physical findings are variable and depend on the PE volume. Generally, findings are undetectable for effusions smaller than 300 ml. Four main types of fluids in the pleural space are serous fluid (hydrothorax), blood (hemothorax), lipid (chylothorax), and pus (pyothorax or empyema). PE develops in 30%–40% of patients with bacterial pneumonia. Those with bacterial pneumonia, especially that caused by *Streptococcus pneumoniae*, have a high predilection for complications. These can include bacteremia and multilobar involvement. Moreover, aerobic Gram-negative bacilli and anaerobic organisms are common causes of empyema [86].

Diagnosis

The initial step in analyzing pleural fluid is to determine whether PE is a transudate or an exudate. The clinical presentation should direct the biochemical and microbiological studies of pleural fluid. The minimal amount of pleural fluid needed for basic diagnostic purposes is 20 ml; if possible, 60 ml should be obtained for diagnostic studies.

If the clinical presentation is highly suggestive of transudative PE, protein and LDH levels should be determined initially. If the patient has undergone diuretic therapy, the pleural albumin level should be determined simultaneously. Concomitant serum total protein, LDH, and, if indicated, serum albumin levels should be measured. If transudative effusion is diagnosed, no further tests are needed. Exudative PE requires further laboratory investigation. Cytological analysis is strongly recommended for patients with a history of undiagnosed exudative PE, suspected malignancy, or *Pneumocystis carinii* infection, or exudative PE with normal fluid glucose and amylase levels [86, 87].

Additional studies should be requested on the basis of the gross appearance of the pleural fluid or when a specific condition is suspected. The gross appearance of the pleural fluid, as well as results of certain laboratory studies, may provide useful diagnostic information (Table 7). Laboratory results can aid in narrowing the differential diagnosis of exudative PE.

Table 7. Clinical significance of pleural fluid characteristics

Characteristic	Significance
Bloody	Most likely an indication of malignancy in the absence of trauma, can also indicate pulmonary embolism, infection, pancreatitis, tuberculosis, mesothelioma, or spontaneous pneumothorax
Turbid	Possible increased cellular content or lipid content
Yellow or whitish, turbid	Presence of chyle, cholesterol, or empyema
Brown	Rupture of amebic liver abscess into the pleural space (amebiasis with a hepatopleural fistula)
Black	Aspergillus involvement of pleura
Yellow-green with debris	Rheumatoid pleurisy
Highly viscous	Malignant mesothelioma (due to increased levels of hyaluronic acid) long-standing pyothorax
Putrid odor	Anaerobic infection of pleural space
Ammonia odor	Urinothorax
Purulent	Empyema
Yellow and thick, with metallic sheen	Effusions rich in cholesterol (long-standing chyliform effusion, e.g., tuberculous or rheumatoid pleuritis)

Imaging studies. This step is the most important in the PE evaluation. Common imaging studies used to confirm PE are chest radiography, ultrasonography, and CT scan [82–87]. Chest radiography is the primary diagnostic tool because of its availability, accuracy, and low cost. It can be used to determine the cause of PE (enlarged cardiac silhouette, underlying lung, parenchymal disease). The most common radiological appearance is blunting of the costophrenic angle and/or sulci. Upright postero-anterior or antero-posterior radiographs may not show lateral costophrenic angle blunting until 250–500 ml of fluid is present. Lateral radiographs show blunting of the posterior costophrenic angle and the posterior gutter when as little as 175–200 ml of fluid is present. Bilateral decubitus radiographs are recommended, especially with larger effusions.

The location of the PE can help in the differential diagnosis. Atypical chest radiographic presentations are possible. When an air-fluid level is present in the pleural space, the following must be considered: bronchopleural fistula, pneumothorax, trauma, presence of gas-forming organisms, diaphragmatic hernia, fluid-filled bullae or lung cysts, and rupture of the esophagus into the pleural space. Diaphragmatic hernias can be excluded or confirmed with the administration of GIT contrast material.

Ultrasonography can be used to detect as little as 5–50 ml of pleural fluid, with 100% sensitivity for effusions of 100 ml or more [86]. It aids in the identification of loculated PE and the differentiation of pleural fluid from pleural fibrosis, thickening, and parenchymal consolidation. It can help localize the diaphragm if pleural or parenchymal disease obscures it. Unlike CT, ultrasonography is rapid and available at the bedside.

Chest CT scanning permits imaging of the entire pleural space, pulmonary parenchyma, and mediastinum simultaneously. CT scans reveal early stage pleural abnormalities. Contrast-enhanced scans can depict multiple loculations and localizing PEs, differentiate between lung consolidation and PE, cystic lesions and solid lesions, necrotic areas, pleural thickening, nodules, masses, or rounded atelectasis, and peripheral lung abscess versus loculated empyema. It also provides information on the extent of the tumor [85, 86].

Invasive diagnostic procedures. After the presence of PE is established, the cause should be identified. This step can be critical because unnecessary invasive procedures cause morbidity and mortality. When a decision is made to investigate the cause of PE, thoracentesis is the first-line invasive diagnostic procedure [86]. Thoracentesis also can be used as a therapeutic modality.

Thoracentesis is the least-invasive procedure and is relatively safe. For stable and asymptomatic patients in whom PE most likely is caused by viral pleurisy, a systemic disease, thoracic or abdominal surgery, or childbearing, thoracentesis may not be indicated, or can be deferred. In this situation, therapy for the specific cause should be initiated, and if no improvement occurs after a few days, diagnostic thoracentesis should be performed.

Thoracentesis is also indicated in cases in which the specific cause of PE is unknown or has never been investigated, or when the thickness of the free pleural fluid level is more 10 mm on the lateral decubitus radiograph. In addition, thoracentesis is indicated if the patient has respiratory compromise, hemodynamic instability, or massive effusion with contralateral mediastinal shift. After thoracentesis, and regardless of its success, chest radiography is recommended to rule out a subsequent pneumothorax. Pneumothorax is the most common complication (incidence 3%–20% with unguided thoracentesis, 2%–7% with ultrasonographic guidance) and is operator dependent. Other complications include subcutaneous hematoma, infection of the pleural space or soft tissue overlying the thoracentesis site, pain at the site, cough, chest pain, hemothorax, vasovagal reflex, re-expansion pulmonary edema, hypovolemia, hypoxemia, splenic or hepatic laceration, hemoperitoneum, and adverse reactions to the local anesthetics. Definite indications to tube thoracostomy include empyema, hemothorax, large pneumothorax, and parapneumonic PE.

Treatment

Most commonly, PE is an incidental finding in a stable patient. Patients with a toxic condition, respiratory distress, or cardiovascular instability require emergency medical services more often. As with any other life-threatening condition, direct initial management is stabilization of the airway to ensure adequate oxygenation and ventilation [84].

On the basis of presentation, patients with PE may be stable, requiring hospital admission, stable, not requiring hospital admission, or unstable. Stable patients who do not require admission include those in whom the clinical circumstances clearly explain PE and/or prior investigations of the cause were performed, PEs are typical of the disease or asymptomatic, and diagnostic or therapeutic thoracentesis is not required.

Stable patients requiring admission include most patients with PE thicker than 10 mm on the lateral decubitus radiograph. Such patients include those with no prior history of PE, patients with parapneumonic PE who do not appear to have a toxic condition, and patients with a prior history of PE who have a change in their usual symptoms or effusion. Although these patients are not in acute respiratory distress, diagnostic thoracentesis is imperative. For parapneumonic PE, delay in diagnostic thoracentesis and antibiotic therapy can be detrimental. Simple parapneumonic PE has a great potential to become complicated or empyema. Antimicrobial therapy alone is not sufficient for complicated parapneumonic PE or empyemas; they require tube thoracostomy and antibiotics [84].

Unstable patients include those with a toxic appearance, respiratory distress, or cardiovascular compromise due to PE. The initial treatment focus should be stabilizing the airway and circulation. Infected pleural fluid with bronchopleural fistula is considered a medical emergency. Bronchopleural fistula should be suspected when a patient with PE produces a larger amount of sputum than expected from associated pulmonary disease. The presence of an air-fluid level in the pleural space on upright radiographs suggests bronchopleural fistula. Patients with this require immediate diagnostic thoracentesis and antibiotics [84, 85].

In any patient with chest-penetrating or non-penetrating trauma, hemothorax should be suspected. Traumatic hemothorax is an indication for the insertion of a large-bore chest tube. Antibiotics and diuretics are commonly used in the initial management of PE. An empiric systemic antibiotic coverage should be initiated in infections or potentially septic conditions (parapneumonic PE, empyemas, esophageal perforation, hemothorax, IA abscesses). Generally, initial antibiotics used should have a broad spectrum of coverage for both aerobic and anaerobic micro-organisms. Most commonly, two antimicrobial agents are necessary to ensure adequate coverage [83–85]. Various effective combinations exist; one of these is a third-generation cephalosporin (cefotaxime) and clindamycin. If the patient is a nursing home resident, a cephalosporin with enhanced antipseudomonas activity is recommended. In children, a monotherapy usually is sufficient.

Wound Infections

These are very frequent after a surgical procedure. The dependency of the infection rate on the type of surgery is reflected in the overall differences in expected infection rates in the different surgical departments, from a low of 2% in plastic surgery, to 3%–5% in orthopedics and vascular surgery, to a high of 9%–27% in general surgery and urology [88, 89]. Surgical wound infections (WIs) can prolong hospitalization by 5–20 days and substantially increase the cost of care [89]. A simple method to evaluate the probability that WI will develop involves classifying the wound according to the scheme illustrated in Table 8.

Risk factors

Surgical WIs occur whenever the combination of microbial concentrations and the virulence is sufficiently large to overcome the local host defense mechanisms and establish progressive growth [88–94]. It is immediately evident that different types of surgical procedures, involving a greater or lesser degree of contamination, are then associated with different probability of developing WIs.

Table 8. Classification of surgical wounds

Clean wounds	Infection risk of about 1-5%. Prophylactic antibiotics are not indicated in clean surgery if the patient has no host risk factors. Factors suggesting the need for prophylaxis are remote infection, diabetes, at least 3 concomitant medical diagnoses. Additive risk factors are, also, abdominal operations and operations expected to last longer than 2 h. Prostheses implants are clean procedures, some of which require antibiotic prophylaxis. Inguinal hernia repair with biomaterials does not benefit from antibiotic prophylaxis
Clean-contaminated wounds	10% or lower risk of infection. Clean-contaminated surgery usually requires prophylaxis
Contaminated wounds	10-20% risk of infection. This type of surgery needs prophylaxis. Biliary, hepatobiliary, and pancreatic operations usually meet the criteria of clean-contaminated wounds. In biliary tract procedures, prophylaxis is required only for cases at high risk of contamination: bile obstruction, jaundice, stones in common duct, reoperation, and cholecystitis. Prophylaxis is always required in hepatobiliary and pancreatic surgery because these operations are long. In gastroduodenal operations the risk is low if gastric acidity is normal, and bleeding, cancer, gastric ulcer, and obstruction are absent. Colorectal procedures are usually contaminated cases. The unique goal of prophylaxis includes the preoperative reduction of bacterial concentration in feces. In association with mechanical bowel preparation, prophylaxis is used in major elective abdominal procedures (i.e., vascular graft) to prevent bacterial translocation from the gut
Infected wounds	Risk of infection of about 20-50%. They meet the following criteria: acute bacterial inflammation encountered, without pus; transection of clean tissue for the purpose of surgical access to a collection of pus; traumatic wound with retained ischemic tissues, foreign bodies, fecal contamination, or delayed treatment. The right treatment is to administer antibiotic therapy, not as prophylaxis, because infection is already present

Several patient factors, besides the type of procedure and the operator skill, are important in affecting the probability of incurring a postoperative WI. One factor is the age of the patient: the higher the age, the higher the incidence. Another factor is the period of hospital stay before surgery: patient with a hospitalization of more than 12 days are more liable to develop an infected wound, showing that a relationship is likely between the incidence of infection and the hospital environment and bacterial flora [91, 92].

Factors Involved in Development of WI

It is clear that the mechanism whereby a patient develops WI is linked to three critical elements. These are represented by the closed space, the infectious agent, which must be present in sufficient numbers and with sufficient virulence, and the susceptible host.

Injury produces enclosed environments, due to pockets of extravasated blood, necrotic tissue, infarcted areas, foreign bodies, and prostheses. The environment in these enclosed spaces soon becomes hypoxic, hypercarbic, and acidic, favoring bacterial growth. In abdominal surgery, GIT represents a huge reservoir of potentially pathogenic bacteria, and recently it has hypothesized that it could act as an undrained abscess, causing infection and MOF [88, 93].

Any infectious agent can contaminate a closed space, but relatively few cause infection. *Streptococcus* spp. invade even minor breaks in the skin and spread through connective tissue planes and lymphatics. *Staphylococcus* spp. are less invasive but more pathogenic. *Pseudomonas* spp. and *Serratia* spp. are often seen as opportunistic invaders. Many fungi and parasites may cause abscesses or sinus, and they are typical of the immunocompromised patient. Anaerobes, such as *Bacteroides* spp., and peptostreptococci are more frequently isolated because of improvements in culture techniques. Post-surgical WI is a multimicrobial disease and unfortunately many bacteria act in synergism [94].

Finally, there are host-dependent factors predisposing to the development of post-surgical infections. Among these are diabetes, severe trauma, burns, malnutrition, cancer, hematological disorders, transplantation, and immunosuppressive drugs. In many patients, these factors are believed to be primarily responsible for a decreased reactivity to delayed hypersensitivity antigens, creating an anergic state associated with an increased incidence of infectious complications. Considering these three elements, it is easier to understand the cycle. Immunosuppression and anergy are very common in a surgical patient; they lead to infection, and the infection itself can deteriorate the immune system.

Treatment

Since infectious complications in surgical patients are responsible for prolonged wound healing, disability, and even death, and since the patient's quality of life can be affected or even permanently altered by them, with huge socioeconomic costs, it is important to prevent them as far as possible.

The importance of the nutritional status is emphasized by the higher incidence of infectious and other surgical complications in malnourished patients. Among several indices of nutritional status, the prognostic nutritional index (PNI), which includes the serum albumin value, is correlated with the probability of infection after surgery. For values of PNI above 50% there is a high risk of postoperative complications. For values between 40% and 49% there is an intermediate risk and for values below 40% there is a low risk. Furthermore, it has been observed that perioperative administration of supplemental oxygen is a practical method of reducing the incidence of surgical WIs [95].

Antibiotic Prophylaxis

The first important point about antibiotic prophylaxis is the timing of its administration [90, 91]. It has been shown that administration of antibiotics just before, during, and up to 3 h after surgery effectively prevents WIs. Many studies have demonstrated that prophylactic antibiotics are most useful if given to patients before contamination has occurred. The most relevant protective effect was observed when antibiotic was given so that good tissue levels were present at the time of the procedure and for the first 3–4 h after the surgical incision. A practical approach would then contemplate administering a single preoperative dose, followed by an intraoperative dose if the procedure lasts longer than 3 h or twice the half-life of the antibiotic, and massive hemorrhage occurs during surgery [88].

Principles of the proper prophylaxis of WIs include the selection of bactericidal antibiotics effective against likely pathogens. It has been shown that single-agent prophylaxis is almost always effective in the majority of clinical situations, provided that the half-life of the antibiotic is long enough to maintain adequate tissue levels throughout the operation and that the dose is equal to a full therapeutic i.v. dose. Recommended antibiotics for prophylaxis of WIs caused by Gram-positive and Gram-negative aerobic bacteria are cefazolin (1 g i.v./i.m.) or vancomycin (1 g i.v.) in patients allergic to cephalosporins. First-generation cephalosporins, such as cefazolin, are a good choice because they are not expensive, have a low rate of allergic responses, and have a broad spectrum of activity against likely aerobic pathogens. Prophylaxis against both Gram-negative aerobes and anaerobes includes clindamycin or metronidazole plus tobramycin, or a single broad-spectrum agent like cefoxitin or cefotetan. Gram-negative anaerobes (*Bacteroides* spp.) are of GIT origin and are synergistic with Gram-negative aerobes in causing infections after GIT surgical procedures. Although the problem is still debated, the combination of two antibiotics is in general more powerful than a single broad-spectrum agent active against both bacterial components [88, 91].

A second point concerns the cases for which the described antibiotic prophylaxis is indicated. In general, an approach like that outlined above is indicated for GIT and anorectal surgery, biliary tract surgery, vaginal hysterectomy, insertion of artificial devices, or for prolonged (more than 3 h) clean surgery. In contaminated or dirty surgery, appropriate therapy should be started as soon as possible. The correct treatment is to administer antibiotic therapy, not as prophylaxis, because infection is already present [88].

In relation to operative contamination and increasing risk of WI, the classification of operative wound includes the four categories mentioned above. This is the most widely applied classification of surgical procedures in terms of contamination and probability that a WI will develop; this risk is about 5%, 10%, 15%, and 30% for the four reported classes, respectively [88].

Urinary Tract Infections

UTI is defined as the presence of high concentrations of bacteria and leucocytes in the presence of symptoms [96, 97] (Chapter 1). Successful management includes proper specimen collection, use of immediately available laboratory testing for presumptive diagnosis, appreciation of epidemiological and host factors that may identify patients with clinically inapparent upper UTI, and selection of appropriate antimicrobial therapy with recommendations for follow-up care [98–100].

Pathophysiology

The urinary tract is normally sterile. Uncomplicated UTI involves the urinary bladder in a host without underlying renal or neurological disease. The clinical entity is termed cystitis and represents bladder mucosal invasion, most often by enteric coliform bacteria (*E. coli*) that inhabit the periurethral vaginal introitus and ascend into the bladder via the urethra. Sexual intercourse may promote this migration, and cystitis is common in otherwise healthy young women [99]. Urine is generally a good culture medium; factors unfavorable to bacterial growth include a low pH (5.5 or less), a high concentration of urea, and the presence of organic acids derived from a diet that includes fruits and protein.

Frequent and complete voiding has been associated with a reduction in the incidence of UTI [100–104]. Normally, a thin film of urine remains in the bladder after emptying, and any bacteria present are removed by the mucosal cell production of organic acids. If the mechanisms of the lower urinary tract fail, upper tract or kidney involvement occurs and is termed pyelonephritis. Host defenses at this level include local leukocyte phagocytosis and renal production of antibodies that kill bacteria in the presence of complement.

Complicated UTI occurs in the setting of underlying structural, medical, or neurological disease [100]. Patients with a neurogenic bladder or bladder diverticulum and postmenopausal women with bladder or uterine prolapse have an increased frequency of UTI due to incomplete bladder emptying. This eventually allows residual bacteria to overwhelm local bladder mucosal defenses. The high urine glucose content and the defective host immune factors in patients with diabetes mellitus also predispose to infection.

Frequency and Mortality/Morbidity

An estimated 11% of women in the United States report at least one physician-diagnosed UTI per year, and the lifetime probability that a woman will have a UTI is 60% [105]. Although simple cystitis may resolve spontaneously, effective treatment lessens the duration of symptoms and reduces the incidence of progression to upper UTI. Pyelonephritis is associated with substantial morbidity [102–104], including systemic effects such as fever, vomiting, dehydration, and loss of vasomotor tone resulting in hypotension. Complications include acute papillary necrosis with possible development of ureteral obstruction, septic shock, and perinephric abscess. Chronic pyelonephritis may lead to scarring with diminished renal function.

Younger patients have the lowest rates of morbidity and mortality. Unfortunately, despite appropriate intervention, 1%–3% of patients with acute pyelonephritis die. Factors associated with unfavorable prognosis are general debility and old age, renal calculi or obstruction, recent hospitalization or instrumentation, diabetes mellitus, sickle cell anemia, underlying carcinoma, intercurrent chemotherapy, or chronic nephropathy.

The largest group of patients with UTI is adult women. The incidence increases with age and sexual activity. Rates of infection are high in post-menopausal women because of bladder or uterine prolapse causing incomplete bladder emptying, loss of estrogens with attendant changes in vaginal flora, loss of lactobacilli, which allows periurethral colonization with Gram-negative aerobes, such as E. coli, and higher likelihood of concomitant medical illness, such as diabetes. UTI is unusual in males younger than 50 years, and symptoms of dysuria and frequency are usually due to urethral or prostatic infection. In older men, however, the incidence of UTI rises because of prostatic obstruction or subsequent instrumentation.

Symptoms and Physical Findings

The classical symptoms of UTI in the adult are dysuria with accompanying urinary urgency and frequency. A sensation of bladder fullness or lower abdominal discomfort is often present. Bloody urine (hemorrhagic cystitis) is reported in as many as 10% of cases of UTI in otherwise healthy women. Fevers, chills, and malaise may be noted, although these are associated more frequently with pyelonephritis. Most adult women with simple lower UTI have suprapubic tenderness with no evidence of vaginitis, cervicitis, or pelvic tenderness. The patient with pyelonephritis usually appears ill and, in addition to fever, sweating, and prostration, is usually found to have flank tenderness.

Diagnosis

If UTI is suspected, the initial test of choice is urinalysis. The midstream-voided technique is as accurate as catheterization if proper technique is followed. Pyuria, as indicated by a positive result of the leukocyte esterase dip test, is found in the vast majority of patients with UTI.

However, low-level pyuria [6-20 WBCs per high-power field (HPF) on a centrifuged specimen] may be associated with an unacceptable level of false-negative results with the leukocyte esterase dip test. In the female with appropriate symptoms and examination findings suggestive of UTI, urine microscopy may be indicated despite a negative result of the leukocyte esterase dip test.

Current emphasis in the diagnosis of UTI rests with the detection of pyuria. As noted, a positive leukocyte esterase dip test suffices in most instances. According to Stamm and Hooton [104], levels of pyuria as low as 2-5 WBCs per HPF in a centrifuged specimen are important in the female with appropriate symptoms. The presence of bacteriuria is as significant.

A positive result on the nitrate test is highly specific for UTI, typically because of urease-splitting organisms, such as *Proteus* spp. and, occasionally, *E. coli*; however, it is very insensitive as a screening tool, as only 25% of patients with UTI have a positive nitrate test result. Low-level or, occasionally, frank hematuria may be noted in otherwise typical UTI; however, its positive predictive value is poor.

Historically, the definition of UTI was based on the finding by culture of 100,000 colonies/ml of a single organism. If a patient has had a UTI within the last month, the same organism probably causes relapse. Relapse represents treatment failure [96]. Reinfection occurs in 1-6 months and usually is due to a different organism (or serotype of the same organism).

In the vast majority of patients with UTI, no imaging studies are indicated. If findings are suggestive of nephrolithiasis complicating the presentation, an intravenous pyelogram (IVP) or renal ultrasonography should be performed to exclude the possibility of obstruction or hydronephrosis [101–103]. Recent studies with dynamic helical CT scan are proving that this study provides information similar to that yielded by IVP without the need for dye injection. Dynamic CT scans also can serve as a convenient screen for abdominal aortic aneurysm masquerading as UTI or renal colic.

Additional testing may be indicated if the diagnosis is in doubt. For example, a pelvic ultrasound scan may be indicated in a young woman with pelvic tenderness, cervical discharge, and unilateral adnexal tenderness; a CT scan may be indicated in the elderly patient whose presentation is not typical for UTI but who has abdominal pain, lower abdominal tenderness, and pyuria.

Catheterization is indicated if the patient cannot void spontaneously, if the patient is too debilitated or immobilized, or if obesity prevents the patient from obtaining a suitable specimen. Although less common than in older men, postvoiding residual urine volume, measurable by catheterization, may reveal urinary retention in a host with a defective bladder-emptying mechanism.

Treatment

Oral therapy with an antibiotic effective against Gram-negative aerobic coliform bacteria, such as E. coli, is the principal treatment intervention in patients with UTI. The patient with an uncomplicated presumed lower UTI or simple cystitis with symptoms of less than 48 h duration may be treated with one of the following agents for a total of 3 days: (1) co-trimoxazole; (2) ciprofloxacin or similar fluoroquinolone; (3) nitrofurantoin macrocrystals; and (4) amoxicillin/clavulanate [100]. The clinical management of UTI is complicated by the increasing incidence of infections caused by strains of E. coli that are resistant to commonly used antimicrobial agents [106]. In recent studies, the rate of resistance to trimethoprim-sulfamethoxazole among E. coli isolates from women with UTI ranged from 15% to 22% [106].

Pregnant, otherwise healthy women with no evidence of upper UTI may be treated with a 2-week course of a cephalosporin [102, 103]. Pregnant patients should be treated for all episodes of pyuria or bacteriuria, regardless of whether they have symptoms.

Ambulatory younger women who present with signs and symptoms of pyelonephritis may be candidates for outpatient therapy. They must be otherwise healthy and must not be pregnant. They must be treated initially with vigorous oral or i.v. fluids, antipyretic pain medication, and a dose of parenteral antibiotics. Studies have shown that outpatient therapy for selected patients was as safe as, and much less expensive than, inpatient therapy for a comparable group of patients.

The decision regarding admission of a patient with acute pyelonephritis is dependent on age, host factors, such as immunocompromising chemotherapy or chronic diseases, known urinary tract structural abnormalities, renal calculi, recent hospitalization, or urinary tract instrumentation. Initial treatment should include i.v. antibiotic therapy (co-trimoxazole, which is directed at coliform Gram-negative bacteria, third-generation cephalosporin, or an aminoglycoside), adequate fluid resuscitation to restore effective circulating volume and generous urinary volumes, and antipyretic pain medications [100]. In the patient with a complicated UTI, coverage for unusual or multiple antibiotic-resistant organisms, such as P. aeruginosa, must be considered.

References

1. Bosscha K, van Vroonhoven JMV, van der Werken C (1999) Surgical management of severe secondary peritonitis. Br J Surg 86:1371–1377
2. Sganga G, Brisinda G, Castagneto M (2001) Peritonitis: priorities and management strategies. In: van Saene HKF , Sganga G, Silvestri L (eds) Infection in the critically ill: an ongoing challenge. Springer-Verlag, Berlin Heidelberg New York, pp 23–33
3. Sganga G (2000) Sepsi addominali chirurgiche e insufficienza multiorgano (MOFS). Edizioni Systems Comunicazioni, Milan
4. Bone RG, Balk RA, Cerra FB, Dellinger RP, Fein AM, Knaus WA, Schein RM, Sibbald WJ (1992) Definitions for sepsis and organ failure and guidelines for the use of innovative therapies in sepsis. The ACCP/SCCM Consensus Conference Committee. American College of Chest Physicians/Society of Critical Care Medicine. Chest 101:1644–1655
5. Parrillo JE (1993) Pathogenetic mechanisms of septic shock. N Engl J Med 328:1471–1477
6. Meakins JL, Solomkin JS, Allo MD, Dellinger EP, Howard RJ, Simmons RL (1984) A proposed classification of intraabdominal infections. Stratification of etiology and risk for future therapeutic trials. Arch Surg 119:1372–1378
7. Finegold SM (1982) Microflora of the gastrointestinal tract. In: Wilson SE, Finegold SM, Williams RA (eds) Intra-abdominal infection. McGraw-Hill, New York, pp 1–22
8. Krepel CJ, Gohr CM, Edmiston CE, Condon RE (1995) Surgical sepsis: constancy of antibiotic susceptibility of causative organisms. Surgery 117:505–509
9. Sganga G, Brisinda G, Castagneto M (2000) Nosocomial fungal infections in surgical patients: risk factors and treatment. Minerva Anestesiol 66 [Suppl 1]:71–77
10. Wheeler AP, Bernard GR (1999) Treating patients with severe sepsis. N Engl J Med 340:207–214
11. Mannick JA, Rodrick ML, Lederer JA (2001) The immunologic response to injury. J Am Coll Surg 193:237–244
12. Knoferl MW, Angele MK, Diodato MD, Schwacha MG, Ayala A, Cioffi WG, Bland KI, Chaudry IH (2002) Female sex hormones regulate macrophage function after trauma-hemorrhage and prevent increased death rate from subsequent sepsis. Ann Surg 235:105–112
13. Sganga G, van Saene HKF, Brisinda G, Castagneto M (2001) Bacterial translocation. In: van Saene HKF, Sganga G, Silvestri L (eds) Infection in the critically ill: an ongoing challenge. Springer-Verlag, Berlin Heidelberg New York, pp 35–45
14. Soares-Weiser K, Paul M, Brezis M, Leibovici L (2002) Antibiotic treatment for spontaneous bacterial peritonitis. BMJ 324:100–102
15. Solomkin JS, Wilson SE, Christou NV, Rotstein OD, Dellinger EP, Bennion RS, Pak R, Tack K (2001) Results of a clinical trial of clinafloxacin versus imipenem/cilastatin for intraabdominal infections. Ann Surg 233:79–87
16. Wittmann DH, Bergstein JM, Frantzides CT (1991) Calculated empiric antimicrobial therapy for mixed surgical infections. Infection 19 [Suppl 6]:345–350
17. Wittmann DH, Schein M, Condon RE (1996) Management of secondary peritonitis. Ann Surg 224:10–18
18. Hopkins JA, Wilson SE, Bobey DG (1994) Adjunctive antimicrobial therapy for complicated appendicitis: bacterial overkill by combination therapy. World J Surg 18:933–938
19. Cohen J (2000) Combination antibiotic therapy for severe peritonitis. Lancet 356:1539–1540

20. Holzheimer RG, Dralle H (2001) Paradigm change in 30 years peritonitis treatment. A review on source control. Eur J Med Res 6:161–168
21. Jimenez MF, Marshall JC (2001) Source control in the management of sepsis. Intensive Care Med 27:S49–S62
22. Rivers E, Nguyen B, Havstad S, Ressler J, Muzzin A, Knoblich B, Peterson E, Tomlanovich M (2001) Early goal-directed therapy in the treatment of severe sepsis and septic shock. N Engl J Med 345:1368–1377
23. Platell C, Papadimitriou JM, Hall JC (2000) The influence of lavage on peritonitis. J Am Coll Surg 191:672–680
24. Sganga G, Brisinda G, Castagneto M (2002) Trauma operative procedures: timing of surgery and priorities. In: Gullo A (ed) Critical care medicine. Springer-Verlag, Berlin Heidelberg New York, pp 447–467
25. Levison MA, Zeigler D (1991) Correlation of APACHE II score, drainage technique and outcome in postoperative intra-abdominal abscess. Surg Gynecol Obstet 172:89–94
26. Baril NB, Ralls PW, Wren SM, Selby RR, Radin R, Parekh D, Jabbour N, Stain SC (2000) Does an infected peripancreatic fluid collection or abscess mandate operation? Ann Surg 231:361–367
27. Brisinda G, Maria G, Ferrante A, Civello IM (1999) Evaluation of prognostic factors in patients with acute pancreatitis. Hepatogastroenterology 46:1990–1997
28. Baron TH, Morgan DE (1999) Acute necrotizing pancreatitis. N Engl J Med 340:1412–1417
29. Beger HG, Rau B, Mayer J, Pralle U (1997) Natural course of acute pancreatitis. World J Surg 21:130–135
30. Bradley EL III (1993) A clinically based classification system for acute pancreatitis: summary of the International Symposium on Acute Pancreatitis, Atlanta, Ga, September 11 through 13, 1992. Arch Surg 128:586–590
31. Marotta F, Geng TC, Wu CC, Barbi G (1996) Bacterial translocation in the course of acute pancreatitis: beneficial role of nonabsorbable antibiotics and lactitol enemas. Digestion 57:446–452
32. Foitzik T, Fernandez-del Castillo C, Ferraro MJ, Mithofer K, Rattner DW, Warshaw AL (1995) Pathogenesis and prevention of early pancreatic infection in experimental acute necrotizing pancreatitis. Ann Surg 222:179–185
33. Isenmann R, Schwarz M, Rau B, Trautmann M, Schober W, Beger HG (2002) Characteristics of infection with *Candida* species in patients with necrotizing pancreatitis. World J Surg 26:372–376
34. Bradley EL III (1994) Surgical indications and techniques in necrotizing pancreatitis. In: Bradley EL III (ed) Acute pancreatitis: diagnosis and therapy. Raven, New York, pp 105–117
35. Paye F, Rotman N, Radier C, Nouira R, Fagniez PL (1998) Percutaneous aspiration for bacteriological studies in patients with necrotizing pancreatitis. Br J Surg 85:755–759
36. Rau B, Pralle U, Mayer JM, Beger HG (1998) Role of ultrasonographically guided fine-needle aspiration cytology in diagnosis of infected pancreatic necrosis. Br J Surg 85:179–184
37. Mithofer K, Fernandez-del Castillo C, Ferraro MJ, Lewandrowski K, Rattner DW, Warshaw AL (1996) Antibiotic treatment improves survival in experimental acute necrotizing pancreatitis. Gastroenterology 110:232–240
38. Sainio V, Kemppainen E, Puolakkainen P, Taavitsainen M, Kivisaari L, Valtonen V, Haapiainen R, Schroder T, Kivilaakso E (1995) Early antibiotic treatment in acute necrotising pancreatitis. Lancet 346:663–667
39. Luiten EJ, Hop WC, Lange JF, Bruining HA (1995) Controlled clinical trial of selective decontamination for the treatment of severe acute pancreatitis. Ann Surg 222:57–65

40. Luiten EJ, Hop WC, Lange JF, Bruining HA (1997) Differential prognosis of gram-negative versus gram-positive infected and sterile pancreatic necrosis: results of a randomized trial in patients with severe acute pancreatitis treated with adjuvant selective decontamination. Clin Infect Dis 25:811–816

41. Pederzoli P, Bassi C, Vesentini S, Campedelli A (1993) A randomized multicenter clinical trial of antibiotic prophylaxis of septic complications in acute necrotizing pancreatitis with imipenem. Surg Gynecol Obstet 176:480–483

42. Ho HS, Frey CF (1997) The role of antibiotic prophylaxis in severe acute pancreatitis. Arch Surg 132:487–493

43. Bassi C, Falconi M, Talamini G, Uomo G, Papaccio G, Dervenis C, Salvia R, Minelli EB, Pederzoli P (1998) Controlled clinical trial of pefloxacin versus imipenem in severe acute pancreatitis. Gastroenterology 115:1513–1517

44. McClave SA, Snider H, Owens N, Sexton LK (1997) Clinical nutrition in pancreatitis. Dig Dis Sci 42:2035–2044

45. Kalfarentzos F, Kehagias J, Mead N, Kokkinis K, Gogos CA (1997) Enteral nutrition is superior to parenteral nutrition in severe acute pancreatitis: results of a randomized prospective trial. Br J Surg 84:1665–1669

46. Windsor AC, Kanwar S, Li AG, Barnes E, Guthrie JA, Spark JI, Welsh F, Guillou PJ, Reynolds JV (1998) Compared with parenteral nutrition, enteral feeding attenuates the acute phase response and improves disease severity in acute pancreatitis. Gut 42:431–435

47. Bozzetti F, Braga M, Gianotti L, Gavazzi C, Mariani L (2001) Postoperative enteral versus parenteral nutrition in malnourished patients with gastrointestinal cancer: a randomised multicentre trial. Lancet 358:1487–1492

48. Warshaw AL (2000) Pancreatic necrosis. To debride or not to debride—that is the question. Ann Surg 232:627–629

49. Buchler MW, Gloor B, Muller CA, Friess H, Seiler CA, Uhl W (2000) Acute necrotizing pancreatitis: treatment strategy according to the status of infection. Ann Surg 232:619–626

50. Farkas G, Marton J, Mandi Y, Szederkenyi E (1996) Surgical strategy and management of infected pancreatic necrosis. Br J Surg 83:930–933

51. Ashley SW, Perez A, Pierce EA, Brooks DC, Moore FD, Whang EE, Banks PA, Zinner MJ (2001) Necrotizing pancreatitis. Contemporary analysis of 99 consecutive cases. Ann Surg 234:572–580

52. Gloor B, Muller CA, Worni M, Stahel PF, Redaelli C, Uhl W, Buchler MW (2001) Pancreatic infection in severe pancreatitis. The role of fungus and multiresistant organisms. Arch Surg 136:592–596

53. Doglietto GB, Gui D, Pacelli F, Brisinda G, Bellantone R, Crucitti PF, Sgadari A, Crucitti F (1994) Open vs closed treatment of secondary pancreatic infection. A review of 42 cases. Arch Surg 129:689–693

54. Kriwanek S, Gschwantler M, Beckerhinn P, Armbruster C, Roka R (1999) Complications after surgery for necrotising pancreatitis: risk factors and prognosis. Eur J Surg 165:952–957

55. Dervenis C, Bassi C (2000) Evidence-based assessment of severity and management of acute pancreatitis. Br J Surg 87:257–258

56. Tsiotos GG, Luque-de Leon E, Sarr MG (1998) Long-term outcome of necrotizing pancreatitis treated by necrosectomy. Br J Surg 85:1650–1653

57. del Castillo CF, Rattner DW, Makary MA, Mostafavi A, McGrath D, Warshaw AL (1998) Debridement and closed packing for treatment of necrotizing pancreatitis. Ann Surg 228:676–684

58. Farkas G (2000) Pancreatic head mass: how can we treat it? Acute pancreatitis: surgical treatment. JOP J Pancreas 1 [Suppl 3]:138–142

59. Mithofer K, Mueller PR, Warshaw AL (1997) Interventional and surgical treatment of pancreatic abscess. World J Surg 21:162–168

60. Widdison AL, Karanjia ND (1993) Pancreatic infection complicating acute pancreatitis. Br J Surg 80:148–154

61. Lumsden A, Bradley EL III (1990) Secondary pancreatic infections. Surg Gynecol Obstet 170:459–467

62. Aranha GV, Prinz RA, Greenlee HB (1982) Pancreatic abscess: an unresolved surgical problem. Am J Surg 144:534–538

63. Warshaw AL, Jin G (1985) Improved survival in 45 patients with pancreatic abscess. Ann Surg 202:408–417

64. Ross Carter C, McKay CJ, Imrie CW (2000) Percutaneous necrosectomy and sinus tract endoscopy in the management of infected pancreatic necrosis: an initial experience. Ann Surg 232:175–180

65. Kjossev KT, Losanoff JE (2001) Laparoscopic treatment of severe acute pancreatitis. Surg Endosc 15:1239–1240

66. Freeny PC, Hauptmann E, Althaus SJ, Traverso LW, Sinanan M (1998) Percutaneous CT-guided catheter drainage of infected acute necrotizing pancreatitis: techniques and results. AJR Am J Roentgenol 170:969–975

67. Baron TH, Morgan DE (1997) Organized pancreatic necrosis: definition, diagnosis, and management. Gastroenterol Int 10:167–178

68. Clancy CJ, Nguyen MH, Morris AJ (1997) Candidal mediastinitis: an emerging clinical entity. Clin Infect Dis 25:608–613

69. Gamlin F, Caldicott LD, Shah MV (1994) Mediastinitis and sepsis syndrome following intubation. Anaesthesia 49:883–885

70. Isaacs L, Kotton B, Peralta MM Jr, Shekar R, Meden G, Brown LA, Raaf JH (1993) Fatal mediastinal abscess from upper respiratory infection. Ear Nose Throat J 72:620–622

71. Becker M, Zbaren P, Hermans R, Becker CD, Marchal F, Kurt AM, Marre S, Rufenacht DA, Terrier F (1997) Necrotizing fasciitis of the head and neck: role of CT in diagnosis and management. Radiology 202:471–476

72. Brunelli A, Sabbatini A, Catalini G, Fianchini A (1996) Descending necrotizing mediastinitis. Surgical drainage and tracheostomy. Arch Otolaryngol Head Neck Surg 122:1326–1329

73. Corsten MJ, Shamji FM, Odell PF, Frederico JA, Laframboise GG, Reid KR, Vallieres E, Matzinger F (1997) Optimal treatment of descending necrotising mediastinitis. Thorax 52:702–708

74. Baldwin RT, Radovancevic B, Sweeney MS (1992) Bacterial mediastinitis after heart transplantation. J Heart Lung Transplant 11:545–549

75. El Oakley RM, Wright JE (1996) Postoperative mediastinitis: classification and management. Ann Thorac Surg 61:1030–1036

76. Milano CA, Kesler K, Archibald N (1995) Mediastinitis after coronary artery bypass graft surgery. Risk factors and long-term survival. Circulation 92:2245–2251

77. Brook I, Frazier EH (1996) Microbiology of mediastinitis. Arch Intern Med 156:333–336

78. Shaffer HA Jr, Valenzuela G, Mittal RK (1992) Esophageal perforation. A reassessment of the criteria for choosing medical or surgical therapy. Arch Intern Med 152:757–761

79. Loop FD, Lytle BW, Cosgrove DM (1990) J Maxwell Chamberlain memorial paper. Sternal wound complications after isolated coronary artery bypass grafting: early and late mortality, morbidity, and cost of care. Ann Thorac Surg 49:179–187

80. Gadek JE, DeMichele SJ, Karlstad MD (1999) Effect of enteral feeding with eicosapen-taenoic acid, gamma-linolenic acid, and antioxidants in patients with acute respira-tory distress syndrome. Enteral Nutrition in ARDS Study Group. Crit Care Med 27:1409–1420

81. Weinzweig N, Yetman R (1995) Transposition of the greater omentum for recalcitrant median sternotomy wound infections. Ann Plast Surg 34:471–477

82. Andrews CO, Gora ML (1994) Pleural effusions: pathophysiology and management. Ann Pharmacother 28:894–903

83. Bartter T, Santarelli R, Akers SM (1994) The evaluation of pleural effusion. Chest 106:1209–1214

84. Fenton KN, Richardson JD (1995) Diagnosis and management of malignant pleural effusions. Am J Surg 170:69–74

85. Kennedy L, Sahn SA (1994) Noninvasive evaluation of the patient with a pleural effu-sion. Chest Surg Clin N Am 4:451–465

86. Light RW (1995) Pleural diseases, 3rd edn. Williams and Wilkins, New York

87. Sahn SA (1988) State of the art. The pleura. Am Rev Respir Dis 138:184–234

88. Sganga G, Brisinda G, Castagneto M (2001) Practical aspects of antibiotic prophylaxis in high-risk surgical patients. In: Saene HKF van, Sganga G, Silvestri L (eds) Infection in the critically ill: an ongoing challenge. Springer-Verlag, Berlin Heidelberg New York, pp 47-58

89. Kurz A, Sessler DI, Lenhardt R (1996) Perioperative normothermia to reduce the inci-dende of surgical-wound infection and shorten hospitalization. N Engl J Med 334:1209–1215

90. Sganga G (2002) New perspectives in antibiotic prophylaxis for intra-abdominal sur-gery. J Hosp Inf 50[Suppl A]:S17–S21

91. Classen DC, Evans RS, Pestotnik A (1992) The timing of prophylactic administration of antibiotics and the risk of surgical-wound infection. N Engl J Med 326:281–287

92. Nathens AB, Marshall JC (1999) Selective decontamination of the digestive tract in surgical patients. A systematic review of the evidence. Arch Surg 134:170–176

93. Silvestri L, Mannucci F, van Saene HKF (2000) Selective decontamination of the dige-stive tract: a life-saver. J Hosp Infect 45:185–190

94. van Saene HKF, Silvestri L, de la Cal M (2000) Prevention of nosocomial infections in the intensive care unit. Curr Opin Crit Care 6:323–329

95. Greif R, Akca O, Horn EP, Kurz A, Sessler DI (2000) Supplemental perioperative oxy-gen to reduce the incidence of surgical-wound infection. N Engl J Med 342:161–167

96. Jancel T, Dudas V (2002) Management of uncomplicated urinary tract infections. West J Med 176:51–55

97. Larcombe J (1999) Urinary tract infection in children. BMJ 319:1173–1175

98. Ellis AK, Verma S (2000) Quality of life in women with urinary tract infections: is benign disease a misnomer? J Am Board Fam Pract 13:392–397

99. Hooten TM, Scholes D, Stapleton AE (2000) A prospective study of asymptomatic bac-teriuria in sexually active young women. N Engl J Med 343:992–997

100. Howes DS, Young WF (2000) Urinary tract infections. In: Tintinalli A (ed) Emergency medicine. A comprehensive study guide. McGraw-Hill, New York, pp 625–631

101. Leibovici L, Greenshtain S, Cohen O, Wysenbeek AJ (1992) Toward improved empiric management of moderate to severe urinary tract infections. Arch Intern Med 152:2481–2486

102. Millar LK, Wing DA, Paul RH, Grimes DA (1995) Outpatient treatment of pyeloneph-ritis in pregnancy: a randomized controlled trial. Obstet Gynecol 86:560–564

103. Safrin S, Siegel D, Black D (1988) Pyelonephritis in adult women: inpatient versus out-

patient therapy. Am J Med 85:793–798
104. Stamm WE, Hooton TM (1993) Management of urinary tract infections in adults. N Engl J Med 329:1328–1334
105. Foxman B, Barlow R, D'Arcy H, Gillespie B, Sobel JD (2000) Urinary tract infection: self-reported incidence and associated costs. Ann Epidemiol 10:509–515
106. Manges AR, Johnson JR, Foxman B, O'Bryan TT, Fullerton KE, Riley LW (2001) Widespread distribution of urinary tract infections caused by a multidrug-resistant Escherichia coli clonal group. N Engl J Med 345:1007–1013

Chapter 18

Infection on the Neonatal and Pediatric Intensive Care Units

A.J. Petros, V. Damjanovic, A. Pigna, J. Farias

Current Concept of Infections on Neonatal and Pediatric Intensive Care Units

Neonatal Intensive Care Unit

Infections in neonates requiring intensive care are unique in each of the essential elements of the pathogenesis of infection, i.e., the potential pathogen and its source, the mode of transmission, and the susceptible host. The pathogen, e.g., hepatitis B virus, or potential pathogen, e.g. *Escherichia coli,* is closely related to its source and mode of transmission. Many micro-organisms are present in the maternal birth canal (the source). They are most commonly *Streptococcus agalactiae, E. coli, Herpes simplex* virus, *Listeria monocytogenes,* and *Candida albicans.* One or more of these micro-organisms can be vertically transmitted from the mother to the neonate. When this type of infection occurs the infection will always be present in the 1st week of the neonate's life (early onset). Different micro-organisms are acquired on the neonatal intensive care unit (NICU). In general, these are coagulase-negative staphylococci (CNS), aerobic Gram-negative bacilli (AGNB) (mainly *Klebsiella* species and *Pseudomonas aeruginosa*), *Staphylococcus aureus,* and *Candida* species. The sources of these micro-organisms acquired on the NICU are mainly other neonates who carry the micro-organisms and/or who are infected with them. Staff on the NICU, mothers, contaminated materials, and equipment (environment) constitute uncommon sources. Although these micro-organisms can be transmitted from one neonate to another via equipment, the hands of healthcare workers are the main mode of transmission on the NICU [1]. Infections due to micro-organisms acquired on the unit are usually of late onset, following an episode of carriage.

The incidence of infection is higher in the neonatal period than at any time in life. Neonates, particularly preterm, are extremely susceptible to infection. Low birth weight is the single most important risk factor for infection in neonates [2].

The reasons for this increased susceptibility include immaturity of the immune system, poor surface defenses, lack of resistance to colonization [3, 4], invasive devices, and usage of broad-spectrum antibiotics. Increased susceptibility to carriage and infection in preterm neonates is the main factor that facilitates transmission of potential pathogens and subsequent outbreaks of infection on the NICU [1]. Moreover, preterm neonates can be susceptible to new and unknown potential pathogens such as *Hansenula anomala*, a saprophytic yeast known as a contaminant in the brewing industry. This newly recognised potential pathogen caused an outbreak of carriage and infection that lasted for 13 months on the Mersey regional NICU [5].

Pediatric Intensive Care Unit

The identical concept of three elements, including potential pathogen, its source, mode of transmission, and susceptible host, applies to the patients admitted to the pediatric intensive care unit (PICU). Recent epidemiological studies in children who required a prolonged PICU admission demonstrated that two-thirds of all infections diagnosed were due to micro-organisms present in the patient's admission flora [6, 7, 9]. These infections were practically all within a week of PICU admission. Infections due to micro-organisms acquired on the unit, and subsequently carried, invariably occurred after 1 week. The three main micro-organisms causing infections within the 1st week are CNS, *S. aureus,* and *C. albicans*. After 1 week the two main micro-organisms are *S. aureus* and *P. aeruginosa*. Unlike neonates, maternal flora is not the source of micro-organisms acquired on a PICU. It is invariably the other patients who function as a major source.

The length of stay in the NICU is substantially longer than that on the PICU (median of 13 versus 6.5 days) [4, 7, 8]. An extensive literature search showed that outbreaks are more common in NICU than PICU (Chapter 13). Finally, lower overall mortality rates of 5% [9] support the observation that children on a PICU are less susceptible hosts compared with the 10% mortality in neonates requiring intensive care on the NICU [4].

Magnitude of the Problem

Neonatal Intensive Care

The overall infection rates in neonates whilst on intensive care vary between 15% and 20%. This is equal to rates reported for adult medical and surgical units and higher than most pediatric units [10]. The main site of infection is the bloodstream, followed by the lower airways.

In a multicenter study of NICUs in Oakland, New Haven in 1994 Beck-Sague et al. [11] reported that nosocomial bloodstream infection occurred at a rate of 5% when surveillance cultures were performed and was actually half that reported in studies reporting the rate of all infections. Bloodstream infections can account for 50% of all infections on the NICU. Lower airway infections occur in approximately 3% of neonates whilst on the NICU [12]. The main organisms are viruses, *S. aureus,* and AGNB.

The survival benefit of intensive care in neonates has significantly increased over the last 25 years. In a 2-year study from New York (1977–1978), the mortality for early onset sepsis in neonates of less than 1,000 g was 53.4%; mortality was 20.3% for late-onset sepsis [13]. Ten years later, a 5-year study from Oxford (1982–1986) reported mortality figures of 28% and 4% for early and late-onset sepsis in neonates, respectively [2]. Recent data from a Dutch NICU show a mortality of less than 10% in a 1-year study (1997) in 436 neonates of about 2,000 g [4].

Pediatric Intensive Care

Nosocomial infection in the PICU is an important cause of morbidity and mortality in ventilated children. Bloodstream and lower airway infections are most common and are almost always due to prolonged use of devices. The incidence of bloodstream infection is reported at 10.6–46.9/1,000 catheter-days [14]. The incidence of lower airways infection is 6.5–20.2/1,000 ventilation-days.

Bloodstream infections. In a recent report from a mixed PICU in Birmingham United Kingdom [15], where all children admitted were included, the incidence of bloodstream infection was 10.6/1,000 patient-days. Consequently the group as a whole was less ill and stayed for a median of 3 days. The larger denominator of >12,000 patient-days also dilutes the real infection rate. Of the microorganisms causing positive blood cultures, 62% were Gram-positive bacteria, mainly CNS, *S. aureus,* and enterococci, 32% were AGNB, and the remainder were yeasts.

In a recent study from Liverpool (UK) comprising 1,241 children requiring a median of 8 days' ventilation, the overall infection rate was 41.9% [9]. Viral infection accounted for 14.5% and bacterial/yeast infections for 33%. The incidence of bloodstream infection was 20.1/1,000 patient-days. The infection rate due to microorganisms acquired while on the PICU was 13.3%; 4% of admitted children developed infections due to resistant micro-organisms. The causative micro-organisms were CNS, enterococci, *Pseudomonas* spp., *S. aureus,* and yeasts.

A study from London (UK) reported an incidence of bloodstream infection of 46.9/1,000 patient-days in a subset of 103 children with a median time of 6 days of line in situ [16]. The causative organisms were CNS, *S. aureus, Candida albicans,* and *Klebsiella* species.

Lower airway infections. In a pediatric trauma unit the rate of lower airway infections was 5.5% [17]. The most common organisms were *S. aureus, Haemophilus influenzae, Enterobacter,* and *Pseudomonas* spp. [17]. In the Liverpool study the overall airway infection rate was 10.6%, with a rate of 9.1 episodes/1,000 patient-days [9]. The three main organisms were *S. aureus, P. aeruginosa,* and *H. influenzae.*

The magnitude of the problem can be assessed in a different way, based upon the carrier state (Chapter 5). Endogenous infection must be distinguished from exogenous infection. Endogenous infection is one caused by potential pathogens previously carried by the patient. If the potential pathogen was present on admission then the infection due to this potential pathogen is called primary endogenous. This type of infection tends to occur early, within the 1st week. If the infection is due to a potential pathogen acquired on the unit, after going through the carriage phase, then the infection is termed secondary endogenous. Infections caused by micro-organisms not carried by the patient are termed exogenous. Obviously surveillance cultures are indispensable for this classification [6, 9].

Some micro-organisms cause more serious clinical disease than others. This differential pathogenic effect can be used to develop a pathogenicity index for an individual micro-organism, in a specific organ system, in a particular homogeneous population for which surveillance cultures are useful [18]. The ratio of the number of ICU patients infected by a particular micro-organism and the number of patients simply carrying that organism in their throat and/or gut is defined as the intrinsic pathogenicity index for a particular micro-organism. Indigenous flora, including anaerobes, will rarely cause infections in the lower airways of patients requiring ventilation for more than 3 days, despite being carried in high concentrations. This is because they have intrinsic pathogenicity index values of between 0.01 and 0.03. Low-level pathogens, including viridans streptococci, enterococci, and CNS, are also carried in high concentrations in the oropharynx by a substantial percentage of ICU patients and are unable to cause lower airway infections. High-level pathogens such as *S. pyogenes* and *Salmonella* have an intrinsic pathogenicity index approaching 1.0, and disease manifests itself in virtually all oropharyngeal and gut carriers. The concept of carriage recognizes about 15 potentially pathogenic micro-organisms with intrinsic pathogenicity indices of between 0.1 and 0.3. These consist of the 6 "community" or "normal" micro-organisms *S. pneumoniae, H. influenzae, Moraxella catarrhalis, E. coli, S. aureus,* and *C. albicans,* present in previously healthy individuals, and 9 "hospital" or "abnormal" bacteria carried by patients with either an acute or chronic underlying condition, namely *Klebsiella,*

Proteus, Morganella, Enterobacter, Citrobacter, Serratia, Pseudomonas, Acinetobacter spp., and methicillin-resistant *S. aureus* (MRSA). The overall mortality on our PICU is in the range of 5%, but the mortality rate rises to 10% in the subset of children who require prolonged mechanical ventilation [9].

Pathogenesis

Figure 1 describes the pathogenesis of infection in neonates and children requiring intensive care. Practically all infections in these two groups are endogenous in origin. Therefore patients infect themselves with micro-organisms that they carry. A recent study in 400 children, requiring ventilation on a PICU, demonstrated that 90% of all lower airway infections were endogenous; 80% of lower airway infections were primary endogenous, 10% secondary endogenous, and the remaining 10% were exogenous [6].

Bloodstream infections occur due to translocation. Micro-organisms in the terminal ileum in overgrowth ($\geq 10^5$ micro-organisms/ml) migrate into the bloodstream [19]. This mechanism applies to *S. agalactiae, S. aureus,* and

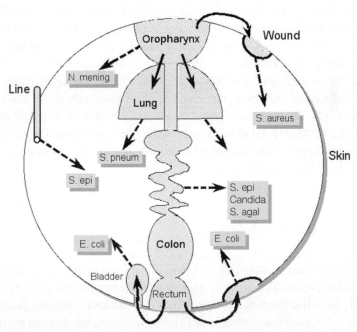

Fig. 1. Schematic representation of the digestive tract, illustrating that the throat and gut are the major internal sources of potential pathogens causing endogenous infections of blood, lower airways, bladder, and wounds (*CNS*, coagulase-negative staphylococci, *S. agal*, *Streptococcus agalactiae*)

Candida species. Recently it has been demonstrated that in neonates and children staying longer that 1 week on the NICU or PICU, CNS and AGNB cause septicemia due to translocation [20].

Lower airway infections are caused by micro-organisms carried in the oropharynx that then migrate into the lower airways. In a previous healthy child, *S. pneumoniae, H. influenzae,* and *S. aureus* cause bacterial lower airway infections. Whilst AGNB and MRSA are causative organisms in children with conditions that require intensive care for longer than 1 week.

Bladder infections are, in general, endogenous due to migrating fecal bacteria. Wound infections of the head, neck, and thorax are, in general, caused by oral bacteria, whilst wound infections between the waist and knee are caused by gut bacteria.

Exogenous infections, defined as infections caused by micro-organisms not carried by the patient, vary between 5% and 25%. They are a particular problem in patients with tracheostomies, leading to lower airway infections of exogenous pathogenesis [21]. Children with wounds, particularly burns, are at high risk of exogenous colonization and infection [9]. Up to 16% of bloodstream infections have an exogenous pathogenesis following contamination of an indwelling intravascular device [19]. Gastrostomies can also be considered as a wound and recurrent exogenous colonization/infection is not uncommon in children with such devices [9]. To identify an exogenous infection, surveillance samples of throat and rectum are indispensable. Blood cultures or lower airway secretions are positive for a potential pathogen that is not present in throat and or rectal cultures.

Risk factor analysis invariably includes low birth weight, the administration of total parenteral nutrition, the presence of invasive indwelling devices, including endotracheal tubes, mechanical ventilation, length of stay, and prior use of antibiotics [2, 22, 23]. All these factors reflect the severity of illness and are difficult to modify in order to control infection. Risk factor analysis cannot easily contribute to infection control.

Diagnosis of Infection

Infection is a microbiologically proven, clinical diagnosis of local and/or general inflammation. The signs of generalized infections in neonates, e.g., septicemia, are often non-specific and may be clinically indistinguishable from those of non-infectious conditions [2]. For instance, the clinical picture of respiratory distress in early onset sepsis may be identical to hyaline membrane disease. Furthermore, the clinical diagnosis of local infection such as meningitis may not differ from that of systemic sepsis without meningeal involvement.

However, infections in the PICU are more specific and further description of local and general infection is related to pediatric patients.

Pneumonia

Microbiologically proven pneumonia requires (1) the presence of new or progressive pulmonary infiltrates on a chest X-ray for ≥48 h *and* (2) purulent tracheal aspirate *and* (3) fever ≥38.5°C *and* (4) leukocytosis (WBC >12,000/ml) or leukopenia (WBC <4,000/ml) *and* (5) tracheal aspirate ≥10^5 colony forming units (CFU) of potentially pathogenic micro-organism/ml *or* bronchoalveolar lavage (BAL) yielding ≥10^4 CFU/ml.

Clinical diagnosis only requires criteria 1-4 above *and* sterile BAL or tracheal aspirate.

Tracheitis/Bronchitis

Diagnosis of tracheitis/bronchitis requires (1) purulent tracheal aspirate *and* (2) fever ≥38.5°C *and* (3) leukocytosis (WBC >12,000/ml) or leukopenia (WBC <4,000/ml) *and* (4) tracheal aspirate yielding ≥10^5 CFU/l. Most importantly, the chest X-ray is normal.

Systemic Inflammatory Response Syndrome

The diagnosis of systemic inflammatory response syndrome (SIRS) requires clinical signs of generalized inflammation caused by micro-organisms and/or their products, including at least three of the following: fever, temperature instability, lethargy, poor perfusion, and hypotension.

Bloodstream Infections

The diagnosis of bloodstream infections requires SIRS with a positive blood culture from either a peripheral vein or an intravascular device.

Intra-abdominal infection

This is defined as an infection of an abdominal organ and of the peritoneal cavity (peritonitis), with local signs such as abdominal tenderness and generalized symptoms including fever and leukoyctosis. Peritonitis can be a localized or a generalized infection of the peritoneal cavity. Following ultrasonography and/or computed tomography and/or laparotomy, the diagnosis is confirmed by the isolation of micro-organisms of ≥3+ or ≥10^5 CFU/ml and ≥2+ leukoyctes in the diagnostic sample [24].

Urinary Tract Infection

Infection of the urinary tract most often involves the bladder. The common features of dysuria, supra-pubic pain, frequency, and urgency, are often not assessable in PICU patients. Therefore the diagnosis of cystitis is based upon freshly obtained catheter urine containing ≥10^5 CFU/ml of urine and ≥5 WBC/high-power light microscopy field.

Wound Infection

Wound infection is diagnosed by purulent discharge from wounds, a culture yielding ≥3+ or ≥10^5 CFU/ml of pus, and signs of local inflammation. The isolation of skin flora is considered to be contamination.

Prevention

Beside the five infection control interventions (Chapter 10), there is only evidence of effectiveness for two antibiotic maneuvers that prevent infection on the NICU and PICU; surgical prophylaxis [25–27] and selective decontamination of the digestive tract (SDD) (Table 1) [28–32].

Table 1. Cardiac and general surgical prophylaxis and prevention protocol for selective decontamination of the digestive tract (*ICU* intensive care unit, *MRSA* methicillin-resistant *Staphylococcus aureus*, *AGNB* aerobic Gram-negative bacilli)

Surgical prophylaxis	Total daily dose (mg/kg)			
	<7 days	>7 days	1 month to 12 years	>12 years
Cardiac				
Teicoplanin	16 then 8		20 then 10 then 6	400 mg then 200 mg
Netilmicin	3<2 kg 6>2 kg	6	6	200 mg
General				
Cefotaxime	100	150	100-200	6–12 g
Metronidazole	22.5	22.5	22.5	1.5 g
Gentamicin	3<2 kg 6>2 kg	6<2 kg 7.5>2 kg	7.5	3-5

cont. →

Table 1 *cont.*

Selective decontamination of digestive tract	Total daily dose (4 daily)		
	<5 years	5–12 years	>12 years
Oropharynx			
AGNB: polymyxin E with tobramycin		2 g of 2% paste/gel	
Yeasts: amphotericin B or nystatin (units)		2 g of 2% paste/gel	
MRSA: vancomycin		2 g of 4% paste/gel	
Gut			
AGNB: polymyxin E (mg)	100	200	400
with tobramycin (mg)	80	160	320
Yeasts: amphotericin B (mg)	500	1,000	2,000
or nystatin	2×10^6	4×10^6	8×10^6
MRSA: vancomycin (mg)	20-40/Kg	20-40/Kg	500-2,000

Therapy	Total daily dose (mg/kg)			
	<7 days	>7 days	1 month to 12 years	>12 years
1. Neonatal ICU				
Ampicillin: active against *L. monocytogenes* and *S. agalactiae*	50	100		
Gentamicin: AGNB (see below)				
2. Pediatric ICU				
Cefotaxime: 'community' + 'hospital' microbes except *P. aeruginosa*	100	150	100-200	6-12g
Ceftazidime:				
P. aeruginosa	60	90	100–150	6–9 g
Gentamicin: AGNB	3<2 kg 6>2 kg	6<2 kg 7.5>2 kg	7.5	3–5
Cephradine: *S. aureus*	50	50	100	4g
Vancomycin: MRSA	15 then 20	15 then 30	45	2g
Amphotericin B: yeasts, fungi (lipophilic)	1-3	1-3	1-3	1-3

Cardiac Surgical Prophylaxis

The aim of prophylactic antibiotics in cardiac surgery is to prevent infections of the heart and mediastinal incision. The main micro-organisms causing endocarditis include CNS, viridans streptococci, and enterococci. Less common are AGNB and yeasts. S. aureus both sensitive and resistant to methicillin are the main cause of mediastinal wound infections. A commonly used combination of antimicrobials prior to cardiac surgery is a glycopeptide and an aminogylcoside. A glycopeptide such as teicoplanin covers all streptococci and staphylococci, whilst an aminoglycoside such as netilmicin is active against AGNB that may translocate following gut ischemia. Short-term prophylaxis of three doses is normally administered, one immediately prior to surgery to achieve high tissues levels and two further doses 8 h apart. Under certain circumstances, such as a chest splinted open because of cardiac edema, these antibiotics may be continued for 5 days, although there is no evidence to support this practice.

General Surgical Prophylaxis

The type of antimicrobial prescribed depends on the proposed surgery and the associated risk of contamination. Clean, sterile procedures do not need antibiotic cover, whereas clean procedures with the likelihood of contamination need cover with one antimicrobial, such as cefotaxime. If there is likely to be fecal contamination, then an aminoglycoside such as gentamicin is also necessary to cover AGNB and enterococci. Finally, if the surgical procedure is likely to be associated with ischemia and possible necrotic tissue, then metronidazole should be added to the prophylactic regimen. Again three doses will suffice.

Selective Decontamination of the Digestive Tract

SDD is a prophylactic intervention designed to prevent early and late infection in the critically ill child, requiring more than 1 week of intensive care (Chapter 14). There are four randomized controlled trials [28–32] that demonstrate a significant reduction in infectious morbidity. With an overall mortality of approximately 10%, a reduction in mortality is harder to demonstrate than in adults. A huge sample size would be necessary. However, in adults, where the overall mortality is approximately 30%, it has been possible to demonstrate a significant reduction of 22% [33–35].

There is a particular indication for SDD on the NICU, namely in the control of an outbreak of infection. Ten years ago, SDD with nystatin was used to control a Candida parapsilosis outbreak on the Mersey regional NICU. Of 106 neonates who carried the outbreak strain, 76 received nystatin in the throat and gut during the 12-month open trial. Six neonates developed fungemias. Once the carriage rate fell from 50% to 5%, no new cases of systemic *Candida* infection were observed. This was the first report of the SDD intervention to control an outbreak of infection on the NICU [36].

Treatment

Neonatal Intensive Care Unit

Early onset infections that occur on the NICU maybe due to *L. monocytogenes* and/or *S. agalactiae*. Ampicillin is the most active antibiotic against these two micro-organisms, which are acquired from the mother, and is combined with gentamicin to cover AGNB and *S. aureus*. Late-onset infections are treated as described in Table 2.

Table 2. Flow diagram for the treatment of an infection

DAY ONE: ABSENCE OF KNOWLEDGE OF CAUSATIVE MICROORGANISM				
EMPIRICAL TREATMENT:	CEFOTAXIME combined with GENTAMICIN if seriously ill			

DAY TWO: PRESUMPTIVE IDENTIFICATION OF CAUSATIVE MICROORGANISM				
TAILORED TREATMENT:				
NORMAL POTENTIAL PATHOGEN			ABNORMAL POTENTIAL PATHOGEN	
S. pneumoniae	*S. aureus*	*Candida* species	Aerobic Gram-negative bacilli	*Pseudomonas* species
STOP Gentamicin	STOP Cefotaxime/Gentamicin	STOP Cefotaxime/Gentamicin	CONTINUE Cefotaxime/Gentamicin	REPLACE Cefotaxime with Ceftazidime
MONOTHERAPY Cefotaxime	MONOTHERAPY Cephadrine	MONOTHERAPY Amphotericin B		

DAY THREE:	CLINICAL IMPROVEMENT

DAY FIVE:	STOP OR CHANGE ANTIMICROBIAL TREATMENT	
	STOP	CHANGE
	Improved after careful clinical, radiological, and microbiological evaluation	Not improved after careful clinical, radiological, and microbiological evaluation

Pediatric Intensive Care Unit

When a child is admitted to the PICU with a severe infection, a decision as to which antimicrobial is to be used has to be made. Antimicrobials are used in combination due to the severity of the child's illness. Our experience over 20 years leads us to the choice of cefotaxime and gentamicin. This choice is empirical due to the absence of any knowledge regarding the causative micro-organism, although reasonable assumptions can be made on the presentation of the child. For example, a child with meningococcal disease requires only cefotaxime. Metronidazole can be added in case of presumed anaerobic involvement. When a presumptive identification of the micro-organism can be made, the physician can then tailor therapy. Cefotaxime/gentamicin can be replaced by cephradine in the case of an infection due to *S. pneumoniae, S. pyogenes,* and *S. aureus.* When *P. aeruginosa* is isolated, ceftazidime should replace cefotaxime and gentamicin should be continued. Yeast infections require liposomal amphotericin B in place of cefotaxime/gentamicin (Table 2). The efficacy of the antimicrobial treatment can be monitored using C-reactive protein levels, in addition to the clinical, radiographic, and microbiological variables. Providing the antimicrobials used are correct, the child will improve within 3 days. In our experience a short 5-day course of intravenous antibiotics is as effective as a course of 2 weeks or more (Chapter 12). After 5 days the child is monitored for signs of infection. When there are no signs of infection, antibiotics are discontinued. Should there be no improvement after 5 days, a change in antibiotic regimen is necessary.

Metronidazole is given only for 3 days. The antifungal agent, liposomal amphotericin B, is given for 3 weeks and may be discontinued once the C-reactive protein level is normal. Systemic antimicrobials are combined with enteral SDD agents to guarantee the prevention of potential pathogens becoming resistant to the systemic agents.

References

1. Damjanovic V, van Saene HKF (1998) Outbreaks of infection in a neonatal intensive care unit. In: van Saene HKF, Silvestri L, de la Cal MA (eds) Infection control in the intensive care unit. Springer, Milan, pp 237–248
2. Isaacs D, Moxon ER (1991) Neonatal infections. Butterworth-Heinemann, Oxford
3. van Saene HKF, Leonard EM, Shears P (1989) Ecological impact of antibiotics in neonatal units. Lancet II:509–510
4. de Man P, Verhoeven BAN, Verburgh HA et al (2000) An antibiotic policy to prevent emergence of resistant bacilli. Lancet 355:973–978
5. Murphy N, Damjanovic V, Hart CA et al (1986) Infection and colonisation of neonates by *Hansenula anomala.* Lancet I:291–293

6. Silvestri L, Sargison RE, Hughes J et al (2002) Most nosocomial pneumonias are not due to nosocomial bacteria in ventilated patients. Evaluation of the accuracy of the 48h time cut-off using carriage as the gold standard. Anaesth Intensive Care 30:275–282

7. Petros AJ, O'Connell M, Roberts C et al (2001) Systemic antibiotics fail to clear multi-drug-resistant *Klebsiella* from a paediatric ICU. Chest 119:862–866

8. Goldmann DA, Leclair J, Macone A (1978) Bacterial colonization of neonates admitted to an intensive care environment. J Pediatr 2:288–293

9. Sarginson RE, Taylor N, Reilly N, Baines PB, van Saene HKF (2004) Infection in prolonged pediatric critical illness: a prospective four year study based on knowledge of the carrier state. Crit Care Med 32:839–847

10. Baltimore RS (1998) Neonatal nosocomial infections. Semin Perinatol 22:25–32

11. Beck-Sague CM, Azimi P, Fonseca SN et al (1994) Bloodstream infections in neonatal intensive care unit patients: results of a multicenter study. Pediatr Infect Dis J 13:1110–1116

12. Gaynes RP, Martone WJ, Culver DH, Grace Emori T et al (1991) Comparison of rates of nosocomial infections in neonatal intensive care units in the United States. Am J Med 91 [Suppl 3B]:192–196

13. La Gamma EF, Drusin LM, Mackles AW et al (1983) Neonatal infections. An important determinant of late NICU mortality in infants less than 1,000g at birth. Am J Dis Child 137:838–841

14. Richards MJ, Edwards JR, Culver DH, Gaynes RP and the National Nosocomial Infections Surveillance System (1999) Nosocomial infection in pediatric intensive care units in the United States. Pediatrics 103:e39

15. Gray J, Gossain S, Morris K (2001) Three-year survey of bacteraemia and fungemia in a pediatric intensive care unit. Pediatr Infect Dis J 20:416–421

16. Pierce CM, Wade A, Mok Q (2000) Heparin-bonded central venous lines reduce thrombotic and infective complications in critically ill children. Intensive Care Med 26:967–972

17. Patel JC, Mollitt DL, Pieper P, Tepas III JJ (2000) Nosocomial pneumonia in the pediatric trauma patient: a single center's experience. Crit Care Med 28:3530–3533

18. Leonard EM, van Saene HKF, Stoutenbeek CP et al (1990) An intrinsic pathogenicity index for micro-organisms causing infections in a neonatal surgical unit. Microb Ecol Health Dis 2:151–157

19. van Saene HKF, Taylor N, Donnell SC et al (2003) Gut overgrowth with abnormal flora: the missing link in parenteral nutrition-related sepsis in surgical neonates. Eur J Clin Nutr 57:548–553

20. Donnell SC, Taylor N, van Saene HKF et al (2002) Infection rates in surgical neonates and infants receiving parenteral nutrition: a five year prospective study. J Hosp Infect 52:273–280

21. Morar P, Singh V, Makura Z et al (2002) Differing pathways of lower airway colonization and infection according to mode of ventilation (endotracheal vs tracheostomy). Arch Otolaryngol Head Neck Surg 128:1061–1066

22. Singh-Naz N, Sprague BM, Patel K, Pollack MM (2000) Risk assessment and standardized nosocomial infection rate in critically ill children. Crit Care Med 28:2069–2075

23. Mahieu LM, De Muynck AO, De Dooy JJ et al (2000) Prediction of nosocomial sepsis in neonates by means of a computer-weighted bed side scoring system (NOSEP score). Crit Care Med 28:2026–2033

24. A'Court CH, Garrard CS, Crook D et al (1993) Microbiological lung surveillance in mechanically ventilated patients, using non-directed bronchial lavage and quantitative culture. Q J Med 86:635–638

25. Petros AJ, Marshall JC, van Saene HKF (1995) Should morbidity replace mortality as an endpoint for clinical trials in intensive care? Lancet 345:369-371
26. Kaiser AB (1986) Antimicrobial prophylaxis in surgery. N Engl J Med 315:1129-1138
27. Infection in Neurosurgery Working Party of the British Society for Antimicrobial Chemotherapy (1994) Antimicrobial prophylaxis in neurosurgery and after head injury. Lancet 344:1547-1551
28. Zobel G, Kuttnig, Grubbauer HM et al (1991) Reduction of colonization and infection rate during pediatric intensive care by selective decontamination of the digestive tract. Crit Care Med 19:1242-1246
29. Smith SD, Jackson RJ, Hannakan CJ et al (1993) Selective decontamination in pediatric liver transplants. Transplantation 55:1306-1309
30. Ruza F, Alvarado F, Herruzo R et al (1998) Prevention of nosocomial infection in a pediatric intensive care unit (PICU) through the use of selective decontamination. Eur J Epidemiol 14:719-727
31. Barret JP, Jeschke MG, Herndon DN (2001) Selective decontamination of the digestive tract in severely burned pediatric patients. Burns 27:439-445
32. www.nhsald02/therapeutic-guideline
33. Krueger WA, Lenhart FP, Neeser G et al (2002) Influence of combined intravenous and topical antibiotic prophylaxis on the incidence of infections, organ dysfunctions, and mortality in critically ill surgical patients: a prospective, stratified, randomized, double-blind, placebo-controlled clinical trial. Am J Respir Crit Care Med 166:1029-1037
34. de Jonge E, Schultz JM, Spanjaard L et al (2003) Effects of selective decontamination of the digestive tract on mortality and acquisition of resistant bacteria in intensive care: a randomized controlled trial. Lancet 362: 1011-1016
35. Liberati A, D'Amico R, Pifferi S et al (2004) Antibiotic prophylaxis to reduce respiratory tract infections and mortality in adults receiving intensive care [Cochrane Review]. In: The Cochrane Library, Issue 1, Chichester, UK, John Wiley
36. Damjanovic V, Connolly CM, van Saene HKF et al (1993) Selective decontamination with nystatin for the control of a *Candida* outbreak in the neonatal intensive care unit. J Hosp Infect 24:245-259

Immediate Adequate Antibiotics Control Morbidity and Mortality in Patients with Pancreatitis, Extensive Burns, Trauma, Exacerbated Chronic Obstructive Pulmonary Disease, or Liver Transplantation

I. Alía, M. A. de la Cal, E. Cerdá, H. K.F. van Saene

Introduction

Infections in patients admitted to intensive care units (ICUs) can be classified according to the patient´s "carrier status" [1, 2]. This status is conferred when the same strain of a potentially pathogenic micro-organism (PPM) is isolated from two or more consecutive pharyngeal or rectal samples. The study of the digestive tract flora in intensive care patients has shown that large proportions of infections in critically ill patients are caused by micro-organisms previously present within the digestive tract. Therefore, such infections have been referred to as endogenous infections. Primary endogenous infection is defined as an infectious process produced by PPM present in the oropharynx and/or rectum at the time of admission to the ICU. Secondary endogenous infection is defined as an infectious process produced by PPM not present in the oropharynx and/or rectum at the time of admission to the ICU, but which was present at these sites in a sample collected prior to the development of the infection. Between 50% and 60% of all infections among patients admitted to the ICU correspond to primary endogenous infections [3–6] and develop in the first 8–9 days after admission to the ICU [5, 6].

The severity of the underlying disease determines the type of PPM found in the oropharynx and gut of patients on admission to the ICU. In previously healthy individuals not hospitalized before admission to the ICU, primary endogenous infections are caused by community or normal flora (*Streptococcus pneumoniae, Haemophilus influenzae, Moraxella catarrhalis, Escherichia coli,* methicillin-sensitive *Staphylococcus aureus, Candida spp.*), since such patients are only exceptionally carriers of aerobic Gram-negative bacilli (AGNB) within the oropharynx. A study of 120 healthy subjects showed the frequency of AGNB carriers to be 6.6% [7]. In contrast, patients with chronic disorders (e.g., chronic bronchitis, diabetes, alcoholics) or patients who have been in hospital for a number of days carry AGNB in the oropharynx or rectum with a frequency dependent upon the severity of the underlying disease. The frequency of Gram-negative bacilli in the oropharynx of patients with severe chronic obstructive pulmonary disease (COPD) was 33%—a figure that decreased to 8% among patients with only moderate COPD [8]. Therefore, in previously ill patients or individuals referred from other services or hospitals, primary endogenous infections are caused by normal community or abnormal hospital flora (*Klebsiella spp., Proteus spp., Morganella spp., Citrobacter spp., Enterobacter spp., Serratia spp., Acinetobacter spp., Pseudomonas spp.,* and methicillin-resistant *S. aureus*).

Systemic antibiotic prophylaxis is given to prevent infections by PPM that are present in the oropharynx or gastrointestinal tract on admission to the ICU. An antibiotic used for systemic prophylaxis should have a spectrum covering both "community" micro-organisms and "hospital" PPM, without affecting the indigenous flora.

This chapter addresses the microbiology of the infections diagnosed in both previously healthy patients admitted to the ICU and patients with chronic underlying diseases. For this purpose, homogeneous populations have been selected, such as trauma and burn patients, patients admitted with acute pancreatitis, patients admitted for exacerbations of a chronic illness such as COPD, and patients admitted after liver transplantation. Additionally, data will be presented showing that parenteral antimicrobials administered early upon ICU admission are useful for the prevention of primary endogenous infections.

Patients with Acute Necrotizing Pancreatitis

The natural course of acute necrotizing pancreatitis comprises two phases. The first 14 days are characterized by a systemic inflammatory response syndrome, produced by the release of inflammatory mediators [9, 10]. The second phase starts approximately 2 weeks after the onset of the disease and involves the development of complications related to infection of the necrotic pancreatic tissues. The latter have been described as diffuse or focal areas of non-viable pancreatic parenchyma together with necrotic peripancreatic fat [11]. Necrotizing pancreatitis is diagnosed when double-phase computed axial tomography (CT) shows the absence of intravenous contrast uptake in over 30% of the pancreatic region, or the presence of focal pancreatic parenchymal zones of more than 3 cm in size and without contrast uptake [12]. The frequency of pancreatic necrosis among patients with acute pancreatitis varies considerably in the literature from 9% to 42% [13–18]. In patients with pancreatic necrosis, the appearance of persistent leukocytosis and fever in the absence of an established septic focus, with an increase in C-reactive protein above 150 mg/l or the appearance of signs of renal, pulmonary, or cardiovascular dysfunction, is suggestive of possible necrotic tissue infection [14–16, 18–22]. Infection of pancreatic necrosis occurs in 30%–70% of patients with necrotizing pancreatitis and

Table 1. Frequency of necrotic tissue infection in necrotizing pancreatitis and its relation to patient mortality

Author	Patients	Necrotic tissue infection n (%)[a]	Mortality among patients with infection	Mortality among patients without infection
Ashley et al. [13]	1,110 with acute pancreatitis	34 (35%)	12%	11%
Bradley and Allen [14]	194 with acute pancreatitis	27 (71%)	15%	0%
Paye et al. [15]	269 with acute pancreatitis	31 (44%)	-	-
Garg et al. [16]	169 with acute pancreatitis	27 (41%)	52%	10%
Beger et al. [17]	114 with necrotizing pancreatitis	45 (39%)	38%	9%
Büchler et al. [18]	204 with acute pancreatitis	29 (34%)	24%	2%
Pederzoli et al. [23]	148 with necrotizing pancreatitis	93 (63 %)	29%	16%
Howard et al. [24]	62 with necrotizing pancreatitis and surgery	20 (32%)	50%	25%
Isenmann et al. [25]	273 with necrotizing pancreatitis	85 (31%)	-	-
Luiten et al. [26]	102 with severe acute pancreatitis	29 (28%)	52%	19%
Le Mée et al. [27]	43 with necrotizing pancreatitis and organ dysfunction	27 (63%)	33%	6%
Ala-Kokko et al. [28]	67 with necrotizing pancreatitis	25 (37%)	36%	14 %

[a]Growth of micro-organisms in pancreatic tissue obtained by fine-needle aspiration under ultrasound or computed tomography (CT) guidance, or in tissue obtained at laparotomy, or CT visualization of extraintestinal gas

constitutes the main risk factor for mortality (Table 1). The incidence of infection varies depending on the duration of the pancreatitis, and the majority of patients with necrotizing pancreatitis develop infection around the 3rd week of the disease. Beger et al. [17] cultured necrotic material obtained at the time of surgery in 114 patients with acute necrotizing pancreatitis. The prevalence of infection was 24% in patients undergoing surgery during the first 7 days, 36% in the 2nd week, 71% in the 3rd week, and 32% after 4 weeks. Büchler et al. [18] prospectively studied 86 patients with necrotizing pancreatitis receiving early antibiotic treatment with imipenem/cilastatin for 14 days. Twenty-seven patients developed infection of the pancreatic necrosis at a mean time of 21 days (range 10–48 days). In the study by Schwarz et al. [29] fine-needle biopsies of the necrotic areas were performed on days 1, 3, 5, 7, and 10 in 26 patients with acute necrotizing pancreatitis. The necrosis became infected after a median time of 9.5 days in patients receiving prophylactic antibiotic treatment and 10 days in patients without antibiotic treatment.

The infection of necrotic pancreatic tissue is diagnosed when gas is visualized in the peripancreatic collections, or micro-organisms are grown in necrotic tissue samples obtained by percutaneous needle aspiration under ultrasound or CT guidance [30]. Rau et al. [19] reported a sensitivity and specificity of 88% and 90%, respectively, for the diagnosis of pancreatic necrosis infection when percutaneous aspiration of the necrotic zone was performed under ultrasound guidance. Büchler et al. [18] found a sensitivity of 96% and a specificicity of 92% when using CT-guided fine-needle aspiration. The growth of micro-organisms in the necrotic pancreatic tissue samples has been considered an indication for surgery [31, 32].

Experimental studies have shown that bacterial translocation of PPM from the intestine is the main cause of infection in necrotizing pancreatitis [33–35]. Hence, the bacterial spectrum of pancreatic necrosis infection comprises AGNB and anaerobes. In a study of 90 patients with severe acute pancreatitis from whom oropharyngeal and rectal swabs were obtained upon admission to the ICU and subsequently twice a week, 15 patients who developed pancreatic necrosis infection by AGNB also showed gut carriage of the same bacteria prior to the development of the infection [36].

The microbiology of pancreatic necrosis infection mainly involves AGNB (Table 2), although in some series 40%–50% of the micro-organisms isolated are Gram positive [18–20, 28].

Pancreatic necrosis infection due to AGNB was associated with increased mortality, but not with infection by Gram-positive bacteria, mainly coagulase-negative staphylococci and enterococci, which showed a mortality similar to that observed in patients without infection of the necrotic parenchyma [20]. This is probably because most Gram-positive infections were caused by S. epidermidis or enterococci, which are less pathogenic than AGNB. In contrast, a

Table 2. Microbiology of pancreatic necrosis infection

Author	No. patients/no. micro-organisms	Mono-microbial infection	Poly-microbial infection	Pseudomonas spp.	Enterobacteriaceae	Staphylococcus aureus/epidermidis	Streptococcus faecalis	Fungi
Ashley et al. [13]	30/-	-	-	-	-	33%	-	3%
Paye et al. [15]	9/13	-	-	3 (23%)	5 (39%)	3 (23%)	-	-
Beger et al. [17]	45/75	87%	13%	5 (7%)	33 (44%)	4 (5%)/1 (1%)	6 (8%)	3 (4%)
Büchler et al. [18]	28/47	30%	70%	2 (4%)	10 (22%)	17 (36%)	6 (13%)	8 (17%)
Pederzoli et al. [23]	93/-	-	-	15%	20%	14%/-	7%	7%
Howard et al. [24]	20/39	40%	60%	4 (10%)	18 (46%)	3 (8%)	6 (15%)	4 (10%)
Ala-Kokko et al. [28]	25/43	-	-	5 (12%)	12%	-/22 (51%)	3 (7%)	1 (2%)
Rau et al. [19]	29/32	79%	21%	1 (3%)	16 (50%)	5 (16%)/-	7 (22%)	3 (9%)
Luiten et al. [20]	29/112	-	-	13 (12%)	38 (34%)	8 (7%)/21 (19%)	19 (17%)	12(11%)
Pederzoli et al. [37]	15/32	40%	60%	4 (13%)	15 (47%)	-	7 (22%)	4 (13%)
Bassi et al. [38]	13/18	-	-	2 (11%)	6 (34%)	5 (28%)/-	1 (5%)	4 (22%)

Finnish study [28] recently reported that mortality among patients with pancreatic necrosis infection due to *S. epidermidis* is significantly greater than in patients with necrotic pancreatic tissue infected by other micro-organisms (36% versus 13%). There is evidence from the literature that pancreatic necrosis infection by *S. epidermidis* is associated with an open surgical technique. In this Finnish study [28], all patients with necrotizing pancreatitis in which necrotic tissue resection was performed using the "open packing" technique (i.e., leaving the abdominal wall open to perform daily necrotic tissue resections) showed growth of *S. epidermidis* in pancreatic tissue. In a Dutch study [39], *S. epidermidis* was also the micro-organism most frequently isolated from necrotic pancreatic tissue cultures in patients undergoing the open packing surgical technique.

A number of experimental and clinical studies have demonstrated the efficacy of prophylactic antimicrobial therapy in reducing infection among patients with acute pancreatitis [21, 22, 26, 29, 40, 41]. A meta-analysis of randomized trials published between 1966 and 1997 evaluated prophylactic antibiotic treatment in patients with acute pancreatitis [42]. Of the eight studies identified, three were carried out in the 1970s among patients with acute pancreatitis of only limited severity and treated with ampicillin. The studies conducted in the 1990s included patients with severe necrotizing pancreatitis receiving broad-spectrum antibiotics. The meta-analysis showed a significant decrease in mortality associated with antibiotic use: 7% among the patients receiving antibiotics versus 13% among the control group. There was no effect on mortality in the three studies using ampicillin. Another meta-analysis of randomized trials published between 1966 and 2000 evaluated the effect of prophylactic treatment with antibiotics other than ampicillin [43]. Six trials were identified. One study compared prophylaxis with two different drugs [38], and two studies enrolled patients without pancreatic necrosis confirmed by abdominal CT [26, 41]. Subsequently, these three trials were excluded from the analysis. The meta-analysis showed a non-significant reduction in the development of pancreatic necrosis infection (12% absolute reduction, with 95% confidence interval -2.4% to 26.4%), and a significant decrease in mortality (12.3%, 95% confidence interval 2.7%–22%).

Our group has conducted a meta-analysis of the six trials published until 2001, evaluating the effect of antibiotic prophylaxis in patients with necrotizing acute pancreatitis or severe acute pancreatitis (Table 3). A significant reduction was found in both the infection of necrotic pancreatic tissue (relative risk 0.50, 50% confidence interval 0.32–0.72) and mortality (relative risk 0.48, 95% confidence interval 0.29–0.80) using a fixed-effects model based on the Mantel-Haenszel method. The number of patients needed to treat to save a life is nine.

Total parenteral nutrition (TPN) has been the standard practice for providing nutritients to patients with severe acute pancreatitis. Enteral nutrition (EN)

Table 3. Randomized trials evaluating the effect of prophylactic antibiotic treatment in patients with necrotizing acute pancreatitis or severe acute pancreatitis

Author (reference)	Patients	Antibiotic treatment	Necrosis infection	Mortality
Sainio et al. [21]	60 patients with severe necrotizing alcohol-induced pancreatitis	Three doses of 1.5 g cefuroxime per day intravenously until clinical recovery and fall to normal of C-reactive protein concentration. If moderately raised CRP cefuroxime was continued for 14 days (two doses of 250 mg/day by mouth)	Treatment group: 9/30 (30 %), control group: 12/30 (40%)	Treatment group: 1/30 (3%), control group: 7/30 (23%)
Nordback et al. [22]	90 patients with necrotizing pancreatitis (32 of the 90 patients enrolled were excluded after randomization)	Imipenem 1 g intravenously three times a day (duration of treatment is not stated)	Treatment group: 2/25 (8 %), control group: 14/33 (42%)	Treatment group: 2/25 (8%), control group: 5/33 (15%)
Luiten et al. [26]	102 patients with clinical signs of severe acute pancreatitis (Imrie Score ≥3 and/or Blathazar grade D or E on CT findings)	Selective decontamination with administration of colistin sulfate, amphotericin, and norfloxacin by mouth and smeared along the upper and lower gums every 6 hours, and in a rectal enema every day. Cefotaxime was given intravenously every 8 h until Gram-negative bacteria were eliminated from the oral cavity and rectum (average 7.4 days)	Treatment group: 9/50 (18 %), control group: 20/52 (38%)	Treatment group: 11/50 (22 %), control group: 18/52 (35%)

cont. →

Table 3 *cont.*

Author (reference)	Patients	Antibiotic treatment	Necrosis infection	Mortality
Pederzoli et al. [37]	72 patients with necrotizing pancreatitis	0.5 g of imipenem given intravenously every 8 h for 14 days	Treatment group: 5/33 (15 %), control group: 10/41 (24%)	Treatment group: 4/33 (12%), control group: 3/41 (7%)
Delcenserie et al. [41]	23 patients with acute pancreatitis with two or more fluid collections demonstrated by CT	Ceftazidime 2 g every 8 h and amikacin 7.5 mg/kg every 12 h and metronidazole 0.5 g every 8 h for 10 days	Treatment group: 0/11 (0%), control group: 4/12 (33%)	Treatment group: 1/11 (9%), control group: 3/12 (25%)
Schwarz et al. [29]	26 patients with acute necrotizing pancreatitis	Twice daily 200 mg ofloxacin and twice daily 500 mg metronidazole intravenously for 10 days	Treatment group: 8/13 (61%), control group: 7/13 (54%)	Treatment group: 0/13 (0%), control group: 2/13 (15%)

has the advantage of being less expensive and having the potential for protecting the gut barrier. The effectiveness and safety of EN compared with TPN has not been adequately evaluated in patients with acute severe pancreatitis. There is a clinical trial of small sample size that compared early enteral feeding with a semi-elemental diet through a nasoenteric tube placed distal to the ligament of Treitz with TPN delivered through a central venous catether in 38 patients with acute necrotizing pancreatitis [44]. The use of EN was associated with a significant reduction of septic complications: 5 patients had 6 septic complications in the EN group and 10 patients had 10 septic complications in the TPN group. Two patients in the EN group developed infected pancreatic necrosis or pancreatic abscess, whilst 4 patients in the TPN group developed septic pancreatic complications.

Burn Patients

Infection is the most important cause of death among burn patients. The incidence of nosocomial infections was prospectively studied in 52 patients admitted to a burn unit during a 6-month period between 1991 and 1992 [45]. In total, 36 nosocomial infections were documented in 26 patients (50%)—pneumonia being the most common infection. A causative micro-organism was identified in 15 of the 22 cases of pneumonia, S. aureus being isolated in 6 cases. The predominance of S. aureus causing infection in burn patients was in accordance with a previous study in which 90 infections occurred in 40 (34%) of 116 burn patients over a 12-month period [46]. The most common infections were pneumonia and infection of the burn wounds (22 and 21 infections, respectively), and S. aureus was identified as the causative micro-organism in 37% of the infections. Nasal carriage of S. aureus on admission was identified as a risk factor for the development of sepsis due to this PPM. The most recent study on the incidence of infections in burn patients was performed in a Swedish University Hospital over a 3-year period (1993–1995) [47]. Of the 230 burn patients consecutively included in the study, 83 (36%) developed a total of 176 infections—infection of the burn wound being the most common (107 infections in 72 patients). There were 17 episodes of pneumonia in 14 patients at a median of 3 days after admission. Of the 17 pneumonia episodes, 13 were bacterial and were mainly caused by S. pneumoniae (6 cases) and S. aureus (3 cases).

The digestive tract flora constitutes an important reservoir of PPM in burn patients [48]. Recently, our group has shown that pneumonia in burn patients is an endogenous problem [6]. We observed 37 cases of pneumonia in 27 of 56 patients with burns of more than 20% of total body surface area. Of the pneumonias, 57% were primary endogenous and were diagnosed within 1–4 days of admission. The micro-organisms responsible for the 21 cases of primary endogenous pneumonia were *S. aureus* (11 cases), *S. pneumoniae* (6 cases), *H. influenzae* (6 cases), methicillin-resistant *S. aureus* (1 case), *Acinetobacter* spp. (1 case), and *P. mirabilis* (1 case). There were 14 cases of secondary endogenous pneumonia due to methicillin-resistant *S. aureus* (10 cases), *P. aeruginosa* (3 cases), and *E. cloacae* (1 case). Of the 37 episodes of pneumonia, 35 (95%) were caused by micro-organisms already present in the oropharynx or rectum of the patients on admission to the ICU, or that were acquired during treatment on the ICU but before the diagnosis of pneumonia. This suggests that prophylactic selective digestive decontamination (SDD) may be effective in reducing the incidence of pneumonia in this type of patient.

A total of 31 patients with burns of ≥30% of total body surface area and receiving SDD were compared with an historical group of 33 patients with burns of similar extent and treated in the same ICU before the introduction of SDD [49]. The frequency of gastric carriage of *Pseudomonas spp.* and enterobacteria was 12% and 51%, respectively, in the group of patients not receiving SDD, versus 0% and 23%, respectively, in the SDD group. There were 9 respiratory tract infections in the control group—the most frequent causal micro-organism being *S. aureus* (6 cases)—whilst in the SDD group there were only 2 respiratory tract infections, caused by *S. aureus*.

To date there is only one randomized trial assessing the efficacy of SDD in burn patients [50]. A significant reduction in both mortality and primary endogenous infections was reported. The number of deaths during the treatment in the burn unit was 5 of 53 patients in the SDD group and 15 of 54 patients in the placebo group (relative risk 0.33 with 95% confidence interval 0.13–0.85). The incidence of pneumonia was significantly higher in the placebo group: 30.8 per 1,000 ventilator-days versus 17 per 1,000 ventilator-days. Primary endogenous pneumonias were completely prevented using SDD, whilst there were 17 primary endogenous pneumonias in the placebo group, mainly due to *S. aureus*, *H. influenzae*, and *S. pneumoniae*.

Trauma Patients

Lower airway infections are a particular problem in trauma patients, especially in those with a decreased level of consciousness. A study of 161 polytraumatized patients showed a 42% incidence of pneumonia in comatose subjects (Glasgow Coma Score <9) versus only 13% in the non-comatose patients [51]. Different studies have demonstrated that 20%–40% of patients with head injuries requiring intensive care develop pneumonia in the first 4–5 days after the start of mechanical ventilation [52–57]. The high prevalence of pneumonia in head injury patients may be due to continuous aspiration of the oropharyngeal contents towards the lower airways secondary to the glottic dysfunction found in comatose patients. Stoutenbeek et al. [58] was the first to report *S. pneumoniae, H. influenzae* and *S. aureus* as the major etiological agents of pneumonia in traumatized and comatose patients. This has since been confirmed by other authors, who also showed that pneumonia in the traumatized patient is basically an endogenous problem [51, 53–55].

Forty-four trauma patients requiring intensive care following head injuries or stroke were included in a prospective study in Spain [53]. Samples from the nasopharynx, gastric juice, and trachea were obtained within the first 24 h after intubation, together with protected bronchial catheter brush samples on a daily basis for the first 4 days and subsequently every 72 h, until extubation, death, or the development of pneumonia. Tracheal colonization on admission was detected in 58% of patients, nasal or pharyngeal colonization in 57%, and gastric colonization in 44%. *S. aureus, S. pneumoniae,* or *H. influenzae* was isolated in 61% of the tracheal aspirates, 50% of the nasal or pharyngeal samples, and in 53% of the bronchial samples. The percentage of samples positive for AGNB varied between 10% and 22%. Over the following days, the frequency of colonization by PPM increased to 91%, mainly due to AGNB obtained from the tracheal aspirates. The diagnosis of pneumonia was confirmed in 19 (40%) of the 48 patients; 9 episodes in the first 4 days (early onset pneumonia) and the other 10 cases after 4 days (late-onset pneumonia). The micro-organisms causing early onset pneumonia were invariably community bacteria (3 *S. aureus,* 2 *S. pneumoniae,* 2 *H. influenzae,* 1 *E. coli*), whilst AGNB were mainly involved in late-onset pneumonia (4 *P. aeruginosa,* 2 *E. cloacae,* 1 *E. coli,* 1 *S. aureus*). Of the 8 micro-organisms causing "early" pneumonia, 6 were carried in the oropharynx at the start of the study, i.e., primary endogenous pathogens, and 7 of the 8 micro-organisms causing "late" pneumonia were first acquired and carried in the oropharynx during the follow-up period prior to the development of pneumonia, i.e., secondary endogenous development.

Colonization of the lower airways with *S. aureus, S. pneumoniae,* or *H. influenzae* in the first 24 h after intubation was shown to be an independent factor associated with the development of "early" pneumonia (odds ratio 28.9, 95% confidence interval 1.59–52.5) [54]. That study included 100 patients with head injuries and a Glasgow Coma Score ≤ 12 who were intubated on admission to the ICU or in the Emergency Service. A tracheal aspirate was obtained in the first 24 h post intubation, together with a sample of lower airway secretions obtained via bronchial minilavage at the time when pneumonia was suspected. Colonization of the lower airway was observed in 68 patients, with the isolation of *S. aureus, S. pneumoniae,* or *H. influenzae* from 71% of the tracheal aspirate samples. Pneumonia was diagnosed in 26 patients on a mean of 3 days after admission—*S. aureus, S. pneumoniae,* or *H. influenzae* being the causative agents in 87% of cases. Moreover, 73% of the patients with pneumonia had tracheal colonization on admission by the same PPM that subsequently produced pneumonia. Finally, the frequency of pneumonia was lower among the patients who had received prophylactic antibioticcs (11% versus 60%).

Similar to burn patients [46], the nasal carrier state of *S. aureus* was a risk factor for pneumonia due to this micro-organism during hospitalization in patients with head injuries [55].

In patients with head injuries or central nervous system involvement due to other etiologies, systemic antibiotic treatment after intubation or the use of SDD has been shown to be effective in reducing the incidence of pneumonia [56, 57, 59].

The same group from Spain studied 105 patients with head injuries or stroke and a Glasgow Coma Score ≤12 who required mechanical ventilation for more than 72 h [57]. The patients were randomly assigned to receive 3 g of intravenous cefuroxime (two doses of 1.5 g given 12 h apart) (n=53) or no cefuroxime (control, n=52). Seventeen patients in the control group received antibiotics for surgical prophylaxis for 3.5±1.8 days. Pulmonary infection was suspected in 52 patients, and in 37 a microbiological diagnosis of pneumonia was established—the most frequently isolated micro-organisms being *S. aureus* (30%), *H. influenzae* (23%), and *S. pneumoniae* (11%). The incidence of pneumonia was significantly lower among the patients who received cefuroxime (23% versus 48%).

A French randomized clinical trial was conducted to assess the efficacy of SDD on infection in 124 neurosurgical patients [56]. Patients in the treatment group received four times daily a suspension of polymyxin, tobramycin, and amphotericin through the nasogastric tube, the same antibiotics plus vancomycin in the oral cavity, and no parenteral prophylactic antibiotic. The study included 66 individuals with head injuries. The frequency of pneumonia in the group receiving SDD (n=64) was 24%, versus 42% in the 60 patients administered placebo. In the patients with head injuries, a significant reduction in the incidence of pneumonia was observed (22% in the SDD group versus 58% in the placebo group). Another French study evaluated the efficacy of SDD in the prevention of nosocomial infections in 148 trauma patients intubated within less than 24 h [59]. Of the 148 trauma patients, 130 patients had head trauma. The SDD protocol consisted of a suspension of colistin sulfate, gentamicin, and amphotericin B instilled through the nasogastric tube and in the nares four times daily, and of an oral gel containing 2% of the same antibiotics applied along the gums four times daily. No parenteral antibiotics were given. The episodes of bronchopneumonia were significantly reduced with SDD (25% in the SDD group and 51% in the placebo group, P=0.01). However, the duration of mechanical ventilation, the length of ICU stay, and the mortality did not differ.

A multicenter study was performed in 17 hospitals in Europe, Australia, and

New Zealand that enrolled 405 patients admitted to the ICU within 24 h of non-penetrating blunt trauma with a Hospital Trauma Index/Injury Severity Score (HTI-ISS) ≥16 and mechanical ventilation [60]. Patients were randomly assigned to receive either SDD or standard treatment. The SDD regimen consisted of a 10-ml suspension of polymyxin E, tobramycin, and amphotericin B administered through the nasogastric tube four times a day. A paste containing 2% of each polymyxin E, tobramycin, and amphotericin B was applied to the buccal mucosa four times a day, and cefotaxime was administered intravenously at a dose of 1 g every 6 h for 4 days. The overall infection rate was significantly reduced from 61% in the control group to 49% in the treatment group (P=0.014). The pneumonia rate was reduced from 23% to 9% (P<0.001) and the tracheobronchitis rate from 40% to 26% (P=0.002). No differences in mortality, duration of mechanical ventilation, and duration in ICU stay were observed.

In a meta-analysis of 33 trials involving more than 5,500 patients on the efficacy of SDD on respiratory tract infections, a subanalysis was performed of the studies in trauma patients [61]. A significant reduction in respiratory tract infection was found both when prophylaxis was given with a combination of topical and systemic antibiotics (odds ratio 0.38, 95% confidence interval 0.29–0.50) and, to a lesser extent, when administering prophylaxis with topical antibiotics only (odds ratio 0.60, 95% confidence interval 0.46–0.79).

Patients with Exacerbations of COPD

Of all patients who require mechanical ventilation for more than 24 h in the ICU, 10%–50% are individuals who have been hospitalized because of exacerbation of COPD [62, 63]. The exacerbation of COPD is characterized by the following signs and symptoms: increased tracheobronchial secretions or changes in sputum characteristics, increased frequency of cough, increased dyspnea, and an absence of acute changes on chest X-rays [64].

In patients with COPD, the exacerbation of the disease has been usually considered the result of a viral or bacterial infection. The studies using quantitative cultures of lower airway samples obtained by protected bronchial brush sampling or bronchoalveolar lavage (BAL) have demonstrated PPM in sufficient concentration to cause infection in approximately 50% of patients with COPD exacerbation [65–68]. However, the role of bacterial infection in the etiology of COPD exacerbation is still under debate, since many patients have PPM in their respiratory secretions even in the stable phases of the disease [66, 69, 70], and these same micro-organisms may be present at the time of exacerbation or may actually be the cause of the exacerbation. The issue is whether the presence of PPM in respiratory secretions indicates chronic colonization or whether these micro-organisms are the cause of COPD exacerbation.

Different authors have described the micro-organisms colonizing the lower airways in patients with COPD, and have shown that the most frequent micro-organisms are *S. pneumoniae* and *H. influenzae*. AGNB are infrequent in patients with non-severe COPD. In a study of 18 patients with stable COPD who required bronchoscopy for different reasons (moderate hemoptysis in 11 cases, suspected bronchiectasia in 3, and chest X-ray alterations in 4), protected bronchial brush samples were obtained [69]. Fifteen patients (83%) had growth of $\geq 10^2$ CFU/ml. However, of the 27 micro-organisms isolated, only 5 were PPM (Table 4). In a similar study of 52 patients, 46 (88%) had growth of $\geq 10^2$ CFU/ml in bronchial brush samples or $\geq 10^3$ CFU/ml in BAL [70]. However, in only 17 patients were the micro-organisms PPM—most species belonging to the community flora (Table 4). In 20 patients hospitalized due to COPD exacerbation, a growth of $\geq 10^2$ CFU/ml in protected bronchial brush sampling was found in 18 (90%) patients, although of the 41 micro-organisms isolated, only 18 were potentially pathogenic [71] (Table 4). From a group of 29 patients with COPD exacerbation who were not hospitalized but gave consent to bronchoscopy, and from 40 patients with stable COPD who were not in hospital but required bronchoscopy, bronchial brush samples were quantitatively cultured [66]. PPM grew in $\geq 10^3$ CFU/ml in 10 of the 40 (25%) patients with stable COPD, and in 15 (52%) of the 29 patients with COPD exacerbation. *H. influenzae* and *S. pneumoniae* were predominant (Table 4). A similar study in 16 patients with stable COPD and in 40 patients with COPD exacerbation reported micro-organisms at $\geq 10^3$ CFU/ml in 4 (16%) of the stable patients and in 21 (84%) of the patients with exacerbation of the disease [67].

Two studies have analyzed the role of bacterial infection in patients requiring mechanical ventilation due to COPD exacerbation on the ICU. The first study [65] involved 54 patients with COPD who required mechanical ventilation due to hypercapnic respiratory failure in the first 24 h after hospital admission and who had received no antibiotic treatment in the preceding 10 days. Quantitative culture of the protected bronchial brush samples showed growths of $\geq 10^2$ CFU/ml of 44 micro-organisms in 27 (50%) patients. Of the 44 micro-organisms, 39 were potentially pathogenic (Table 4). The second study [68] evaluated the lower airway flora in 50 patients requiring mechanical ventilation due to COPD exacerbation. Although 21 of the 50 patients had received antibiotic treatment before obtaining the protected bronchial brush samples, growth of $\geq 10^2$ CFU/ml of 26 PPM was present in 23 (46%) patients, and 11 non-pathogens in 8 patients. Of the 26 PPM, 8 (31%) were AGNB (Table 4).

Patients admitted to hospital with COPD exacerbation receive antibiotics in 80% of cases [72]. However, the efficacy of antibiotics in COPD exacerbation is under debate. The unnecessary prescription of antibiotics can lead to the emergence of antimicrobial resistance and may put the patient at risk of adverse

Table 4. Potentially pathogenic micro-organisms (PPM) isolated from the lower airways of patients with chronic obstructive pulmonary disease (COPD) (*AGNB* aerobic Gram-negative bacteria)

Author	Patients	No. PPM and diagnostic method	*H. influenzae* or *parainfluenzae*	*S. pneumoniae*	*S. aureus*	AGNB	*Pseudomonas stenotroph.* spp.
Cabello et al. [69]	18 patients with stable COPD	5 PPM with growth $\geq 10^2$ CFU/ml in protected bronchial brush sampling	2 (40%)	2 (40%)	1 (20%)	-	-
Soler et al. [70]	52 patients with stable COPD	21 PPM with growth $\geq 10^2$ CFU/ml in protected bronchial brush sampling		18 (86%)			3 (14%)
Martinez et al. [71]	20 patients with exacerbated COPD	18 PPM with growth $\geq 10^2$ CFU/ml in protected bronchial brush sampling	5 (28%)	9 (50%)	-	-	1 (6%)
Monsó et al. [66]	29 patients with exacerbated COPD	17 PPM with growth $\geq 10^3$ CFU/ml in protected bronchial brush sampling	10 (59%)	3 (18%)	-	-	2 (12%)
Pela et al. [67]	40 patients with exacerbated COPD	15 PPM with growth $\geq 10^3$ CFU/ml in protected bronchial brush sampling	1 (7%)	10 (67%)	-	1 (7%)	1 (7%)
Fagon et al. [65]	54 patients with exacerbated COPD and mechanical ventilation	39 PPM with growth $\geq 10^2$ CFU/ml in protected bronchial brush sampling	17 (44%)	7 (18%)	4 (10%)	5 (13%)	3 (8%)
Soler et al. [68]	50 patients with exacerbated COPD and mechanical ventilation	26 PPM with growth $\geq 10^2$ CFU/ml in protected bronchial brush sampling	10 (38%)	4 (15%)	-	1 (4%)	7 (27%)

reactions or interactions with the other pharmacological treatments. Ten place-bo-controlled clinical trials have been published in the English literature between 1957 and 1999, assessing the efficacy of antibiotic treatment in patients with exacerbations of COPD but without pneumonia. Five of these studies were conducted before 1990, and evaluated antibiotics that are no longer in use. Moreover, the main study variables were not relevant from the clinical perspective, but included changes in fever, characteristics and volume of secretions, spirometric indices, or blood gas recordings. Two studies showed that in patients treated with antibiotics a more rapid reduction in sputum purulence and fever occurred [73].

A meta-analysis of randomized trials comparing treatment with antibiotics or placebo in patients with COPD exacerbation, and published between 1955 and 1994, has been published [74]. The meta-analysis includes nine studies, of which four were conducted in hospitalized patients. The authors reported a benefit in peak expiratory flow of 10.75 l/min (95% confidence interval 4.96–16.54 l/min).

The marginal benefits obtained in some clinical trials do not allow the generalization of such results to patients admitted to the ICU. An analysis has recently been performed of the efficacy of antibiotic treatment in patients with COPD exacerbation requiring mechanical ventilation, in the context of a randomized clinical trial comparing treatment for 10 days with ofloxacin (n=45) or placebo (n=45) [75]. The hospital mortality rate was 4% in the ofloxacin group and 22% in the placebo group, while the need for additional antibiotic treatment reached 7% in the ofloxacin group and 36% in the placebo series. The authors found the development of pneumonia to be associated with increased mortality (31% and 8% in the patients with and without pneumonia, respectively). It is quite plausible that the benefit of antibiotics was mainly associated with prevention of the development of pneumonia in the first 7 days among the patients requiring endotracheal intubation (83% in the ofloxacin group versus 85% in the placebo series).

Patients Undergoing Liver Transplantation

Infection remains a significant cause of morbidity and mortality in liver transplant recipients. Bacterial and fungal infection rates in the first 30 days after transplantation vary between 40% and 80% [76–79]. The largest European series detailing bacterial and fungal infections after liver transplantation is an English study of 284 consecutive adult patients undergoing orthotopic liver transplantation because of acute liver failure (n=51) or chronic liver disease (n=233) [76]. Patients were studied prospectively for evidence of infection and routine samples of blood, bile, urine, drain fluids, and sputum or endotracheal aspirates were collected on days 1, 3, and 7 after transplantation. There were 222 episodes of bacterial infection occurring before day 28 after transplantation in 122 (43%) patients. Wound infection was the most frequent infection (n=55), followed by bacteremia (n=44), respiratory tract infection (n=34), and urinary tract infection (n=31). The most common bacterial pathogens were *S. aureus* (n=48, causative agent in 44% of wound infections), *Enterococcus faecium* (n=39, causative agent in 20% of wound infections), coagulase-negative staphylococcus (n=32, causative agent in 23% of bacteremias), *Klebsiella* spp. (n=27, causative agent in 16% of bacteremias, 20% of pneumonias, 19% of urinary tract infections), and *E. faecalis* (n=21, causative agent in 22% of urinary tract infections). Fifty-three patients (19%) of this series had received antibiotics pre transplantation for a median of 3 days. Logistic regression analysis showed that pre-transplantation antibacterials had a protective effect for the development of bacterial infection (odds ratio 0.89, 95% confidence interval 0.81–0.99).

It is believed that most infections in patients receiving liver transplantation are endogenous. Therefore, eliminating the PPM from the gastrointestinal tract in these patients by SDD seems to be a sensible measure to prevent infection.

The effect of SDD on the frequency of post-liver transplant infection has been the subject of six randomized controlled trials (RCT) [77-82]. The first clinical trial [77] from Birmingham in the UK involved 59 adults with chronic liver disease who were randomly assigned to receive one of two antibiotic regimens: (1) SDD group (n=27) received amphotericin, polymyxin E, and tobramycin administered as a flavored suspension and as a gel base for oral application started at home as soon as a donor liver became available and before admission into the hospital; (2) control group (n=32) only received oral nystatin from the time of surgery. Both groups received cefotaxime and ampicillin intravenously for 48 h after liver transplantation. Patients in the SDD group received the antimicrobial mixture to the gut through a nasogastric tube and in the oropharyngeal cavity postoperatively for a mean of 12 days. Seven patients were excluded from the analysis (1 control and 5 SDD patients died preoperatively, 1 SDD patient withdrew from the study). The number of patients with infections was significantly lower in the SDD group: 3 of 21 (14%) versus 12 of 31 (39%). The most notable difference was the absence of respiratory tract infections in the SDD group, whilst there were 8 respiratory infections in the control group. Five control patients died before hospital discharge and all the SDD group survived until they were discharged home.

The second clinical trial comparing systemic antibiotic prophylaxis with systemic antibiotic prophylaxis plus SDD in liver transplant recipients was performed at the University of Chicago Hospital and involved 69 pediatric and adult patients with underlying liver disease [78]. Patients were randomly assigned to receive one of two regimens of perioperative antibiotic prophylaxis: (1) control group consisted of intravenous cefotaxime and ampicillin administered 30 minutes before surgery, every 6 h intraoperatively, and then every 8 h thereafter for 48 h; (2) SDD group consisted of ampicillin and cefotaxime administered as in the control group, and a suspension of gentamicin, polymyxin E, and nystatin given orally or through a nasogastric tube every 6 h, and a paste containing 2% of the aforementioned antibiotics applied to the buccal mucosa every 6 h while the patient was in the ICU receiving respiratory support. Of the 36 patients in the SDD group, 28 reported taking their antibiotic regimen before transplantation for a mean of 14 days and 26 of these patients received the SDD regimen for at least 3 days before transplantation. The total number of isolates of AGNB from surveillance cultures was 40 for the 26 SDD patients given the regimen ≥3 days before transplantation, 16 for the 10 SDD patients given the regimen ≤2 days before transplantation, and 159 for the 33 control patients. There was no statistically significant difference between the two groups in the proportion of patients with bacterial and/or fungal infections during the first 28 days after transplantation: 39% (14/36) in the SDD group and 33% (14/33) in the control group. Overall mortality during hospitalization was 8% among SDD patients and 9% among control patients. When SDD patients who received the regimen ≥3 days before transplantation were compared with control patients, rates of infections caused by AGNB were significantly reduced (0 infections in 26 SDD patients versus 7 infections in 33 control patients).

The third RCT was a placebo-controlled study [79]. This trial included 89 adult patients undergoing elective orthotopic transplantation of the liver in two university hospitals in The Netherlands that were randomly assigned to receive placebo or SDD regimen as soon as they were accepted for transplantation. Patients undergoing SDD received preoperatively 400 mg of norfloxacin orally once daily and lozenges, containing colistin, tobramycin, and amphotericin B, four times daily. Postoperatively, they received a suspension containing colistin, tobramycin, and amphotericin B, four times daily through the nasogastric tube, combined with an oral paste containing a 2% solution of the same antibiotics until the 30th postoperative day. Patients receiving placebo had a similar regimen with placebo drugs. Perioperative antibiotic prophylaxis was started at the induction of anesthesia and continued for 48 h with intravenous cefotaxime (1 g every 8 h) and tobramycin (4 mg/kg every 24 h). There were 31 patients who stopped the study medications before their transplantation (16 in the SDD group and 15 in the placebo group) and 3 patients died during surgery or immediately thereafter, leaving 55 patients for the final analysis (26 receiving SDD, 29 receiving placebo). Colonization with AGNB was significantly reduced in the rectum and urine but not in the throat, sputum, and bile in patients undergoing SDD. The percentage of patients acquiring a bacterial or fungal infection in the 1st month after transplantation was 84.5% in the SDD group and 86% in the placebo group. There was no statistically significant difference in the mean number of infections per patient (1.77±0.28 in the SDD group and 1.93±0.31 in the placebo group). Although the total number of infections was similar in both groups, infections involving AGNB were significantly lower in the SDD group (10 episodes in placebo group and 1 episode in SDD group).

In the fourth American RCT from Jacksonville, Florida 80 candidates for liver transplantation were randomly assigned to an SDD protocol consisting of gentamicin 80 mg, polymyxin 100 mg and nystatin 2 million units [37 patients] or to nystatin alone [43 patients] four times a day [80]. When intubation was necessary for respiratory support, SDD was administered by nasogastric tube and a paste [Orabase], containing either 2% gentamicin, 2% polymyxin E, and 2% nystatin, or 2% nystatin alone, was applied to the lingual and buccal mucosa every 6 h. In addition, all participants received ceftizoxime [1g], IV, every 8 h, beginning immediately before liver transplantation and continuing for 48 h thereafter. The enteral antimicrobials were given from the time of randomisation through to day 21 after liver transplantation. No significant difference in the proportion of patients with infection was found between the group receiving SDD [12/37, 32.4%] and the group receiving nystatin alone [12/43, 27.9%]. However, of the 12 infected patients on nystatin 8 developed infections with potential pathogens including AGNB, yeast and *S.aureus*. Amongst the 12 SDD patients only one developed a pseudomonal cholangitis, whilst the other 7 were invariably infected with low level pathogens coagulase-negative staphylococci and enterococci. There were two deaths in each group.

The fifth RCT was performed in Berlin [Germany] and included 95 patients [81]. Three groups were compared: Group 1 received standard formula and SDD [n = 32]; Group 2 fiber-containing formula and living *Lactobacillus plantarum* 299 [n = 32]; and Group 3 fiber-containing formula and heat-killed *L. plantarum* 299. SDD consisted of 100 mg of polymyxin E sulphate, 80 mg of tobramycin and 500 mg of amphotericin B given orally four times a day for 6 weeks, postoperatively. The patients did not receive oropharyngeal decontamination using the paste with 2% of polymyxin, tobramycin and amphotericin B. They all received parenteral antibiotics including ceftriaxone [2 g twice daily] and metronidazole [500 mg twice daily] 30 minutes before surgery and until two days after surgery. Surveillance cultures were not part of the protocol. Fifteen patients receiving SDD [48%] developed infection, whilst only 4 [13%] in Group 2 and 11 [34%] in Group 3. The difference was statistically significant between Groups 1 and 2 [p = 0.017]. Cholangitis and pneumonia were the most frequent infections, and enterococci and coagulase-negative staphylococci were the predominant bacteria in all 3 groups. AGNB were isolated twice [*E. coli*] in patients receiving SDD, and on two occasions [*E. coli*, *Klebsiella*] in the placebo group. There were no patients with yeast infections.

Finally, the sixth RCT was performed in the paediatric transplant unit of Pittsburgh in the USA [82]. A total of 36 children were randomised in 2 groups:

SDD with polymyxin E, tobramycin and amphotericin B versus control. The children allocated to the test group received both oropharyngeal with 2% paste and gastrointestinal decontamination with suspension. Both SDD and control groups received parenteral antibiotics cefotaxime and ampicillin the day of the transplant and postoperatively for a minimum of 5 days. Surveillance cultures of throat and rectum were regularly obtained. There were significantly fewer patients with AGNB-infections in the SDD group: 3/18 patients [11%] versus 11/18 patients [50%] in the control group [p<0.001]. Mortality was not statistically different in the two group: 2 patients on SDD died, and 3 in the control group.

Summary

Infection of the necrotic tissue occurs in almost 40% of patients with necrotizing pancreatitis and is associated with a mortality that varies from 30% to 50%. Translocation of AGNB present in overgrowth in the terminal ileum is the main cause of infection in necrotizing pancreatitis. Because infection of necrotic tissue may have already occurred during the 1st week of the disease, antibiotic prophylaxis should be administered as soon as possible after admission. A number of randomized trials have demonstrated that prophylactic antibiotic treatment in patients with necrotizing pancreatitis reduces the occurrence of infection and the mortality. The administration of non-absorbable enteral antimicrobials erradicates AGNB from the gastrointestinal tract. To provide additional cover during establishment of decontamination of the digestive tract with enteral antibiotics, a short-term systemic prophylaxis with an antibiotic with adequate coverage against AGNB and S. aureus should be also implemented. The optimal duration of the systemic antibiotic treatment has not been established, but in almost all the clinical trials parenteral antimicrobials were administered for 10–14 days.

Infection is the main cause of death in burn patients, the burn wound and the respiratory tract being the most common sites of infection. Pneumonia in burn patients is an endogenous problem that it is mainly due to community micro-organisms. The only randomized clinical trial evaluating the efficacy of prophylactic antibiotic treatment administered immediately after admission to the burn unit has demonstrated that a regimen combining SDD with non-absorbable antibiotics administered during the ICU stay and intravenous cefotaxime during the first 4 days significantly reduces both mortality and primary endogenous infections in burn patients.

Trauma patients, especially those with a decreased level of consciousness, are very prone to develop pneumonia. Different studies have demonstrated that

20%–40% of patients with head injury requiring intensive care develop pneumonia in the first days after the start of mechanical ventilation. The microorganisms causing pneumonia in trauma patients are carried in the oropharynx prior to the development of pneumonia. Respiratory tract infections appearing in the 1st week after ICU admission are mainly caused by community bacteria, whilst AGNB are involved in late-onset pneumonias. Randomized clinical trials have demonstrated a significant reduction in the incidence of pneumonia in head trauma patients with the administration of either a short course of intravenous cefuroxime immediately upon ICU admission or SDD with or without parenteral antimicrobials. However, no effect on mortality, duration of mechanical ventilation, and duration of ICU stay has been shown in these clinical trials.

The lower respiratory tract is colonized by PPM in sufficient concentration to cause infection in almost 50% of patients with COPD exacerbation. Although *S. pneumoniae* and *H. influenzae* are the most frequent micro-organisms in patients with severe COPD requiring mechanical ventilation, AGNB may represent one-third of the PPM isolated in the lower airways. Randomized clinical trials on the effect of antimicrobial treatment in patients with non-severe exacerbations of COPD have failed to demonstrate relevant clinical benefit. However, in patients with COPD exacerbation requiring mechanical ventilation, treatment with ofloxacin for 10 days has been associated with a significant reduction in hospital mortality.

Two-thirds of liver transplant recipients will develop bacterial infections in the 30 days following transplantation. Gram-positive cocci are the causative agents in more than one-half of these infections. A number of studies have demonstrated that SDD is an effective measure to reduce the gastrointestinal overgrowth of AGNB in liver transplant recipients when it is started before transplantation. Randomized trials evaluating the effect of SDD on infection in liver transplant patients have consistently shown that the development of infections by AGNB is significantly reduced when SDD has been administered before transplantation and during the following 2 or 3 weeks. The effect of SDD on the overall incidence of infection and mortality in patients undergoing liver transplantation should be assessed in randomized trials with adequate sample size [83, 84].

References

1. van Saene HKF, Damjanoviç V, Murray AE, de la Cal MA (1996) How to classify infections in intensive care units–the carrier state. A criterion whose time has come? J Hosp Infect 33:1–12
2. de la Cal MA, Cerdá E (1997) Vigilancia y control de infecciones en las unidades de cuidados intensivos: tasas, resistencias y estado de portador. Enferm Infecc Microbiol

Clin 15:47–52
3. Murray AE, Chambers JJ, van Saene HF (1998) Infections in patients requiring ventilation in intensive care: application of a new classification. Clin Microbiol Infect 4:94–99
4. Silvestri L, Monti Bragadin C, Milanese M (1999) Are most ICU infections really nosocomial? A prospective observational cohort study in mechanically ventilated patients. J Hosp Infect 42:125–133
5. Silvestri L, Sarginson RE, Hughes J, Milanese M, Gregori D, van Saene HKF (2002) Most nosocomial pneumonias are not due to nosocomial bacteria in ventilated patients. Evaluation of the accuracy of the 48 h time cut-off using carriage as the gold standard. Anaesth Intensive Care 30:275–282
6. de la Cal MA, Cerdá E, García-Hierro P et al (2001) Pneumonia in patients with severe burns. A classification according to the concept of the carrier state. Chest 119:1160–1165
7. Mobbs KJ, van Saene HKF, Sunderland D, Davies PDO (1999) Oropharyngeal gram-negative bacillary carriage. A survey of 120 healthy individuals. Chest 115:1570–1575
8. Mobbs KJ, van Saene HKF, Sunderland D, Davies PD (1999) Oropharyngeal gram-negative bacillary carriage in chronic obstructive pulmonary disease: relation to severity of disease. Respir Med 93:540-545
9. Norman J (1998) The role of cytokines in the pathogenesis of acute pancreatitis. Am J Surg 175:76–83
10. Gloor B, Reber HA (1998) Effects of cytokines and other inflamatory mediators on human acute pancreatitis. J Intensive Care Med 13:305–312
11. Bradley EL (1993) A clinically based classification system for acute pancreatitis. Arch Surg 128:586–590
12. Balthazar EJ, Robinson DL, Megibow AJ (1990) Acute pancreatitis: value of CT in establishing prognosis. Radiology 174:331–336
13. Ashley SW, Perez A, Pierce EA et al (2001) Necrotizing pancreatitis. Contemporary analysis of 99 consecutive cases. Ann Surg 234:572–580
14. Bradley EL, Allen K (1991) A prospective longitudinal study of observation versus surgical intervention in the management of necrotizing pancreatitis. Am J Surg 161:19–25
15. Paye F, Rotman N, Radier C, Nouira R, Fagniez PL (1998) Percutaneous aspiration for bacteriological studies in patients with necrotizing pancreatitis. Br J Surg 85:755–759
16. Garg PK, Khanna S, Bohidar NP, Kapil A, Tandon RK (2001) Incidence, spectrum and antibiotic sensitivity pattern of bacterial infections among patients with acute pancreatitis. J Gastroenterol Hepatol 16:1055–1059
17. Beger HG, Bittner R, Block S, Buchler M (1986) Bacterial contamination of pancreatic necrosis. Gastroenterology 91:433–438
18. Büchler MW, Gloor B, Müller CA, Friess H, Seiler CA, Uhl W (2000) Acute necrotizing pancreatitis: treatment strategy according to the status of infection. Ann Surg 232:619–626
19. Rau B, Pralle U, Mayer JM, Beger HG (1998) Role of ultrasonographically guided fine-needle aspiration cytology in the diagnosis of infected pancreatic necrosis. Br J Surg 85:179–184
20. Luiten EJ, Hop WC, Lange JF, Bruining HA (1997) Differential prognosis of gram-negative versus gram-positive infected and sterile pancreatic necrosis: results of a randomized trial in patients with severe acute pancreatitis treated with adjuvant selective decontamination. Clin Infect Dis 25:811–816
21. Sainio V, Kemppainen E, Puolakkainen P et al (1995) Early antibiotic treatment in acute necrotising pancreatitis. Lancet 346:663–667

22. Nordback I, Sand J, Saaristo R, Paajamen H (2001) Early treatment with antibiotics reduces the need for surgery in acute necrotizing pancreatitis. A single-center randomised study. J Gastrointest Surg 5:113–120
23. Pederzoli P, Bassi C, Vesentini S et al (1990) Retroperitoneal and peritoneal drainage and lavage in the treatment of severe necrotizing pancreatitis. Surg Gynecol Obstet 170:197–203
24. Howard TJ, Wiebke EA, Mogavero G et al (1995) Classification and treatment of local septic complications in acute pancreatitis. Am J Surg 170:44–50
25. Isenmann R, Rau B, Beger HG (1999) Bacterial infection and extent of necrosis are determinants of organ failure in patients with acute necrotizing pancreatitis. Br J Surg 86:1020–1024
26. Luiten EJT, Hop WCJ, Lange JF, Bruining HA (1995) Controlled clinical trial of selective decontamination for the treatment of severe acute pancreatitis. Ann Surg 222:57–65
27. Le Mée J, Paye F, Sauvanet A et al (2001) Incidence and reversibility of organ failure in the course of sterile or infected necrotizing pancreatitis. Arch Surg 136:1386–1390
28. Ala-Kokko TI, Tieranta N, Laurila J, Syrjala H (2001) Determinants of ICU mortality in necrotizing pancreatitis: the influence of *Staphylococcus epidermidis*. Acta Anaesthesiol Scand 45:853–857
29. Schwarz M, Isenmann R, Meyer H, Beger HG (1997) Antibiotic use in necrotizing pancreatitis. Results of a controlled study. Dtsch Med Wochenschr 122:356–361
30. Gergof SG, Banks PA, Robbins AH et al (1987) Early diagnosis of pancreatic infection by computed tomography-guided aspiration. Gastroenterology 93:1315–1320
31. Beger HG, Rau B, Isenmann R (2001) Prevention of severe change in acute pancreatitis: prediction and prevention. J Hepatobiliary Pancreat Surg 8:140–147
32. Dervenis C, Bassi C (2000) Evidence-based assessment of severity and management of acute pancreatitis. Br J Surg 87:257–258
33. Widdison AL, Karanjia ND, Reber HA (1994) Routes of spread of pathogens into the pancreas in a feline model of acute pancreatitis. Gut 36:1306–1310
34. Foitzik T, Fernández del Castillo C, Ferraro MJ, Mlthöfer K, Rattner DW, Warshaw AL (1995) Pathogenesis and prevention of early pancreatic infection in experimental acute necrotizing pancreatitis. Ann Surg 222:179–185
35. Gianotti L, Munda R, Alexander JW, Tchervenkov JI, Babcock GF (1993) Bacterial translocation: a potential source for infection in acute pancreatitis. Pancreas 8:551–558
36. Luiten EJT, Hop WC, Endtz HP, Bruining HA (1998) Prognostic importance of gram-negative intestinal colonization preceding pancreatic infection in severe acute pancreatitis. Results of a controlled clinical trial of selective decontamination. Intensive Care Med 24:438–445
37. Pederzoli P, Bassi C, Vesentini S, Campedelli A (1993) A randomised multicenter clinical trial on antibiotic prophylaxis of septic complications in acute necrotizing pancreatitis with imipenem. Surg Gynecol Obstet 176:480–483
38. Bassi C, Falconi M, Talamini G, Uomo G, Papaccio G, Dervens C et al (1998) Controlled clinical trial of pefloxacin versus imipenem in severe acute pancreatitis. Gastroenterology 115:1513–1517
39. Bosscha K, Hulstaert PF, Hennipman A et al (1998) Fulminant acute pancreatitis and infected necrosis: results of open management of the abdomen and "planned" reoperations. J Am Coll Surg 187:255–262
40. Gianotti L, Munda R, Gennari R, Pyles T, Alexander JW (1995) Effect of different regimens of gut decontamination on bacterial translocation and mortality in experimental acute pancreatitis. Eur J Surg 161:85–92

41.   Delcenserie R, Yzet T, Ducroix JP (1996) Prophylactic antibiotics in treatment of severe acute alcoholic pancreatitis. Pancreas 13:198–201

42.   Golub R, Siddiqi F, Pobl D (1998) Role of antibiotics in acute pancreatitis: a meta-analysis. J Gastrointest Surg 2:496–503

43.   Sharma VK, Howden CW (2001) Prophylactic antibiotic administration reduces sepsis and mortality in acute necrotizing pancreatitis: a meta-analysis. Pancreas 22:28–31

44.   Kalfarentzos F, Kehagias J, Mead N, Kokkinis K, Gogos CA (1997) Enteral nutrition is superior to parenteral nutrition in severe acute pancreatitis: results of a randomized prospective trial. B J Surg 84:1665–1669

45.   Wurtz R, Karajovic M, Dacumos E, Jovanovic B, Hanumadas M (1995) Nosocomial infections in a burn intensive care unit. Burns 21:181–184

46.   Taylor GD, Kibsey P, Kirkland T, Burroughs E, Tredget E (1992) Predominance of staphylococcal organisms in infections occurring in a burns intensive care unit. Burns 18:332–335

47.   Appelgren P, Björnhagen V, Bragderyd K, Jonson CE, Ransjo U (2002) A prospective study of infections in burn patients. Burns 28:39–46

48.   van Saene HFK, Nicolai JPA (1979) The prevention of wound infections in burn patients. Scand J Plast Reconstr Surg Hand Surg 13:63–67

49.   Mackie DP, van Hertum WAJ, Schumburg T, Kuijper EC, Knape P (1992) Prevention of infection in burns: preliminary experience with selective decontamination of the digestive tract in patients with extensive injuries. J Trauma 32:570–575

50.   Cerdá E, de la Cal MA, García-Hierro P, Gómez-Santos D, Negro E, Lorente JA, Ballesteros D (2001) La descontaminación digestiva selectiva reduce la mortalidad en los enfermos con quemaduras graves. Med Intensiva 26:152

51.   Rello J, Ausina V, Castella J, Net A, Prats G (1992) Nosocomial respiratory tract infections in multiple trauma patients. Influence of level of consciousness with implications for therapy. Chest 102:525–529

52.   Hsieh AH, Bishop MJ, Kubilis PS, Newell DW, Pierson DJ (1992) Pneumonia following closed head injury. Am Rev Respir Dis 146:290–294

53.   Ewig S, Torres A, El-Ebiary M et al (1999) Bacterial colonization patterns in mechanically ventilated patients with traumatic and medical head injury. Am J Respir Crit Care Med 159:188–198

54.   Sirvent JM, Torres A, Vidaur L, Armengol J, de Batlle J, Bonet A (2000) Tracheal colonisation within 24 h of intubation in patients with head trauma: risk factor for developing early-onset ventilator-associated pneumonia. Intensive Care Med 6:1369–1372

55.   Campbell W, Hendrix E, Schwalbe R, Fattom A, Edelman R (1999) Head-injured patients who are nasal carriers of *Staphylococcus aureus* are at high risk for *Staphylococcus aureus* pneumonia. Crit Care Med 27:798–801

56.   Korinek AM, Laisne MJ, Nicolas MH, Raskine L, Deroin V, Sanson-Lepors MJ (1993) Selective decontamination of the digestive tract in neurosurgical intensive care unit patients: a double-blind, randomised, placebo-controlled study. Crit Care Med 21:1466–1473

57.   Sirvent JM, Torres A, El-Ebiary M, Castro P, de Batlle J, Bonet A (1997) Protective effect of intravenously administered cefuroxime against nosocomial pneumonia in patients with structural coma. Am J Respir Crit Care Med 155:1729–1734

58.   Stoutenbeek CP, van Saene HK, Miranda DR, Zandstra DF, Langrehr D (1987) The effect of oropharyngeal decontamination using topical nonabsorbable antibiotics on the incidence of nosocomial respiratory tract infections in multiple trauma patients. J Trauma 27:357–364

59.   Quinio B, Albanèse J, Bues-Charbit M, Viviand X, Martin C (1996) Selective decontamination of the digestive tract in multiple trauma patients. A prospective double-

blind, randomized, placebo-controlled study. Chest 109:765–772

60. Stoutenbeek CP, van Saene HKF, Little RA, Whitehead A for the working group on selective decontamination of the digestive tract (2005) The effect of selective decontamination of the digestive tract on mortality in multiple trauma patients. Intensive Care Med (in press)

61. D′Amico R, Pifferi S, Leonetti C et al (1998) Effectiveness of antibiotic prophylaxis in critically ill adult patients: systematic review of randomised controlled trials. BMJ 316:1275–1285

62. Esteban A, Anzueto A, Alía I et al (2000) How is mechanical ventilation employed in the intensive care unit? An international utilization review. Am J Respir Crit Care Med 161:1450–1458

63. Esteban A, Anzueto A, Frutos F et al (2002) Characteristics and outcomes in adult patients receiving mechanical ventilation. A 28-day international study. JAMA 287:345–355

64. American Thoracic Society (1987) Standards for the diagnosis and care of patients with chronic obstructive pulmonary disease (COPD) and asthma. Am Rev Respir Dis 136:225–244

65. Fagon JY, Chastre J, Trouillet JL et al (1990) Characterization of distal bronchial micro-flora during acute exacerbation of chronic bronchitis. Am Rev Respir Dis 142:1004–1008

66. Monso E, Ruiz J, Rosell A et al (1995) Bacterial infection in chronic obstructive pulmonary disease. A study of stable and exacerbated outpatients using the protected specimen brush. Am J Respir Crit Care Med 152:1316–1320

67. Pela R, Marchesani F, Agostinelli C et al (1998) Airways microbial flora in COPD patients in stable clinical conditions and during exacerbations: a bronchoscopic investigation. Monaldi Arch Chest Dis 53:262–267

68. Soler N, Torres A, Ewig S et al (1998) Bronchial microbial patterns in severe exacerbations of chronic obstructive pulmonary disease (COPD) requiring mechanical ventilation. Am J Respir Crit Care Med 157:1498–1505

69. Cabello H, Torres A, Celis R et al (1997) Bacterial colonization of distal airways in healthy subjects and chronic lung disease: a bronchoscopic study. Eur Respir J 10:1137–1144

70. Soler N, Ewig S, Torres A, Filella X, Gonzalez J, Zaubet A (1999) Airway inflammation and bronchial microbial patterns in patients with stable chronic obstructive pulmonary disease. Eur Respir J 14:1015–1022

71. Martinez JA, Rodriguez E, Bastida T, Bugés J, Torres M (1994) Quantitative study of the bronchial bacterial flora in acute exacerbations of chronic bronchitis. Chest 105:976

72. Smith JA, Redman P, Woodhead MA (1999) Antibiotic use in patients admitted with acute exacerbation of chronic obstructive pulmonary disease. Eur Respir J 13:835–838

73. Russon RL, D'Aprile M (2001) Role of antimicrobial therapy in acute exacerbations of chronic obstructive pulmonary disease. Ann Pharmacother 35:576–581

74. Saint S, Bent S, Vittinghoff E, Grady D (1995) Antibiotics in chronic obstructive pulmonary disease exacerbations. A meta-analysis. JAMA 273:957–960

75. Nouira S, Marghli S, Belghith M, Besbes L, Elatrous S, Abroug F (2001) Once daily oral ofloxacin in chronic obstructive pulmonary disease exacerbation requiring mechanical ventilation: a randomised placebo-controlled trial. Lancet 358:2020–2025

76. Wade JJ, Rolando N, Hayllar K, Philpott-Howard J, Casewell MW, Williams R (1995) Bacterial and fungal infections after liver transplantation: an analysis of 283 patients. Hepatology 21:1328–1336

77. Bion JF, Badger I, Crosby HA et al (1994) Selective decontamination of the digestive

tract reduces gram-negative pulmonary colonization but not systemic endotoxemia in patients undergoing elective liver transplantation. Crit Care Med 22:40–49

78.   Arnow PM, Carandang GC, Zabner R, Irwin ME (1996) Randomized controlled trial of selective bowel decontamination for prevention of infections following liver transplantation. Clin Infect Dis 22:997–1003

79.   Zwaveling JH, Maring JK, Klompmaker IJ et al (2002) Selective decontamination of the digestive tract to prevent postoperative infection: a randomized placebo-controlled trial in liver transplant patients. Crit Care Med 30:1204–1209

80.   Hellinger WC, Yao JD, Alvarez S et al (2002) A randomized, prospective, double-blinded evaluation of selective bowel decontamination in liver transplantation. Transplantation 73:1904-1909

81.   Rayes N, Seehofer D, Hansen S et al (2002) Early enteral supply of lactobacillus and fiber versus selective bowel decontamination: a controlled trial in liver transplant recipients. Transplantation 74:123-127

82.   Smith SD, Jackson RJ, Hannakan CJ et al (1993) Selective decontamination in pediatric liver transplants. A randomized, prospective study. Transplantation 55:1306-1309

83.   Nathens AB, Marshall JC (1999) Selective decontamination of the digestive tract in surgical patients: a systematic review of the evidence. Arch Surg 134:170-176

84.   Safdar N, Said A, Lucey ML (2004) The role of selective digestive decontamination for reducing infection in patients undergoing liver transplantation: A systematic review and meta-analysis. Liver Transpl 10: 817-827

Chapter 20

Intensive Care Unit Patients Following Transplantation

A. Martínez-Pellús, M. Palomar

Introduction

Solid organ transplantation is a procedure that has become common in recent years and constitutes the only therapeutic option available to patients with advanced and irreversible organ failure. Although the surgical technique is standard, these patients may present complex postoperative conditions (including blood clotting disorders, hemodynamic instability, etc.) related to phenomena derived from ischemia/reperfusion of the implanted organ. These require close monitoring. This has led to an increase in the number of these patients admitted to intensive care units (ICU). In these cases, rejection and infection are the two sides of the scales whose needle is immunosuppression, which requires a strict balance in order to ensure a favorable prognosis in the long term. During the immediate postoperative period in the ICU, some of these patients require prolonged ventilatory assistance and diagnostic and therapeutic instrumentation that puts them at risk for infections, favored by the immunosuppression required to avoid rejection. At this early stage, infection is the most frequent problem [1] and the one with the greatest influence on prognosis [2], amply surpassing the surgical complications described above [3] as the cause of mortality. For this reason, exhaustive prevention protocols have been designed. The risk is so high that prophylaxis must be maintained for prolonged periods, until a situation of minimum immunosuppression is reached. If, in spite of everything, an infection occurs, it will pose a serious problem, which will lead to hospitalization and to the use of complex diagnostic techniques and broad-range antibiotic treatments. In this case, patients who have previously received a transplant may need to be admitted to the ICU, depending on the seriousness of an infection and the requirement for special hemodynamic or respiratory support measures.

Postoperative monitoring and the handling of a late infection that may endanger the life of the transplant recipient represent a serious challenge for intensivists when establishing diagnostic protocols that will reduce the empiricism of the initial treatment to the minimum, and therapeutic patterns based on updated information about the predominant pathogens in a particular service, as well as their sensitivity pattern.

The main objective in the case of a transplant recipient is, therefore, to prevent infection (or to treat it quickly and efficiently), while maintaining an adequate state of immunosuppression to avoid the rejection of the implanted organ. The difficulty lies in the combination of two factors: the continuous and intense exposure of the transplant recipient to a great variety of potentially infectious agents (viruses, fungi, community and hospital pathogens, endogenous and exogenous flora, etc.) and what is known as the "net state of immunosuppression" [4], influenced by the alterations produced by immunosuppressive medication on the inflammatory response and by invasive perioperative instrumentation. The environmental exposure of the transplant recipient occurs both in the community and in the hospital. Respiratory viruses, food infections, fungi, and mycobacteria (as primary infection or reactivation) [5] are unusual community pathogens among immunocompetent patients that can produce devastating symptoms in transplant recipients. The reactivation of latent infections, due to immunosuppression, is also frequent. There is relative consensus regarding immunosuppression regimens, and they always include steroids, together with cyclosporine, tacrolimus, and mycophenolate or azathioprine, in different combinations. The evidence shows that all of these drugs can be associated with infections caused by opportunistic pathogens such as *Pneumocystis carinii* and *Aspergillus* (steroids), the replication of latent viruses (cyclosporine and tacrolimus), and cytomegalovirus (CMV) and bacterial infections (mycophenolate). They are most effective after several months of treatment, and this allows us to establish a certain timetable for the appearance of specific infections, depending on the duration and level of immunosuppression (Fig. 1). Exceptions to this timetable suggest either excessive environmental exposure or excessive immunosuppression. This "expected" sequence of infections in a transplant recipient also serves to guide the preventive measures taken against them.

In the period immediately following the transplant (the 1st month), when the highest probability of hospitalization in the ICU occurs, the infections that usually appear are similar in their localization (surgical wounds, catheter-related bacteremias, urinary tract infections, etc.) to those suffered by immunocompetent patients that have undergone surgery. They are produced by typical nosocomial pathogens (*Staphylococcus aureus*, coagulase negative staphylococcus, aerobic gram-negative bacilli), to which fungi are progressively added. Prophylaxis should be aimed at these "expected" micro-organisms, bearing in mind that these patients may have been hospitalized previously or have had long preoperative stays, and thus may carry multi-resistant hospital flora

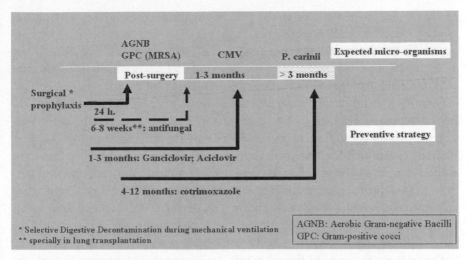

Fig. 1. Timing of infectious complications and sugested preventive measures after transplantation

including *Pseudomonas*, methicillin-resistant *S. aureus* (MRSA), and *Aspergillus*. Preventive measures based on selective decontamination of the digestive tract (SDD) using polymyxin, tobramycin, and amphotericin B, in throat and gut have proved useful in preventing infection in patients that have undergone orthotopic liver transplantation (OLT).

After the 1st month, CMV is the main pathogen involved, especially in previously seropositive patients, or in seronegative patients who have received an organ from a seropositive patient. Infection with CMV is one of the most important causes of morbidity and mortality in solid organ transplants, and it encourages the appearance of other opportunistic infections. It is also associated with the risk of chronic rejection, due to vascular injury of the immune type. For these reasons, this field is one of the most widely documented in terms of the effectiveness of prophylactic measures. In a controlled study, the administration of ganciclovir to cardiac transplant patients (5 mg/kg per 12 h from day 1 to day 14 after the transplant, followed by 6 mg/kg per 24 h 5 days a week until day 28) achieved a significant decrease in CMV disease (9% versus 46% in the placebo group) [6]. In another study with patients that received antilymphocyte antibodies to prevent rejection, low doses of ganciclovir (pre-emptive therapy) reduced the risk of developing disease from 65% to less than 20% [7]. A recent systematic review of this issue [8] concluded that prophylactic acyclovir or ganciclovir is associated with a significant reduction of CMV infection compared with placebo or untreated patients [relative risk 0.62, 95% confidence interval (CI) 0.53–0.73, $p<0.001$]. There were no proven effects on the incidence of rejection or on mortality rates. This infection, although potentially serious, rarely require hospitalization in the ICU. In the long term, patients with chronic rejection, who need severe and sustained immunosuppression, may develop opportunistic infections (*P. carinii*, *Listeria monocytogenes*, *Nocardia asteroides*, *Aspergillus*, *Cryptococcus neoformans*) [4], which require prolonged prophylaxis using trimethoprim-sulfamethoxazole and antifungal medication.

Any of the infections described above can pose a serious problem for immunodepressed patients, hence preventive measures must begin at the routine pre-transplant examination, in order to define the most appropriate prophylactic strategies. Together with a rigorous epidemiological survey (environmental exposure to "unusual" pathogens, childhood vaccinations, previous surgery, relapsing infections, antibiotic consumption, etc.), the recipient must undergo a tuberculin test and serology to detect CMV, Epstein-Barr virus, *Toxoplasma gondii*, and lues (both in the donor and in the recipient). If the tuberculin test is positive, the measures to be taken are controversial, due to the potential hepatotoxicity of the tuberculostatics and their interference with the pharmacokinetics of cyclosporine and tacrolimus. If clinical and X-ray examinations are performed every 6 months, no prophylaxis is needed. In patients with risk factors (earlier tuberculosis, family contact, malnutrition, radiological suspicions, etc.), a 9- to 12-month cycle of isoniazid may be suggested. If not already vaccinated, vaccination against tetanus, diphtheria, mumps, influenza, pneumococcus, *Haemophilus influenzae* type B, and hepatitis B must be given [9] before the transplant, since vaccination with live organisms after the transplant may trigger an infection or favor the rejection of the organ. If the recipient is seronegative for varicella zoster, he or she must be immunized before the transplant, although there are doubts regarding the effectiveness of the vaccine [10]. Other prophylactic measures are well established. Thus, the use of trimethoprim-sulfamethoxazole in a single daily dose for 4–12 months after the transplant has practically eliminated *P. carinii* and reduced infections by *L. monocytogenes*, *N. asteroides*, and *T. gondii* in high-risk patients, such as those undergoing a cardiac transplant [11]. Attempts must be made to eradicate infections that are present in the preoperative period (like spontaneous peritonitis in a cirrhotic patient). In the case of carriage of *Pseudomonas* or *Aspergillus* in patients with cystic fibrosis who are to receive a lung transplant it is necessary to start broad spectrum coverage before surgery. Some studies have shown a significant decrease in *Aspergillus* infections among patients with lung or cardiac transplants that were administered aerosolized amphotericin B as prophylaxis [12]. However, it is difficult to determine the best approach when the fungus is detected in a respiratory sample, since it may indicate simple colonization [13]. A recent study that attempted to establish the predictive value of the isolation of *Aspergillus* in diagnostic samples showed that the detection of more than two colonies in two or more sites correlated with invasive disease [14].

The most frequent infections among transplant recipients are bacteremias and lung infections, with clinical and radiological results that may be atypical, so that invasive diagnostic procedures and computed tomographic scans are frequently required. Acute processes with consolidation suggest a bacterial infection (including *Legionella*), while edema-like diffuse infiltrates are usually viral. Sub-acute or chronic processes are usually due to fungi, *Nocardia*, tuberculosis, *P. carinii*, and viruses. To treat infections in transplant recipients, the antibiotics with the least-toxic effects and the lowest interference with immunosuppressive drugs are β-lactams, fluoroquinolones, and fluconazole.

Bone Marrow Transplants

Although, technically speaking, bone marrow transplants are limited to the intravenous infusion of hematopoietic stem cells to try to recover bone marrow function [15], they require the previous administration of high doses of radiotherapy, chemotherapy, or both, until the patient's own cellular activity is completely abolished, thus keeping the remains of active cells in the recipient's immune system from destroying the implanted cells. This pretransplant treatment causes severe neutropenia, while injuring the integrity of the mucous barriers and favoring bacterial translocation from the digestive tract. Hence, besides complications due to immunological phenomena (graft-versus-host disease, hepatic vein occlusive disease, or rejection), the most frequent problem among these patients, and the one that leads to the highest mortality rates, is infection [16]. It is accepted that a bone marrow recipient needs at least 24 months to become immunocompetent, so long as immunosuppression is not maintained for any reason including graft-versus-host disease or rejection. This period may be longer for allogeneic transplants.

As in solid organ transplants, prophylaxis for a bone marrow recipient must begin with a rigorous pretransplant evaluation to rule out active or latent infections. The variety of infections that may affect these patients (bacteria, viruses, fungi) makes it difficult to plan preventive strategies. During the 1st month after the transplant, phagocyte deficit and the loss of the barrier effect provided by mucous membranes constitute the main risk, together with instrumentation (tubes, venous catheters, etc.). If steroids are not required for other reasons, this critical period may last 3-4 weeks, until achieving neutrophil levels >500 mm^3 and the recovery of phagocytosis. Infections during this period tend to develop without an evident primary focus, requiring immediate antibiotic treatment, which must therefore be empirical [17]. Bacterial and fungal infections are the most frequent. Although many are of intestinal origin [18], general prevention measures do not include parenteral and enteral SDD antibiotics in asymptomatic neutropenic patients, due to the lack of randomized controlled trials

(RCT). Some studies of fluoroquinolones as a prophylactic measure during neutropenia following a bone marrow transplant have shown a decrease in the incidence of bacteremia without any effect on mortality [19]. When considering a prophylaxis protocol, the antibiotics should be adjusted according to the patterns of sensitivity of the most common pathogens in a particular service or hospital, bearing in mind the relative prevalence of fluoroquinolone-resistant S. aureus, S. pneumoniae, and Escherichia coli, and the appearance of vancomycin-resistant enterococci and staphylococci. The extensive use of these antibiotics should therefore be avoided.

The routine use of fluconazole as a prophylactic measure has significantly reduced fungal infections (Candida), producing a favorable impact on mortality [20]. An increase in infections by species of Candida other than albicans (C. krusei, C. glabrata) has been related to this prophylaxis [21]. Surveillance cultures could be useful in deciding when to administer fluconazole to patients with prolonged neutropenia. A study of this type showed that patients with low counts of Candida in pharyngeal swabs (<10 CFU) and faecal cultures (<10^3 CFU/g of feces) did not present systemic candidiasis. However, 19% of those with one high count and 86% of those whose counts were both high had fungemia [22].

Unfortunately, no reports have been published on the use of SDD in this field. Its use would seem justified in the early phase of the transplant, in view of the expected pathogens (aerobic gram-negative bacilli and fungi). The low number of bone marrow recipients seen in the ICU (always due to established septic problems) and the fact that SDD is practically limited to the area of intensive care may help to explain this lack of studies.

Between 30 and 100 days after the transplant, the most serious and frequent infection is interstitial pneumonia, which develops as an acute respiratory distress syndrome and is usually due to CMV [23]. In two comparative studies of similar design, one with a placebo group [24] and another with an untreated group [25], of asymptomatic patients with positive CMV cultures of bronchoalveolar lavage fluid, urine, or blood, the administration of ganciclovir in doses of 5 mg/kg, twice a day (for 1–2 weeks), followed by one dose per day (5–7 days a week), up to 100 days after the transplant, resulted in a significant decrease in the incidence of CMV disease and mortality, with few side effects.

In the late phase (>100 days), prophylactic measures are recommended against encapsulated pathogens (S. pneumoniae, H. influenzae, and N. meningitidis) only in allogeneic transplant recipients with a chronic form of graft-versus-host disease requiring treatment with cyclosporine or tacrolimus. Vaccines (pneumococcus and H. influenzae) have a potential benefit, so they should be given 12 and 24 months after the transplant. Growth factors (GM-CSF and G-CSF) must be administered, especially when there is pronounced neutropenia.

Liver Transplant

Since it entered general use in the mid 1970s as the only therapeutic option for patients with massive liver tumors [26], OLT has become one of the most widespread surgical procedures in the treatment of diffuse hepatopathy of fatal evolution (cirrhosis, acute liver failure, deposit diseases, etc.). Advances in surgery and ample experience in immunosuppression have turned OLT into a procedure that, in selected patients, provides long-term survival rates of over 80%, with a practically normal quality of life. The trade-off is a life-long dependency on immunosuppressive treatment, with the inherent risk of suffering opportunistic infections, which are especially frequent in the post-surgical period. Their incidence is described as higher than in other diagnostic groups of ICU patients [1]. However, study of the 119 patients that received transplants in our hospital over the past 3 years shows a global incidence of infection of 14%. This is similar to that of other seriously ill post-surgical patients at our service, with an absolute predominance of bacterial infections (92%) over candidiasis (6%) and viral infections (2%) (Table 1). Infection risk factors in a univariate analysis were: acute liver failure as the reason for OLT, APACHE II on admission, the need to maintain mechanical ventilation for reasons other than anesthesia, early reintervention for any reason, and the duration of mechanical ventilation, urinary catheter, and central venous catheter (Table 2). In a regression analysis, the only factors related to infection were acute liver failure as the reason for the transplant [odds ratio (OR) 11.5, 95% CI 1.8–73] and early reintervention (OR 26.3, 95% CI 5.8–119). Stays in the ICU and mortality were strongly influenced by infection.

The complexity of the surgical technique and, especially, the fact that the transplanted organ must inevitably undergo more or less prolonged times of cold ischemia, with the consequent reperfusion after the implant, have led many centers to monitor the immediate postoperative condition of these patients in ICUs. This would explain why OLT is the only kind of transplant in which studies of SDD as a prophylactic measure against infection have been carried out. For over 10 years, different authors have reported the effectiveness of SDD in reducing infection by aerobic gram-negative bacilli and fungi in OLT. In an open study, Wiesner et al. [27] found a significant decrease in intestinal colonization by aerobic gram-negative bacilli and *Candida* after administering polymyxin, gentamicin, and nystatin orally for 3 days to patients waiting to receive an OLT. The prophylaxis was continued for 21 days, and no episode of infection by aerobic gram-negative bacilli was documented in the 1st month after the transplant. When SDD was discontinued, 90% of the patients were recolonized by aerobic gram-negative bacilli and 35% by *Candida* within a 5-day period. In a later study of 145 patients without a control group, the same

Table 1. Characteristics of infectious episodes

	Total
patients	21/119 (17.6%)
episodes	60

Type of infection		Microbiological isolates
VAP	3	*A.baumannii; S. pneumoniae; Aspergillus*
SB	1	*S. pneumoniae*
LRTI	4	*Pseudomonas aeruginosa* (3); MRSA
UTI	5	3 *E.coli* (3); *Serratia marcescens*; *E. faecalis*
SB	1	*Serratia marcescens*
PB	13	CNS (7); *E.coli* (2); *E. faecalis*; Alpha streptococci; *Bacteroides fragilis*; *S.pneumoniae*
CVC	18	CNS (9); *A.baumannii* (2); *E.faecalis* (2); AGNB (2); MRSA; *Serratia marcescens*; *Candida albicans*
SB	7	CNS (3); MRSA; *E. faecalis*; *Serratia marcescens*; *A. baumannii*
Peritonitis	3	*E. faecalis*; *C. albicans* + *E. faecalis*; *E.coli*
SB	1	*E. faecalis*
Surgical wound	2	Alpha streptococci; *E.coli*
Other	2	CMV; *A. baumannii*

VAP: ventilator associated pneumonia; LRTI: lower respiratory tract infecion; UTI: urinary tract infection; CVC: central venous catheter; PB: primary bacteremia; SB: secondary bacteremia; CNS: coagulase negative staphylococci; MRSA: methicilin resistant *S. aureus*; CMV: Cytomegalovirus; AGNB: aerobic Gram negative bacilli

authors [28] recorded only five infections with aerobic gram-negative bacilli and one case of systemic candidiasis. This study used pharyngeal application of the same antibiotics during mechanical ventilation and systemic antibiotics for the first 2 days after surgery. Six RCTs evaluated the effect of SDD. In a pediatric population, Smith et al. [29] found a decrease in the incidence of infection from 50% to 11% ($p<0.001$) when they compared patients receiving standard prophylaxis with systemic antibiotics with others who also received SDD during the postoperative period. In another study, Bion et al. [30] described a significant decrease in lung infections following SDD. There was no difference in endotoxemia. This deserves comment, since in this study SDD began in the postoperative period, and it has been proven that the eradication of aerobic gram-negative bacilli as a source of endotoxin requires a minimum of 3 days of SDD [31, 32]. Arnow et al. reported no statistically significant benefit of SDD

Table 2. Risk factors for infection in 119 liver transplant patients

| | Infection | | |
	Yes (%)	no (%)	p
n	21 (17.6)	98 (82.4)	
Age	55+-10	50+-11	0.093
M/F	12/9	71/27	0.23
Cirrhosis	16 (76)	93 (95)	0.015
Acute liver failure	5 (24)	5 (5)	0.01
Hepatocarcinoma	2 (9)	8 (8)	1
Alcohol abuse	6 (28.5)	38 (38.7)	0.46
Unscheduled surgery	9 (43)	5 (5)	0.0001
APACHE II (admission)	16+-6	11+-5	0.007
Mechanical ventilation	12 (57)	15 (15)	0.0001
Early rejection	8 (38)	20 (20)	0.095
ICU stay	31+-16	5.3+-3.6	0.001
Mortality	8 (38)	5 (5)	0.0001

[33]. A subgroup analysis found that patients receiving SDD for 3 or more days before transplantation had a lower incidence of overall infection and of infection at intra-abdominal, surgical or respiratory sites and in the blood stream caused by aerobic gram- negative bacilli (0 versus 21%, $p<0,05$). In a fourth RCT, Hellinger found that there was no statistically significant difference between the two groups with regard to infection and mortality [34]. Again, of the bacterial pathogens causing infection, one (11%) was an aerobic gram-negative bacillus in the SDD group and four (33%) were aerobic gram-negative bacilli in the test group. The Dutch RCT of Zwaveling reports significantly less infections due to aerobic gram-negative bacilli and yeasts in patients receiving SDD [35]. In the sixth German RCT, there were two infections due to aerobic gram-negative bacilli in both the tests and control group [36]. There are two meta-analysis of 3 and 4 RCTs respectively, showing a beneficial effect of SDD on infections due to aerobic gram-negative bacilli and yeasts [37, 38]. However, the effect of SDD on overall infections was limited due to a higher rate of minor infections caused by enterococci and coagulase-negative staphylococci in the patients receiving SDD [39].

Fungal infection is one of the most frequent infections among patients who have undergone OLT, with incidences of up to 40% in some series, most due to

Candida species. Functional disruption of the intestine and translocation phenomena would be involved in this process [18]. The most important studies of prophylaxis in this field are limited to the use of systemic antifungals in comparative studies with placebo. Two studies of similar design by Tollerman et al. [41, 42] (1 mg/kg per day of ambisone versus placebo) provide contradictory results. The first [40] found no significant differences in fungal infections, while the second [41] showed a significant reduction (0% versus 13%, $p<0.001$). Mortality within a 30-day period was similar in both groups. In another double-blind study comparing fluconazole (400 mg/day for 10 weeks) with placebo in 212 transplant recipients, Winston et al. [42] found a significant decrease in fungal infections (43% versus 9%, $p<0.001$), both in superficial mycoses (28% versus 4%, $p<0.001$) and in invasive mycoses (23% versus 6%, $p<0.001$). Two studies in which SDD, including nystatin, was used [43, 44] showed an incidence of fungal infections of only 11%, with a very low rate of *Candida* infection, which would suggest that SDD has a protective effect, although none of these studies had a control group. The additional advantage of SDD using polymyxin/tobramycin/amphotericin B, would be the simultaneous prevention of bacterial infections, pneumonia and bacteremia, during the postoperative period in the ICU. SDD regimens should be adapted to the most common pathogens in each service, bearing in mind their resistance patterns (MRSA, *Pseudomonas*, multiresistant aerobic gram-negative bacilli). As in the other transplants ganciclovir is the drug with the best cost-effectiveness ratio for the prevention of CMV infection in OLT.

Surgical prophylaxis, in the absence of data about previous colonization or infection by problem pathogens, is well standardized. A 24-h cover with second-generation cephalosporines might be enough to prevent infection problems related to the surgery.

An additional factor that may lead to postoperative infections among OLT patients is a prolonged stay in an area of high environmental exposure to potential pathogens and multiple instrumentation, like the ICU. A recent study of factors that influence the short-term prognosis of a liver transplant concludes that, given a similar age of recipient and donor, pretransplant functional stage, time of cold ischemia, and intraoperative bleeding, those patients who stayed in the ICU > 3 days showed a higher mortality rate (19.5% versus 2%, $p<0.001$) and a greater number of infectious episodes (41.5% versus 11%, $p<0.001$) than those who were there for less than 3 days [45]. This study, despite being retrospective, is interesting because it demonstrates the risk of a prolonged hospitalization in the ICU, and it underlines the importance of early extubation, supported by vigorous physiotherapy measures (in the pre- and postoperative periods) and the quick removal of venous lines and drainages. In another observational study, mortality rates within 30 days among liver transplant recipients with fever who were admitted to the ICU were significantly higher (34% versus 5%) than those of similar patients treated on a hospital ward [46]. Finally, such simple measures as early and continuous posture changes, in order to avoid atelectasis and other problems related to prolonged immobilization, have also proven successful in the prevention of respiratory tract infections in the post-transplant period [47].

Conclusion

Patients who require a solid organ transplant or a bone marrow transplant are at high risk of infection, both in the short and in the long term, depending on the severity of immunosuppression before surgery. Measures to minimize this problem have gradually increased and, generally have proven successful. The main objective to be considered in a global infection prevention plan is to achieve the shortest possible postoperative stay in the ICU, to establish quick weaning programs, the removal of tubes and drainages, and intensive physiotherapy. The observation that the pathogens involved at this early stage (1st month) are similar to those found in other post-surgical patients admitted to the ICU could justify the use of SDD as prophylaxis. This might be especially important while the patient is undergoing invasive instrumentation (mechanical ventilation, central catheters) or until a situation of minimal immunosuppression is reached (monotherapy with cyclosporine). The growing incidence of fungal infection (mainly *Candida*), promoted in these cases by the use of steroids in immunosuppression protocols, would support this indication. For liver transplants, there are studies that show a protective effect, both of the systemic antifungals (fluconazole) and of the enteral non-absorbable antifungals as part of SDD. The risk of selection of *Candida* species other than *albicans* that are resistant to azole antifungals, observed with the use of fluconazole, does not seem very likely with the use of enteral amphotericin B. Other measures, like the systematic use of trimethoprim-sulfamethoxazole, have practically eliminated *P. carinii* as a pathogen among these patients. Ganciclovir has proven to be a valid strategy to prevent CMV infection in transplant recipients. Criticism that prophylactic measures do not influence mortality rates should not deprive these patients of the potential benefit of avoiding infection. A study designed to solve this controversy once and for all would need a complex design and a huge sample size. This makes it unlikely that it will ever be performed.

In the medium or long term, the problem of prevention depends on the patient's willingness to maintain a prophylactic regimen for long periods, together with the risk of toxicity, interaction with immunosuppression, and selection of resistant pathogens. Educational programs and the greater participation of the patients themselves in the decision making would be ideal to achieve this goal.

References

1. Wade JJ, Rolando N, Hayllar K et al (1995) Bacterial and fungal infections after liver transplantation: an analysis of 284 patients. Hepatology 21:1328–1336
2. Paya CV, Hermans PE, Washington JA et al (1989) Incidence, distribution and outcome of episodes of infection in 100 orthotopic liver transplantations. Mayo Clin Proc 64:555–564
3. Scharschmidt BF (1984) Human liver transplantation: analysis of data on 540 patients from four centers. Hepatology 4:958–1018
4. Rubin RH (1994) Infection in the organ transplant recipient. In: Rubin RH, Young LS (eds) Clinical approach to infection in the compromised host, 3rd edn. Plenum, New York, pp 629–705
5. Hadley S, Karchmer AW (1995) Fungal infections in solid organ transplant recipients. Infect Dis Clin North Am 9:1045–1074
6. Merigan TC, Renlund DG, Keay S et al (1992) A controlled trial of ganciclovir to prevent cytomegalovirus disease after heart transplantation. N Eng J Med 326:1182–1186
7. Hibberd PL, Tolkoff-Rubin NE, Conti D et al (1995) Preemptive ganciclovir therapy to prevent cytomegalovirus disease in cytomegalovirus antibody-positive renal transplant recipient: a randomized controlled trial. Ann Intern Med 123:18–26
8. Couchoud C (2001) Cytomegalovirus prophylaxis with antiviral agents for solid organ transplantation. Cochrane Database of Systematic Reviews. Issue 4
9. Hibberd PL, Rubin RH (1990) Approach to immunization in the immunosuppressed host. Infect Dis Clin North Am 4:23–27
10. White CJ (1997) Varicella-Zoster virus vaccine. Clin Infect Dis 24:753
11. Orr KE, Gould FK, Short G et al (1994) Outcome of *Toxoplasma gondii* mismatches in heart transplant recipients over a period of 8 years. J Infect 29:249–253
12. Reichenspurner H, Gamberg P, Nitschke M et al (1997) Significant reduction in the number of fungal infections after lung, heart-lung, and heart transplantation using aerosolized amphotericin B prophylaxis. Transplant Proc 29:627–628
13. Westney GE, Kesten S, De Hoyos A et al (1996) *Aspergillus* infection in single and double lung transplant recipients. Transplantation 61:915–919
14. Brown RS, Lake JR, Katzman BA et al (1996) Incidence and significance of *Aspergillus* cultures following liver and kidney transplantation. Transplantation 61:666–669
15. Armitage JO (1994) Bone marrow transplantation. N Engl J Med 330:827–838
16. Kernan NA, Bartsch G, Ash RC et al (1993) Analysis of 462 transplantations from unrelated donors facilitated by the National Marrow Donor Program. N Engl J Med 328:593
17. Hughes WT, Armstrong D, Bodey GP et al (1997) 1997 Guidelines for the use of antimicrobial agents in neutropenic patients with unexplained fever. Clin Infect Dis 25:551
18. Cole GT, Halawa AA, Anaissie EJ (1996) The role of the gastrointestinal tract in the hematogenous candidiasis: from the laboratory to bedside. Clin Infect Dis 22 [Suppl 2]:S73–S88
19. Cruciani M, Rampazzo R, Malena M et al (1996) Prophylaxis with fluoroquinolones for bacterial infection in neutropenic patients: a meta-analysis. Clin Infect Dis 23:795
20. Marr KA, Siedel K, Slavin MA et al (2000) Prolonged fluconazole prophylaxis is associated with persistent protection against candidiasis-related death in allogenic marrow transplant recipients: long-term follow-up of a randomized, placebo-controlled trial. Blood 96:2055
21. Abi-Said D, Anaissie E, Uzun O et al (1997) The epidemiology of hematogenous candidiasis caused by different *Candida* species. Clin Infect Dis 24:1122

22. Guiot HFL, Fibbe WE, Van't Wout JW (1996) Prevention of invasive candidiasis by flu-conazol in patients with malignant hematological disorders and a high grade of can-dida colonisation (abstract). Abstracts of the 36th Interscience Conference on Antimicrobial Agentes and Chemotherapy. New Orleans, LM33

23. Wingard JR, Mellits ED, Sostrin MB et al (1988) Interstitial pneumonitis after alloge-nic bone marrow transplantation: nine-year experience at a single institution. Medicine (Baltimore) 67:175–186

24. Goodrich JM, Mori M, Gleaves CA et al (1991) Early treatment with gancyclovir to prevent cytomegalovirus disease after allogenic bone marrow transplantation. N Engl J Med 325:1601–1607

25. Schmidt GM, Horak DA, Niland JC et al (1991) A randomized, controlled trial of prophylactic ganciclovir for cytomegalovirus pulmonary infections in recipients of allogenic bone marrow transplants; The City of Hope-Standford-Syntex CMV Study Group. N Engl J Med 324:1005–1011

26. Maddrey WC, van Thiel DH (1988) Liver transplantation: an overview. Hepatology 8:948–959

27. Wiesner RH, Hermans PE, Rakela J et al (1988) Selective bowel decontamination to decrease gram-negative aerobic bacterial and *Candida* colonization and prevent infec-tion after orthotopic liver transplantation. Transplantation 45:570–574

28. Wiesner RH (1990) The incidence of gram-negative bacterial and fungal infection in liver transplant patients treated with selective decontamination. Infection 18 [Suppl 1]:S19–S21

29. Smith SD, Jackson RJ, Hannakan CJ et al (1993) Selective decontamination in pediatric liver transplants. A randomized prospective study. Transplantation 55:1306–1309

30. Bion JF, Badger I, Crosby HA et al (1994) Selective decontamination of the digestive tract reduces gram-negative pulmonary colonization but not systemic endotoxemia in patients undergoing elective liver transplantation. Crit Care Med 22:40–49

31. van Saene JJM, Stoutenbeek CP, van Saene HKF et al (1996) Reduction of the intesti-nal endotoxin pool by three different SDD regimens in human volunteers. J Endotoxin Res 3:337–343

32. Oudemans-van Straaten HM, van Saene HKF, Zandstra DF (2003) Selective deconta-mination of the digestive tract: use of the correct antibiotics is crucial. Crit Care Med 31:334-335

33. Arnow PM, Carandang GC, Zabner R, Irwin ME (1996) Randomized controlled trial of selective bowel decontamination for prevention of infections following liver tran-splantation. Clin Infect Dis 22:997-1003

34. Hellinger WC, Yao JD, Alvarez S et al (2002) A randomized, prospective, double-blin-ded evaluation of selective bowel decontamination in liver transplantation. Transplantation 73:1904-1909

35. Zwaveling JH, Maring JK, Klompmaker IJ et al (2002) Selective decontamination of the digestive tract to prevent postoperative infection: a randomized placebo-controlled trial in liver transplant patients. Crit Care Med 30:1204-1209

36. Rayes N, Seehofer D, Hansen S et al (2002) Early enteral supply of lactobacillus and fiber versus selective bowel decontamination: a controlled trial in liver transplant reci-pients. Transplantation 74:123-127

37. Nathens AB, Marshall JC (1999) Selective decontamination of the digestive tract in surgical patients: a systematic review of the evidence. Arch Surg 134:170–176

38. Safdar N, Said A, Lucey MR (2004) The role of selective digestive decontamination for reducing infection in patients undergoing liver transplantation: a systematic review and meta-analysis. Liver Transpl 10:817-827

39. van Saene HKF, Zandstra DF (2004) Selective decontamination of the digestive tract: rationale behind evidence-based use in liver transplantation. Liver Transpl 10:828-833

40. Tollerman J, Ringden O (1993) Double-blind randomized trials with AmBisome as prophylaxis in bone marrow and liver transplant patients. Transplantation 12 [Suppl 4]:S151-S152

41. Tollerman J, Hockerstedt K, Erickzon BG et al (1995) Liposomal amphotericin B prevents invasive fungal infections in liver transplant recipients. A randomized, placebo-controlled study. Transplantation 59:45-50

42. Winston DJ, Pakrasi A, Busuttil RW (1999) Prophylactic fluconazole in liver transplant recipients. A randomized, double-blind, placebo-controlled trial. Ann Intern Med 131:729-737

43. Patel R, Portela D, Bradley AD et al (1996) Risk factors of invasive *Candida* and non-*Candida* infections after liver transplantation. Transplantation 62:926-934

44. Singh N, Gayowsky T, Wagener MM et al (1997) Invasive fungal infections in liver transplant recipients receiving tacrolimus as primary immunosuppressive agent. Clin Infect Dis 24:179-184

45. Mor E, Cohen J, Erez E et al (2001) Short intensive care unit stay reduces septic complications and improves outcome after liver transplantation. Transplant Proc 33:2939-2940

46. Singh N, Chang FY, Gayowski T et al (1999) Fever in liver transplant recipient in the intensive care unit. Clin Transplant 13:504-511

47. Whiteman K, Nachtmann L, Kramer D et al (1995) Effects of continuous lateral rotation therapy on pulmonary complications in liver transplant patients. Am J Crit Care 4:133-139

Chapter 21

Clinical Virology in NICU, PICU and Adult ICU

C.Y.W. Tong, S. Schelenz

Introduction

The role of viruses in causing nosocomial infections has not been well recognized until recently. In healthy individuals, most viral infections are self-limiting. They are therefore not perceived as important in terms of morbidity and mortality. Traditionally, viral infections were difficult to diagnose due to the lack of rapid and specific diagnostic tests. Even when disease due to a specific virus was evident, no specific treatment or intervention was available. This led to difficulties in both case ascertainment and outbreak control.

This perception of viral infection is now changing. Advances in medicine have led to a large number of immunocompromised patients who are susceptible to infection including severe viral infections. Many such patients are cared for in intensive care units (ICU) and in turn become an infectious hazard for other vulnerable patients. Health care workers can acquire common viral infections from the community and spread them to susceptible patients in the ICU. Patients in neonatal ICU (NICU) and pediatric ICU (PICU) are most susceptible, because of the lack of prior immunity against many viruses circulating in the community. With the availability of rapid antigen detection methods and other molecular diagnostic tests, many viral infections can now be diagnosed rapidly. Rapid and accurate typing of viral strains using DNA techniques can help to identify the source of outbreaks. Also, specific post-exposure prophylaxis and treatment are now available for many important nosocomial viral infections.

In this chapter, we will discuss some of the important viruses that are associated with nosocomial infections in the ICU. These viruses are categorized according to their most common mode of transmission (Table 1). Due to the special concern of rabies and Creutzfeldt-Jakob disease in ICU, a section on rare nervous system infection is included. General measures to prevent cross-infection for each virus are summarized in Table 2.

Table 1. Mode of transmission of viral infections in intensive care units (ICU)

	Respiratory route	Fecal-oral route	Blood and body fluid	Direct contact/ fomites
Respiratory syncytial virus	+++	-	-	++
Parainfluenza viruses	+++	-	-	++
Influenza viruses	+++	-	-	++
Adenovirus	+++	++	-	+++
Varicella-zoster virus (Chickenpox)	+++	-	-	++
Rotavirus	+	+++	-	++
Norovirus	++	+++	-	++
Enterovirus	-	+++	-	++
Hepatitis A virus	-	+++	+/-	++
Hepatitis B virus	-	-	+++	-
Hepatitis C virus	-	-	++	-
Human immunodeficiency virus	-	-	++	-
Hemorrhagic fever viruses	+/-	-	++++	+++
Cytomegalovirus	-	-	+	++
Herpes simplex virus	-	-	-	++
Varicella-zoster virus (zoster)	-	-	-	++
Rabies	-	-	-	+/-
Transmissible spongiform encephalopathies (TSE)	-	-	+/-	++

- unlikely
+/- possible
+ common
(the number of + is an arbitrary indicator of transmissibility)

Viruses Transmitted by the Respiratory Route

Respiratory Syncytial Virus (RSV)

Respiratory syncytial virus (RSV) belongs to the *Paramyxoviridae* family, genus *Pneumovirus* and is a major cause of lower respiratory tract infections in young children and infants. Other vulnerable patients are the immunocompromised, the elderly and those with chronic pulmonary disease. Severely infected young infants (< 1 year) often present with bronchiolitis, pseudo-croup or pneumonia. They are the most common group that would require intensive care. In the United States, bronchiolitis due to RSV results in an average of 31 hospital admissions per 1000 children aged less than 1 year per annum [1].

Table 2. Infection control measures for the prevention of viral infections

Virus	Isolation or cohorting*	Hand washing	Apron /gown+	Gloves	Masks /goggles	Incubation	Duration of infectivity
Respiratory syncytial virus (RSV) [16]	✔ II	✔ IA	✔ IB	✔ IA		2–8 days	48 h before symptoms and 7 days from onset; longer in immunocompromised (up to 30 days)
Parainfluenza viruses	✔	✔	✔	✔		2–4 days	As long as symptoms last
Influenza viruses [16]	✔ (Negative pressure) IB (II)	✔	✔	✔	✔ IB	1–4 days	Prodromal phase and 3 days after onset
Adenovirus	✔	✔	✔	✔		5–10 days	As long as symptoms last
Varicella-zoster virus (Chickenpox) [23]	✔ (Negative pressure) (IB)	✔	✔			10–21 days	2 days before first vesicle until all lesions are crusted
Rotavirus	✔	✔	✔	✔		2–3 days	Up to 4-7 days after onset of illness
Norovirus [28]	✔ IB	✔ IA	✔ IB	✔ IB		15–48 h	Up to 48 h after becoming symptom free
Enterovirus		✔	✔	✔		2–25 days	7 –14 days from onset of illness; asymptomatic shedding common

cont. →

Table 2 *cont.*

Virus	Isolation or cohorting*	Hand washing	Apron /gown+	Gloves	Masks /goggles	Incubation	Duration of infectivity
Hepatitis A virus	✓	✓	✓	✓		2–6 weeks	Infectious 1 week before onset of illness, infectivity declines rapidly after onset of illness
Hepatitis B virus		✓		✓		2–3 months	As long as patient is viremic
Hepatitis C virus		✓		✓		2–3 months	As long as patient is viremic
Human Immuno-deficiency virus (HIV)		✓		✓		3–6 weeks from primary infection	Indefinitely although viral load may be controlled by antiretroviral therapy
Viral hemorrhagic fever viruses	✓ (High security isolation)	✓	✓	✓	✓	3–21 days	High infectivity during illness
Cytomegalovirus (CMV)		✓	✓ (con-genital CMV)	✓ (con-genital CMV)		3–6 weeks from primary infection	Congenital infection – from birth. Asymptomatic shedding common
Herpes simplex virus (HSV)		✓		✓		Often due to reactivation	Until lesions have healed
Varicella-zoster virus (shingles)	✓	✓	✓	✓		Often due to reactivation	Until vesicles crusted over

cont. →

Table 2 *cont.*

Virus	Isolation or cohorting*	Hand washing	Apron /gown+	Gloves	Masks /goggles	Incubation	Duration of infectivity
Rabies virus	✓	✓	✓	✓	✓	2–8 weeks or longer	Duration of illness
Transmissible spongiform encephalopathy		✓				Indeterminate (congenital CMV)	Duration of illness

* In standard isolation, patients should be in single room or cohorted

+Gowns and gloves should be for single use

√ indicates that the practice is recommended. Categorization of recommendations (definitions based on Ref [16]) are listed with reference where available - **IA:** Strongly recommended for all hospitals and strongly supported by well-designed experimental or epidemiological studies; **IB:** Strongly recommended for all hospitals and viewed as effective by experts in the field. These recommendations are based on strong rationale and suggestive evidence, even though definitive scientific studies may not have been performed; **II:** Suggested for implementation in many hospitals. These recommendations may be supported by suggestive clinical or epidemiological studies, a strong theoretical rationale, or definitive studies applicable to some but not all hospitals

The incidence of RSV is seasonal in temperate climates and hospital admissions usually peak during winter months. There have been several reports of nosocomial transmission of RSV in ICU, with the majority of outbreaks occurring in PICU [2]. However, viral pneumonias, including RSV, should also be suspected in adult ICU patients not responding to antibiotics [3, 4].

RSV can be transmitted directly by large droplets during close contact with infected individuals or indirectly by contaminated hands, fomites, and environmental surfaces [5]. Staff may also acquire infection from patients and transmit the virus to other patients.

RSV binds to bronchoepithelial cells via its outer glycoprotein G and fuses with the cell glycoprotein forming the typical syncytial giant cells. It then replicates in the epithelial cells causing edema, inflammation, necrosis and small airway obstruction. The infection is limited to the respiratory tract and respiratory secretions are thought to be the only body fluid containing infectious virus.

The incubation period is 2-8 days and virus shedding can be detected a few days prior to the onset of symptoms, and continues for a further 7-10 days. Immunocompromised patients are less able to control viral replication and therefore excrete the virus for longer.

The gold standard diagnosis of RSV is tissue culture isolation of the virus from nasopharyngeal aspirate or bronchoalveolar lavage fluid. This takes at least 7–10 days and is therefore not suitable for infection control purposes. In contrast, antigen detection systems using direct or indirect immunofluorescence or enzyme immunoassays (EIA) can provide same-day results with good sensitivity and specificity. These are frequently used to help the grouping of infected infants on PICU. Detection of RSV RNA using reverse transcriptase-polymerase chain reaction (RT-PCR) could be more sensitive. However, this remains a research tool at present as it is a more time-consuming procedure and is generally not available for routine use.

As RSV has a high rate of nosocomial transmission, it is important to identify infected patients and to apply effective infection control procedures (Table 2). Recent studies have demonstrated that the combination of cohort nursing and the wearing of gloves and gowns significantly reduce the cross-infection rate of RSV [6]. Hand washing with liquid soap or aqueous antiseptic solution (Table 3) should be reinforced, as it is the single most important procedure in the prevention of nosocomial infections. One study demonstrated that the use of goggles covering the eyes or nose was associated with a decrease in pediatric nosocomial RSV infections [7]. This may be due to a reduction of transmission of RSV in health care staff [8]. However, the practicality of routinely wearing masks and goggles presents a problem and is generally not recommended.

The treatment of RSV infection is mainly supportive, including oxygen, ventilation and bronchodilatory drugs. The guanosine analogue anti-viral agent ribavirin has been used in severe cases when given by aerosol. However, a recent

Table 3. Activity of hand-hygiene antiseptic agents against viruses [25] (*QAC* quaternary ammonium compounds)

Agent	Activity	Speed of action
Alcohols	Excellent	Fast
Chlorhexidine	Excellent	Intermediate
Iodine compounds	Excellent	Intermediate
Iodophores	Good	Intermediate
Phenol derivatives	Fair	Intermediate
Triclosan	Excellent	Intermediate
QAC	Fair	Slow

meta-analysis of infants treated with aerosol ribavirin showed no evidence of a significant benefit [9]. One study has shown that severely immunocompromised adults may benefit from a combination of ribavirin and intravenous γ-globulin [10]. Pregnant staff or visitors should avoid the patient during the period the drug is aerosolized since ribavirin is potentially teratogenic.

At present there is no safe and effective vaccine to prevent RSV infection. Passive immunization using RSV immune globulin or humanized monoclonal antibodies (palivizumab) has been used to prevent serious RSV disease in high-risk patients (e.g., premature babies or those with cardiac anomalies) or to limit further nosocomial spread [11].

Recently, a new paramyxovirus known as the Human metapneumovirus (HMPV) was identified which shares the same spectrum of clinical illness as RSV. The significance of this new virus and its control is unclear at present, but it is likely that general infection control measures against RSV would be effective against HMPV.

Parainfluenza Viruses

Parainfluenza viruses belong to the family of *Paramyxoviridae*. There are four human parainfluenza types (type 1 and 3, genus *Paramyxovirus* and type 2 and 4, genus *Rubulavirus*). Infections with parainfluenza type 1 and 2 are seasonal with a peak in autumn affecting mainly children between six months and six years of age. Clinically they often present with croup or a febrile upper respiratory illness. In contrast, parainfluenza type 3 is endemic throughout the year and infects mostly young infants in the first 6 months up to two years of age, often with bronchiolitis and pneumonia. In immunocompromised adults such as stem cell transplant recipients, parainfluenza type 3 is associated with a high mortality. Such patients often present with severe pneumonia and many would require admission to ICU.

The incubation time of parainfluenza is 2-8 days and patients are infectious for 1-4 days prior to the onset of symptoms and may last as long as 14 days. The route of transmission is thought to be via droplets or indirect person-to-person contact. The diagnosis can be confirmed by rapid antigen detection using immunofluorescence of nasopharyngeal aspirates or bronchoalveolar lavage fluid.

Parainfluenza infections are usually self-limiting and the management is mainly supportive care. Intravenous, oral or aerosol ribavirin has been used in severely immunocompromised adults infected with parainfluenza type 3 virus. There is at present little evidence that the use of ribavirin alters patient outcome.

Nosocomial transmission is often due to parainfluenza virus type 3 and has been documented in NICU [12]. Infection control precautions are the same as for RSV (Table 2). Hand washing and change of gowns are the most effective measures to control nosocomial spread [13].

Influenza Viruses

Influenza viruses belong to the family of *Orthomyxoviridae* and are classified into type A, B and C. Clinically influenza infection is characterised by abrupt onset of fever, sore throat, myalgia, cough, headache and malaise. Young children may develop croup, pneumonia or middle ear infection. More severe disease and high mortality can be seen in the elderly, immunocompromised, those with pre-existing chronic heart or lung disease. This is often due to secondary bacterial infection with *Staphylococcus aureus*, *Streptococcus pneumoniae* or *Haemophilus influenzae*.

Influenza has a short incubation time of 1-4 days. The virus is transmitted via droplets and patients are infectious during the prodromal phase up to three days after onset of symptoms. Rapid diagnosis can be made by detection of antigen in respiratory secretions using immunofluorescence or EIA.

The risk of nosocomial transmission in hospitals is well documented and there have been reports of outbreaks in NICU [14, 15]. Admission of adult patients with influenza to ICU is often the result of severe secondary bacterial infection, by which time influenza virus is no longer shed from upper respiratory secretions.

Influenza A but not type B can be treated with the M2 protein inhibitors amantadine or rimantadine that lessens the severity of the illness if started early. Recently, a new class of neuraminidase inhibitors (zanamivir and oseltamivir), active against both influenza A and B has been introduced. Infection control measures are similar to those for RSV (Table 2). The United States Centers for Disease Control (CDC) guidelines for the prevention of nosocomial pneumonia recommend that infected patients should be placed into a single room or cohorted with re-inforcement of hand washing and the wearing of gloves and gowns [16]. The primary focus of efforts to prevent and control nosocomial influenza is the vaccination of high-risk patients and front line health care workers, including ICU staff, before the influenza season begins. The prophylactic use of amantadine or neuraminidase inhibitors may also help to reduce transmission during an outbreak. However, vaccination remains the most efficient and cost-effective means of disease control.

Adenovirus

Adenovirus comprises of numerous serotypes and belongs to the family of *Adenoviridae*, genus *Mastadenovirus*. The virus multiplies in the pharynx, conjunctiva or small intestine and has a short incubation time (5-8 days). Clinically the infection is localized and presents often with pharyngitis and conjunctivitis or gastroenteritis depending on the serotype. However, in young infants and immunocompromised patients adenovirus can cause severe pneumonia. The diagnosis can be confirmed by detection of viral antigen using immunofluorescence or EIA or the detection of viral DNA using PCR.

In respiratory infections, the virus spreads via droplets or through contaminated hands or fomites. Nosocomial adenovirus infections have been reported and can be a particular problem in neonatal units [17]. It is important to adhere to strict infection control procedures to prevent nosocomial spread (Table 2). Adenovirus is susceptible to the antiviral agent cidofovir *in vitro*. There are isolated case reports of the successful use of cidofovir in severe adenovirus infection [18].

Varicella Zoster Virus - Chickenpox

Primary varicella zoster virus (VZV) infection causes chickenpox. This is a common self-limiting childhood infection characterized by a mild fever and a generalised vesicular rash. However, adults, smokers or the immunocompromised may develop severe disease including pneumonia, encephalitis or hemorrhagic fulminating varicella and require ICU admission. Chickenpox is highly infectious and can be transmitted via inhalation of respiratory secretions or by direct contact of vesicular lesions. Patients are likely to be infectious 48 hours before the appearance of the rash until the last lesion has crusted over. A rapid diagnosis of chickenpox can be made by electron microscopy or immunofluorescence of scrapings from the vesicle base. A person who has had chickenpox in the past does not develop the infection again, but the latent virus may reactivate as zoster. In the absence of a clear history of previous chickenpox, prior exposure can be determined by the presence of serum VZV IgG antibodies.

The immediate management of exposed susceptible patients is important (Fig. 1). Airborne nosocomial outbreaks of chickenpox in hospitals have been reported [19]. Although it is rare for chickenpox cases to be admitted to adult

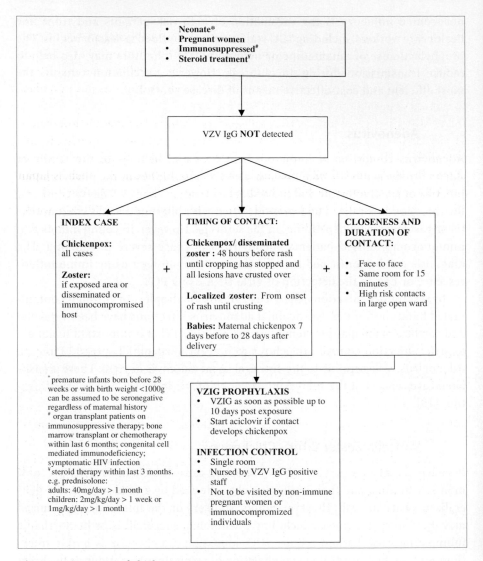

Fig.1. Management of chickenpox or zoster exposure

or pediatric ICU, there may be patients, staff or visitors attending the unit incubating the virus putting non-immune patients at risk. Several outbreaks of chickenpox in NICU due to such circumstances have been reported [20-22]. It is therefore important to apply strict infection control procedures in order to reduce transmission of this highly contagious virus (Table 2). Infected patients need to be isolated immediately, preferably in rooms with negative pressure [23] and exposed patients and staff investigated for immune status (Fig. 1). Susceptible staff should be excluded from contact with high-risk patients for 8-21 days postexposure.

Neonates born to mothers who develop chickenpox within 7 days of delivery are highly susceptible due to the lack of maternal antibodies and can develop severe VZV infection. In such cases, varicella-zoster immune globulin (VZIG) prophylaxis of the neonate is recommended to reduce the severity of infection. The baby should be isolated and the above precautions put into place to minimize nosocomial transmission.

Most cases of childhood chickenpox do not require treatment. However, in severe cases (e.g. pneumonitis, disseminated disease and those requiring hospitalization), intravenous aciclovir (5–10 mg/kg 8 hourly) is the treatment of choice. A live attenuated VZV vaccine is available. Some countries, such as Japan and USA, practise universal childhood vaccination against VZV, whilst others, such as the UK, aim at targeted vaccination of non-immune health care workers to limit nosocomial infection.

Viruses Transmitted by the Fecal-Oral Route

Rotavirus

Rotavirus (Family *Reoviridae*, genus R*otavirus*) is a significant cause of nosocomial gastroenteritis. It generally coincides with community outbreaks of infection and peaks in winter and early spring months in temperate climate countries. Using a definition of hospitalisation for 48 hours or more before onset of illness, a recent study involving three European countries found between 49% and 63% of pediatric nosocomial gastroenteritis positive for rotavirus with an incidence of 1–2.3 per 1000 hospital days [24]. The median hospitalization time ranged from 4 to 7 days before onset of symptoms and resulted in prolongation of hospitalization from 1.5 to 4.5 days. National differences in incidence and severity could be related to variation in facilities for grouping and isolating patients. Significantly, between 10% and 23% were in premature infants, where severe complications like necrotizing enterocolitis and intestinal perforation is commonly reported. Very low birth weight infants (< 1500 g) are at the highest risk of severe infection. A rare complication of rotavirus encephalopathy has also been reported and in some cases may be associated with hemophagocytic lymphohistiocytosis. Sick infants with complications have a high mortality. They require intensive care and could in turn be the source of nosocomial infection in ICU. Nosocomial rotavirus infections in adults have also been reported and could potentially cause serious complications, in particular in immunocompromised patients. Hence, it is necessary to investigate stool samples for rotavirus (and/or other viral agents) in any ICU patients with diarrhea by direct electron microscopy or antigen detection EIA. Adherence to infection control policy, attention to handhygiene with the use of antiseptic agents effective against viruses (Table 3) [25], and the practice of enteric precautions (Table 4) can help to stop an outbreak.

Table 4. General measures to control outbreaks of viral gastroenteritis [28]

- Hand washing (with liquid soap) or hand decontamination (with aqueous antiseptic or alcohol-based hand-rub) after contact

- Wear gloves and aprons when contact with stool or vomitus is likely

- Isolate symptomatic individuals (particularly those with uncontrolled diarrhea, patients with incontinence and children)

- Avoid unnecessary movement of patients to unaffected areas

- Staff that have worked in affected areas must not work in unaffected areas within 48 h

- Exclude symptomatic staff from duty until symptom free for 48 h

- If many patients are involved and no further isolation facilities are available, close the unit to new admissions or transfer until 72 h after the last new case

- Terminal cleaning of the cleaned environment, use freshly prepared hypochlorite (1,000 ppm) on hard surfaces

- Caution visitors and emphasize hand hygiene

Norovirus (Formerly Norwalk-Like Viruses)

Noroviruses belong to the family of *Caliciviridae*. They were known previously as Norwalk-like viruses or by their electron microscopic appearance as "small round structured viruses" (SRSV). Noroviruses are the most common cause of outbreaks of gastroenteritis in hospitals. There are two genogroups, both are highly infectious and can be transmitted by the faecal-oral route as well as by aerosols [26]. A recent study suggests that person-to-person spread is the main source of hospital outbreaks [27]. Despite numerous reports of nosocomial infections, Noroviruses have not been reported to cause outbreaks in ICU. This is probably due to the relatively short and acute illness and that most patients do not have severe symptoms that require intensive care. However, they can theoretically be introduced into any clinical areas by patients, visitors or staff. Norovirus infection can be diagnosed in fecal material by direct electron microscopy, antigen detection EIA or by the use of RT-PCR. A detail description of prevention measures has been described [28]. Vigorous and meticulous carrying out of standard enteric precautions is required to contain an outbreak (Tables 3 and 4).

Enteroviruses

Enteroviruses belong to the family of *Picornaviridae* and comprise nearly 70 different serotypes including polioviruses, coxsackie A and B viruses, echoviruses and the newer 'numbered enteroviruses'. They are transmitted by the fecal route and are significant causes of nosocomial infection, particularly in NICU. Infection could be introduced to the ICU through perinatal infection of a neonate or by members of staff. Outbreaks involving up to 23 neonates have been reported [29] and an attack rate of 29% was reported in one outbreak [30]. Enterovirus infection could present as neonatal sepsis, meningo-encephalitis, myocarditis, hepatitis or gastroenteritis. Necrotizing enterocolitis with pneumatosis intestinalis is a known complication in neonates. Some enteroviruses such as enterovirus 71 can cause severe and fatal illness in older children. With the global eradication of polioviruses in sight, poliomyelitis is unlikely to be a significant problem. However, vaccine-associated paralysis could be a problem in unimmunized adults. Health care workers in PICU who may be in contact with live vaccine poliovirus-shedding infants should ensure that they are immunized.

One of the main obstacles in infection control is the frequent delayed diagnosis of enterovirus. Although most enteroviruses grow rapidly in cell culture, some grow poorly and some not at all. Molecular techniques have revolutionized the diagnosis and management of outbreaks. RT-PCR has been used in the rapid diagnosis of enteroviruses and direct PCR product sequencing has successfully identified a concurrent outbreak of two different enteroviruses [29]. Hand washing (with liquid soap) or hand decontamination (aqueous antiseptic or alcohol based hand-rub, Table 3) is the most important measure during an outbreak and has been used successfully on its own to contain the infection [30] Cohorting, source isolation and screening are other measures frequently used. Clearance of the virus by the host is antibody mediated and many have advocated the use of normal human immunoglobulin [31]. Pleconaril is a new antiviral agent specifically designed for the *Picornaviridae* family. It has been used as an investigative drug or on compassionate basis in a number of cases with some success [32].

Hepatitis A Virus

Hepatitis A virus (family *Picornaviridae*, genus *hepatovirus*) belongs to the same family as enteroviruses and is usually transmitted via the fecal-oral route. Nosocomial transmission of hepatitis A virus is well documented. An outbreak in an adult ICU was reported to have occurred as a result of inadequate precautions taken while handling bile of a patient not suspected to be incubating hepatitis A [33]. Most other outbreaks occurred in PICU or NICU. Attack rates in contacts varied from between 15% and 25%. Risk factors included handling soiled bed pad, nappies, or gowns of the index patient [34], failure to wash hands after treating the index case for apnea or bradycardia [35] and eating in the ICU [36]. These factors all pointed to inadequate handwashing and subsequent oral contamination as the route of transmission. A case-control study also suggested that hepatitis A was transmitted among infants by nurses [37]. In NICU, vertical transmission [35] and blood transfusion [38] have been implicated as the cause of infection in the index neonate(s). The effect of nosocomial hepatitis A infection varies from asymptomatic infection to a classical presentation with acute hepatitis. Diagnosis is by serological detection of hepatitis A-specific IgM. RT-PCR can help to identify early infection or in difficult cases such as those with immunodeficiency. Sequencing of PCR products is useful in establishing epidemiological links during outbreaks. The use of normal human immunoglobulin (HNIG) has been successfully used for post-exposure prophylaxis to control outbreaks. There is now increasing evidence that hepatitis A vaccine can be used for prophylaxis if the contact occurs within 7 days from onset of illness in the primary case [39]. However, children < 2 years old should receive HNIG.

Viruses Transmitted by Blood and Body Fluid

The most commonly encountered nosocomial blood-borne viruses are hepatitis B virus (HBV), hepatitis C virus (HCV) and human immunodeficiency virus (HIV). The main risks are transmission from patients to health care workers. However, transmissions between patients and from health care workers to patients have been reported.

The best way to prevent occupational exposure of blood-borne viruses is to practice "universal precautions". Blood and body fluids (Table 5) from any

Table 5. Body fluids that may pose a risk for hepatitis B virus (HBV), hepatitis C virus (HCV) and human immunodeficiency virus (HIV)

Amniotic fluid
Breast milk
Cerebrospinal fluid
Exudate from burns or skin lesions
Pericardial fluid
Peritoneal fluid
Pleural fluid
Saliva after dental treatment
Synovial fluid
Unfixed tissues or organs
Any other fluid if visibly blood stained

Note: Saliva, urine, or stool that are not blood stained are not considered as high risk for blood-borne viruses

patients, whether or not there are identifiable risk factors, should be considered as potentially at risk. This would encourage good and safe practice and would help to prevent unnecessary accidents. Physical isolation of patients with blood-borne virus infection is generally not necessary unless there is profuse uncontrolled bleeding. Infection control teams should adopt a proactive approach to educate and prevent sharps injury (Table 6). There should also be specific instructions on how to deal with blood and body fluid exposure (Table 7).

Table 6. "Sharps" safety educational points (adapted from the Infection Control Team guidelines of Guys and St. Thomas' Hospital Trust, London, UK):

- Never re-sheath needles
- Dispose of all sharps in an approved container (UN 3291 compliant)
- Dispose of sharps at the point of use
- If carried, sharps must be placed in a tray
- Do not overfill sharps bins – dispose of sharps bins when 3/4 full

Table 7. Actions to be taken immediately after a blood/body fluid exposure (adapted from the Infection Control Team guidelines of Guys and St. Thomas' Hospital Trust, London, UK)

1. Rinse area thoroughly under running water

2. If a wound, wash site with liquid soap, encourage the wound to bleed, and apply a waterproof dressing (if appropriate)

3. Report it immediately to:
   a. Your supervisor (or Line Manager)
   b. Occupational Health or Accident and Emergency

4. Document incident by completing an incident form with source name and details

Hepatitis B Virus

HBV is the most infectious of the three common blood-borne viruses. The risk of transmission depends on the viral load of the source patient. An HBV carrier with HBeAg tends to have a high viral load and therefore more infectious than carriers without HBeAg. Estimates of infectivity range from 2% (HBeAg absent) to 40% (HBeAg present) [40]. All health care workers should be immunized against HBV. Management in relation to HBV after a significant blood/body fluid exposure depends on the vaccination status of the recipient (Table 8) [41].

Table 8. HBV prophylaxis after significant blood/body fluid exposure [41]

Recipients	Source HBsAg negative	Source HBsAg unknown	Source HBsAg positive
≤ 1 dose of HB vaccine	Initiate vaccination	Accelerated course of HB vaccine[a]	HBIG[b], accelerated course of HB vaccine[a]
≥ 2 doses of HB vaccine (anti-HBs level not known)	Complete course of vaccination	One dose of vaccine	One dose of vaccine followed by another dose 1 month later
Vaccine responder	Consider booster	Consider booster	Consider booster
Vaccine non-responder	Consider booster	HBIG[b], consider booster	HBIG[b], consider booster

[a]An accelerated course of vaccine consists of doses spaced at 0, 1, and 2 months.
[b]HBIG – Hyperimmune hepatitis B globulin (500 iu intramuscularly within 48 h of exposure)

Hepatitis C Virus

HCV is probably the commonest blood-borne virus encountered in western countries. In the United Kingdom, over a 3-year period, 462 incidences of occupational exposures to HCV were reported in comparison with 293 of HIV and 151 of HBV [42]. Follow-up studies of health care workers who sustained a percutaneous exposure to blood from a patient known to have HCV infection have reported an average incidence of seroconversion of 1.8% (range 0%–7%) [43]. No vaccine or post-exposure prophylaxis was available to prevent HCV transmission. However, there is some evidence that early interferon treatment after seroconversion is of benefit [44]. Actions to be taken after blood/body fluid exposure depends on the HCV status of the source (Table 9) [45].

Human Immunodeficiency Virus

The average risk of HIV transmission after percutaneous exposure to HIV-infected blood is about 0.3%. After muco-cutaneous exposure the risk is estimated to be less than 0.1%. Up to the end of 1999, worldwide 102 confirmed and 217 probable cases of occupational acquisition of HIV were reported. A case-control study [46] identified four factors associated with increased risk of transmission:

- Deep injury
- Visible blood on the device that caused the injury
- Injury with a needle that has been placed in a source patient's artery or vein
- Terminal HIV-related illness in the source patient

Table 9. Actions to be taken after blood/body fluid exposure in relation to HCV [45]

Hepatitis C status of source	Actions
Anti-HCV negative	Consider testing source for HCV RNA if the source is known to be immunocompromised or if acute infection is suspected, otherwise **reassure**
Anti-HCV unknown	**Low risk:** anti-HCV at 24 weeks **High risk:** manage as known infected source
Anti-HCV positive	1. Test source for HCV RNA 2. Follow-up at 6 weeks for HCV RNA 3. Follow-up at 12 weeks for HCV RNA and anti-HCV 4. Follow-up at 24 weeks for anti-HCV

This study also showed that the use of zidovudine prophylaxis reduces the risk of transmission by 80%. Post-exposure prophylaxis should therefore be offered to all health care workers who have a significant exposure to blood or body fluid from a patient known to be or at high risk of HIV infection. Various post-exposure prophylaxis options are available depending on national recommendations, and usually include a combination of zidovudine, lamivudine, and a protease inhibitor such as indinavir or nelfinavir. This should be started as soon as possible after exposure and continued for 4 weeks.

Viral Hemorrhagic Fevers

Viral hemorrhagic fevers (VHFs) are severe and life-threatening diseases caused by a range of viruses. They are either zoonotic or arthropod-borne infections and are often endemic in certain parts of the world (Table 10). They are often highly infectious through close contact with infected blood and body fluid and therefore pose a significant risk of hospital-acquired infection. Since many patients with VHF present with shock and require vigorous supportive treatment, it is a potential problem in ICU. The major viruses of concern are Marburg virus, Ebola virus, Rift Valley fever virus, Lassa virus, Crimean Congo hemorrhagic fever virus and Hantaan virus (MERLCH). Yellow fever and Dengue may also be a problem, although their transmission usually requires an insect vector. The incubation period for these VHFs ranges from 3 to 21 days. Initial symptoms are often non-specific, but could eventually lead to hemorrhage and shock. Any febrile patient who has returned from an endemic area of one of the VHF agents or has a history of contact with cases suspected to have VHF within 3 weeks should be considered at risk. However, malaria should always be excluded. A risk assessment needs to be performed and any patient known or strongly suspected to be suffering from VHF should be admitted to a

Table 10. Main viruses responsible for viral hemorrhagic fevers

Virus	Geographic distribution	Reservoir	Vector
Marburg and Ebola	Sub-Sahara Africa	Unknown	Unknown
Rift Valley Fever	Mainland Africa	Sheep, cattle	Mosquito
Lassa	West Africa	Rodents	None
Crimean Congo hemorrhagic fever	East and West Africa, North and Central Asia, Middle East, India and Pakistan, Balkans, West China	Cows, hares, hedgehogs, birds	Ticks
Hantaan	Asia	Rodents	None
Dengue	Asia, Caribbean, Pacific West Africa	Human	Mosquito
Yellow fever	Africa, South America	Monkey/human	Mosquito

high security infectious disease unit that is designated to manage these patients [47]. While awaiting transfer to a secure unit, such patients should be placed in a negative pressure room with strict source isolation. Specimens for patient management should be processed in a high security laboratory designated for category 4 pathogens. The etiological agent can be established using serology, isolation and PCR in designated specialized laboratories. All areas and materials in contact with infected patients should be autoclaved, incinerated, or treated with hypochlorite (10,000 ppm of available chlorine). If the patient dies, the body should be placed in a sealable body bag, sprayed, or wiped with hypochlorite. Individuals who have been in contact with a case of VHF should be put under surveillance for 3 weeks. There are reported successes of the use of intravenous ribavirin in some cases of VHFs (Lassa, Crimean Congo hemorrhagic fever, and Hantaan). Apart from yellow fever, no vaccine is available.

Cytomegalovirus

Cytomegalovirus (CMV) is a ubiquitous virus from the *Herpesviridae* family. It is spread by direct contact with body fluid such as urine, saliva, blood, semen, and vaginal secretion. In a hospital setting, it can be transmitted by blood transfusion or organ transplantation. Most individuals acquire infection in early childhood and the reported seroprevalence in adults ranges from 50% to

100%. Following primary infection, CMV persists in a latent form and asymptomatic reactivation is common. Increase in mortality has been reported in ICU patients who had CMV reactivation, some of whom were symptomatic [48].

One particular concern is primary infection of pregnant women. Up to 40% of pregnant women with primary infection transmit CMV to the fetus, but only 10%-15% of these develop clinically apparent disease. In addition, a further 5%–15% of asymptomatic but infected infants may develop long-term sequelae such as deafness. Despite a lot of concern about nosocomial CMV infection, particularly in NICU, there is little evidence to show that the risk to health care workers who attend to children is higher than others. Screening of asymptomatic pregnant health care workers is therefore not warranted. DNA analysis should be used in a suspected case of hospital-acquired infection, as the infection could have been acquired from family and community rather than from the hospital. Nevertheless, epidemiological clusters of CMV infections have been reported in NICU [49]. To prevent cross infection in ICU, standard blood and body fluid precautions are sufficient. Since all children, not only those diagnosed to have congenital CMV infection, may be shedding CMV, universal precaution is necessary. To avoid introducing CMV infection through blood transfusion, NICU should use blood from CMV-seronegative donors or leukocyte-depleted blood.

Viruses Transmitted by Direct Contact

Varicella Zoster Virus - Shingles

Shingles or zoster is the result of the reactivation of latent VZV in the dorsal root or cranial nerve ganglia. The clinical presentation is a painful vesicular eruption covering the affected dermatome(s). The clinical diagnosis can be confirmed rapidly by immunofluorescence, electron microscopy, culture, or PCR of the cellular material obtained from a vesicular scraping. The infection is usually self-limiting. However, in severe disease or in the immunocompromised, multi-dermatome zoster or disseminated infection could occur. Such cases should be managed as if they were chickenpox and respiratory precautions for infection control have to be enforced.

Patients or staff with classical shingles are contagious from the day of the rash until the lesions are crusted over. There is some risk of nosocomial transmission if the lesions are in exposed areas of the body and in those who are immunocompromised. Cases of hospital-acquired chickenpox due to exposure to an immunocompromised patient with shingles have been reported [50]. Non-immune (VZV-IgG negative) patients or staff with no history of chickenpox are susceptible if they have close contact with shingles. They should be managed as described for chickenpox contact (Fig. 1).

Herpes Simplex Virus (HSV)

The herpes simplex viruses (HSV) consist of two types: HSV-1 and HSV-2. They are members of the *Herpesviridae* family. Clinically they most commonly manifest with oral (predominantly HSV-1) or genital (predominantly HSV-2) ulcerations/vesicles. Other presentations include keratitis, encephalitis, herpetic whitlow or neonatal infection. Reactivation is common, particularly in ICU settings. The diagnosis can be confirmed rapidly by immunofluorescence, electron microscopy, viral culture, or PCR of vesicle/ulcer scrapings. In the immunocompromised, HSV can cause life-threatening disseminated infection and early treatment with intravenous aciclovir is recommended. It has also been suggested that occult herpes virus reactivation may increase the mortality of ICU patients [51]. However, it is difficult to distinguish between causation and concurrent reactivation in a severely ill patient.

As the infected lesions contain virus there is an increased risk of nosocomial transmission until the lesions have crusted over. Standard isolation precautions should be in place to reduce transmission (Table 2). Patients with active lesions should be nursed away from high-risk groups (i.e. immunocompromised, severe eczema, burns patients, or neonates). As patients can be asymptomatic secretors, health care workers should wear gloves when dealing with oral secretions to avoid infections such as herpetic whitlow. Infected staff should cover lesions if possible and should not attend those at risk. Neonatal herpes is usually transmitted from mother to the child at the time of delivery. However, this may not be noticed until the infant develops disease. Universal precautions (in particular hand washing) should always be in place to reduce transmission of infection. Outbreaks of HSV-1 in NICU have been described [52]. In order to contain the outbreak, infected cases should be cohorted and nursed by dedicated staff that will not attend 'non infected' infants.

Rare Nervous System Infection in ICU

Viral nervous system infections are frequently caused by herpesviruses or enteroviruses. These have been dealt with in the previous sections. There are, however, two further rare causes of nervous system infection, which may be of concern, in terms of infection control, in the ICU.

Rabies Virus

Rabies virus is a *Lyssavirus* belonging to the family of *Rhabdoviridae*. Rabies is usually transmitted to humans via the bite of an infected animal, usually a dog. Cases of transmission by bats have also been reported. The incubation period is long (average 4-12 weeks, but up to 2 years). However, only 40% of exposed people develop disease. The virus spreads from the wound to the central nervous system via the nerves and can be present in saliva, skin, eye, and brain tissue. Clinically the infection may present in two different forms. The 'furious' form of rabies is characterized by muscular contractions, convulsions, and tremor, whereas the 'dumb' rabies presents with ascending flaccid paralysis, sensory disturbance, slurred speech, and difficulty with swallowing and breathing. There is no specific treatment and the infection is almost always fatal. The diagnosis can be confirmed by demonstrating the virus directly in brain tissue or corneal swab by RT-PCR or by immunofluorescence detection of antigen in skin biopsies from the nape of the neck. Due to the severe and paralyzing condition, patients may be admitted to ICU. So far, the only cases of human-to-human transmission of rabies were through corneal transplants taken from infected donors. However, there is a theoretical risk of nosocomial infection to health care workers. It is therefore recommended that any health care worker with a significant exposure (e.g., splash of secretion onto mucosa or broken skin) should receive rabies vaccine and specific immunoglobulins [41]. Organs from patients with suspected rabies or an undiagnosed encephalopathy should not be used for transplantation.

Transmissible Spongiform Encephalopathies

These include Creutzfeldt-Jacob disease (CJD), variant CJD, fatal familial insomnia, and Gerstmann-Sträussler-Scheinker syndrome. Transmissible spongiform encephalopathy is thought to be caused by self-replicating proteins termed prions, which accumulate in the central nervous system causing fatal disease. The incubation is over several years (>10) and patients develop a progressive dementia. Magnetic resonance imaging, electroencephalography and 14-3-3 protein in the cerebrospinal fluid are useful diagnostic investigations in suspected cases. However, the diagnosis is often only confirmed by post-mortem histology of brain or tonsil tissue. Human-to-human transmission of CJD has occurred due to contaminated pituitary growth hormone, corneal transplants, dura mater grafts, and surgical instruments. Various tissue and body fluids are thought to carry a different risk of infectivity (Table 11).

Table 11. Tissue infectivity of variant Creutzfeldt-Jacob disease (vCJD) [53]:

High risk	Medium risk	Low risk	Negligible risk
Brain tissue	Appendix	Blood	Urine
Spinal cord	Tonsils		Feces
CSF	Spleen		Saliva
Optic nerve			
Retina			

Generally, there is little risk for health care workers and isolation precautions such as masks and gowns are unnecessary for routine care. Universal precautions should be in place and practised. Special precautions are required for handling high-risk specimens (e.g., central nervous or eye tissue and cerebrospinal fluid and procedures (e.g., lumbar puncture). The United Kingdom Department of Health has set out guidelines for health care workers regarding CJD [53]. As prions are extremely resistant to conventional autoclaving and most disinfectants, special precautions must be taken and contaminated instruments and medical devices should not be reprocessed. Since CJD can be transmitted by organ transplantation, organs from patients with suspected CJD or an undiagnosed encephalopathy should not be used for transplantation.

Conclusions

There are increasing number of reports of outbreaks or cross-infection of viruses in the ICU. However, very little evidence-based practice is available in the literature. Intensivists should be on the alert for nosocomial viral infections and should work closely with clinical virologists. Better epidemiological studies are necessary to determine the best infection control practice in ICU.

Acknowledgements. We thank Dr. David Treacher and Mr. David Tucker for reviewing the manuscript and for their comments and advice.

References

1. Shay DK, Holman RC, Newman RD, Liu LL, Stout JW, Anderson LJ (1999) Bronchiolitis-associated hospitalisations among US children, 1980-1996. JAMA 282:1440–1446
2. Thorburn K, Kerr S, Taylor N, van Saene HKF (2004) RSV outbreak in a paediatric intensive care unit. J Hosp Infect 57:194–201
3. Guidry GG, Black-Payne CA, Payne DK, Jamison RM, George RB, Bocchini JA Jr (1991) Respiratory syncytial virus infection among intubated adults in a university medical intensive care unit. Chest 100:1377–1384
4. Holladay RC, Campbell GD Jr (1995) Nosocomial viral pneumonia in the intensive care unit. Clin Chest Med 16:121–133
5. Blydt-Hansen T, Subbarao K, Quennec P, McDonald J (1999) Recovery of respiratory syncytial virus from stethoscopes by conventional viral culture and polymerase chain reaction. Pediatr Infect Dis J 18:164–165
6. Madge P, Paton JY, McColl JH, Mackie PL (1992) Prospective controlled study of four infection control procedures to prevent nosocomial infection with respiratory syncytial virus. Lancet 340:1079–1083
7. Gala CL, Hall CB, Schnabel KC, Pincus PH, Blossom P, Hildreth SW, Betts RF, Douglas

RG Jr (1986) The use of eye-nose goggles to control nosocomial respiratory syncytial virus infection. JAMA 256:2706–2708

8. Agah R, Cherry JD, Garakian AJ, Chapin M (1987) Respiratory syncytial virus (RSV) infection rate in personnel caring for children with RSV infections. Routine isolation procedure vs routine procedure supplemented by use of masks and goggles. Am J Dis Child 141:695–697

9. Randolph AG, Wang EE (1996) Ribavirin for respiratory syncytial virus lower respiratory tract infection. Arch Pediatr Adolesc Med 150:942–947

10. Falsey AR, Walsh EE (2000) Respiratory syncytial virus infection in adults. Clin Microbiol Rev 13:371–384

11. Cox RA, Rao P, Brandon-Cox C (2001) The use of palivizumab monoclonal antibody to control an outbreak of respiratory syncytial virus infection in a special care baby unit. J Hosp Infect 48:186–192

12. Moisiuk SE, Robson D, Klass L, Kliewer G, Wasyliuk W, Davi M, Plourde P (1998) Outbreak of parainfluenza virus type 3 in an intermediate care neonatal nursery. Pediatr Infect Dis J 17:49–53

13. Nichols WG, Corey L, Gooley T, Davis C, Boeckh M (2001) Parainfluenza virus infections after hematopoietic stem cell transplantation: risk factors, response to antiviral therapy, and effect on transplant outcome. Blood 98:573–578

14. Cunney RJ, Bialachowski A, Thornley D, Smaill FM, Pennie RA (2000) An outbreak of influenza A in a neonatal intensive care unit. Infect Control Hosp Epidemiol 21:449–454

15. Munoz FM, Campbell JR, Atmar RL, Garcia-Prats J, Baxter BD, Johnson LE, Englund JA (1999) Influenza A virus outbreak in a neonatal intensive care unit. Pediatr Infect Dis J 18:811–815

16. Centres for Disease Control and Prevention (1997) Guidelines for the prevention of nosocomial pneumonia. MMWR Morb Mortal Wkly Rep 46:1–79

17. Piedra PA, Kasel JA, Norton HJ, Garcia-Prats JA, Rayford Y, Estes MK, Hull R, Baker CJ (1992) Description of an adenovirus type 8 outbreak in hospitalized neonates born prematurely. Pediatr Infect Dis J 11:460–465

18. Legrand F, Berrebi D, Houhou N, Freymuth F, Faye A, Duval M, Mougenot JF, Peuchmaur M, Vilmer E (2001) Early diagnosis of adenovirus infection and treatment with cidofovir after bone marrow transplantation in children. Bone Marrow Transplant 27:621–626

19. Gustafson TL, Lavely GB, Brawner ER Jr, Hutcheson RH Jr, Wright PF, Schaffner W (1982) An outbreak of airborne nosocomial varicella. Pediatrics 70:550–556

20. Friedman CA, Temple DM, Robbins KK, Rawson JE, Wilson JP, Feldman S (1994) Outbreak and control of varicella in a neonatal intensive care unit. Pediatr Infect Dis J 13:152–154

21. Gustafson TL, Shehab Z, Brunell PA (1984) Outbreak of varicella in a newborn intensive care nursery. Am J Dis Child 138:548–550

22. Stover BH, Cost KM, Hamm C, Adams G, Cook LN (1988) Varicella exposure in a neonatal intensive care unit: case report and control measures. Am J Infect Control 16:167–172

23. Burns SM, Mitchell-Heggs, Carrington D (1998) Occupational and infection control aspects of varicella. A review prepared for the UK advisory group on chickenpox on behalf of the British Society for the study of Infection. J Infect 36 [Suppl 1]:73–78

24. Frühwirth M, Heininger U, Ehlken B, Petersen G, Laubereau B, Moll-Schüler I, Mutz I, Forster J (2001) International variation in disease burden of rotavirus gastroenteritis in children with community- and nosocomially acquired infection. Pediatr Infect Dis J 20:784–791

25. Boyce JM, Pittet D. (2002) Guideline for hand hygiene in health-care settings. Recommendations of the Healthcare Infection Control Practices Advisory Committee and the HICPAC/SHEA/APIC/IDSA Hand Hygiene Task Force. Society for Healthcare Epidemiology of America/Association for Professionals in Infection Control/Infectious Diseases Society of America. MMWR Recomm Rep 51:1–45

26. Marks PJ, Vipond IB, Carlisle D, Deakin D, Fey RE, Caul EO (2000) Evidence for airborne transmission of Norwalk-like virus (NLV) in a hotel restaurant. Epidemiol Infect 124:481–487

27. Lopman BA, Adak GK, Reacher MH, Brown DWG (2003) Two epidemiologic patterns of Norovirus outbreaks: surveillance in England and Wales, 1992-2000. Emerg Infect Dis 9:71–77

28. Chadwick PR, Beards G, Brown D, Caul EO, Cheesbrough J, Clarke I, Curry A, O'Brien S, Quigley K, Sellwood J, Westmoreland D (2000) Management of hospital outbreaks of gastro-enteritis due to small round structured viruses. J Hosp Infect 45:1–10

29. Takami T, Sonodat S, Houjyo H, Kawashima H, Takei Y, Miyajima T, Takekuma K, Hoshika A, Mori T, Nakayama T (2000) Diagnosis of horizontal enterovirus infections in neonates by nested PCR and direct sequence analysis. J Hosp Infect 45:283–287

30. Isaacs D, Dobson SR, Wilkinson AR, Hope PL, Eglin R, Moxon ER (1989) Conservative management of an echovirus 11 outbreak in a neonatal unit. Lancet 8637:543–545

31. Wreghitt TG, Sutehall GM, King A, Gandy GM (1989) Fatal echovirus 7 infection during an outbreak in a special care baby unit. J Infect 19:229–236

32. Aradottir E, Alonso EM, Shulman ST (2001) Severe neonatal enteroviral hepatitis treated with pleconaril. Pediatr Infect Dis J 20:457–459

33. Hanna JN, Loewenthal MR, Negel P, Wenck DJ (1996) An outbreak of hepatitis A in an intensive care unit. Anaesth Intensive Care 24:440–444

34. Burkholder BT, Coronado VG, Brown J, Hutto JH, Shapiro CN, Robertson B, Woodruff BA (1995) Nosocomial transmission of hepatitis A in a pediatric hospital traced to an anti-hepatitis A virus –negative patient with immunodeficiency. Pediatr Infect Dis J 14:261–266

35. Watson JC, Fleming DW, Borella AJ, Olcott ES, Conrad RE, Baron RC (1993) Vertical transmission of hepatitis A resulting in an outbreak in a neonatal intensive care unit. J Infect Dis 167:567–571

36. Drusin LM, Sohmer M, Groshen SL, Spiritos MD, Senterfit LB, Christenson WN (1987) Nosocomial hepatitis A infection in a paediatric intensive care unit. Arch Dis Child 62:690–695

37. Klein BS, Michaels JA, Rytel MW, Berg KG, Davis JP (1984) Nosocomial hepatitis A. A multinursery outbreak in Wisconsin. JAMA 252:2716–2721

38. Noble RC, Kane MA, Reeves SA, Roeckel I (1984) Posttransfusion hepatitis A in a neonatal intensive care unit. JAMA 252:2711–2715

39. Crowcroft NS, Walsh B, Davison KL, Gungabissoon U on behalf of PHLS advisory committee on vaccination and immunisation (2001) Guidelines for the control of hepatitis A virus infection. Commun Dis Public Health 4:213–227

40. Gerberding JL (1995) Management of occupational exposures to blood-borne viruses. N Engl J Med 332:444–451

41. Salisbury DM, Begg NT (eds) (1996) Immunisation against infectious disease. HMSO ISBN 0-11-321815-X, London, UK

42. Evans B, Duggan W, Baker J, Ramsay M, Abiteboul D on behalf of the occupational exposure surveillance advisory group (2001) Exposure of healthcare workers in England, Wales, and Northern Ireland to bloodborne viruses between July 1997 and June 2000: analysis of surveillance data. BMJ 322:397–398

43. Centers for Disease Control and Prevention (1997) Notice to readers recommenda-

tions for follow-up of health-care workers. MMWR Morb Mortal Wkly Rep 46:603-606
44. Jackel E, Cornberg M, Wedmeyer H, Santantonio T, Mayer J, Zankel M, Pastore G, Dietrich M, Trautwein C, Manns MP for the German acute hepatitis C therapy group (2001) Treatment of acute hepatitis C with interferon alfa-2b. N Engl J Med 345:1452-1457
45. Ramsay ME (1999) Guidance on the investigation and management of occupational exposure to hepatitis C. Commun Dis Public Health 2:258-262
46. Cardo D, Culver DH, Ciesielski CA et al. (1997) A case control study of HIV seroconversion in health care workers after percutaneous exposure. N Engl J Med 337:1485-1490
47. ACDP (1996) Management and control of viral haemorrhagic fevers. London Stationery Office, London, United Kingdom
48. Heininger A, Jahn G, Engel C, Notheisen T, Unertl K, Hamprecht K (2001) Human cytomegalovirus infections in nonimmunosuppressed critically ill patients. Crit Care Med 29:541-547
49. Aitken C, Booth J, Booth M, Boriskin Y, Testard H, Kempley S, Breuer J (1996) Molecular epidemiology and significance of a cluster of case of CMV infection occurring on a special care baby unit. J Hosp Infect 34:183-189
50. Juel-Jensen BE (1983) Outbreak of chickenpox from a patient with immunosuppressed herpes zoster in hospital. B Med J 286:60
51. Cook CH, Yenchar JK, Kraner TO, Daives EA, Ferguson RM (1998) Occult herpes family viruses may increase mortality in critically ill surgical patients. Am J Surg 176:357-360
52. Hammberg O, Watts J, Chernesky M, Luchsinger I, Rawls W (1983) An outbreak of herpes simplex virus type 1 in an intensive care nursery. Pediatr Infect Dis J 2:290-294
53. Advisory Committee on Dangerous Pathogens (ACDP)/Spongiform Encephalopathy Advisory Committee (SEAC) (1998) Transmissible spongiform encephalopathy agents: safe working and the prevention of infection. HMSO, Department of Health, London, United Kingdom

Chapter 22

AIDS Patients in the Intensive Care Unit

L. Alvarez-Rocha, P. Rascado-Sedes, J. Pastor-Benavent, F. Barcenilla-Gaite

Introduction

The first cases of acquired immunodeficiency syndrome (AIDS) were reported in the summer of 1981, in American young homosexual males. Two years later, the virus responsible for the disease, known as human immunodeficiency virus (HIV-1), was identified. Although this agent causes the vast majority of cases, a variant of this virus (HIV-2) was later isolated in patients from or epidemiologically linked to West Africa. From its onset, the epidemic of HIV/AIDS has shown continuous growth beyond all predictions. According to the Joint United Nations Program on HIV/AIDS (UNAIDS), at the end of 1999, about 56 million people worldwide had been infected, of which, 20 million had died [1]. The problem is particularly worrying in developing countries, where 95% of the HIV-infected people live, especially in Sub-Saharan Africa, with a mean prevalence of 8.8% in the adult population (it has been estimated that 25.3 million people infected by HIV were living in this area at the end of 2000). In contrast, in North America and Western Europe together, at the end of 2000 the infected population was 1.46 million. In addition, the development of preventive programs and the availability of highly active antiretroviral therapy (HAART) in industrialized countries has determined a change in the pattern of the epidemic: not only is the growth of the epidemic slower but survival of infected patients is also increasing. In Spain, according to data from the Health Department (http://www.msc.es/sida), the infection rate has decreased from 187.6 per million in 1994 to 58.9 in 2000.

The HIV/AIDS epidemic is a major health problem, with high morbidity, mortality, and costs produced by a chronic and ultimately fatal disease. It also has a great socio-economic impact, since HIV infection affects mainly young productive adults. Likewise, the disease affects individuals belonging to high economic and educational classes, at least in the first stages, although later it persists in the most-vulnerable classes. This epidemic has therefore led to a significant reduction in life expectancy, even to the appearance of a negative demographic growth, and to an important decrease of the gross domestic product in countries with a greater incidence of the disease.

HIV/AIDS and the Intensive Care Unit

Patients with HIV infection are admitted to intensive care units (ICUs) for monitoring and vigilance, or for advanced life support; but a non-negligible number of patients can be admitted to these units due to causes unrelated to the infection. In the last 3 years, only 33% of HIV/AIDS patients were admitted to our unit due to conditions directly associated with the disease, while the other conditions were not associated (trauma, coronary syndromes, drug overdose, etc.) (unpublished data).

The presence of HIV-infected patients in ICUs varies widely depending on the area being considered and the type of hospital [2]. In some units, this group of patients can reach more than 33% of all admissions [3]. Overall, of all HIV-infected patients admitted to a hospital, about 4%–12% will require ICU care [4, 5].

The improvement of preventive and therapeutic options has prolonged the life of HIV/AIDS patients, and has changed the spectrum of diseases that cause hospitalization. At the beginning of the epidemic, more than two-thirds of ICU admissions were due to respiratory failure, especially secondary to *Pneumocystis carinii* pneumonia (PCP) [6, 7]. However, in the last few years only 38%–49% of admissions were due to respiratory failure [3–5] (Table 1), and 37%–45% of these were caused by PCP [3–5, 8]. Bacterial pneumonia is becoming the leading cause of respiratory failure leading to ICU admission (47%–53%), but other etiologies, such as tuberculosis, toxoplasmosis, or Kaposi sarcoma (KS), still represent a significant minor proportion [3, 8]. Neurological problems (11%–27%), sepsis (10%–15%), and several types of cardiac manifestations (5%) are other frequent reasons for ICU admission [3–5, 8]. Toxoplasmosis is the major cause of cerebral dysfunction in this group of patients (62% of cases of central nervous system disease in the series of Casalino et al. [3]), although tuberculosis, cryptococcosis, bacterial meningitis, cerebral lymphoma, or progressive multifocal leukoencephalopathy (PML) are also reported with variable frequencies [9]. Sepsis and septic shock are mainly of pulmonary origin and bacterial etiology [10, 11]. In the series of Rosenberg et al. [11], pneumonia caused 65% of episodes of sepsis, and in 45% of infections a bacterial agent was identified, although in this study and in others, other micro-organisms were found, such as *P. carinii*, *Mycobacterium tuberculosis*, cytomegalovirus (CMV), *Cryptococcus neoformans*, and *Toxoplasma gondii*. The most common cardiac manifestations in HIV/AIDS patients are pericarditis,

Table 1. Reasons for intensive care unit (ICU) admission among HIV/AIDS patients[a]

	% of Admissions
Respiratory failure	38.4–49.2
Neurological disease	11.1–26.8
Severe sepsis	10.2–58.1
Gastrointestinal bleeding	6.3–6.5
Cardiac disease	4.5–7.9
Drug overdose	2.3–5.3
Metabolic disturbance	1.6–1.7
Trauma	1.1–2.9
Miscellaneous	2–9.3

[a]From references [4–6, 12]. The intervals are the extreme values reflected in the references

myocarditis, dilated cardiomyopathy, endocarditis, neoplasms, and cardiac drug toxicity [12]. Some of the most frequent infectious agents associated with cardiac disease are *Staphylococcus aureus*, *Streptococcus viridans*, *Salmonella*, *M. tuberculosis*, *T. gondii*, and *C. neoformans*, and the most common neoplasms are KS and lymphoma [3, 12].

Finally, during the first stage of the epidemic, the observed mortality among AIDS patients admitted to the ICU was high. Wachter et al. [6] and Schein et al. [7] reported a mortality of 69% and 77% respectively, which increased to 87% and 91% in patients who developed acute respiratory failure. These poor outcomes changed physicians' attitudes to these patients, and it was thought that ICU admission was generally futile and mechanical ventilation was rarely indicated. This led to the search for new therapeutic options outside the ICU. However, introduction of antiretroviral therapy and the availability of better options for prevention and management of opportunistic infection, especially PCP, with the use of co-trimoxazole and corticosteroids, have changed the prognosis and management of HIV/AIDS infection. In several recent series [3–5], in-ICU and in-hospital mortality among HIV/AIDS patients admitted to the ICU ranged between 21% and 24% and between 30% and 39%, respectively. The 1-year survival was 27%–28% [3, 4, 13]. These rates are comparable to those observed in high-risk non-HIV-infected patients admitted to the ICU (severe sepsis, the elderly, patients needing cardiopulmonary resuscitation, bone marrow transplantation recipients) [3]. According to these data, admission of HIV/AIDS patients to the ICU should not be considered futile, although more studies are needed to evaluate the impact of HAART.

We must bear in mind that the outcome varies with the cause of ICU admission [3–5, 8, 10, 11]. In-hospital mortality is 44%–93% in patients admitted due to severe sepsis/septic shock, 26%–46% in those with acute respiratory failure, 32%–41% in those with central nervous system dysfunction, and 6%–69% in those with cardiac involvement. Multiple risk factors have been identified in several studies, with independent association with mortality in HIV/AIDS patients admitted to the ICU (APACHE/SAPS scores, need for mechanical ventilation, and duration, diagnosis of PCP, patients coming from a hospital ward, serum albumin level less than 25 g/l, CD4+ count less than $50x10^6/l$, functional status, weight loss, HIV disease stage, duration of AIDS, etc.) [3–5, 8, 11] (Table 2). As a general rule, as reported by Casalino et al. [3], short-term in-ICU and in-hospital outcome is determined by the severity of the acute disease and health status prior to admission, whereas long-term outcome depends mainly on those variables reflecting the stage of HIV infection. However, to date, no single factor or combination of factors has been able to reasonably predict after-ICU survival. For example, Nickas and Wachter [4] reported an in-hospital mortality of 39% in a group of patients with very high mortality predicted on a theoretical basis (CD4+ cells count less than $50x10^6/l$, serum albumin level less than 25 g/l, and mechanical ventilation). Therefore, caution must be used when evaluating these markers for a particular case.

Table 2. Factors influencing in-ICU/in-hospital mortality among HIV/AIDS patients admitted to the ICU (multivariate analysis)[a]

	Odds ratio
Functional status (>2)	1.82
AIDS diagnosis in ICU	1.62
AIDS diagnosis prior to ICU	2.63
Time since AIDS diagnosis (>360 days)	1.91
Albumin level	0.39 per 10 g/l increase
Serum albumin <25 g/l	3.06
APACHE II score >17	3.41
APACHE III score >80	3.1
SAPS I score >12	1.62
Mechanical ventilation requirement	4.3–19.2
Acute respiratory distress syndrome in ICU	14.0
Bacterial cause of infection	1.3
Pneumonia	1.9
Pneumocystis carinii pneumonia diagnosis	2.4–4.5

[a]From references [4, 5, 9, 12]. Only statistically significant results are presented. Functional status assessed by a modified Karnofsky index (see reference [4]). The intervals are the extreme values reflected in the references

Pathogenesis

HIV infection is a consequence of viral infection and replication inside cells bearing CD4+ receptors (CD4+ T lymphocytes and, in minor proportion, macrophages and dendritic cells) and then cell destruction. Besides CD4+, other co-receptors (mainly CCR5 and CXCR4) are needed for virus internalization [14].

Among all branches of the immune system, T cell-mediated immunity plays a pivotal role in control of HIV infection. However, unlike in other viral infections, the immune response is unable to control the disease [15]. This seems to be due to the defective response of HIV-infected (CD4+) and non-infected (CD8+) T lymphocytes.

The average time from HIV infection to the development of AIDS is 8–10 years. However, there is a small proportion of patients not following this usual evolution, and the study of these individuals has been essential for knowledge of the immunity to HIV [14–17]. Asymptomatic patients with a normal CD4+ cell count, a low or undetectable viral burden despite long-term HIV infection, and no treatment are known as non-progressors and represent 5%–10% of HIV-infected patients. In addition, there are some exposed yet uninfected individuals despite repeated exposure to HIV. Finally, those who develop AIDS in the first 5 years after HIV infection are known as rapid progressors.

In the first days to weeks after HIV primary infection, a high level of viremia is observed, together with an important immune system activation, essentially represented by T lymphocytes, with a partial control of viral replication [14, 15]. After a few weeks or months, a rapid decrease in viremia occurs, followed by a return of T lymphocyte count to near-normal levels. The patient enters a prolonged asymptomatic stage with a balance between viral production and destruction, despite detectable viral burden. The progression of the disease is characterized by a continuous increase in viral burden and a decrease in T lymphocyte CD4+ (T-helper cells) count, and finally, appearance of severe immunosuppression [14, 15, 17].

After activation induced by viral antigens, T cells release several cytokines, in particular interleukin-2 (IL-2), which in turn stimulate the CD8+ T lymphocytes (T cytotoxic cells). These are the effector arm of cellular immunity, with the ability to recognize and lyze cells expressing foreign proteins. During HIV infection, HIV-specific CD8+ T lymphocytes proliferate, and these cells, with a broad spectrum of antiviral activity, play an essential role in controlling the disease [14, 15]. However, HIV selectively infects and destroys activated CD4+ T lymphocytes, and this depletion of T-helper cells diminishes the subsequent immune response. It is well known that CD4+ T lymphocytes are important for the initiation of the response, for the maintenance of memory and maturation of the functions of CD8+ T lymphocytes [15, 17].

HIV-specific CD8+ T cells exert a broad spectrum of antiviral activities. They produce a protein, perforin, which together with the granzymes, are essential for the lysis of infected cells [15]. They influence viral replication through the production of several cytokines. Some of these, such as interferon-γ (IFN-γ), inhibit replication, while others, such as tumor necrosis factor-α (TNF-α), can up-regulate HIV replication [15, 16]. They can also interfere with viral replication through the production of chemokines that limit, by competition or down-regulation, interaction of HIV with cell co-receptors [15]. RANTES (regulated on activation normal T expressed and secreted), MIP-1 α (macrophage inflammatory protein), and MIP-1 β block the CCR5 co-receptor. SDF-1 (stromal cell-derived factor) is the natural ligand for CXCR4 co-receptor.

Humoral immunity also plays a role in the defense against HIV, but is not well defined [14]. Although some data support a protective function of anti-HIV antibodies, as in the case of a possible decrease in perinatal transmission in the presence of maternal antibodies [18], or a potential protection of some health care workers by neutralizing antibodies [19], current evidence is not enough to state a crucial importance of humoral immunity in the control of the disease [20, 21]. Antibodies against HIV can be detected 2–3 weeks after the primary infection, but even in their presence, viral replication continues. Only when the infection is well established, sometimes even in the final stages, are HIV-neutralizing antibodies present [14, 21]. Together with their neutralizing function, they can complement other defensive mechanisms, namely complement and cellular immunity [14, 21].

Finally, several local factors, not well defined yet, are involved in the defense against HIV [14–16]. The presence of sexually transmitted diseases and lack of circumcision are known to be associated with a higher risk of infection. Dendritic cells, which take antigens in the periphery and transport them to lymph nodes, where T lymphocytes are activated, may play a role during the primary infection of the mucosa. In addition, the presence of CD8+ T lymphocytes and HIV-specific IgA antibodies can also help to control the viral burden in the genital tract.

Despite the deployment of such an important defense system, HIV continues to replicate and therefore the disease progresses [14–17, 20]. The mechanisms (not well characterized) seem to be multiple, namely mutations in *gag*, *pol*, and *env* genes, a decrease of HIV-specific CD8+ T lymphocytes due to clonal deletion, and persistence of the virus in immune-privileged sites (central nervous system, eye, testis, dendritic cells, and infected memory T cells).

Antiretroviral Therapy

The introduction of HAART in 1996 has turned HIV infection, formerly a fatal disease, into a chronic process with a survival of several decades. At the end of the 1990s, the mortality of patients with CD4+ counts of less than $100 \times 10^6/l$ was approximately 66% less than in former years [22]. With this type of treatment, based on the use of potent antiretroviral drugs in combination, a favorable response can be elicited in 60%–90% of antiretroviral-naive patients [23].

The main goal of HAART is to achieve a sustained reduction of viral burden to the lowest possible levels and, ideally, a complete viral suppression (HIV-1 RNA plasma levels under detection limits of 50–20 copies/ml). A rapid reduction (a few months) of viral burden under 20 copies/ml is related to a long-term response [24].

Current recommendations to start treatment for HIV infection are mainly based on viral burden and CD4+ T lymphocyte level [22, 23, 25]. However, all symptomatic patients should be treated, regardless of the viral burden or CD4+ T cell level. Patients with CD4+ cells less than $200 \times 10^6/l$, even if asymptomatic, should also be treated. Treatment can be postponed in asymptomatic patients with CD4+ levels greater than $350 \times 10^6/l$. In asymptomatic patients with CD4+ levels between 200 and $350 \times 10^6/l$, the decision to treat should be based on the rate of lymphocyte decrease, viral burden, and the preference of the patient. Sex is not a determinant of decision to treat.

Three groups of antiretroviral agents are currently in use, exerting activity on two HIV enzymes (reverse transcriptase and protease). The first group is that of the nucleoside reverse transcriptase inhibitors (NRTIs), comprising DDI, 3TC, D4T, DDC, and AZT. Another group is the non-nucleoside reverse transcriptase inhibitors (NNRTIs), including delavirdine, efavirenz, and nevirapine. The last group, the protease inhibitors (PIs), includes amprenavir, indinavir, nelfinavir, ritonavir, and saquinavir.

Current recommendations for initial combination antiretroviral therapy are the following [22, 23, 25]: two NRTIs plus one PI; two NRTIs plus one NNRTI; two PIs plus one or two NRTIs; one PI plus one NNRTI, with or without one or two NRTIs; three NRTIs. Regimens including PIs have the advantage of a high potency and the evidence of long-term efficacy (more than 3 years). However, there are also several drawbacks, such as their complexity, their toxic effects (metabolic, cardiovascular, etc.), and the possible appearance of cross-resistance within PIs, thus limiting the use of these drugs in future regimens. Non-PI combinations offer the advantage of sparing the most potent drugs; however, although initial efficacy seems to be similar, it has not been proved in the long term; in addition, resistance can appear more rapidly, and their toxic effects are not negligible. Therefore, treatment must be individualized, taking into consideration the advantages and disadvantages for each particular case.

Despite the efficacy of the treatment, HIV replication in latently infected resting T lymphocytes and other long-lived cell populations has been demonstrated. Even in patients with an undetectable viral burden for a long time, plasma HIV-1 RNA rebounds can occur after interruption of antiretroviral therapy [23, 25]. Thus, it seems unlikely that antiretroviral therapy alone can eradicate HIV.

Current research is directed at the design of more potent drugs, with less toxicity, which are better tolerated, and also with different targets (fusion inhibitors). At the same time, much work is in progress to increase the activity of antiretroviral therapy (hydroxyurea, cyclosporine) and to improve immunity against HIV (cytokine therapy, vaccines) [22, 25].

Opportunistic Infections

The introduction of HAART with at least three antiretroviral drugs has resulted in a major change in the prognosis and management of HIV infection. The incidence of some opportunistic infections (OI), such as PCP, disseminated *Mycobacterium avium* complex (MAC), or CMV, has been drastically reduced. Similarly, a decrease has been observed in other conditions, for which no effective treatment was available, such as KS, PML, and cryptosporidiosis [26].

OI are present in patients not receiving HAART or in those with failure of therapy. Likewise, immediately after starting antiretroviral therapy, a paradoxical increase of OI is observed, because the immune system has not yet recovered or due to the appearance of the so-called immune reconstitution syndrome (IRS). It has been reported that in some cases 2 weeks are enough to recover the immune response against OI [27]. IRS especially presents in severely immunosuppressed patients in the first 12–16 weeks after starting HAART, and is characterized by a severe inflammatory response. With effective antiretroviral therapy, with an adequate immunological and virological response, IRS determines the presence of clinical manifestations in patients with latent infections or a paradoxical deterioration of a patient with an OI under treatment. This syndrome has been reported in CMV, MAC, and *M. tuberculosis*, among others, as well as with PML and KS [28]. Treatment for IRS is not well defined, but steroids or non-steroidal anti-inflammatory drugs can be useful in severe cases, together with HAART and the corresponding etiological therapy for OI [26, 28]. In the rest of the chapter we shall review some of the OI that can cause admission to ICU among AIDS patients.

P. carinii

This is an eukaryotic micro-organism considered to be a fungus closely related to *Ascomycetes*. At present, several lines of evidence suggest that re-infection is a major cause of PCP in immunosuppressed individuals [29], presenting typically as a pneumonia in HIV-infected patients, while extrapulmonary disease is generally associated with the use of prophylactic inhaled pentamidine [30]. The risk of PCP markedly increases with CD4+ counts of less than $200 \times 10^6/l$ (relative risk 4.9 versus CD4+ count greater than $200 \times 10^6/l$) [31].

The course of the disease is generally insidious and the usual symptoms include fever, dry cough, and dyspnea. The characteristic radiographic findings of PCP are fine, bilateral perihiliar interstitial shadowing. However, chest radiographs can be normal or reveal pneumothorax, solitary nodules, or upper lobe shadowing. Use of inhaled pentamidine as prophylaxis has been associated with atypical radiographic findings [29]. High-resolution computed tomography (CT) is more sensitive than plain chest films for the diagnosis of PCP, with the typical findings being a mosaic pattern of ground-glass shadowing.

The gold standard for the diagnosis of PCP is detection of the micro-organism in respiratory tract samples. Since *P. carinii* cannot be cultured, diagnosis is made through direct observation of the organism by light microscopy or using monoclonal antibodies techniques. Fibrobronchoscopic bronchoalveolar lavage (BAL), with a diagnostic confirmatory rate of 79%–98%, is the reference technique for collecting samples [31], and when combined with transbronchial biopsy has a diagnostic yield near to 100% [32]. Induced sputum is an alternative to BAL, with a sensitivity of 55%–95% [31]. Studies based on induced sputum show a low sensitivity and poor diagnostic yield. In addition, use of the polymerase chain reaction (PCR) offers the possibility of improving the yield of non-invasive samples. However, PCR at present can only be considered a research tool, and it remains to be determined whether it will prove more cost-effective than BAL.

The main prognostic marker in PCP is blood oxygen level at the time of diagnosis. Patients with a PO_2 less than 70 mmHg or an alveolar-arterial gradient greater than 35 mmHg have an elevated risk of death, and their condition must be considered as moderate to severe.

The treatment of choice in all cases of PCP is trimethroprim-sulfamethoxazole (TMP-SMX) for 21 days [29, 32, 33] (Table 3). If a favorable response is observed, therapy can be continued via the oral route. Adverse events are frequent (rash, fever, liver enzyme elevation, neutropenia, thrombocytopenia, erythema multiforme, or renal toxicity), precluding treatment in 25%–50% of patients [32]. Given the high therapeutic efficacy of TMP-SMX, treatment must be continued as long as side effects are of moderate intensity, and desensitization is recommended in cases of hypersensitivity. When side effects are severe, alternative treatments include IV pentamidine and IV trimetrexate plus folinic acid (Table 3). Pentamidine can produce hypoglycemia, pancreatitis, diabetes

On the other hand, incidence of bacteremia among AIDS patients is also higher than in the general population; the usual agents are *S. pneumoniae, S. aureus, S. epidermidis, P. aeruginosa, H. influenzae,* and *Salmonella spp.* Pneumonia, followed by gastrointestinal infection and catheters, is the most frequent source [48]. Treatment of bacterial infection is not different in AIDS patients from immunocompetent patients.

Other Infections

Mycobacterial diseases [*Mycobacterium tuberculosis, Mycobacterium avium complex* (MAC)] are other OI that have experienced a resurgence with the AIDS epidemic. The progression rate of tuberculosis from latent infection to active disease is higher in the HIV-positive population (10% each year versus 5% after 2 years) [49]. The evolution is different depending on the country being analyzed. In Spain, tuberculosis still represents 40% of the initial AIDS-defining diseases, whereas MAC disease is of minor relevance [26, 28, 49]. These diseases, especially MAC, appear in stages of severe immunosuppression (CD4+ count less than $50x10^6$/l). The clinical presentation is generally atypical, as fever of unknown origin, extrapulmonary manifestations, or even as an immune reconstitution syndrome [26, 28, 49]. Pulmonary disease is generally seen in patients with higher CD4+ counts [28, 49]. A high index of suspicion is necessary, as diagnosis can be difficult. Tuberculosis skin testing can be negative in up to 40% of individuals with the disease [26, 28, 49]. Introduction of clarithromycin and azithromycin has produced a major change in treatment/prophylaxis of MAC disease [26, 28] (Table 3). Therapy for tuberculosis in AIDS patients does not differ significantly from that in the general population [28, 49, 50] (Table 3). However, it is necessary to know the frequent interactions of tuberculostatic agents with antiretroviral drugs, which may force changes in therapy, such as substituting rifampin for rifabutin, among others [28, 49, 50].

References

1. Gayle HD, Hill GL (2001) Global impact of human immunodeficiency virus and AIDS. Clin Microbiol Rev 14:327–335
2. Curtis JR, Bennett CL, Horner RD, Rubenfeld GD, DeHovitz JA, Weinstein RA (1998) Variations in intensive care unit utilization for patients with human immunodeficiency virus-related *Pneumocystis carinii* pneumonia: importance of hospital characteristics and geographic location. Crit Care Med 26:668–675
3. Casalino E, Mendoza-Sassi G, Wolff M, Bedos JP, Gaudebout C, Regnier B, Vachon F (1998) Predictors of short- and long-term survival in HIV-infected patients admitted

to the ICU. Chest 113:421–429

4. Nickas G, Wachter RM (2000) Outcomes of intensive care for patients with human immunodeficiency virus infection. Arch Intern Med 160:541–547

5. Afessa B, Green B (2000) Clinical course, prognostic factors, and outcome prediction for HIV patients in the ICU. The PIP (Pulmonary complications, ICU support, and prognostic factors in hospitalized patients with HIV) study. Chest 118:138–145

6. Wachter RM, Luce JM, Turner J, Volberding P, Hopewell PC (1986) Intensive care of patients with the acquired immunodeficiency syndrome. Outcome and changing patterns of utilization. Am Rev Respir Dis 134:891–896

7. Schein RM, Fischl MA, Pitchenik AE, Sprung CL (1986) ICU survival of patients with the acquired immunodeficiency syndrome. Crit Care Med 14:1026–1027

8. Alves C, Nicolas JM, Miro JM, Torres A, Agusti C, Gonzalez J, Rano A, Benito N, Moreno A, Garcia F, Milla J, Gatell JM (2001) Reappraisal of the aetiology and prognostic factors of severe acute respiratory failure in HIV patients. Eur Respir J 17:87–93

9. Skiest DJ (2002) Focal neurological disease in patients with acquired immunodeficiency syndrome. Clin Infect Dis 34:103–115

10. Thyrault M, Gachot B, Chastang C, Souweine B, Timsit JF, Bedos JP, Regnier B, Wolff M (1997) Septic shock in patients with the acquired immunodeficiency syndrome. Intensive Care Med 23:1018–1023

11. Rosenberg AL, Seneff MG, Atiyeh L, Wagner R, Bojanowski L, Zimmerman JE (2001) The importance of bacterial sepsis in intensive care unit patients with acquired immunodeficiency syndrome: implications for future care in the age of increasing antiretroviral resistance. Crit Care Med 29:548–556

12. Rerkpattanapipat P, Wongpraparut N, Jacobs LE, Kotler MN (2000) Cardiac manifestations of acquired immunodeficiency syndrome. Arch Intern Med 160:602–608

13. Choperena G, Arcega I, Marco P, Alberdi F, Azaldegui F, Alberola I, von Wichman MA (2001) One-year survival of HIV-positive patients admitted to the ICU before the era of combined antiretroviral therapy. Medicina Intensiva 25:263–268

14. Hogan CM, Hammer SM (2001) Host determinants in HIV infection and disease. 1. Cellular and humoral immune responses. Ann Intern Med 134:761–776

15. McMichael AJ, Rowland-Jones SL (2001) Cellular immune responses to HIV. Nature 410:980–987

16. Hogan CM, Hammer SM (2001) Host determinants in HIV infection and disease. 2. Genetic factors and implications for antiretroviral therapeutics. Ann Intern Med 134:978–996

17. McCune JM (2001) The dynamics of CD4+ T-cell depletion in HIV disease. Nature 410:974–979

18. Tranchat C, van de Perre P, Simonon-Sorel A, Karita E, Benchaib M, Lepage P, Desgranges C, Boyer V, Trepo C (1999) Maternal humoral factors associated with perinatal human immunodeficiency virus type-1 transmission in a cohort from Kigali, Rwanda, 1988-1994. J Infect 39:213–220

19. Lathey JL, Pratt RD, Spector SA (1997) Appearance of autologous neutralizing antibody correlates with reduction in virus load and phenotype switch during primary infection with human immunodeficiency virus type 1. J Infect Dis 175:231–232

20. Parren PW, Moore JP, Burton DR, Sattentau QJ (1999) The neutralizing antibody response to HIV-1: viral evasion and escape from humoral immunity. AIDS 13 [Suppl A]:S137–S162

21. Poignard P, Sabbe R, Picchio GR, Wang M, Gulizia RJ, Katinger H, Parren PW, Mosier DE, Burton DR (1999) Neutralizing antibodies have limited effects on the control of established HIV-1 infection in vivo. Immunity 10:431–438

22. Weller IV, Williams IG (2001) ABC of AIDS. Antiretroviral drugs. BMJ 322:1410–1412

Chapter 23

Therapy of Infection

J.H. ROMMES, A. SELBY, D.F. ZANDSTRA

Introduction

The appropriate treatment of an infection in the critically ill requires an understanding of the pathogenesis of infections (Chapter 5). Recent studies [1–6] using surveillance cultures from the throat and rectum to detect carrier states have revealed that infections due to microbial sources external to the patient rarely occur in the 1st week of treatment in the intensive care unit (ICU). The incidence of these types of infection, termed secondary endogenous and exogenous infections, varies between 15% and 40%.

In the case of secondary endogenous infections, potentially pathogenic micro-organisms (PPM), that are within the ICU but are not present in the patient's admission flora, are first acquired in the oropharynx due to transmission via the hands of health care workers. In the critically ill patient, oropharyngeal acquisition invariably leads to abnormal microbial carrier states in the throat, stomach, and gut (termed secondary or super-carriage). The subsequent build up to overgrowth, defined as $\geq 10^5$ PPM/ml of saliva and/or per gram of feces, can then result in colonization and infection of the normally sterile internal organs. This may take a few days. The degree of immunosuppression of the ICU patient determines the day on which colonization leads to an established secondary endogenous infection.

The other type of ICU infection, the exogenous infection, is equally due to breaches of hygiene procedures. Exogenous infections may occur at any time during the patient's treatment on the ICU. The causative bacteria are also acquired on the unit but are never present in the digestive tract of the critically ill. Long-stay patients, particularly those who receive a tracheostomy, are at high risk of exogenous pneumonias. Purulent lower airway secretions yield a PPM never previously carried by the patient in the oropharynx. Although the tracheostomy and the oropharynx both provide routes vulnerable to bacterial

Cultures to Ensure Identification of the Causative Micro-Organisms

Whilst 'empirical' treatment needs to be started immediately [9, 10], before the identity of the micro-organism is known, it is important that the appropriate measures are taken to identify the micro-organism(s) as soon as possible so that modification of the otherwise 'empirical' treatment can be undertaken as necessary. There are local issues as regards the site of infection, but the basic principles are the same. Before antibiotic administration, diagnostic samples of blood, urine, tracheal aspirate, and wounds, together with surveillance samples of the throat and rectum are collected.

Immediate and Adequate Antibiotic Treatment to Sterilize Internal Organs, Including Lungs and Blood

Immediately after obtaining surveillance and diagnostic samples, parenteral antibiotics should be started [9, 10]. Delivery of antibiotics must be reliable and this may only be realistic using parenterally administered antimicrobial agents that can sterilize infected internal organs. Orally administered drugs in critically ill patients are inevitably unpredictable with regards to absorption, due to dysfunction of the gastro-intestinal tract. If the patient was previously in reasonably good health, monotherapy with cefotaxime is sufficient as the patient carries 'normal' flora in the oropharynx and gut (Table 4). Patients who are

Table 4. Proposed strategy for management of suspected pneumonia during mechanical ventilation (*AGNB* aerobic Gram-negative bacilli)

Primary endogenous pneumonia	Secondary endogenous and exogenous pneumonia

PPM imported in patient's flora
A. Normal PPM
B. Abnormal PPM   i. AGNB
     ii. MRSA
     iii. *Pseudomonas* spp.
C. *Legionella, Mycoplasma* species
	PPM acquired on ICU
	
	B. Abnormal PPM i. AGNB
	     ii. MRSA
	     iii. *Pseudomonas* spp.

Antimicrobials
A. Cefotaxime/cephradine
B. (i) Cefotaxime/gentamicin
   (ii) Vancomycin
   (iii) Ceftazidime/gentamicin
C. Macrolides
	Antimicrobials
	Treatment depends on the pattern of resistance
	For sensitive organisms, see B (i–iii) opposite
	For multi-resistant organisms, treatment depends on local sensitivity patterns and antibiotic policy

Duration of treatment 7 days (or 5 days if SDD used simultaneously)	Duration of treatment 7 days (or 5 days if SDD used simultaneously)

admitted with a chronic underlying condition or who are transferred from another hospital or ward are usually carriers of abnormal flora, and hence require the parenteral administration of cefotaxime with gentamicin. In the case of an intra-abdominal infection, gentamicin and metronidazole are added to cefotaxime. Collections of pus, i.e., abscesses, require surgical drainage. On the next day, the clinical microbiologist is able to distinguish 'normal' from 'abnormal' potential pathogens. This information allows the intensivist to adjust the parenteral antimicrobials (Table 4). There is no evidence to support an antibiotic course exceeding 1 week [11].

The Source of Potential Pathogens Causing the Infection—whether Endogenous or Exogenous—Requires Elimination

In endogenous infections, the throat and gut of the critically ill are the *internal* sources of potential pathogens, whilst in exogenous infections the source of PPM is *external*, i.e., outside the patient. Abolishing the source of potential pathogens has two aims: a more rapid recovery of the original infection and the prevention of relapses and/or superinfections.

All patients expected to require a minimum of 3 days of mechanical ventilation, immediately receive selective decontamintion of the digestive tract (SDD) (Chapter 14). Oropharyngeal, gastro-intestinal, and vaginal carriage can be abolished by the administration of the non-absorbable polymyxin E, tobramycin, and amphotericin B (PTA), with the aim of eradicating the *internal* sources. SDD is usually continued until the patient is weaned from the ventilator and extubated. Identification and eradication of an *external* source is often more difficult and requires close cooperation between the intensivists, the nurses, and the infection control team.

Topical Antimicrobials for Delivering High Antibiotic Concentrations Directly to the Site of Infection

The topical application of antimicrobials is safe and contributes to a more-rapid killing of potential pathogens, resulting in cultures of colonized/infected sites becoming sterile earlier. For example, to increase the antimicrobial activity in the lower airway secretions topical therapy using aerosolized antibiotics should be considered [12]. Pastes with polymyxin, tobramycin, and amphotericin B can be applied topically to tracheostomies, gastrostomies, and pressure sores [13]. All topical antimicrobial agents mixed with a translucent gel aquaform can be applied in thin layers over fine mesh gauze to cover, for example, grafted burn wounds [14].

patients with a lower respiratory tract infection [9, 10]. Immediately after obtaining surveillance and diagnostic samples, systemic antibiotics should be started. An aminoglycoside and cefotaxime should provide adequate cover and be supplemented with topical antimicrobials (SDD). Cultures will hopefully follow and identify 'normal' or 'abnormal' PPM. The former can be treated with monotherapy, such as 5 days of cefotaxime. Monotherapy of infections caused by 'abnormal' PPM is associated with the emergence of resistant strains [26–28]. In this situation an aminoglycoside in combination with cefotaxime might be used (Table 4).

The topical application of antimicrobials by nebulization is safe and contributes to a more rapid killing of PPM, resulting in cultures of the tracheal aspirate becoming sterile earlier [12]. To increase the antimicrobial activity in the lower airway secretions, topical therapy, using aerosolized antibiotics, should be considered.

A placebo-controlled trial showed that nebulized delivery of aerosolized antibiotics in combination with systemic antibiotics resulted in a significantly more rapid eradication of aerobic Gram-negative bacilli from the tracheal aspirate [29]. The doses of the different aerosolized antimicrobials are shown in Table 5. Relatively high doses are applied to the airways, as less than 5% of the aerosolized drug reaches the terminal airways [30]. Tracheal aspirate is obtained daily until cultures are negative. To prevent recolonization of the lower airways, the tracheal tube should be replaced after 3 days. Systemic antibiotics and nebulized antimicrobials are discontinued when the cultures are clear; usually this is within 5 days.

Atypical pneumonia. If a patient admitted with a primary endogenous lower respiratory tract infection does not improve on this antibacterial therapy with-

Table 5. Doses of aerosolized antimicrobials

Antimicrobial agent	Dose (mg/5 ml)	Interval (h)
Cefotaxime	500	6
Gentamicin	40	6
Tobramycin	40	6
Ceftazidime	500	6
Cephradine	500	6
Colistin (polymyxin E)	20	6
Amphotericine B	5	6
Vancomycin	250	6

in 24–48 h and all cultures are sterile, the possibility of an atypical pneumonia, e.g., *Legionella pneumophila*, should be considered and investigated [31, 32] (Table 4).

Eradication of the source of the PPM is an important component of an effective treatment of respiratory tract infections. Contaminated ventilators, humidifiers, and sinks are potential sources of external PPM. Breaches of hygiene by care givers, particularly during busy periods, may lead to increased transmission of micro-organisms and a higher exogenous infection rate.

Sepsis

Sepsis is the clinical picture caused by a generalized inflammation due to micro-organisms and/or their toxic products. The clinical diagnosis of sepsis (synonymous with the sepsis syndrome) is based on the following clinical criteria: increased heart rate, tachypnea or impaired gas exchange, fever or hypothermia, symptoms of decreased organ perfusion, and clinical suspicion of an infection. The clinical picture is caused by the release of inflammatory mediators into the circulation, i.e., cytokinemia. Blood cultures are always sterile.

Septicemia and Septic Shock

Septicemia is defined as sepsis combined with a positive blood culture. Septic shock is defined as sepsis in combination with the clinical signs of cardiovascular collapse.

Once the diagnosis of sepsis, septicemia, or septic shock has been made and appropriate cultures taken, immediate combination therapy to provide an adequate spectrum of antibacterial activity should be commenced. This might be a combination of an aminoglycoside with cefotaxime for example. If an intra-abdominal focus is suspected metronidazole is added to this treatment.

The combination does not cover low-level pathogens, including enterococci, and may be ineffective against *P. aeruginosa*. The initial 'empirical' therapy is adjusted according to the results of the diagnostic cultures (Table 4). The source of sepsis should be identified and eliminated as soon as possible. SDD using enteral PTA should be commenced immediately to eradicate small intestinal overgrowth responsible for translocation.

Intra-Abdominal Infection

Intra-abdominal infection is defined as infection of an abdominal organ and the peritoneal cavity (peritonitis) with local signs such as abdominal tenderness and generalized symptoms including fever and leukocytosis. Peritonitis can be a localized or generalized infection of the peritoneal cavity. Following ultrasonography and computed tomography, the diagnosis is confirmed by the isolation of micro-organisms of ≥3+ or ≥10^5 CFU/ml and ≥ 2+ leukocytes in the diagnostic sample. Drainage of the site of infection should be performed as soon as possible by the surgeon or interventional radiologist.

Again the six basic principles should be applied [33, 34].

1. Suitable cultures to ensure later identification of the organism should be taken.
2. A suitable spectrum of systemic antibiotic cover such as an aminoglycoside with cefotaxime and metronidazole should be administered to empirically cover the likely organisms. This empirical therapy is adjusted when results become available.
3. The source should be eradicated with SDD. Eradication of PPM from the gut of patients with peritonitis is difficult due to the absence of motility and the anatomy and physiology is often disturbed due to surgical intervention. Decontamination of the gut in that subset of patients is not impossible but requires commitment and tenacity by the ICU team. Blind loops are decontaminated with SDD suspension containing 40 mg tobramycin, 50 mg polymyxin E, and 500 mg amphotericin B administered via the stoma. In the case of overgrowth in the rectum, i.e., ≥10^5 CFU/ml of PPM, SDD enemas are administered twice daily until surveillance cultures are free from PPM (Chapter 14).
4. During laparotomy and repeat laparotomy the abdominal cavity is extensively rinsed with a disinfecting agent, 2% taurolin [35].
5. All potentially contaminated devices may act as a source of infection and should be removed or replaced.
6. Treatment is evaluated by ongoing surveillance.

Wound Infection

The clinical signs of a wound infection are purulent discharge, redness, swelling, tenderness, and local warmth. The clinical diagnosis is confirmed by the isolation of ≥3 or ≥10^5 micro-organisms and ≥2+ leukocytes in the purulent discharge of the wound [36]. The use of systemic antimicrobial therapy is seldom indicated in the treatment of wound infections, unless symptoms of sepsis, septicemia, or septic shock occur. Local treatment, drainage, debridement, and removal of plastic devices is essential and generally sufficient. Following local treatment the wounds are rinsed twice daily with a disinfectant, 2% taurolin, for 3 days.

Aquaform gel mixed with 2% PTA and/or vancomycin can be applied to colonized/infected wounds [14].

Bloodstream Infection Associated with Contaminated Intravascular Lines

The diagnosis of catheter-related bloodstream infection is based on one of the following [37]: (1) at least two positive blood cultures before catheter removal and persistently negative cultures after removal of the line; (2) isolation of the same micro-organism from two of the following three sites: blood drawn via the suspected line, blood drawn from a peripheral vein, or from the catheter tip; (3) quantitative blood cultures drawn via the central venous line and a peripheral vein reveal the same micro-organism in a ratio of greater than 5:1.

Recommendations vary but some authors suggest that 'it would be unusual for central venous catheters to be left in situ for more than 7 days' [38]. A recent meta-analysis made no specific recommendations but advised randomized trials of catheter management [39].

The only effective treatment of a catheter-related bloodstream infection is removal of the contaminated line. The predominant micro-organisms involved in this type of infection are the low-level pathogens coagulase-negative staphylococci and enterococci. Systemic treatment with antimicrobials is seldom indicated even if PPM such as aerobic Gram-negative bacilli and yeasts are involved in the bloodstream infection. If the diagnosis of catheter-related infection is correct, clinical signs of infection, particularly temperature, will normalize within 24 h.

More complex is the patient with a prosthetic heart valve who develops a catheter-related bloodstream infection. If the signs of infection (fever, increased C-reactive protein, leukocytosis) do not resolve within 24 h of removal of the contaminated catheter, an aggressive approach is indicated. Combination therapy with vancomycin and gentamicin should be commenced. If ultrasonography reveals vegetations, antibiotic treatment should be continued for 3 weeks. If after 3 weeks' treatment clinical evaluation reveals signs of a persistent infection, a second course of antimicrobials is given, often following surgical replacement of the prosthetic heart valve [40].

Urinary Tract Infection

Urinary tract infection is defined as infection of the mucosa of the lower urinary tract, i.e., urethra and bladder. The appearance of turbid urine in the catheter and collecting bag should raise suspicion of a urinary tract infection. Sometimes systemic signs such as fever and leukocytosis may occur, particularly when obstruction or lesions of the bladder are present. In the diagnostic urine sample $\geq 10^5$ CFU of a micro-organism are detected together with $\geq 2+$ leukocytes.

Urinary tract infections in the critically ill are relatively uncommon, in part because most systemic antibiotics are excreted via the kidney, reaching high concentrations in the urine and therefore sterilizing the bladder. When the diagnosis of lower urinary tract infection is made, the combination of an aminoglycoside and cefotaxime should provide reasonably comprehensive cover. An essential part of the treatment is replacement of the urinary catheter after 24 h of treatment.

To prevent new infections the patient is treated with SDD. Vaginal carriage can be the source of PPM causing bladder infections in women. Successful decontamination of the vagina is confirmed by negative surveillance cultures of the vagina. If a patient develops a urinary tract infection with 'abnormal' PPM while the throat and rectum are free of PPM, an external source, such as urinometer, or breaches of hygiene during catheterization must be investigated in order to prevent relapses.

Management of Infections caused by MRSA

The classical SDD protocol comprising parenteral cefotaxime and enteral polymyxin E, tobramycin, and amphotericin B is not designed to control infections by MRSA; for which the addition of enteral vancomycin is required [41–45].

The policy of surveillance cultures of the throat and rectum combined with enteral vancomycin in managing MRSA in 'at risk' patients is analogous to the way in which aerobic Gram-negative bacillary and fungal carriage is managed by the enteral antimicrobials polymyxin E, tobramycin, and amphotericin B. It should be remembered that the principal aim of enteral non-absorbable antimicrobials is the eradication of carriage in overgrowth of potential pathogens, including MRSA. Thus, enteral vancomycin not only eliminates a prime source of endogenous MRSA infection in 'at risk' patients, but also profoundly influences the dissemination and subsequent hand contamination with MRSA, within the ICU.

Table 6 shows the components of the MRSA eradication protocol. These include *surveillance samples* to detect the asymptomatic oropharyngeal and gut carrier. These are crucial in the control of antibiotic resistance. Regular surveillance cultures on admission and throughout treatment on the ICU, e.g., Monday and Thursday, allow the detection of the asymptomatic MRSA carriers at an 'early' stage, allowing the immediate implementation of isolation, barrier precautions, and enteral vancomycin. Relying solely on diagnostic samples of blood, tracheal aspirate, urine, and pus results in an inherent and substantial delay that permits dissemination to other patients and maintains endemicity. A

Table 6. MRSA eradication protocol

I.   Surveillance samples to detect carriers of MRSA
      Obtain swabs from nose, throat and rectum

II.   Enteral/topical vancomycin to eradicate carriage
      1. Treatment of MRSA carrier (5 days)
          a) Nasal carriage: 2% mupirocin cream 4 times a day or 2% vancomycin cream 4
             times a day
          b) Oropharyngeal carriage: 4% vancomycin paste (0.5 g) 4 times a day, or 4% van-
             comycin gel (0.5 g) 4 times a day, or 5 mg vancomycin lozenges 4 times a day
          c) Gastrointestinal carriage: 40 mg/kg per day oral solution in four doses
          d) Skin carriage: 4% chlorhexidine bath/shower on alternate days
      2. Treatment of colonization/infection (3 days)
          a) Tracheostomy, gastrostomy: 4% vancomycin paste 2 times a day; change
             foreign body
          b) Lower airways: nebulized vancomycin 4 mg/kg per dose, 4 times a day diluted
             in normal saline. Patient must receive a dose of nebulized salbutamol prior to
             vancomycin because of the risk of bronchoconstriction reported

III. Limiting use of flucloxacillin to lift selection pressure on MRSA

IV.   High level of anti-staphylococcal hygiene including hand washing and device policy

---

shift from diagnostic towards pre-emptive surveillance samples is required to avoid wasting time in the control of MRSA spread. Nasal surveillance has to be supplemented with digestive tract surveillance, as gut carriage of MRSA cannot be ignored [46].

Enteral/topical vancomycin is used to eradicate carriage. The application of a 4% vancomycin paste or gel has been found to be effective in eradicating oropharyngeal carriage of MRSA; the administration of a vancomycin solution (40 mg/kg per day) through the nasogastric tube readily clears gut carriage. Intranasal mupinocin or vancomycin is indicated to eradicate nasal carriage and 4% chlorhexidine liquid soap is used to clear skin carriage.

   MRSA has an affinity for both intact and damaged skin, particularly when a plastic device such as a tracheostomy or gastrostomy is present [47, 48]. After removal and replacement, a 4% vancomycin paste is required to treat colonization and/or infection. In lower airway colonization/infection, aerosolised vancomycin should be delivered via the endotracheal tube.

Use of flucloxacillin should be limited to lift selection pressure on MRSA. In general, improved antibiotic utilization to limit selective pressure is not that difficult, but unfortunately receives little consideration in therapeutic decision making. Protection of the indigenous flora is required to control the overgrowth of MRSA. Cephradine is preferred as the first line anti-staphylococcal agent, as flucloxacillin disrupts gut ecology to a greater extent than cephradine [49].

A high level of anti-staphylococcal hygiene is important. Improved adherence to infection control practices, in particular hand hygiene, cannot be overstated, to control transmission of MRSA via the hands of carers. It is highly likely that hand washing will be more effective in the prevention of MRSA transmission in units that implement the new approach. Carriers who receive enteral vancomycin have significantly less MRSA on their skin, so the risk of contaminating the carer's hands is less and the level of contamination is lower making hand washing more effective.

Staphylococci, both coagulase positive and negative, have an *affinity for plastic devices*. Most patients who require long-term intensive care have indwelling devices, including intubation tubes, intravascular lines, urinary catheters, tracheostomy and/or gastrostomy. The chance that these devices become contaminated with MRSA is substantial in a patient who is a carrier of MRSA in the nose, throat, gut, and skin [47, 48]. A strict device policy is required on the ICU. Devices are changed immediately if diagnostic samples are positive for MRSA, e.g., in the case of positive tracheal aspirates, the ventilation tube is replaced; in the case of a positive blood culture taken through an indwelling vascular line or a positive vascular catheter site swab, the intravascular lines are removed and replaced.

Evidence for This Protocol

What is the evidence that the above approach of the treatment of infections in critically ill patients is superior to the traditional treatment, i.e., only systemic antimicrobials? There are only three reports available that have evaluated the efficacy of SDD in combination with systemic antimicrobials in primarily infected patients [50–52].

One hundred and thirty-five patients who were all infected on admission to the ICU were randomly assigned to receive SDD in addition to systemic antibiotics versus solely parenteral antibiotics [50]. The design was double-blind, placebo-controlled. There were significantly more infected patients in the placebo group (32/76=42%) compared with the test group (13/59=22%, $P=0.048$). In both groups *Acinetobacter baumannii* caused exogenous lower airway infections: 6 in the SDD group, 12 in the placebo group. All these patients received early tracheostomies.

In total 25 patients with pneumonia due to aerobic Gram-negative bacilli were treated using the full SDD protocol [51]. The lower airways were sterile in 24 patients within a median of 5 days. The cure rate was 96%. Two patients had a relapse. Neither carriage of resistant PPM nor superinfections was observed.

Outcome data retrieved from the Dutch National Database in patients who were admitted with established pneumonia to the ICU show a significant survival benefit in the patients who cared for on ICUs using SDD [52]. The mortality rate was 28.4% in the group of 229 patients with pneumonia on admission and who were treated traditionally, without SDD. In comparison, the death rate was 14.6% in the 103 pneumonia patients treated with both topical and systemic antibiotics (P=0.008). In addition, both ICU stay and hospital stay were significantly shorter in the decontaminated group. These promising results need to be confirmed in properly designed trials.

Safety and Costs of This Protocol

The most recent meta-analysis includes 36 randomized controlled trials in 6,922 patients, and shows that SDD reduces the odds ratio for pneumonia to 0.35 [95% confidence interval (CI) 0.29–0.41] and mortality to 0.78 (95% CI 0.68–0.89) [53]. In order to prevent 1 case of pneumonia 5 ICU patients need to be treated with SDD and 21 ICU patients need to be treated to prevent 1 death. Two recent large randomized controlled trials report an absolute mortality reduction of 8%, corresponding to the treatment of 12 patients with SDD to save 1 life [54, 55]. There was no clinically significant harmful effect of SDD in any of the trials in terms of diarrhea due to *Clostridium difficile*. In addition, the safety of SDD relies on the long-term level of resistance against the SDD antimicrobials remaining low. Antimicobial resistance among aerobic Gram-negative bacilli has never been a problem over a period of 17 years of clinical ICU research. Five SDD studies prospectively evaluated resistance for 2, 2.5, 4, 6, and 7 years [56–60]. No increase in the rate of superinfections due to resistant aerobic Gram-negative bacilli could be demonstrated. The latest randomized controlled trial, evaluating SDD in about 1,000 patients, had significantly fewer carriers of multi-resistant aerobic Gram-negative bacilli in the patients receiving SDD than the control group [55]. Finally, the cost per survivor represents a useful endpoint in any such exercise, and four randomized studies employing this measure found it to be substantially lower in patients receiving SDD than among those managed traditionally [61–64]. This favorable outcome is due to reduced morbidity, less use of systemic antibiotics and blood products, and a higher proportion of survivors.

References

1. Murray AE, Chambers JJ, van Saene HKF (1998) Infections in patients requiring ventilation in intensive care: application of a new classification. Clin Microbiol Infect 4:94–99

2. Silvestri L, Monti Bragadin C, Milanese M et al (1999) Are most ICU-infections really nosocomial? A prospective observational cohort study in mechanically ventilated patients. J Hosp Infect 42:125–135

3. de la Cal MA, Cerda E, Garcia-Hierro P et al (2001) Pneumonia in patients with severe burns. A classification according to the concept of the carrier state. Chest 119:1160–1165

4. Petros AJ, O'Connell M, Roberts C et al (2001) Systemic antibiotics fail to clear multidrug-resistant *Klebsiella* from a paediatric ICU. Chest 119:862–866

5. Silvestri L, Sarginson RE, Hughes J et al (2002) Most nosocomial pneumonias are not due to nosocomial bacteria in ventilated patients. Evaluation of the accuracy of the 48h time cut-off using carriage as the gold standard. Anaesth Intensive Care 30:275–282

6. Sarginson RE, Taylor N, Reilly N et al (2004) Infection in prolonged pediatric critical illness: a prospective four-year study based on knowledge of the carrier state. Crit Care Med 32:839–847

7. Angus DC, Linde-Zwirble WT, Lidicker J et al (2001) Epidemiology of severe sepsis in the United States: analysis of incidence, outcome and associated costs of care. Crit Care Med 29:1303–1310

8. Brawley RL, Weber DJ, Samsa GP et al (1989) Multiple nosocomial infections. Am J Epidemiol 130:769–780

9. Torres A, Aznar R, Gatell JM et al (1990) Incidence, risk and prognosis factors of nosocomial pneumonia in mechanically ventilated patients. Am Rev Respir Dis 142:523–528

10. Alvarez-Lerma F and ICU-Acquired Pneumonia Group (1996) Modification of empiric antibiotic treatment in patients with pneumonia acquired in the intensive care unit. Intensive Care Med 22:387–394

11. Chastre J, Wolff M, Fagon JY et al (2003) Comparison of 8 versus 15 days of antibiotic therapy for ventilator associated pneumonia in adults. A randomised trial. JAMA 290:2588–2598

12. Palmer LB, Smaldone GC, Simon SR et al (1998) Aerolized antibiotics in mechanically ventilated patients: delivery and response. Crit Care Med 26:31–39

13. Morar P, Makura Z, Jones AS et al (2000) Topical antibiotics on tracheostoma prevents exogenous colonization and infection of lower airways in children. Chest 117:513–518

14. Desai MH, Rutan RL, Heggers JP et al (1992) *Candida* infection with and without nystatin prophylaxis. Arch Surg 127:159–162

15. Brown EM (1997) Empirical antimicrobial therapy of mechanically ventilated patients with nosocomial pneumonia. J Antimicrob Chemother 40:463–468

16. A'Court CHD, Garrard CS, Crook D et al (1993) Microbiological lung surveillance in mechanically ventilated patients, using non-directed bronchial lavage and quantitative culture. Q J Med 86:635–648

17. Montravers P, Fagon JY, Chastre J et al (1993) Follow-up protected specimen brushes to assess treatment in nosocomial pneumonia. Am Rev Respir Dis 147:38–44

18. Singh N, Rogers P, Atwood CW et al (2000) Short course empiric antibiotic therapy for patients with pulmonary infiltrates in the intensive care unit: a proposed solution for indiscriminate antibiotic prescription. Am J Respir Crit Care Med 162:505–511

19. Dennesen PJW, van der Ven AJAM, Kessels AGH et al (2001) Resolution of infectious parameters after antimicrobial therapy in patients with ventilator-associated pneumonia. Am J Respir Crit Care Med 163:1371-1375

20. Ledingham IMac, Alcock SR, Eastaway AT et al (1988) Triple regimen of selective decontamination of the digestive tract, systemic cefotaxime and microbiological surveillance for prevention of acquired infection in intensive care. Lancet I:785-790

21. Holzapfel L, Chevret S, Madivier G et al (1993) Influence of long-term oro- or nasotracheal intubation on nosocomial maxillary sinusitis and pneumonia: results of a prospective randomised clinical trial. Crit Care Med 21:1132-1138

22. Rouby JJ, Laurent P, Gosnach M et al (1994) Risk factors and clinical relevance of nosocomial maxillary sinusitis in the critically ill. Am Rev Respir Crit Care Med 150:776-783

23. Ramphal R, Small PM, Shands JW et al (1980) Adherence of *Pseudomonas aeruginosa* to tracheal cells injured by influenza infection or by endotracheal intubation. Infect Immun 27:614-619

24. van Saene HKF, Ashworth M, Petros AJ et al (2004) Do not suction, above the cuff. Crit Care Med 32:2160-2162

25. Torres A, Ewig S (2004) Diagnosing ventilator-associated pneumonia. N Engl J Med 350:433-435

26. Clone LA, Woodward DR, Stolzman DS (1985) Ceftazidime versus tobramycin/ticarcillin in the treatment of pneumonia and bacteremia. Antimicrob Agents Chemother 28:33-36

27. Ewig S, Torres A, El-Ebiary M et al (1999) Bacterial colonization patterns in mechanically ventilated patients with traumatic and medical head injury. Am J Respir Crit Care Med 159:188-198

28. Fink MP, Snydman DR, Niederman MS (1994) Treatment of severe pneumonia in hospitalised patients: results of a multicenter, randomised, double-blind trial comparing intravenous ciprofloxacin with imipenem-cilastin. Antimicrob Agents Chemother 38:547-557

29. Brown RB, Kruse JA, Counts GW (1990) Double-blind study of endotracheal tobramycin in the treatment of gram-negative pneumonia. Antimicrob Agents Chemother 34:269-272

30. Stoutenbeek CP (1987) Infection prevention in intensive care. PhD thesis. Van Denderen BV Groningen, The Netherlands

31. Ortqvist A, Sterner G, Nilsson JA (1985) Severe community-acquired pneumonia: factors influencing need of intensive care treatment and prognosis. Scan J Infect Dis 17:377-386

32. Torres A, Serra-Batles J, Ferrer A et al (1991) Severe community-acquired pneumonia. Am Rev Respir Dis 144:312-318

33. Marshall JC, Innes M (2003) Intensive care unit management of intra-abdominal infection. Crit Care Med 31:2228-2237

34. Lamme B, Boermeester MA, Reitsma JB et al (2002) Meta-analysis of relaparotomy for secondary peritonitis. Br J Surg 89:1516-1524

35. Gormans SP, McCafferty DF, Woolfson AD (1987) Reduced adherence of micro-organisms to human mucosal epithelial cells following treatment with taurolin, a novel antimicrobial agent. J Appl Bacteriol 62:315-320

36. Weber JM, Sheridan RL, Pasternack MS et al (1997) Nosocomial infections in pediatric patients with burns. Am J Infect Control 25:195-201

37. Kurkchubasche AG, Smith MD, Rowe MI (1992) Catheter-sepsis in short bowel syndrome. Arch Surg 127:21-25

38. Elliott TSJ, Faroqui MH, Armstrong RF et al (1994) Guidelines for good practice in central venous catheterisation. J Hosp Infect 28:163–176
39. Cook D, Randolph A, Kemerman P et al (1997) Central venous catheter replacement strategies: a systemic review of the literature. Crit Care Med 25:1417–1424
40. Eykyn SJ (1997) Infective endocarditis: some popular tenets debunked? Heart 77:191–193
41. Silvestri L, Milanese M, Oblach L et al (2002) Enteral vancomycin to control methicillin-resistant *Staphylococcus aureus* outbreak in mechanically ventilated patients. Am J Infect Control 30:391–399
42. de la Cal MA, Cerda E, van Saene HKF et al (2004) Effectiveness and safety of enteral vancomycin to control endemicity of methicillin-resistant *Staphylococcus aureus* in a medical/surgical intensive care unit. J Hosp Infect 56:175–183
43. Silvestri L, van Saene HKF, Milanese M et al (2004) Prevention of MRSA pneumonia by oral vancomycin decontamination: a randomised trial. Eur Respir J 23:921–926
44. Sanchez M, Mir N, Canton R et al (1997) The effect of topical vancomycin on acquisition, carriage and infection with methicillin-resistant *Staphylococcus aureus* in critically ill patients. A double-blind, randomised, placebo-controlled study (abstract). Abstracts of the 37th ICAAC, Toronto, Canada, p 310
45. Solis A, Brown D, Hughes J et al (2003) Methicillin-resistant *Staphylococcus aureus* in children with cystic fibrosis: an eradication protocol. Pediatr Pulmonol 36:189–195
46. Coello R, Jimenez J, Garcia M et al (1994) Prospective study of infection, colonization and carriage of methicillin-resistant *Staphylococcus aureus* in an outbreak affecting 990 patients. Eur J Clin Microbiol Infect Dis 13:74–81
47. Steinberg JP, Clark CC, Hackman BO (1996) Nosocomial and community-acquired staphylococcus bacteremias from 1980 to 1993: impact of intravascular devices and methicillin-resistance. Clin Infect Dis 23:255–259
48. Chang FY, Singh N, Gayowski T et al (1998) *Staphylococcus aureus* nasal colonisation in patients with cirrhosis: prospective assessment of association with infection. Infect Control Hosp Epidemiol 19:328–332
49. de Man P, Verhoeven BA, Verbrugh HA et al (2000) An antibiotic policy to prevent emergence of resistant bacilli. Lancet 355:973–978
50. Hammond JMJ, Potgieter PD (1995) Is there a role for selective decontamination of the digestive tract in primarily infected patients in the ICU? Anaesth Intensive Care 23:168–174
51. Stoutenbeek CP, van Saene HKF, Miranda DR (1986) Nosocomial gram-negative pneumonia in critically ill patients. Intensive Care Med 12:419–423
52. Zandstra DF, van Saene HKF, Bosman RJ (2001) Pneumonia management in the ICU: an integrated approach. In: van Saene HKF, Sganga G, Silvestri L (eds). Infection in the critically ill: an ongoing challenge. Springer Verlag, Milan, pp 1–7
53. Liberati A, D'Amico R, Pifferi S et al (2004) Antibiotic prophylaxis to reduce respiratory tract infections and mortality in adults receiving intensive care. Cochrane Review, The Cochrane Library, Issue 1. Wiley, Chichester
54. Krueger WA, Lenhart FD, Neeser G et al (2002) Influence of combined intravenous and topical antibiotic prophylaxis on the incidence of infections, organ dysfunctions, and mortality in critically ill surgical patients: a prospective, stratified, randomised double-blind, placebo-controlled clinical trial. Am J Respir Crit Care Med 166:1029–1037
55. de Jonge E, Schultz MJ, Spanjaard L et al (2003) Effects of selective decontamination of digestive tract on mortality and acquisition of resistant bacteria in intensive care: a randomised controlled trial. Lancet 362:1011–1016
56. Hammond JMJ, Potgieter PD (1995) Long-term effects of selective decontamination on antimicrobial resistance. Crit Care Med 23:637–645

57.　Stoutenbeek CP, Van Saene HKF, Zandstra DF (1987) The effects of oral nonabsorbable antibiotics on the emergence of resistant bacteria in patients in an intensive care unit. J Antimicrob Chemother 19:513–520

58.　Lingnau W, Berger J, Javorsky F et al (1998) Changing bacterial ecology during a five year period of selective intestinal decontamination. J Hosp Infect 39:195–206

59.　Leone M, Albanese J, Antonini F et al (2003) Long-term (6-year) effect of selective decontamination on antimicrobial resistance in intensive care, multiple-trauma patients. Crit Care Med 31:2090–2095

60.　Tetteroo GWM, Wagenvoort JHT, Bruining HA (1994) Bacteriology of selective decontamination: efficacy and rebound colonisation. J Antimicrob Chemother 34:139–148

61.　Rocha LA, Martin MJ, Pita S (1992) Prevention of nosocomial infections in critically ill patients by selective decontamination of the digestive tract. A randomised, double blind, placebo controlled study. Intensive Care Med 18:398–404

62.　Korinek A, Laisne MJ, Nicolas MH, Raskine L, Deroin V, Sanson-Lepors MJ (1993) Selective decontamination of the digestive tract in neurosurgical intensive care unit patients. A double blind, randomised, placebo controlled study. Crit Care Med 21:1466–1473

63.　Stoutenbeek CP, van Saene HKF, Zandstra DF (1996) Prevention of multiple organ system failure by selective decontamination of the digestive tract in multiple trauma patients. In: Faist E, Baue AE, Schildberg FW (eds) Immune consequences of trauma, shock and sepsis. Pabst, Lengerich, pp 1055–1066

64.　Sanchez Garcia M, Cambronero Galache JA, Lopez Dias J et al (1998) Effectiveness and cost of selective decontamination of the digestive tract in critically ill patients. A randomized, double-blind, placebo-controlled, multicenter trial. Am J Respir Crit Care Med 158:908–916

SECTION FIVE
SPECIAL TOPICS

Chapter 24

SIRS, Sepsis, and MODS

G. Berlot, A. Tomasini, M. Viviani

For decades, a number of different terms, such as sepsis and septicaemia, derived from the ancient Greek term indicating putrefaction, have been used to indicate the clinical conditions associated with severe infections [1]. This lack of uniformity was due to extreme heterogeneity of the infection-related systemic signs and symptoms, ranging from mild fever to severe cardiovascular collapse. As a consequence, although every minimally experienced physician could distinguish between a moderately sick patient with pneumonia and a critically ill patient dying in septic shock, the intermediate degrees of severity were much less well defined. Further confusion was added by the suffix "-aemia", derived from the Greek word indicating the blood; it was generally held that the presence of germs in the bloodstream was the only factor responsible for the disturbances involving the whole organism; only recently has it become clear that (1) these are primarily related to the interaction between the germs and the host's immune system, leading to the production and the release of a host of mediators with either pro- or anti-inflammatory properties, and that (2) this process can occur everywhere in the body, and the resulting systemic disturbances are related to the spillover of these substances from the initial site of reaction [2].

In the late 1980s and in the early 1990s the interest of intensivists was captured by two remarkable developments. First, the basic mechanisms underlying the septic process were elucidated, and a number of endogenous molecules responsible for the related symptoms were isolated; moreover, it became clear that the very same symptoms associated with the most-severe infections could be present in a number of non-infectious conditions, including acute pancreatitis, postoperative status, etc. A systemic inflammatory reaction involving the whole organism appeared as a final common pathway linking both conditions. Second, a number of different molecules aimed at inhibiting the putative mediators of this process became available. Preliminary experimental results in different models of sepsis, as well as in a small number of patients, were encouraging, and large, internationals trials with different molecules were initiated. Consequently, more-precise definitions of the degrees of severity of the infection-related conditions were needed, in order to compare and to track the clinical course of patients enrolled in clinical trials running in different countries and treated with these novel substances. Under the auspices of the American Society of Chest Physicians (ACCM) and of the Society of Critical Care Medicine (SCCM), a consensus conference was then held which ultimately established a number of definitions to describe different clinical settings (Table 1) [2, 3]. At the same time, the definition of multipe organ dysfunction syndrome (MODS) replaced the multiple organ failure (MOF) to indicate that the derangement of two or more organs cannot be considered an all-or-nothing phenomenon, but rather a progressive (and hopefully reversible) loss of function occurring along a continuum.

The proposed definitions were not uniformly accepted and were challenged primarily on the basis of their low diagnostic specificity, as the same symptoms can occur both following severe infections and in non-inflammatory conditions, such as strenuous exercise, drug intoxication, heat stroke, etc [4-6]. Other authors, albeit recognizing their limitations, considered them valuable as they set some standards, thus allowing intensivists from all over the world to use a common language [7, 8].

Recently, several North American and European intensive care societies agreed to revisit the definitions for sepsis and related conditions in a conference including 29 participants. The published document reflected a process whereby a group of experts and opinion leaders revisited the 1992 sepsis guidelines and found that apart from expanding the list of sign and symptoms of sepsis to reflect clinical bedside experience, no evidence exited to support a change to the definitions [9].

In this chapter, the advantages as well as the shortcomings of these definitions will be reviewed and discussed, on the basis of the following questions:
- Do these definitions describe clinical settings with different courses and outcomes?
- Do these definitions reflect different physiopathological conditions?
- Can the diagnostic tools available 10 years ago still be considered valuable to differentiate between infectious and non-infectious conditions?

Put in other words, is it wise to choose among different treatments only relying upon the ACCP- SCCM definitions?

Table 1. ACCP/SCCM Consensus Conference definitions of sepsis, severe sepsis, and septic shock. Modified from reference [3]

Definitions	Features	Possible clinical settings
Systemic inflammatory response syndrome (SIRS)	The systemic inflammatory response to a wide variety of severe clinical insults, manifested by 2 or more of the following conditions: 1. Temperature> 38°C or < 36°C 2. Heart rate> 90 bpm 3. Respiratory rate> 20 breaths/min or $PaCO_2$ < 32 mmHg 4. White blood cell count> 12,000/ml or < 4,000/ml or> 10% immature forms	Acute pancreatitis Status post repair of ruptured aortic aneurysm Acute vasculitis Postoperative status Burns Trauma
Sepsis	The systemic inflammatory response to a documented infection. The clinical manifestations should include 2 or more of the following signs as a result of a clinical infection: 1. Temperature> 38°C or < 36°C 2. Heart rate> 90 bpm 3. Respiratory rate> 20 breaths/min or $PaCO_2$ < 32 mmHg 4. White blood cell count> 12,000/ml or < 4,000/ml or> 10% immature forms	Uncomplicated pneumonia Urinary infections Uncomplicated appendicitis
Severe sepsis	SIRS or sepsis associated with signs of organ dysfunction or hypoperfusion, including, but not limited, to lactic acidosis, hypotension, oliguria or acute deterioration of the mental status	Complicated pneumonia or abdominal infection
Septic shock	Sepsis-induced hypotension unresponsive to fluid resuscitation, along with signs of organ dysfunction, hypoperfusion and hypotension, including, but not limited, to lactic acidosis, hypotension, oliguria or acute deterioration of the mental status	Peritonitis
Multiple organ dysfunction syndrome	Presence of altered organ function in an acutely ill patient such that homeostasis cannot be maintained without intervention	Combined acute respiratory and renal failure

Do these definitions apply to different clinical settings?

The final goals of any classification are (1) to describe individuals or groups characterized by different features; and, possibly, (2) to describe whether and how these differences interact with other variables [i.e., the length of stay (LOS) in the intensive care unit (ICU) or in the hospital, the final outcome, etc]. As far as the ACCP-SCCM classification is concerned, several investigators were able to demonstrate that subjects belonging to different diagnostic groups encountered different clinical courses. In a study involving 2,527 patients, Rangel-Frausto et al. [10] demonstrated several relevant findings. First, the mortality rate was associated with the severity of the systemic disorders, ranging from 3% in patients free from systemic inflammatory response syndrome (SIRS) to 46% in those with septic shock; interestingly, the mortality of patients with SIRS roughly paralleled the number of criteria recorded, being 7% in those with 2 and 10% and 17% in those with 3 or 4 signs, respectively. Second, there was a progression of symptoms, as patients with 2 signs of SIRS developed a third criterion by day 7; furthermore, as many as 32%, 36%, and 45% of patients with 2, 3, or 4 criteria for SIRS developed sepsis within 14 days. The median interval from sepsis to severe sepsis was remarkably shorter, being only 1 day, and that from severe sepsis to septic shock was 28 days. Third, end-organ dysfunctions, including acute respiratory distress syndrome (ARDS), disseminated intravascular coagulation (DIC), and acute renal failure (ARF) were more frequent in patients with severe sepsis and septic shock compared with patients with SIRS and uncomplicated sepsis. Finally, blood cultures (BC) were positive only in 17% of patients with sepsis, 25% of patients with severe sepsis, and 69% of patients with septic shock, further strengthening the concept that viable germs in the bloodstream are not necessary to trigger the inflammatory reaction eventually leading to the septic shock.

In another multicenter study that involved 1,100 patients, Salvo et al. [11] observed that, on admission, 52% of patients could be diagnosed as SIRS, whereas 4.5%, 2.1 %, and 3% belonged to the sepsis, severe sepsis, and septic shock groups, respectively. The mortality rate of patients with septic shock was substantially higher than in the study of Rangel-Frausto et al. [10], peaking at 82%. The causes of this difference are not clear. It is likely however that multiple factors, including a delay in the referral of the enrolled patients to the participating ICU s and an inappropriate choice of the antibiotic treatment, could at least partially account for them. Similar to the previous study, the risk of progression towards septic shock was higher in patients with sepsis and severe sepsis than in patients with SIRS; moreover, patients diagnosed as having severe sepsis or septic shock were sicker, as demonstrated by the higher severity scores. The time-related progression of infection-related systemic disturbances has been reported also by Berlot et al. [12] who observed that the rate of patients dying with sepsis and severe sepsis increased with the LOS in the ICU, whereas the incidence of septic shock remained fairly constant in patients dying during the 2nd week in ICU or later.

Some conclusions can be drawn from these studies, thus answering the question posed in the title of this section. First, the ACCM -SCCM definitions describe fairly accurately patients with different clinical courses and risk of death. Second, the progression from one condition to another is possible, and the corresponding worsening of the clinical conditions is more likely in patients who, at the time of admission, present with sepsis or severe sepsis; however, it should be remembered that there is not a risk-free group. Third, it appears that the longer the LOS in ICU, the higher the risk of developing sepsis and the related consequences, including ARDS, ARF, and DIC. Finally, in a relevant minority of patients with severe sepsis and septic shock, BCs are negative, thus making these diagnostic tools of limited usefulness in those patients who could take the maximal advantage of early and precise antibiotic therapy.

Does these definitions reflect different physiopathological conditions?

Both non-infectious and infectious events can trigger an inflammatory reaction, ultimately leading to MODS. Several lines of evidence suggest that the postinsult inflammatory response, as estimated from the concentration of some mediators involved in the septic process, (1) is more marked in SIRS patients shifting to sepsis than in those recovering from their condition, (2) is more pronounced in septic than in SIRS patients, and (3) in the majority of patients, its persistence is associated with a poor prognosis. Several investigators demonstrated that, in septic patients, persistently elevated levels of inflammatory mediators are associated with the development of MODS and a poor prognosis [13-15]. Similar considerations also apply in circumstances apparently not associated with infections. In a group of patients resuscitated from a cardiac arrest, Geppert et al. [16] observed that (1) SIRS was frequent, being present in 66% of patients, and was unrelated to some variables related to the event, including the duration of the cardiopulmonary resuscitation, the overall dose of epinephrine, and the blood lactate levels, and (2) P-selectin levels were higher in patients with SIRS and even more elevated in those who developed sepsis later. In a group of abdominal postoperative patients, Haga et al. [17] observed that both the number of diagnostic criteria of SIRS, its and duration, and the peak values of the C-reactive protein (CRP) were correlated with some intraoperative variables, including blood loss and the duration of the intervention; moreover, SIRS persisting beyond the 3rd postoperative day was associated with the development of sepsis and MODS. However, since proinflammatory mediators are produced along with substances aimed at blocking their actions, including soluble receptors and cellular receptor blocking agents [18], the existence of a condition defined as a compensatory anti-inflammatory response syndrome (CARS) has been hypothesized, in which blocking agents predominate due to the exhaustion of the inflammatory response [19]. Theoretically, this condition could be at least as harmful as SIRS has been developed and maintained throughout evolution to counteract the spreading of an initial infection, and its blocking could favour an initially circumscribed septic focus.

Can the diagnostic tools available 10 years ago still be considered valuable to differentiate between infectious and non-infectious conditions?

With identical symptoms and biochemical markers, the presence of a suspected or confirmed infection represents .the true border dividing SIRS from sepsis and its more-severe consequences. However, the accuracy of the diagnosis cannot be considered, since a delayed or inappropriate antibiotic treatment, which is not indicated in SIRS but absolutely mandatory in sepsis, has been associated with a poor prognosis. While in many cases an infectious cause of a systemic response can be reliably hypothesized even when a precise identification of the responsible microorganisms is still pending (i.e., faecal peritonitis, urinary tract infections, etc), in other cases the diagnosis is less straightforward. As an example, despite the elevated rate of ventilator-associated pneumonias among critically ill patients, the commonly adopted diagnostic criteria are not sensitive or specific enough to allow a precise diagnosis in 100% of suspected cases [20]. Similar considerations apply to patients with severe sepsis and septic shock, in whom cultures can remain negative in a significant number of cases [21]. Several factors can account for a failed growth of bacteria in the culture media, including a low inoculum, the effect of antibiotics, wrong or untimely sampling, and a poor processing of the sample itself; moreover, the host's response can be caused by the absorption of endotoxin and/or other bacterial byproducts from the intestinal lumen, by the activation of the gut-associated immune cells [21] or by its release following the administration of antibiotics [23].

Since the recent and impressive advances in genetic techniques make it possible to identify bacterial products in biological samples, it has been argued that many cases of SIRS should be re-diagnosed as sepsis or sepsis-related complications and consequentially treated. Cursons et al. [24] used two different techniques of bacterial DNA amplification by means of the polymerase chain reaction (PCR) in 110 critically ill patients with suspected or documented infections, and were able to demonstrate that PCR was positive in 8 patients with negative BC, whereas 7 patients had positive BC but negative PCRs; using a more-refined technique of DNA amplification, in 29 patients with negative BC the PCR was positive. In another study, Sleigh et al. [25] used the amplification of the gene 16S rDNA, which is common to all bacteria, and demonstrated that it was present in the bloodstream of 25 of 121 patients with negative BC. Other false-positives resulted from non-pathogenic microorganisms or from coagulase-negative staphylococci recovered from samples drawn from the indwelling vascular catheters. Other commonly used markers of sepsis and infections such as white blood cell count and temperature, were similar in patients with positive BC and in those with negative BC but in whom the PCR was positive. Despite these encouraging results, some points need to be clarified. First, as stated by Sleigh et al. [25], as many as 40% of PCR-positive blood samples were of doubtful clinical utility, due to different factors, including quality of the sample and the presence of DNA sequences derived from non-pathogenic or contaminant microorganism [26]. With these limitations in mind, the PCR could be valuable especially in those patients in whom the signs of a systemic inflammatory reaction persist despite (1) the negativity of cultures and/or (2) the administration of an apparently appropriate antibiotic treatment, provided that the presence of surgically amenable septic foci has been excluded.

The measurement of blood levels of some mediators involved in the septic process, including tumor necrosis factor (TNF)-α, interleukin (IL)-1, IL-6, IL-1 receptor antagonists, soluble TNF-α receptors, elastase, has been advocated in the monitoring of critically ill septic patients [8, 27]. However, this approach is expensive, time and labour intensive, and in many cases the results are not available rapidly. Moreover, blood levels reflect only part of the burden of mediators, while most of their action is exerted at a tissue levels [28]. More recently, the serial measurements of CRP [29-31] and of procalcitonin (PCT) [32, 33] have been proposed both as a reliable marker of infection and as a diagnostic tool to distinguish SIRS from sepsis. Several investigators demonstrated that although both substances are increased during sepsis, in septic patients PCT levels are higher than CRP [34, 35], its variations are more rapid and consistent with the clinical course, making this mediator a reliable marker of the ongoing process and of the response to treatment. Moreover, CRP increases in minor infections and in non-infectious conditions, including autoimmune and rheumatological disorders, acute coronary events, and malignancies [36-39]. Despite these shortcomings, the measurements of CRP are still valuable, as they are far cheaper than those of PCT, do not require sophisticated laboratory facilities, and the results are rapidly available. Bearing in mind its limitations, serial measurements of CRP have been advocated in the follow-up of critically ill patients with sepsis to evaluate the effects of the treatment [40]. The advantages as well the limitations of the measurement of some septic mediators are shown in Table 2.

Table 2. Advantages and disadvantages of the measurement of some inflammatory mediators in the diagnosis of SIRS and sepsis (*PCT* procalcitonin, *CRP* C-reactive protein)

Marker	Infection-specific	Inflammation-specific	Advantages	Limitations
PCT	4+	1+	Rapid appearance T/2 24 h	Low specificity for focal infections. High specificity for severe sepsis and septic shock Relatively expensive
CRP	2+	2+	Not expensive Widespread availability	Low specificity Slow appearance No correlation with the severity
Cytokines	1+	2+	High sensitivity Rapid appearance	Expensive Time consuming Labour intensive

In conclusion, the diagnostic tools available today allow (1) a good discrimination between SIRS and sepsis, and (2) monitoring of the clinical course and the response to the treatments. In selected cases, one should take advantage of DNA amplification technology to distinguish between the two conditions.

Are these criteria reliable?

The ultimate problem associated with the ACCM-SCCM diagnostic definitions is their reliability to assist in the choice of treatment. Some investigations [6, 10, 11] suggest that the difference between SIRS and sepsis is rather narrow, thus casting serious doubt on the possibility that some "false SIRS" could be rather a "true sepsis". This appears particularly relevant, since in critically ill patients a delay in the appropriate therapy is unavoidably associated with a higher rate of complications and a worse prognosis. From the above studies, it appears that although the ACCP-SCCM definitions describe accurately most of conditions presented by critically ill patients, a grey area persists in which both the clinical signs and the commonly measured biological variables cannot discriminate between non-infectious and infectious source of disturbances [8].

Unfortunately, the threshold for either the administration of antibiotics or the surgical drainage of a septic focus lies in this area. This "twilight zone" can be reduced, but probably not totally eliminated, by the use of new diagnostic tools, including the repeated measurement of selected mediators and the PCR [26, 41, 42].

Conclusions

Despite their introduction into clinical practice nearly 10 years ago and the criticisms raised, the ACCP-SCCM definitions are still widely used throughout the world and seem to be robust, and should remain as described [9]. The main criticism is based on their broadness and consequent lack of specificity, even though signs and symptoms of sepsis [9] are, at the moment, more varied than the initial criteria established in 1991 [2, 3]. It is likely that novel diagnostic approaches based on PCR could enhance the diagnostic sensitivity, thus reducing the grey area between infections and non-infectious conditions. The serial measurements of selected inflammatory mediators, including the CRP and PCT, allow a fairly accurate discrimination between SIRS and sepsis and can constitute a guide for treatment. The future may lie in developing a staging system that will characterize the progression of sepsis including predisposing factors, nature of infection, host response and extent of the resultant organ dysfunction.

References

1. Webster's ninth collegiate dictionary (1991) Merriam -Webster, Springfield, Mass.
2. Bone RC, Balk RA, Cerra FB et al (1992) American College of Chest Physicians/Society of Critical Care Medicine Consensus Conference. Definitions for sepsis and organ failure and guidelines for the use of innovative therapies. Chest 101:1644-1655
3. American College of Chest Physicians-Society of Critical Care Medicine Consensus Conference (1992) Definitions for sepsis and organ failure and guidelines for the use of innovative therapies in sepsis. Crit Care Med 328:864-875
4. Vincent JL (1997) Dear SIRS, I am sorry to say that I don't like you... Crit Care Med 25:372-374
5. Vincent JL, Bihari D (1992) Sepsis, severe sepsis or sepsis syndrome: need for clarification. Intensive Care Med 18:255-257
6. Pittet D, Rangel-Frausto S, Li N et al (1995) Systemic inflammatory response syndrome, sepsis, severe sepsis and septic shock: incidence, morbidities and outcomes in a surgical ICU. Intensive Care Med 21:303-309
7. Dellinger RP, Bone RC (1998) To SIRS with love. Crit Care Med 25:178-179

8. Marik PE (2002) Definitions of sepsis: not quite time to dump the SIRS. Crit Care Med 30:706-708
9. Levy MM, Fink MP, Marshall JC et al (2003) 2001 SCCM/ESICM/ACCP/ATS/SIS International Sepsis Definitions Conference. Crit Care Med 31:1250-1256
10. Rangel-Frausto M, Pittet D, Costigan M et al (1995) The natural history of the systemic inflammatory response syndrome (SIRS). JAMA 273:117-123
11. Salvo I, de Cian W, Musicco M et al (1995) The Italian SEPSIS study: preliminary results on the incidence and evolution of SIRS, sepsis, severe sepsis and septic shock. Intensive Care Med 21[Suppl 2]:S244-S249
12. Berlot G, Dezzoni R, Viviani M et al (1999) Does the length of stay in the intensive care unit influence the diagnostic accuracy? A clinical-pathological study. Eur J Emerg Med 6:227-231
13. Adrie C, Pinsky MR (2000) The inflammatory balance in human sepsis. Intensive Care Med 26:364-375
14. Pinsky MR, Vincent JL, Deviere J et al (1993) Serum cytokine levels in human septic shock-relation to multiple system organ failure and mortality. Chest 103:565-575
15. Meduri GU, Headley S, Kohler G et al (1995) Persistent elevation of inflammatory cytokines predicts a poor outcome in ARDS. Plasma IL-1 beta and IL-6 levels are consistent and efficient predictors of outcome over time. Chest 107:1062-1073
16. Geppert A, Zorn G, Karth GD et al (2000) Soluble selectins and the systemic inflammatory response syndrome after successful cardiopulmonary resuscitation. Crit Care Med 28:2360-2365
17. Haga Y, Beppu T, Doi K et al (1997) Systemic inflammatory response syndrome and organ dysfunction syndrome following gastrointestinal surgery. Crit Care Med 25:1994-2000
18. Poll van der, Deventer SJH van (1999) Cytokines and anticytokines in the pathogenesis of sepsis. Infect Dis Clin North Am 13:413-426
19. Bone RC (1996) Sir Isaac Newton, sepsis, SIRS and CARS. Crit Care Med 24:1125-1136
20. Keenan DP, Heyland DK, Jacka ML et al (2002) Ventilator-associated pneumonia: prevention, diagnosis and therapy. Crit Care Clin 18:107-125
21. Reimer LG, Wilson ML, Weinstein MP (1997) Update on detection of bacteremia and fungemia. Clin Microbiol Rev 10:444-465
22. Deitch E (2002) Bacterial translocation or lymphatic drainage of toxic products from the gut: what is important in human beings? Surgery 131:241-244
23. Maskin B, Fontan PA, Spinedi EG et al (2002) Evaluation of endotoxin release and cytokine production induced by antibiotics in patients with Gram-negative nosocomial pneumonia. Crit Care Med 30:349-354
24. Cursons RTM, Jeyerajah E, Sleigh JW (1999) The use of polymerase chain reaction to detect septicemia in critically ill patients. Crit Care Med 27:937-940
25. Sleigh J, Cursons R, La Pine M (2001) Detection of bacteraemia in critically ill patients using 16S rDNA polymerase chain reaction and DNA sequencing. Intensive Care Med 27:1269-1273
26. Struelens MJ, de Mendonca R (2001) The emerging power of molecular diagnostics: toward improved management of life-threatening infections. Intensive Care Med 27:1696-1698
27. Gramm HJ, Hannemann L (1996) Activity markers for the inflammatory host response and early criteria of sepsis. Clin Int Care 7[Suppl 1]:320-321
28. Cavaillon JM, Munoz C, Fitting C et al (1992) Circulating cytokines: the tip of the iceberg? Circ Shock 38:145-152
29. Dev D, Wallace E, Sankaran R et al (1998) Value of C-reactive protein measurements in exacerbations of chronic obstructive pulmonary disease. Respir Med 92:664-667

30. Erikson S, Granstrom L, Olander B, Wretlind B (1995) Sensitivity of interleukin-6 and C-reactive protein concentrations in the diagnosis of acute appendicitis. Eur J Surg 161:41-45

31. Povoa P, Almeida E, Moreira P et al (1998) C-reactive protein as an indicator of sepsis. Intensive Care Med 24:1052-1056

32. Assicot M, Gendrel D, Carsin H et al (1993) High serum procalcitonin concentrations in patients with sepsis and infection. Lancet 341:515-518

33. Brunkhorst FM, Heinz U, Forcki ZF (1998) Kinetics of procalcitonin in iatrogenic sepsis. Intensive Care Med 24:888-889

34. Ugarte H, Silva E, Mercan D et al (1999) Procalcitonin used as a marker in the intensive care unit. Crit Care Med 27:498-504

35. Selberg O, Hecker H, Martin M et al (2000) Discrimination of sepsis and systemic inflammatory response syndrome by determination of circulating plasma concentration of procalcitonin, protein complement 3a and interleukin-6. Crit Care Med 28:2793-2798

36. Eberhard OK, Haubitz M, Brunkhorst FM et al (1997) Usefulness of procalcitonin for differentiation between activity of systemic autoimmune disease (systemic lupus erythematosus/systemic antineutrophil cytoplasmatic antibody-associated vasculitis) and invasive bacterial infection. Arthritis Rheum 40:1250-1256

37. Schwener V, Sis J, Breitbart A, Andrassy K (1998) CRP levels in autoimmune disease can be specified by measurement of procalcitonin. Infection 26:274-276

38. Lindahl B, Toss H, Siegbahn A et al for the FRISC study group (2000) Markers of myocardial damage and inflammation in relation to long-term mortality in unstable coronary artery disease. N Engl J Med 343:1139-1147

39. Meisner M, Tschaikowsky K, Hutzler A et al (1998) Postoperative plasma concentrations of procalcitonin after different types of surgery. Intensive Care Med 24:680-684

40. Reny JL, Vuagnat A, Ract C et al (2002) Diagnosis and follow up of infections in intensive care patients: value of C-reactive protein compared with other clinical and biological variables. Crit Care Med 30:529-535

41. Zahorec R (2000) Definitions for septic syndrome should be re-evaluated. Intensive Care Med 26:1870

42. Abraham E, Matthay ME, Dinarello CA et al (2000) Consensus conference for sepsis, septic shock, lung injury and acute respiratory distress syndrome. Time for a reappraisal. Crit Care Med 28:232-235

Chapter 25

SIRS/Sepsis: Metabolic and Nutritional Changes and Treatment

F. Iscra, A. Randino

The Metabolic Response of the Host to SIRS/Sepsis

Sepsis, whether due to an infection or as a result of a trauma, generates a potent and serious reaction in the host, with numerous serious metabolic changes. Sepsis, which may manifest itself clinically through one or more symptoms— fever or hypothermia, leukocytosis or leukopenia, tachycardia, tachypnea, or increased respiration rate [1]—is largely due to (apart from a powerful activation of the neuroendocrine system) an increase in the release of cytokines. These substances activate both the inflammatory response and the compensatory anti-inflammatory response systems. The cytokines, that are activated by microbial toxins, and predominantly responsible for inflammation are interleukin-1, tumor necrosis factor, and interleukin-8. Those that induce the anti-inflammatory response are interleukin-6 and interleukin-10 [2, 3].

The systemic inflammatory response can also arise as a result of apparently slight stimuli, including local infections or those that are barely clinically evident, such as ischemia/reperfusion of the gastrointestinal tract [4]. The activation pathways are characterized by the release of counter-regulatory hormones from the hypothalamic-pituitary-adrenal axis, the action of the autonomous nervous system, and by the cellular response that precipitates the release of substances including cytokines, and products of the endothelial cells, including prostaglandin, endothelin, and nitric oxide. Such conditions of double-activation, classic hormonal, and peptidic inflammation can work synergistically; likewise, cytokines and other products can inhibit this axis, depending on the various concentrations and timing. In turn, the action of cytokine-producing cells is regulated by cortisol [5–9].

From the metabolic point of view, a totally undermining process takes place. A hypermetabolic state is observed with a significant increase in VO_2, often under conditions of inadequate oxygen supply [10].

There is also an increase in the flow of glucose towards the glucose-dependent organs or tissues; there is an alteration (often an increase) in lactate production; an increase in neoglucogenesis by amino acids, notably alanine; certain non-essential amino acids such as glutamine become functionally indispensable for the immune system or for the intestinal mucosa; a serious proteolysis in muscle tissue sets in, particularly in skeletal muscle; catecholamines such as circulating adrenaline and noradrenaline released from post-ganglionic sympathetic neurones have a direct effect on increased lipolysis and rising non-esterified fatty acid (NEFA) levels and they reduce peripheral glucose uptake and increase glycerol delivery to the liver [11].

The host's increased energy demands are met by a rapid utilization of glucose. Glycogen soon runs out and in the septic patient, neoglycogenesis is much reduced [12]. The phenomenon is particularly evident in glucose-dependent tissues, particularly "wound tissue"; furthermore, glucose uptake is insulin independent in red and white blood cells and in macrophage-rich tissues [13].

This results in an increase in neoglucogenesis, with an increased flow of amino acids from muscle towards the liver, alanine and glutamine in particular, and end products of urogenesis. Glucose is readily available for use, however the productive pathway is costly in both energetic and functional terms, as in the periphery, essential amino acids such as leucine, isoleucine, and valine are used for energy. This dictates a significant increase in both urea and ammonia levels. The altered homeostasis of carbohydrate metabolism results in an increased production of lactate, skeletal muscle being one of the principal sources.

The critically ill patient often has an increased lactate blood level. It is not clear whether this is due solely to increased production or to reduced clearance. What is certain is that it is linked to the enormous increase in pyruvate production [14, 15].

The etiopathogenesis is probably multifactorial and, in the critically ill patient, apart from the classic anaerobic response due to hypoxia, there is a connection with the action of epinephrine and with the enzymatic inhibition of pyruvic dehydrogenase (PDH1 and 2) [16, 17].

Under conditions of increased liver glucose output, there is a significant associated increase in the transformation of lactic acid for gluconeogenetic purposes [18]. The Cory cycle describes the peripheral production of lactate from glucose originally released by the liver, the transfer of lactate back to the liver, and its glucogenetic conversion to glucose. Two molecules of 3-carbon lactate are needed to produce one molecule of 6-carbon glucose, with energy provided from hepatic oxidation of NEFA. From energy point of view it is clearly an inefficient process, but has the important effect of limiting the breakdown of skeletal muscle to produce glucose during fasting [11]. Hyperlactatemia may no longer be seen only as a prognostic sign [19] but as the result of a generalized inflammatory response and of the activation of an alternative energy pathway, although it is not really energy efficient [20].

Glucose intolerance simultaneously worsens in exactly the same way as insulin resistance. In the first case the normal feedback mechanism is absent, the mechanism by which in the presence of high levels of blood glucose, both exogenous and endogenous, there is no suppression of liver glucose production. There appears to be resistance to insulin at both hepatic and peripheral levels; during insulin infusion, there is neither a reduction in glucose production (hepatic resistance) nor an increase in stimulation of peripheral glucose uptake (peripheral resistance). There is a significant difference in the efficiency of insulin in trauma and sepsis, where the efficiency is reduced by 50%. The reasons for this are not clear, but a cut-off of blood level activity is hypothesized [21].

In the critically ill patient, the activation of the autonomous nervous system with the increased secretion of catecholamines stimulates lipolysis and brings about a significant increase in the release of free fatty acids (FFA).

The function of oxidation of this substrate is to bridge the gap between the total energy demand of the host and that provided by oxidation of carbohydrates. The level of FFA released is much higher than that which can be oxidized. Hence the remaining FFA are stored in the liver or laid down in adipose tissue in the form of triglycerides and very low-density lipoprotein. In the critically ill patient this recycling system can increase by a factor of up to 5 times the physiological rate. Oxidation could be inhibited by the high levels of glucose and insulin, especially during artificial nutrition with glucose and insulin [21].

The nitrogen balance is negative since increased protein degradation is not compensated for by synthesis. This occurs rapidly, as is shown by the elevated rates of leucine oxidation, and can affect all parenchymal structures. In particular, apart from muscle tissue, the gastrointestinal tract, the lungs, and the kidneys are strongly affected [22–24].

This increased degradation is mainly due to the increased flow of amino acids towards the liver. At muscular level, although there is an enormous increase in the neosynthesis of neoglucogenetic amino acids, and alanine in particular, this is not enough to compensate for the losses, and compared with a healthy individual, the production of glutamine markedly drops [25]. Glutamine, the most widespread amino acid in body, becomes functionally essential as demand for it increases dramatically. It is the prime source of energy for high-replication cells, both in the immune system and the intestinal parenchyma. Moreover, it is involved in the formation of arginine, an amino acid essential for the development of lymphocytes and the immune response [26, 27].

Protein synthesis, under the stimulus of cytokines, assumes a central role in production of proteins of the acute phase of the anti-inflammatory response [28]. However, protein synthesis is limited by energy shortfalls and substrates [29].

The main and commonly used protein is C-reactive protein (CRP). CRP is very sensitive and specific and could be considered either as a functional expression of synthesis in the anti-protease protein system, or as a prognostic index [30].

Malnutrition

The use of protein tissue in skeletal muscle as an energy source, together with shortfalls in essential amino acids for neosynthesis of proteins, especially for anti-inflammatory and/or immune purposes, leads to severe protein malnutrition. This situation is frequently accompanied by a sharp imbalance between availability of energy giving substrates and energy demand. The patient is unable to ingest any food and often any kind of exogenous artificial provision is either poor or absent [31].

This results in the rapid onset of energy-protein malnutrition, which can cause an increase in morbidity and death [32]. It is calculated that over 50% of hospital patients are undernourished or at least show an altered parameter of malnutrition and a high rate of complications [33]. The energy demand of patients with sepsis tends to increase significantly with respect to physiological base levels and varies markedly throughout the course of various clinical conditions (initial sepsis, delayed or septic shock) and is strongly affected by whatever therapy is applied [34, 35].

The infusion of exogenous amines, administered during shock, can increase VO_2 levels by 30%–35%, while mechanical ventilation significantly reduces excessive energy expenditure [36]. Artificial nutrition, and in particular parenteral nutrition, can induce significant increases in VO_2 and in CO_2 production [37].

Protein demand increases quantitatively, but more importantly there are changes in the qualitative demands. In the critically ill patient, nitrogen losses can reach 4 or 8 times normal levels, depending on whether the patient is septic or suffering from burns [38]. It has been clearly shown that it is impossible to achieve balanced nitrogen levels in the most acute phases of inflammation. The goal here is rather to encourage protein synthesis for immunity and to attenuate muscle catabolism. Massive doses of protein can lead to marked increases in urea and CO_2. Malnutrition can develop in patients who spend long periods in intensive care and, despite metabolic support and adequate protein supply, these subjects still lose considerable amounts of soft tissue and skeletal muscle [39]. A functional shortfall of glutamine has been observed because the synthesis is reduced in stress' conditions. The endocellular glutamine level and reserves are reduced, particularly in the gut for maintaining a constant blood level and the optimal delivery to immunocells [40,41].

Organ Failure: the Gastrointestinal Tract

The gastrointestinal tract is an organ of digestion and absorption that is meta-bolically active and has specific nutrient requirements. In health, it has an addi-tional function as a major barrier, protecting the body from harmful intralumi-nal pathogens and large antigenic molecules.

In disease states, such as sepsis, when the mucosal barrier is compromised, micro-organisms and their toxic products gain access to the portal and sys-temic circulation producing deleterious effects. Under these circumstances, sys-temic inflammatory response syndrome (SIRS) and multiple-organ dysfunction syndrome (MODS) develop, leading to deterioration and death of the patient.

Clinical studies strongly suggest that intestinal barrier dysfunction and increased permeability occur in patients with intestinal inflammation and other diseases associated with increased morbidity and mortality [42]. In this clinical situation, the translocating micro-organisms and toxins activate a sys-temic inflammatory cascade and promote organ dysfunction and failure.

Factors that favor the development of sepsis syndromes include changes in the luminal micro-environment, perfusion and oxygen deficit, ischemia/reper-fusion injury, malnutrition, and hepatic dysfunction.

The development of paralytic ileus and the formation of a blind loop allow stagnation of the intraluminal contents, creating favorable conditions for micro-bial overgrowth. The use of parenteral antibiotics causes a reduction in the normal indigenous flora and a subsequent overgrowth of potentially pathogenic micro-organisms. The mucosa at the tip of the villi is particularly prone to ischemia due to the counter-current exchange mechanism of the vessels, and occurs when there is shunting of blood under low-flow conditions. Shock states have a detrimental effect on the immune and hepatic cells, reducing their capacity to clear bacteria and endotoxins.

Intestinal ischemia may develop as a result of poor extraction and utiliza-tion of nutrients by the intestine despite normal oxygen content and delivery [43]. When ischemia is relieved by perfusion or resuscitation, oxygen-derived free radicals are generated by the xanthine oxidase pathway and cause direct injury to the lipid membranes of the cells and hyaluronic acid of their basal membrane [44]. There is a growing body of evidence that shows that mast cells recruit neutrophils, and together these cells contribute to the pathogenesis of ischemia/reperfusion in the intestine and maintain local and systemic inflam-mation by releasing mediators [45]. Malnutrition and total parenteral nutrition may cause atrophy of the enterocytes and a reduction in IgA antibody produc-tion [46]. Hyperbilirubinemia is often present in sepsis. It represents a direct toxic effect on liver parenchymal cells, causing inflammation in the portal tri-ads and intrahepatic cholestasis. It may be exacerbated by hypovolemia, the use of parenteral nutrition, drugs, and excessive hemolysis [47].

The immune compartment in the gut-associated lymphoid tissue, which includes the oral cavity, the small intestine, and the colon, is a dynamic and highly complex group of specialized structures and cell types. This structure includes Peyer's patches, mesenteric lymph nodes, and intestinal lamina propria, and contains a population of cells consisting of both effector and regulatory subsets of T lymphocytes, B lymphocytes, macrophages, mast cells, dendritic cells, natural killer cells, neutrophils, and eosinophils. While epithelial cells and enterocytes maintain the integrity of the mucosal barrier, the gastrointestinal mucosal immune system maintains a balance, protecting the host against potential pathogens crossing mucosal barriers and providing immune tolerance against food antigens and normal intestinal flora. The normal state of the intestine is controlled inflammation in the presence of systemic suppression. While T lymphocytes and B lymphocytes are in an activated state in the normal gut, they are systemically suppressed (Chapter 2).

If remote injury affects splanchnic blood flow to the gut, gut injury may occur from cytokines and mediators from remote sites, as well as from the influx of neutrophils and monocytes from the blood into gut tissue that is ischemic/reperfused. All these factors may contribute to gut dysfunction in the critically ill patient [48].

Artificial Nutritional Support

Metabolic and nutritional support has been shown to be indispensable in treating critically ill patients, reducing deterioration. This practice has become more widespread over recent years and has become a true therapy with indications and complications. It has never been shown that artificial nutrition results in a significant reduction in mortality [49]. Over the last few years, the amount of exogenous energy administered to critically ill patients has been reduced, as one realised that hyperalimentation was not able to suppress intense protein catabolism and caused numerous complications. These included raised excessive energy expenditure, increased CO_2 output, and respiratory complications linked to lipid infusion [49, 50].

A calculation of basal energy expenditure can be performed with the help of the Harris-Benedict regression, corrected for whatever pathological variation is present. This kind of evaluation is not always reliable in critically ill patients because of the obvious difficulty of assessing an accurate body weight. Edema and hyperhydration are two factors that can give a false reading for body weight, which is one of the fundamental components of the Harris-Benedict regression [51]. Indirect calorimetry, a non-invasive system, is a useful and accurate method for determining energy expenditure. By means of analysis of respiratory gases it is possible to determine the energy expenditure at the bedside of the mechanically ventilated critically ill patient. In our experience, which is similar to that in the literature, this value does not exceed 30 kcal/kg per day either in sepsis or trauma [52, 53].

Fundamentally it is believed that the exogenous caloric contribution must not exceed 35 kcal/kg per day and that as a general guide, a supply of 25–30 kcal/kg per day for males and 20–25 kcal/kg per day for females is recommended. However, particular attention must be paid to elderly patients, where a reduction in the external supply of 15%-20% is recommended compared with that used in younger subjects [54].

A recent meta-analysis shows that a higher lipid concentration can cause deterioration and complications [55]. It has been shown that long-chain fats/lipids given intravenously reduce reticuloendothelial function, neutrophil function, and suppress the relationship between T-helper and T-suppressor lymphocytes [55]. Furthermore, they cause alterations in the lung and promote susceptibility to infection [56]. In patients with acute respiratory distress syndrome there is a reduction in oxygenation index and a significant increase in shunt fraction [57].

Such a condition could be attributed to a higher prostaglandin output and the consequent hypoxic vasoconstriction mechanism. Medium-chain lipids, which could potentially have an advantageous effect in septic patients, for example giving good and rapid oxygenation and rapid clearance, in practice do not provide any real advantage either given in isolation or alongside long-chain lipids [58]. Furthermore, the glycose system, poor in lipids, compared with the mixed diet, seems to favor a better anabolism [59]. In practice, during the acute phase of shock, we must bear in mind that a minimum dose of around 150–180 g/day of glucose is necessary to support glucose-dependent tissues, and subsequently diets with 70%-80% of the necessary caloric contribution administered as glucose gives the best results. It has been shown that the exogenous protein contribution is fundamental in guaranteeing protein synthesis for both pro- and anti-inflammatory activity. This avoids protein autodigestion that can develop in patients with infections. The nitrogen contribution seems to have a minimum threshold of 0.1 g/kg per day, although the best results are obtained at over 0.2 g/kg per day. At this level we find not only a significant improvement in nitrogen balance, but above all in nitrogen retention. Above values of 0.2 g/kg per day, these are no significantly different results. The ideal exogenous protein quantity for critically ill patients should always be 0.16 g N/kg per day and not over 0.24 g N/kg per day. Quantities that exceed these values do not give advantages in terms of improved nitrogen balance or better protein synthesis, and bring higher risks of kidney overload [60–62].

It has been shown that critically ill patients receiving parenteral nutrition have a higher rate of infection compared with those treated with early enteral feeding, even excluding infections associated with the central venous catheter [63]. Many clinical and economic comparisons of the two methods have shown the greater advantages of artificial nutrition administered by means of a nasal stomach tube, jejunally, or by other more invasive methods such as jejunostomy or percutaneous endoscopic gastrostomy. We must remember that the minimum doses for an enteral diet (300–500 kcal/day) can avoid intestinal hypotrophy, maintain splanchnic flow, and optimize the immune response and that enteral artificial nutrition is possible in anesthetized or paralyzed patients even for extended periods or those in prone position [64].

The use of total parenteral nutrition solutions is indicated when enteral nutrition is contraindicated in case of intestinal occlusions, jejuno-ileal fistulas at high flow (>0.5 l/h), serious non-hypovolemic intestinal ischemias, intestinal insufficiency due to massive resectioning, or absorption deficit.

Some patients with a functioning gastrointestinal tract are intolerant of enteral support or rather do not receive a sufficient calorie-protein input. In this case nutritional therapy may indicate a combination of available techniques (enteral nutrition plus parenteral nutrition by central venous catheter or given peripherally), allowing a sufficient calorie-protein support.

Patients with vomiting or bleeding in the upper digestive tract can be treated by means of a different enteral access (probe positioned in the duodenum or into the jejunum by means of an endoscope or by gravity, with two-way probes that allow one part for drainage of gastric material and the other for infusion of substances into the jejunum), surgical jejunostomy [65–67].

The importance of maintaining intestinal function under highly stressful conditions such as sepsis has been demonstrated to improve the clinical condition and prognosis of patients. The role of the intestine as an organ with a powerful immune action has been clearly demonstrated. One potential benefit for critically ill patients is the proposed use of enteral solutions enriched with high immune system-impact amino acids such as arginine and glutamine, and with substances with an anti-inflammatory action such as $\Omega 3$ fatty acids, nucleotides, and antioxidants. Some recent meta-analyses have reported encouraging results in terms of minor infections and reduction of stay in both intensive care unit and hospital. No significant reduction in mortality rates has been shown [68–70].

These results, although undoubtedly positive, are open to discussion.
- There are often mixed groups of patients, probably with different metabolic profiles (patients with emergency medical diagnoses, with trauma or postoperative scheduled surgery intervention, or emergencies).
- There are often variations in the methodology and quality of the work under examination.

- The authors of meta-analyses use different criteria to those used in the original studies.
- The outcomes are not always completely accepted.
- There are various interpretations of the intention-to-treat analysis, in that many patients do not receive the prescribed enteral support.
- The constituents of the diet are often mixed and the individual effects of the components are impossible to distinguish.

In a recent paper the ICU and hospital mortality were calculated in three of the largest ICU studies using the same nutritional formula that has proven successful in reducing infection in surgical patient. The mortality risk and benefits should be looked at using the decision to feed (intention to treat) as one does in practice. The two largest studies with hospital mortality data, using the same immunonutrient feed showed a significant excess mortality (odds ratio OR 1.45, 95% confidence interval [CI], 1.06-2.11; p=0.02). In the septic subgroup the hospital mortality was 25% in Impact fed patients (11/44) vs. 8.9% in control fed patients (4/45) (p=0.04) [71].

In a multicentre study of patients with sepsis, a significant reduction in mortality rate was shown in treated patients, especially those in the APACHE 2 range between 10 and 15 points, and in the number of episodes of bacteremia and nosocomial infections [72]. The Zaloga analysis on timing shows that early enteral support is more efficient compared with later support in terms of infectious and non-infectious complications [73]. The attempt to treat inflammation that flares up in critical patients is at the center of an original contribution on the effects of immunostimulants and antioxidants given enterically. Ω3 fatty acids show a minor platelet activation, thrombogenetic activity, and induce less cytokine release than n6 fatty acids. Gadek et al. [74] showed that the group treated with enteral solution enriched with eicosapentaenoic acid, γ-linolenic acid and antioxidants had a significant improvement in gaseous exchange, with a reduced time of mechanical ventilation, reduced time in intensive care, and a lower incidence of renewed organ insufficiency [74]. Glutamine is often deficient in supplements for critically ill patients. The rationale for early administration of glutamine in order to stimulate the immune response and prevent complications is very persuasive. However, the results of small clinical trials are contradictory and have not always included critically ill patients. The true mechanism of action has not really been clarified, neither has the best and most efficient means of administration [27, 58].

Several possible mechanisms can be advocated, including:
- metabolic: protein synthesis, carbon and nitrogen interorgan transporter, gluconeogenetic precursor, ammoniogenesis
- immunologic: replication of immune cells, T cell helper function and responsiveness, synthesis of immunoglobulin A
- antioxidant: glutathione synthesis, precursor of taurine

References

1. American College of Chest Physicians/Society of Critical Care Medicine Consensus Committee (1992) Definitions for sepsis and organ failure and guidelines for the use of innovative therapies in sepsis. Crit Care Med 20:864–890
2. Moldawer LL (1994) Biology of proinflammatory cytokines and their antagonist. Crit Care Med 22:S3–S7
3. Marshall JC (2001) Inflammation, coagulopathy, and the pathogenesis of multiple organ dysfunction syndrome. Crit Care Med 29:S99–S106
4. Michie HR(1996) Cytokines and the acute catabolic state. In: Revhaug A (ed) Acute catabolic state. Springer Verlag, Berlin Heidelberg New York
5. Reichlin S (1993) Neuroendocrine-immune interactions. N Engl J Med 329:1246–1253
6. Foster AH (1996) The early endocrine response in injury. In: Revhaug A (ed) Acute catabolic state. Springer Verlag, Berlin Heidelberg New York, pp 35–78
7. Lavery GG, Glover P (2000) The metabolic and nutritional response to critical illness. Curr Opin Crit Care 6:233–238
8. Kinney JM (1995) Metabolic responses of the critically ill patient. Crit Care Clin 11:569–585
9. Imura H, Kukata J (1994) Endocrine-paracrine interaction in communication between the immune and endocrine system. Activation of the hypothalamic-pituitary-adrenal axis in inflammation. Eur J Endocrinol 130:32–38
10. Russel JA, Phang PT (1995) The oxygen delivery/consumption controversy: approaches to management of critically ill. Am J Respir Crit Care Med 149:533–537
11. Heller SR, Robinson RTC (1999) Glucose metabolism In: Jenkins RC, Ross RJM (eds) The endocrine response to acute illness. Karger, Basel, pp 4–23
12. Saeed M, Carlson GL, Little RA et al (1999) Selective impairment of glucose storage in human sepsis. Br J Surg 86:813–821
13. Meszaros K, Lang CH, Bagby GJ et al (1987) Contribution of different organs to increased glucose consumption after endotoxin administration. J Biol Chem 262:10965–10970
14. Levy B, Sadoune LO, Gelot AM (2000) Evolution of lactate/pyruvate and arterial ketone body ratios in the early course of catecholamine-treated septic shock. Crit Care Med 28:114-119
15. Vary TC, Drnevich D et al (1995) Mechanisms regulating skeletal muscle glucose metabolism in sepsis. Shock 6:403–410
16. Vary TC, Siegel JH, Nakatani T et al (1986) Effect of sepsis on activity of PDH complex in skeletal muscle and liver. Am J Physiol 250:E634–E640
17. James JH, Luchette FA, McCarter F et al (1999) Lactate is an unreliable indicator of tissue hypoxia in injury or sepsis. Lancet 354:505–508
18. Wolfe RR, Burke J (1978) Effect of glucose infusion on glucose and lactate metabolism in normal and burned guinea pigs. J Trauma 18:800–805
19. Weil MH, Afifi AA (1970) Experimental and clinical studies on lactate and pyruvate as indicators of severity of acute circulatory failure. Circulation 16:989–1001
20. Lehninger AL, Bioenergetics NY et al (1986) Lactate production under fully aerobic condition: the lactate shuttle during rest and exercise. Fed Proc 45:2924–2929
21. Wolfe RR (1999) Sepsis as a modulator of adaptation to low and high carbohydrate and low and high fat intakes. Eur J Clin Nutr 53:S136–S142
22. Hourami H, William PE, Morris et al (1990) Effect of insulin-induced hypoglycemia on

protein metabolism in vivo. Am J Physiol 259:E342–E350

23. Iscra F, Biolo G et al (2001) Lung vs. skeletal muscle amino acid flow in septic ARDS patients. Intensive Care Med 27:S243

24. Tessari P, Garibotto G et al (1996) Kidney, splanchnic and leg protein turnover in human. J Clin Invest 98:1481–1492

25. Biolo G, Fleming R et al (2000) Inhibition of muscle glutamine formation in hypercatabolic patients. Clin Sci (Colch) 99:189–194

26. Bode BP, Pan M et al (1996) Glutamine, the gut, and the acute catabolic state. In: Revhaug A (ed) Acute catabolic state. Springer Verlag, Berlin Heidelberg New York,pp 103–114

27. Andrews FJ, Griffths RD (2002) Glutamine–essential for immune nutrition in the critically ill. Br J Nutr 87 [Suppl 1]:3–8

28. Sganga G, Siegel JH et al(1985) Reprioritization of hepatic plasma protein release in trauma and sepsis. Arch Surg 120:187–199

29. Biolo G, Toigo G et al(1997) Metabolic response to injury and sepsis: changes in protein metabolism. Nutrition 13:S52–S57

30. Povoa P, Almeida E et al (1998) C-reactive protein as an indicator of sepsis. Intensive Care Med 24:1052–1056

31. Lynn ML, Zhong J et al (2000) The effect of nutritional supplementation on survival in seriously ill hospitalized adults: an evaluation of the SUPPORT data. J Am Geriatr Soc 48:S33–S38

32. Giner M, Laviano A et al (1996) In 1995 a correlation between malnutrition and poor outcome in critically ill patients still exists. Nutrition 12:23–29

33. Naber THF, Schermer T et al (1997) Prevalence of malnutrition in non surgical hospitalized patients and its association with disease complication. Am J Clin Nutr 66:1232–1239

34. Uehara M, Plank LD et al (1999) Components of energy expenditure in patients with severe sepsis and major trauma: a basis for clinical care. Crit Care Med 27:1295–1302

35. Moriyama S, Okamoto K et al (1999) Evaluation of oxygen consumption and resting energy expenditure in critically ill patients with SIRS. Crit Care Med 27:2133–2136

36. Chiolero R, Bracco D et al (1993) Does indirect calorimetry reflect energy expenditure in the critically ill patient In: Wilmore DW,Carpentier YA (eds) Metabolic support of the critically ill patient. Springer-Verlag, Berlin Heidelberg New York, pp 95–118

37. Pitkanen O, Takala J et al (1993) Nutrition status, severity of illness and thermogenic response to parenteral nutrition. Nutrition 9:411–417

38. Elwyn DH (1987) Protein metabolism and requirement in the critically ill patient. Crit Care Clin 3:57–69

39. Monk DN, Plank LD et al (1996) Sequential changes in the metabolic response in critically injured patients during the first 25 days after blunt trauma. Ann Surg 223:395–405

40. Souba WW, Herskovitz K et al (1990) The effects of sepsis and endotoxinemia on gut glutamine metabolism. Ann Surg 211:543–551

41. Souba WW, Smith RJ et al (1985) Glutamine metabolism by the intestinal tract. J Parenter Enteral Nutr 9:608–617

42. Rowlands BJ, Gardiner KR (1998) Nutritional modulation of gut inflammation. Proc Nutr Soc 57:395–401

43. Fiddian-Green RG (1992) The role of the gut in shock and resuscitation. Clin Intensive Care 3:395–401

44. Parks DA, Bulkley GB et al (1982) Ischaemia injury in the cat small intestine: role of

superoxide radicals. Gastroenterology 82:9–15

45. Kubes P (1996) Mast-cell and neutrophils in intestinal ischemia/reperfusion. In: Rombeau JL, Takala J (eds) Gut dysfunction in critical illness. Springer Verlag, Berlin Heidelberg New York, pp 102–113

46. Reynolds JV, O'Farrelly C, Feighery C, Murchan P, Leonard N, Fulton G, O'Morian C, Keane FB, Tanner WA (1996) Impaired gut barrier function in malnourished patients. Br J Surg 83:1288–1291

47. Rowlands BJ, Soong CV et al (1999) The gastrointestinal tract as a barrier in sepsis. Br Med Bull 55:196–211

48. Mc Vay LD (1996) Immunology of the gut. In: Rombeau JL, Takala J (eds) Gut dysfunction in critical illness. Springer Verlag, Berlin Heidelberg New York, pp 76–101

49. Heyland DK, McDonald S et al (1998) Total parenteral nutrition in the critically ill patient. A meta-analysis. JAMA 280:2013–2019

50. Heymfield SB (1984) Respiratory, cardiovascular and metabolic effects on enteral hyperalimentation: influence of formula dose and composition. Am J Clin Nutr 40:116–130

51. Harris JA, Benedict FC (1919) A biometric study of basal metabolism in man. Carnegie Institute of Washington, DC

52. Iscra F, Romano E et al (1986) Calorific assessment of multiple trauma patients. Clin Nutr 5 [Suppl]:144

53. Iscra F, Berlot G et al (1990) Metabolic and nutritional aspects of COPD patients in ICU. Intensive Crit Care Med 1103

54. Working Group on Nutrition and Metabolism EISCM (1998) Enteral nutrition in intensive care patients: a practical approach. Intensive Care Med 24:848–860

55. Seidner DL, Masioli EA et al (1989) Effects of long chain triglyceride emulsions on reticuloendothelial function in humans. J Parenter Enteral Nutr 13:614–619

56. Battistella FD, Widergren JT et al (1997) A prospective, randomized trial of intravenous fat emulsion administration in trauma victims requiring total parenteral nutrition. J Trauma 43:52–58

57. Sukner U, Katz DP et al (2001) Effects of intravenous fat emulsion on lung function in patients with ARDS or sepsis. Crit Care Med 29:1569–1574

58. Nitenberg G (2000) Nutritional support in sepsis: still skeptical? Curr Opin Crit Care 6:253–256

59. Iapichino G, Raddrizzani D (1993) Anabolic drive in critically ill patients: pros and cons of a prevailing glucose system. In: Wilmore DW, Carpentier YA (eds) Metabolic support of the critically ill patient. Springer Verlag, Berlin Heidelberg New York, pp 137–156

60. Ishibashi N, Plank LD et al (1998) Optimal protein requirements during the first 2 weeks after the onset of critical illness. Crit Care Med 26:1529–1535

61. Larsson J, Lennmarken C et al (1990) Nitrogen requirement in severely injured patient. Br J Surg 77:413–416

62. Burstein S, Elwyn DH et al (1989) Nitrogen balance in energy metabolism, indirect calorimetry and nutrition. Williams and Wilkins, Baltimore, pp 85–118

63. Moore FA, Feliciano DV et al (1992) Early enteral feeding, compared with parenteral, reduces postoperative septic complications. The results of a meta-analysis. Ann Surg 216:172–183

64. van der Voort PHJ, Zandstra DF (2001) Enteral feeding in the critically ill: comparison between the supine and prone position. A prospective crossover study in mechanically ventilated patients. Crit Care 5:216–220

65. Iscra F, Randino A et al (1999) TPN vs TEN in critically ill patients. In: Guarnieri G,

Iscra F (eds) Metabolism and artificial nutrition in the critically ill. Springer Verlag, Milan, pp 115–124

66. Zaloga G (1993) Parenteral vs enteral nutrition. In: Wilmore DW, Carpentier YA (eds) Metabolic support of the critically ill patient. Springer Verlag, Berlin Heidelberg New York, pp 267–293

67. Kirby DF, Kudsk KA (2000) Obtaining and maintaining access for nutrition support. In: Pichard C, Kudsk KA (eds) From nutrition support to pharmacological nutrition in the ICU. Springer Verlag, Berlin Heidelberg New York, pp 125–137

68. Heys SD et al (1999) Enteral nutrition supplementation with key nutrients in patients with critical illness and cancer: a meta-analysis of randomized controlled clinical trials. Ann Surg 229:467–477

69. Beale RJ, Bryg DJ et al (1999) Immunonutrition in the critically ill: a systematic review of clinical outcome. Crit Care Med 27:2799–2805

70. Heyland DK, Novak F et al (2001) Should immunonutrition become routine in critically ill patients? JAMA 286:944–953

71. Griffiths RD (2003) Specialized nutrition support in critically ill patients. Curr Opin Crit Care 9:249–259

72. Galban C, Montejo JC et al (2000) An immune-enhancing enteral diet reduces mortality rate and episodes of bacteremia in septic intensive care unit patients. Crit Care Med 28:643-648

73. Marik PE, Zaloga GP (2001) Early enteral nutrition in acutely ill patients: a systematic review. Crit Care Med 29:2264-2270

74. Gadek JE, DeMichele SJ et al (1999) Effect of enteral feeding with eicosapentaenoic acid, γ-linolenic acid and antioxidants in patients with ARDS. Crit Care Med 27:1409–1420

75. Preiser JC, Wernerman J (2003) Glutamine, a life-saving nutrient, but why? Crit Care Med 31:2555–2556

76. Novak F, Heyland DK, Avenell A (2002) Glutamine supplementation in serious illness: A systematic review of the evidence. Crit Care Med 30:2022–2029

77. Garrel D, Patenaude J, Nedelec B et al (2003) Decreased mortality and infectious morbidity in adult burn patients given glutamine supplements: a prospective, controlled, randomized clinical trial. Crit Care Med 31:2444–2449

78. Nathens AB, Neft MJ, Jurkovich GJ et al (2002) Randomized, prospective trial of antioxidant supplementation in criticaly ill surgical patients. Ann Surg 236:814–822

79. Caparros T, Lopez J, Grau T (2001) Early enteral nutrition in criticaly ill patients with a high-protein diet enriched with arginine, fibre, and antioxidant compared with a standard high-protein diet: the effect on nosocomial infections and outcome. J Parenter Enteral Nutr 25:299–308

80. Lovat R, Preiser JC (2003) Antioxidant therapy in intensive care. Curr Opin Crit Care 9:266–270

81. Capes SE, Hunt D, Malmberg K et al (2000) Stress hyperglycemia and increased risk of death after myocardial infarction in patients with and without diabetes: A systematic overview. Lancet 355:773–778

82. Dandona P, Aljada A, Mohanty P et al (2001) Insulin inhibits intranuclear nuclear factor kappaB and stimulates kappaB in mononuclear cells in obese subjects: Evidence for an antiinflammatory effect? J Clin Endocrinol Metab 86:3257–3265

83. Ferrando AA, Chinkes DL, Wolf SE et al (1999) A submaximal dose of insulin promotes net skeletal muscle protein synthesis in patients with severe burns. Ann Surg 229:11–18

84. van den Berghe G, Wouters PJ, Weekers F et al (2001) Intensive insulin therapy in cri-

tically ill patients. N Engl J Med 345:19–1359

85.   van den Berghe G, Wouters PJ, Bouillon R et al (2003) Outcome benefit of intensive insulin therapy the critically ill:Insulin dose versus glycemic control. Crit Care Med 31:359–366

86.   Svensson S, Svedjeholm R, Ekroth R et al (1990) Trauma metabolism and the heart: Uptake of substrates and effects of insulin early after cardiac operations. J Thorac Cardiovasc Surg 99:1063–1073

87.   Fath-Ordoubadi F, Beatt KJ (1997) Glucose -insulin- potassium therapy for treatment of acute myocardial infarction: An overview of randomized placebo-controlled trials. Circulation 96:1152–1156

Gut Mucosal Protection in the Critically Ill Patient. Towards an Integrated Clinical Strategy

D.F. ZANDSTRA, P.H.J. VAN DER VOORT, K. THORBURN, H.K.F. VAN SAENE

Introduction

Traditionally, the critically ill patient is considered at risk for the development of stress ulcer-related bleeding (SURB) from the intestinal canal. Back diffusion of H^+ is considered the most important mechanism in the etiology of SURB [1]. The routine administration, in the intensive care unit (ICU), of specific prophylaxis using antacids, histamine$_2$ (H_2) receptor antagonists, and cytoprotectives has been practiced over the past 30 years. Several meta-analyses have shown a reduction from 15% to 5% in SURB after administration of antacids and H_2 receptor antagonists [2–5].

Despite the reduced incidence of SURB, overt SURB contributes to both morbidity and mortality [6]. The risk of death is increased only when the bleeding occurs more than 4 weeks after ICU admission, which suggests a different pathophysiology for early and late-onset bleeding [7]. Early bleeding is associated with acute hemodynamic disturbances, such as shock and incomplete resuscitation, whereas late bleeding is due to sepsis and multiple organ dysfunction syndrome.

Magnitude of the Problem

The reported incidence of SURB in adult patients who do not receive prophylaxis has also fallen from 60% (1978) to 0.65% in 1994 [8]. Since 1994 the incidence of SURB has remained constant (1%–5%), irrespective of whether the patient received prophylaxis or not [8]. Reduction of mortality has never been demonstrated using any prophylactic regimen [9, 10].

Pathogenesis of SURB in the Critically Ill

The pathogenesis of SURB is complex. Under normal conditions the mucosa is protected against potentially aggressive factors (e.g., gastric acid, pepsin, and bile) by a mucus layer. The most important mechanisms involved are vascular injury, gastric acid, ischemia, sepsis, endotoxin and inflammation in serious infection, *Helicobacter pylori* gastritis, and parenteral feeding.

Vascular Injury

Time sequence studies in animal experiments have shown that vascular injury is the rate-limiting step in the pathogenesis of mucosal injury caused by various substances. Vascular injury of the superficial mucosal capillaries may lead to a reduced or even absent blood flow, with subsequent edema and congestion of the mucosal layer. Whilst the blood supply remains intact, the self-restoring capacity of the mucosal layer is enormous. When the vascular injury is minimal or absent, the lesions of the epithelial surface are covered by migrating cuboidal cells within 60 min [11].

Gastric Acid

The back diffusion of H^+ ions was considered to be of the utmost importance in the development of SURB [1]. Recent work questions the pivotal role of gastric acid in the pathogenesis of SURB. A recent meta-analysis showed that ranitidine is no better than placebo in reducing the incidence of SURB [12]. H_2 receptor antagonists are contraindicated in the critically ill as they contribute to infection [13]. The H_2 receptors are not located on the acid-producing cells of the stomach, but on the surface of the immune-competent cells in the mucosal lining [14]. These immune cells orchestrate the local immune system in the gut ("enteric minibrain"). H_2 receptor antagonists downregulate the gut immune system, explaining the higher incidence of infections [13].

Critically ill patients often have gastric exocrine failure, with a subsequent gastric pH>4 [15]. SURB is frequently observed in this particular condition where the critically ill are unable to produce gastric acid, therefore gastric acid can be considered as a secondary factor in the pathogenesis of SURB. The primary step is impairment of the mucosal barrier functions due to ischemia.

Ischemia

Mucosal ischemia plays a key role in the pathogenesis of SURB [16, 17]. Mucosal cell ischemia occurs during shock, sepsis, and endotoxemia. The fundus and corpus of the stomach are particularly sensitive to ischemia. Mucosal cells do not have the ability to store glycogen as an energy substrate. During ischemia these cells cannot maintain cellular function by anaerobic glycolysis [18]. The reduced splanchnic blood flow leads to a decreased oxygen delivery and energy deficit that causes impairment of the barrier function of the mucosa. The back-diffusion of acid may occur, with subsequent mucosal damage and erosions or ulcers.

Hypovolemia, low cardiac output, and vasoconstrictive medication may all reduce splanchnic perfusion. Hypovolemia, particularly in surgical patients, is associated with an increased risk of gastrointestinal complications [19, 20]. There is a relationship between endotoxemia and the central venous pressure [21]. Mechanical ventilation on its own is associated with impaired intestinal perfusion in a high percentage of patients and may lead to impaired oxygenation [20]. Circulation therapy aimed at adequate microcirculation (flow), rather than blood pressure, remains crucial in the prevention of SURB.

Ischemia of the mucosa may persist due to arterio-venous shunting in the submucosa. Consequently, reperfusion injury may occur. Several experimental studies have shown that the oxygen radical scavengers attenuate the mucosal damage [22, 23].

Sepsis

The link between SURB and infection becomes increasingly clear in clinical practice. The incidence of SURB was 20% in patients with ineffectively treated pneumonias, whereas it was less than 10% in adequately treated patients [24]. Therefore pneumonia can be considered a major factor in the pathogenesis of SURB. Ventilator-associated pneumonia in the critically ill patient can effectively be prevented by selective decontamination of the digestive tract [25]. The potential role of sepsis in the pathogenesis of coagulation disorders that impact on SURB should be emphasized [10].

Experimental studies that focused on the role of sepsis in the pathogenesis of SURB are scarce. However, clinical experience shows that sepsis is the most important risk factor of SURB [7]. Various mechanisms are involved.

1. The release of vasoactive substances, including serotonin, histamine, adrenaline, and noradrenaline, promotes vasoconstriction following the release of endotoxin.
2. Hemodynamic changes may cause hypotension during the early phase of sepsis and may lead to a redistribution of blood flow between and within organs [26]. During sepsis, a substantial deficit in nutrient flow to the mucosa has been observed despite fluid resuscitation [27]. Increased arterio-venous shunting may cause tissue hypoxemia irrespective of increased blood flow [28].

Endotoxin and Inflammation in Serious Infections

Many clinical conditions are associated with increased intestinal permeability and may lead to endotoxemia, which is related to the degree of permeability [21]. Increased permeability can be prevented by vasodilators and adequate intravascular volume [21].

This inflammatory insult involves the activation of leukocytes, which may then adhere to the endothelium of the venular side of the microcirculation. This may block the microcirculation by means of subsequent stasis and ulceration [29].

Serious infections such as pneumonia have been shown to result in high levels of interleukin-6 and tumor necrosis factor. These inflammatory mediators increase the expression of adhesion molecules on the endothelium and on the leukocyte [30]. The expression of the adhesion molecules can be prevented by the use of steroids. Several anti-inflammatory agents reduce mucosal damage by preventing leukocyte adherence to the venular endothelium [31, 32].

There is good evidence for the role of activated leukocytes in the development of SURB. Steroids prevent the adhesion of leukocytes and thereby mucosal damage. Although steroids were believed to promote SURB, risk analysis failed to substantiate this [10].

Gastritis by *H. pylori*

H. pylori infection is the most important factor in the pathogenesis of gastric and duodenal ulceration in the non-ICU patient. In this population the prevalence of *H. pylori* infection is about 30%. The potential role of *H. pylori* infections in the pathogenesis of SURB in critically ill patients was investigated in detail in our unit [33–37].

The following endpoints were studied: (1) a new method for the detection of *H. pylori* in mechanically ventilated patients using a urea breath test; (2) the incidence of *H. pylori* infection in patients requiring acute admission to the ICU using the urea breath test and serology; (3) the impact of parenteral and enteral antibiotics of selective digestive decontamination on the eradication of *H. pylori*; (4) the incidence and risk factors of mucosal damage on admisson to the ICU by direct endoscopy; (5) *H. pylori* infection as an occupational hazard on the ICU.

Serological tests are unreliable for identifying *H. pylori* infections in the ICU patient. The laser-assisted ratio analyzer (LARA) ^{13}C-urea breath test (Alimenterics, N.J., USA) is a more reliable method for the detection of *H. pylori* infections in the ventilated patient [34]. The incidence of *H. pylori* infections in acutely admitted ICU patients is 40% [33]. A relationship was found between the degree of gastric mucosal lesions on admission to the ICU and the presence of an active infection [35].

Antimicrobials may also be effective in the treatment of *H. pylori* infection of the gastric mucosa, e.g., enteral non-absorbable antibiotics have been shown to control *H. pylori* infections in the critically ill [36]. Selective decontamination of the digestive tract reduces SURB, in part via elimination of *H. pylori*. Transmission of *H. pylori* from infected patients to nursing staff has been shown in our study [37].

Feeding

Enteral feeding has been shown to reduce infectious morbidity [38]. The delay in starting enteral feeding promotes mucosal vasoconstriction due to a reduced synthesis of prostaglandins. Stressful conditions combined with food deprivation have been shown to increase the incidence of ulceration. Enteral feeding protects the mucosa by (1) neutralization of acid, (2) stimulation of perfusion, and (3) intraluminal substrate as fuel for the colonic mucosal cell. Three studies show that enteral feeding has a beneficial effect on the incidence of stress ulceration [39–41]. However, enteral feeds administered too early could theoretically increase the risk of SURB, as the microcirculation is still impaired in the acute shock phase. Increased metabolism combined with impaired energy supply may increase ischemia.

Clinical Approach to Control SURB

The decreased incidence of SURB in patients without prophylaxis is due to improved ICU treatment over the last decades. The main factors are optimization of the microcirculation, effective infection control, early enteral feeding, and control of inflammation/infection due to *H. pylori*.

Aggressive correction of hypovolemia is achieved by adequate fluid replacement and by the prevention of vasoconstriction, using vasodilators. Vasoconstricting agents should be administered cautiously. The treatment of low cardiac output syndrome is based on the administration of inodilators following diagnosis. Steroids prevent the release of adhesion molecules. In this way leukocytes do not adhere to the endothelium.

H_2 receptor antagonists are contraindicated in the critically ill, as they are risk factors for infection. As the risk of ventilator-associated pneumonia with prolonged mechanical ventilation is increased, and the subsequent hyperinflammatory status predisposes to the development of SURB, the effective prevention of serious infection by selective decontamination of the digestive tract has been shown to reduce the incidence of SURB [42]. Selective decontamination has been shown to significantly reduce infectious morbidity and mortality.

Enteral feeding protects the gut mucosa and contributes to the control of infection. Selective decontamination using enteral and parenteral antibiotics controls *H. pylori* infections. Selective decontamination of the digestive tract clears fecal endotoxin, thus preventing endotoxin absorption and subsequent inflammation. The rapid elimination of the fecal endotoxin pool can also be promoted by the use of prokinetics [43].

Clinical measures are important to optimize microcirculation, to prevent nosocomial infections, and to reduce the state of hyperinflammation, which in turn reduces the incidence of SURB. This strategy, comprising continuous vasodilators to prevent mucosal ischemia, selective decontamination to control infection and to reduce intestinal endotoxin, and steroids to reduce leukocyte adherence, was associated with a SURB incidence of 0.6% in a cohort of critically ill ICU patients needing prolonged mechanical ventilation >48 h over a period of 7 years [35, 42]. These data, in combination with the lack of efficacy of specific prophylaxis in most recent studies, support the concept that SURB prevention is not only a matter of intragastric acid control. The most significant risk factors for SURB are prolonged mechanical ventilation of >48 h and coagulation disorders [10].

Despite decreased incidences of SURB, overt SURB still contributes to both morbidity and mortality [6]. However, this risk of mortality due to bleeding was not constant over time. The risk of death was increased only when bleeding occurred 4 or more weeks after ICU admission. This may reflect the different pathophysiology of late-onset bleeding [7]. Early bleeding results from acute hemodynamic disturbances, such as shock and incomplete resuscitation, whereas late bleeding can be considered the consequence of sepsis and infections, with subsequent microcirculatory insufficiency.

Pediatric Experience

There is a paucity of information concerning the incidence of clinically significant SURB in pediatric practice, with the reported incidence ranging from 0.4% to 1.6% [44, 45]. The basic pathophysiology is similar in children and adults [46]. There is no clear evidence of improvement with prophylaxis [46]. In a large pediatric ICU in Liverpool, there were only 3 cases of clinically important SURB in 3,238 admissions (>85% ventilated), including 772 post cardiopulmonary bypass (personal communication). No prophylaxis is used, but there is a policy of early enteral feeding and SDD.

Conclusions

Over the past 30 years, clinical strategies for the control of SURB have shifted from interventions to neutralize intragastric acid (antacids) and to inhibit acid synthesis (H_2 receptor antagonists) towards maneuvers that aim to maintain and improve microcirculatory perfusion (aggressive circulatory support, including vasodilators). The use of anti-inflammatory drugs for the prevention of microcirculatory sludging is important to maintain adequate microcirculation. Prevention of infection is achieved by selective decontamination of the digestive tract. This therapy also suppresses *H. pylori* gastritis, which plays a role in the pathogenesis of SURB. The implementation of this strategy guarantees a consistently low incidence of <1% of SURB in patients requiring a minimum of 2 days of mechanical ventilation.

Table 1. Protocol for the prevention of stress-ulcer related bleeding

Circulation
    Prevention of microcirculatory stasis by aggressive correction of hypovolemia and of low cardiac output
    Prevention of arterio-venous shunting using vasodilators
    Prevention of corpuscular endothelial adhesion using steroids

Infection prevention
    Prevention of serious infections including pneumonia and septicemia by selective decontamination of the digestive tract and immunonutrition

Intestinal contents
    Reduction of fecal endotoxin using selective decontamination of the digestive tract
    Prevention of stasis of intestinal contents using enema and neostigmine
    Enteral feeding to ensure mucosal energy supply

Control of gastritis due to *Helicobacter pylori*
    Elimination of *Helicobacter pylori* using enteral and parenteral antimicrobials of the selective decontamination of the digestive tract protocol

References

1. Skillman JJ, Gould SA, Chung W et al (1970) The gastric mucosal barrier: clinical and experimental studies in critically ill and normal man, and in the rabbit. Ann Surg 172:564–582
2. Cook DJ, Witt LJ, Cook RJ (1991) Stress ulcer prophylaxis in the critically ill: a meta-analysis. Am J Med 91:519–527

3. Shuman RB, Schuster DP, Zuckerman GR (1987) Prophylactic therapy for stress bleeding: a reappraisal. Ann Intern Med 106:562–567

4. Lacroix J, Infante-Rivard C, Jecinek M et al (1989) Prophylaxis of upper gastrointestinal bleeding in intensive care units. Crit Care Med 17:862–869

5. Tryba M (1991) Der Einfluss praeventiver Massnahmen auf Morbiditaet und Mortalitaet von Intensivpatienten. Anaesthesiol Intensivmed Notfallmed Schmerzther [Suppl] 1:42–53

6. Cook DJ, Griffith LE, Walter S et al (2001) Canadian Critical Care Trials Group. The attributable mortality and length of intensive care unit stay of clinically important gastrointestinal bleeding in critically ill patients. Crit Care 5:368–375

7. Zandstra DF, Stoutenbeek CP, Oudemans-van Straaten HM (1989) Pathogenesis of stress ulcer bleeding. In: van Saene HKF et al. (eds) Update in intensive and emergency medicine. Springer Verlag, Berlin Heidelberg New York p 166–172

8. Zandstra DF (1995) Stress ulceration in the critically ill. Not longer a problem? Proceedings SMART. Springer, Milan, pp 30–32

9. Tryba M (1991) Stress bleeding prophylaxis 1990—a meta-analysis. Clin J Gastroenterol 13 [Suppl 2]:44–55

10. Cook DJ, Fuller HD, Guyatt GH et al (1994) Risk factors for gastrointestinal bleeding in critically ill patients. N Eng J Med 330:377–381

11. Lacey ER, Ito S (1984) Rapid epithelial restitution of the rat gastric mucosa after ethanol injury. Lab Invest 51:573–583

12. Messori A, Trippoli S, Vaiani M et al (2000) Bleeding and pneumonia in intensive care patients given ranitidine and sucralfate for prevention of stress ulcer: meta-analysis of randomized controlled trials. BMJ 321:1103–1106

13. O'Keefe GE, Gentilello LM, Maier RV (1998) Incidence of infectious complications associated with the use of histamine$_2$-receptor antagonists in critically ill trauma patients. Ann Surg 227:120–112

14. Mezey E, Palkovits M (1992) Localisation of targets for anti-ulcer drugs in cells of the immune system. Science 258:1662–1665

15. Stannard VA, Hutchinson A, Morris DL et al (1988) Gastric exocrine failure in critically ill patients: incidence and associated features. BMJ 296:155–156

16. Fiddian-Green RG, McCough E, Pittenger G et al (1983) Predictive value of intramural pH and other risk factors for massive bleeding from stress ulceration. Gastroenterology 85:613–620

17. Hottenrott C, Seufert RM, Becker H (1978) The role of ischaemia in the pathogenesis of stress induced gastric lesions in piglets. Surg Gynecol Obstet 146:217–220

18. Menguy R, Desbaillets L, Masters YF (1974) Mechanisms of stress: influence of hypovolaemic shock on energy metabolism in the gastric mucosa. Gastroenterology 66:46–55

19. Christenson JT, Schmuziger M, Maurice J et al (1994) Gastrointestinal complications after coronary artery bypass grafting. J Thorac Cardiovasc Surg 108:899–906

20. Love R, Choe E, Lipton H et al (1995) Positive end-expiratory pressure decreased mesenteric blood flow despite normalization of cardiac output. J Trauma 39:195–199

21. Oudemans-van Straaten HM, Jansen PG, Velthuis H et al (1996) Endotoxaemia and postoperative hypermetabolism in coronary artery bypass surgery: the role of ketanserin. Br J Anaesth 77:473–479

22. Bhattacharjee M, Bhattacharjee S, Gupta A et al (2002) Critical role of an endogenous gastric peroxidase in controlling oxidative damage in *H. pylori*-mediated and nonmediated gastric ulcer. Free Radic Biol Med 32:731–743

23. Biswas K, Bandyopadhyay U, Chattopadhyay I et al (2003) A novel antioxidant and antiapoptotic role of omeprazole to block gastric ulcer through scavenging of hydroxyl radical. J Biol Chem 278:1099–1001
24. Alvarez Lerma F, ICU Acquired Infection Group (1996) Modification of empiric antibiotic treatment in patients with acquired pneumonia in the ICU. Intensive Care Med 22:387–394
25. Liberati A, D'Amico R, Pifferi et al (2004) Antibiotic prophylaxis to reduce respiratory tract infections and mortality in adults receiving intensive care (Cochrane Review). In: The Cochrane Library, Issue 1. John Wiley and Sons, Chichester, UK
26. Lang CH, Bagby GJ, Ferguson JL et al (1984) Cardiac output and redistribution of organ blood flow in hypermetabolic sepsis. Am J Physiol 246:331
27. Kreimeier U, Yang ZH, Messmer K (1988) The role of fluid replacement in acute endotoxin shock. In: Kox W, Bihari D (eds) Shock and the adult respiratory distress syndrome. Springer Verlag, Berlin Heidelberg New York
28. Bowen JC, LeDoux JC, Harkin GV (1979) Evidence for pathophysiologic arteriovenous shunting in the pathogenesis of acute gastric mucosal ulceration. Adv Shock Res 1:35–42
29. McCafferty DM, Granger DN, Wallace JL (1995) Indomethacin induced gastric injury and leucocyte adherence in arthritic versus healthy rats. Gastroenterology 109:1173–1180
30. Cush JJ, Rothlein R, Lindley HB et al (1993) Increased levels of circulating intercellular adhesion molecules in the sera of patients with rheumatoid arthritis. Arthritis Rheum 36:1098–1102
31. Low J, Grabow D, Sommers C et al (1995) Cytoprotective effects of CI-959 in the rat gastric mucosa; modulation of leukocyte adhesion. Gastroenterology 109:1224–1233
32. Santucci L, Firucci S, Giansanti M et al (1994) Pentoxifylline prevents indomethacin induced acute mucosal damage in rats: role of TNF. Gut 35:909–915
33. van der Voort PH, van der Hulst RW, Zandstra DF et al (2001) Prevalence of Helicobacter pylori infection in stress-induced gastric mucosal injury. Intensive Care Med 27:68–73
34. van der Voort PHJ, van der Hulst RW, Zandstra DF et al (1999) Detection of Helicobacter pylori in mechanically ventilated patients: the LARA-^{13}C-Urea breath test and serology. Clin Intensive Care 10:91–95
35. van der Voort PHJ, van der Hulst RW, Zandstra DF et al (2001) Suppression of Helicobacter pylori infection during intensive care stay: related to stress ulcer-bleeding incidence? J Crit Care 16:182–187
36. van der Voort PHJ, van der Hulst RW,, Zandstra DF et al (2000) In vitro susceptibility of Helicobacter pylori to, and in vivo suppression by antimicrobials used in selective decontamination of the digestive tract. J Antimicrob Chemother 46:803–805
37. van der Voort PHJ, van der Hulst RW, Zandstra DF et al (2001) Gut decontamination of critically ill patients reduces Helicobacter pylori acquisition by intensive care nurses. J Hosp Infect 47:41–45
38. Beale RJ, Bryg DJ, Bihari DJ (1999) Immunonutrition in the critically ill: a systematic review of clinical outcome. Crit Care Med 27:2799–2805
39. Ephgrave KS, Scott DL, Ong A et al (2000) Are gastric, jejunal, or both forms of enteral feeding gastroprotective during stress? J Surg Res 88:1–7
40. Ephgrave KS, Kleiman-Wexler RL, Adair CG (1990) Enteral nutrients prevent stress ulceration and increase intragastric volume. Crit Care Med 18:621–624

41. Raff T, Germann G, Hartmann B (1997) The value of early enteral nutrition in the prophylaxis of stress ulceration in the severely burned patient. Burns 23:313–318

42. Zandstra DF, Stoutenbeek CP (1994) The virtual absence of stress-ulcer related bleeding in ICU patients receiving prolonged mechanical ventilation without any prophylaxis: a prospective cohort study. Intensive Care Med 20: 335–340

43. van der Spoel JI, Oudemans-van Straaten HM, Stoutenbeek CP, Bosman RJ, Zandstra DF (2001) Neostigmine resolves critical illness-related colonic ileus in intensive care patients with multiple organ failure—a prospective, double-blind, placebo-controlled trial. Intensive Care Med 27:822–827

44. Lacroix J, Nadeau D, Laberge S et al (1992) Frequency of upper gastrointestinal bleeding in a pediatric intensive care unit. Critical Care Med 20:35–42

45. Chaibou M, Tucci M, Dugas M-A et al (1998) Clinically significant upper gastrointestinal bleeding in a pediatric intensive care unit: a prospective study. Pediatrics 102:933–938

46. Crill CM, Hak EB (1999) Upper gastrointestinal bleeding in critically ill pediatric patients. Pharmacotherapy 19:162–180

Selective Decontamination of the Digestive Tract: the Role of the Pharmacist

N.J. Reilly, A.J. Nunn, K. Pollock

Introduction

Selective decontamination of the digestive tract (SDD) is a prophylactic strategy aimed at preventing both endogenous and exogenous infections in patients admitted to the intensive care unit (ICU) [1]. Endogenous infections in critically ill patients are invariably preceded by oropharyngeal and gastrointestinal carriage of potentially pathogenic micro-organisms (PPMs). "Community" and "hospital" PPMs (Table 1) carried by the patient upon admission are the causative agents of primary endogenous infections, whilst "hospital" PPMs acquired by the patient during their time on the ICU are responsible for secondary endogenous infections. Exogenous infections are caused by mainly hospital PPMs not carried by the patient at all [2].

The causative bacteria for exogenous infections are also acquired on the unit, but are never present in the throat and/or gut flora of patients [3]. For example, long-stay patients, particularly those who receive a tracheostomy on respiratory units, are at high risk of exogenous, lower airway infections. Purulent lower airway secretions yield a micro-organism that has never been previously carried by the patient in the digestive tract flora, or indeed in their oropharynx. Although both the tracheostomy and the oropharynx are equally accessible for bacterial entry, the tracheostomy tends to be the entry site for bacteria that colonize/infect the lower airways. Within a group of adult ICU patients it has been shown that c. 55% will develop "early" or primary endogenous infections, c. 30% will develop secondary endogenous infections, and will develop exogenous infections.

There are few epidemiological studies on nosocomial infections in ICU (PICU) [4–8] compared with published studies on neonatal and Publications demonstrating the benefits of SDD in the PICU are [9–14]. Two recent meta-analyses, however, have shown the imp that SDD has on morbidity and mortality in adult patients. Th

Table 1. Potentially pathogenic micro-organisms (PPM) causing infection in intensive care unit (ICU) patients

Previously healthy host ("community" PPM)	Host with severe underlying disease ("hospital" PPM)
1. Streptococcus pneumoniae	7. Klebsiella spp.
2. Haemophilus influenzae	8. Proteus spp.
3. Moraxella catarrhalis	9. Morganella spp.
4. Escherichia coli	10. Enterobacter spp.
5. Staphylococcus aureus	11. Citrobacter spp.
6. Candida albicans	12. Serratia spp.
	13. Acinetobacter spp.
	14. Pseudomonas spp.

meta-analysis of the two reviewed 36 randomized SDD trials and concluded that the use of SDD had led to a reduction of lower airway infections and mortality by 65% and 22%, respectively [15]. The second meta-analysis in surgical patients showed that SDD usage led to a reduction in lower airway infection, septicemia, and mortality by 80%, 50%, and 30%, respectively [16]. A recent prospective cohort study on a PICU [17] reported that 61% of their infections were caused by micro-organisms carried by the patients on admission and hence unrelated to the PICU ecology. A low secondary endogenous infection rate of 5% was attributed to the use of SDD and was in line with the results of the two meta-analyses. In this study the exogenous infection rate was 34% and suggested that transmission via hands was a problem in a busy PICU.

The concept of SDD was introduced in the early 1980s by Stoutenbeek et al. [18] and was aimed at controlling the three types of infections (i.e., primary endogenous, secondary endogenous, and exogenous infections) caused by both "community" and "hospital" PPMs, by means of a parenteral antibiotic, a mixture of topical non-absorbable antimicrobials, high levels of hygiene, and surveillance cultures [19, 20]. Due to the lack of commercially available topical formulations, the application of SDD to hospital practice has required a substantial input from pharmacists in both the development and extemporaneous preparation of SDD formulations. This article aims to provide the reader with comprehensive information on the pharmaceutical technology involved in the implementation of SDD and how the role of the pharmacist is essential if this concept is to be successfully utilized to reduce carriage, colonization, and infection rates.

The Use of Non-Absorbable Antimicrobials-the PTA Regimen˙

In healthy individuals host defense mechanisms prevent abnormal carriage in the digestive tract of PPMs, including aerobic gram-negative bacilli (AGNB). However, if host defense mechanisms are impaired in traumatized and infected patients, e.g., after intubation (impaired cilia), urinary catheterization (sphincter breached), or gut paralysis, carriage can lead to colonization and with immunoparalysis to infection [3]. Micro-organisms present in the oropharynx migrate down to the lower airways causing respiratory tract infections and subsequent pneumonia. Those present in the rectum migrate to the urethra and bladder to cause urinary tract infections. Lesions of the head, neck, and thorax can become infected by salivary flora, whilst lesions below the waist are usually infected by fecal flora. Septicemia may follow pneumonia, cystitis, and wound infection by further migration of micro-organisms. Translocation of PPM through the gut mucosal lining may occur, producing systemic infection without the stage of colonization [21–23].

SDD aims to convert the abnormal carrier state into normal carriage, using oral, non-absorbable antimicrobials. It is a method of controlling colonization/infection, moderating the systemic inflammatory response, and containing the spread of multi-resistant micro-organisms. Locally applied oropharyngeal and gastrointestinal antibiotics are directed at eradicating the carriage of PPMs, including *Staphylococcus aureus*, AGNB, and yeasts [24]. Only the use of non-absorbable antimicrobials can guarantee concentrations in the saliva and feces high enough to selectively abolish the carriage of PPMs [25] without influencing the protective anaerobic flora, thereby decreasing colonization resistance. The ideal regimen should use antimicrobials that are non-toxic, inexpensive, palatable, and microbiologically active in the presence of feces, saliva, or antacids [26, 27]. It should be noted that only a parenteral antibiotic can eradicate colonization and infection; enteral agents only prevent carriage [28, 29]. The most widely used SDD regimen is that of the Groningen group [18] who devised a protocol using polymyxin E, tobramycin, and amphotericin B applied as an oral paste and suspension to treat both the throat and gut, respectively. Hence the antimicrobials of this SDD regimen are often referred to in the literature as "PTA" after the initial letters of polymyxin E, tobramycin, and amphotericin B. In the United Kingdom polymyxin E is known as colistin.

There are 14 potential pathogens (Table 1) that can cause serious infection and death during a patient's ICU stay. The rationale behind the use of SDD is to control the three types of infection due to the 14 potential pathogens [19]. The combination of polymyxin E and tobramycin is synergistic against *Proteus* and *Pseudomonas* species. It is the most potent anti-pseudomonal combination associated with an effective clearance of *Pseudomonas* from the gut. Emergence of resistance to polymyxin is rare. Although there are bacteria producing tobramycin-inactivating enzymes, polymyxin is thought to protect tobramycin from being destroyed by these bacterial enzymes [24]. Tobramycin is the preferred aminoglycoside because it is intrinsically most active against *Pseudomonas* and is minimally inactivated by saliva and feces [30]. It also has useful activity against *Staphylococcus aureus* [28]. Both agents absorb endotoxin released by AGNB in the gut. This feature is important because endotoxin can be absorbed from the gut of seriously ill patients producing fever, release of inflammatory mediators, and shock [31]. Amphotericin B is included to prevent overgrowth by yeasts. It is intrinsically the most potent antifungal but there is a high rate of inactivation in the gut requiring the use of high doses [32]. By design, the PTA regimen is inactive against the indigenous flora, such as *Streptococcus viridans*, enterococci, coagulase-negative staphylococci, and anaerobes [28], each of which is necessary for normal physiological gut function.

Indications

In the PICU setting SDD is indicated [33]:
1. In the control of infection—in patients requiring ventilation for more than 3 days SDD reduces the risk of endogenous infections.
2. In the control of inflammation—following cardiac surgery (and particularly cardiopulmonary bypass) patients develop the systemic inflammation response syndrome (SIRS), characterized by high levels of cytokines, leukocytes, and increased C-reactive protein. Polymyxin E and tobramycin neutralize endotoxin and reduce gut overgrowth.
3. To prevent resistance—SDD eradicates multi-resistant micro-organisms detected from surveillance swabs of throat and rectum.

Method of Application

Selective Decontamination of the Oropharynx

SDD gel containing 2% polymyxin, tobramycin, and amphotericin B (PTA) is used. A pea-sized application of gel is evenly smeared in the lower cheeks four times a day. A 5-g tube lasts approximately 5 days.

Selective Decontamination of Gastrointestinal Tract

The antimicrobials are given orally or through the nasogastic tube. When the patient requires gastric suction, the nasogastric tube is clamped and the suction is discontinued for 1 h. When the normal anatomy of the gastrointestinal tract is disrupted (gastro or intestinal fistulae or colostomy), each (blind) loop should be separately treated with approximately half of the oral PTA dose in an adequate volume [33]. Doses of the preparations used are shown in Table 2.

Table 2. Doses for selective decontamination of the digestive tract (SDD) [33]

Over 12 years	Polymyxin E/colistin	100 mg≡3,000,000 units four times daily
	Tobramycin base	80 mg four times daily
	Amphotericin B	500 mg four times daily
	SDD gel	A pea-sized application four times daily
5-12 years	Polymyxin E/Colistin	50 mg≡1,500,000 units four times daily
	Tobramycin base	40 mg four times daily
	Amphotericin B	250 mg four times daily
	SDD gel	A pea-sized application four times daily
1-4 years	Polymyxin E/Colistin	25 mg≡750,000 units four times daily
	Tobramycin base	20 mg four times daily
	Amphotericin B	100 mg four times daily
	SDD gel	A pea-sized application four times daily
Small infants/ neonates	Polymyxin E/Colistin	25 mg≡750,000 units four times daily
	Tobramycin base	20 mg four times daily
	Amphotericin B	100 mg four times daily
	SDD gel	A pea-sized application four times daily

The dose administered is dependent on gut volume
To be administered 30 min before feeds and not with feeds
Sucralfate significantly reduces concentrations of colistin, tobramycin, and amphotericin B, therefore separate administration by 2–4 h [34]
Colistin doses in milligrams are specified as colistin base, where 1 mg=30,000 units. However, colistin should normally be prescribed in units and the appropriate preparation used to give the specified number of units
1 mg tobramycin base is equivalent to 1.5 mg tobramycin sulfate
1 mg colistin base is equivalent to 1.5 mg colistin sulfate

Pharmaceutical Technology

The development of SDD medication has depended upon close collaboration between pharmacists and microbiologists. For decontamination of the gut in the unconscious adult and in children, liquid preparations for administration via a nasogastric tube are required [35]. For decontamination of the oropharynx, formulations covering oral gel and paste, pastilles, and lozenges have been developed and prepared by hospital and academic pharmacists [36]. Solutions or suspensions of the three antimicrobials are used for oral and nasogastric administration [33]. Colonic coated tablets of colistin have also been prepared for positioned release into the colon [37]. No commercial company has yet shown more than a passing interest in the further development, licensing, or marketing of these preparations, and this may have influenced the rate of development of the SDD concept.

Since all preparations are made extemporaneously in the hospital pharmacy or manufacturing units, they are classed as "hospital specials" and as such are unlicensed. In using these unlicensed products in clinical practice, responsibility for safety and efficacy lies with the prescriber and responsibility for quality is with the pharmacist. Ideally, to reduce risks to the patient it would be preferable to use medicines that have been appropriately researched and subjected to the scrutiny of the medicines licensing process. One other problem with extemporaneous production is that in the United Kingdom pharmacy departments are limited in the quantities of products that they can prepare, unless they have a Manufacturer's licence (specials) issued by the Medicines Control Agency (MCA).

Because SDD medication is not commercially available or supported by the usual manufacturers' marketing activity [38], scientific background to the formulations (assay, rheology) is limited. To date little work has been undertaken to develop assays for the PTA ingredients, when combined in mixtures or formulations for local, oral application. Assays should indicate activity of the constituent antimicrobials and therefore a microbiological assay is preferred to techniques such as high-performance liquid chromatography. Suitable microorganisms must be selected for their resistance to the other PTA components, lack of reversion to sensitivity must be demonstrated, and diffusion from the gel to agar plate must be matched to that of standard antimicrobial solutions.

In spite of commercial apathy, hospital-based research is continuing into areas such as modifications to the gel, the development of colonic positioned release products, and the production of placebo products for trial work. It should be noted, however, that the extemporaneous production of SDD formulations does lead to an increase in a hospital pharmacy department's workload and that involvement in research programs requires a considerable amount of research and development work that would be best met by commercial support.

Choice of Formulation

Oropharynx

In order to abolish carriage of PPMs in the oropharynx a contact time of at least 20 min is required for effective decontamination [30, 36]. Pastes, gels, pastilles, and lozenges therefore offer advantages over suspensions, aerosols, and oral rinses, as they have a longer contact time [39]. The ideal formulation for use in the oropharynx should therefore have a prolonged contact time with the oral mucosa, should release the antimicrobials into the oropharynx throughout the contact period, should be pharmaceutically stable, and should be acceptable to the patient [36].

There are four suitable formulations recommended for use in the oropharynx–paste, gel, lozenge, or pastille. It should be noted that the shelf life for these products has been assigned on the basis of *in vivo* microbiological experience and not by traditional pharmaceutical methodology. For use in our PICU, the majority of these preparations are prepared and supplied to us by a specialist hospital pharmacy manufacturing unit at the Western Infirmary in Glasgow, Scotland.

Paste. A paste has advantages in that it is easy to produce, it has good adhesion to the mucosa, it has a prolonged release of medicament, it is stable, and has a well-proven formula [39] (Table 3). Although the paste is effective in the elimination of AGNB, it has several drawbacks. It has an unpleasant taste and appearance and can cause considerable drying of the oral mucosa and it can be difficult to remove, occasionally causing trauma to the mucosa [35]. Because of this it has poor acceptability with patients, staff, and relatives. We restrict the use of the paste to topical applications around tracheostomy and gastrostomy sites, where the adherence and barrier properties of the paste are particularly useful. Application of the topical antimicrobials to tracheostomy sites has been proven to be effective in reducing the exogenous route of colonization [3].

Table 3. Formula for SDD paste [39]

Amphotericin B powder	2 g (adjusted for potency)
Tobramycin sulfate USP	2 g
Colistin sulfate BP	2 g
Liquid paraffin	10 g
Orabase paste (ConvaTec)	to 100 g

Shelf life: 1 month
Do not refrigerate
SDD paste is prepared by mixing each of the antimicrobial powders with 10% w/w liquid paraffin and gradually incorporating Orabase. Vigorous mixing causes the Orabase to crack

Pastille. The advantages of the pastille are that it can be flavored easily, it has good release characteristics, it is easy to use, and it is acceptable to the conscious patient (Table 4). Studies in cancer patients have demonstrated that SDD pastilles are effective in eradicating the carriage of AGNB and yeasts, reducing the incidence of radiation mucositis and yeast stomatitis in these patients [40].

Table 4. Formula of SDD pastille [39]

Gelatin	500 g
Glycerol BP	700 g
Sucrose	100 g
Sodium benzoate	4 g
Distilled water	600 ml
Lemon oil	2 ml
Blackcurrant powder	10 g
Amphotericin B powder	15.88 g (adjusted for potency)
Colistin sulfate BP	12.95 g
Tobramycin sulfate USP	12.95 g

To prepare SDD pastilles soak the gelatin and water and heat to melt. Add most of the glycerol and the other ingredients except the antibiotics and mix well. Heat for 30 min and then add the antibiotics, wetting the amphotericin with glycerin
Shelf life: 6 months
Each pastille weighs 1.5 g and contains 12 mg of amphotericin and 10 mg of tobramycin and colistin

The pastille, however, has limited use as it cannot be used in comatose patients, it has a high sugar content, and therefore cannot be used in diabetics, and it is unsuitable for young children [34]. It is difficult to produce, as many hospital pharmacy departments do not have appropriate facilities, and therefore this preparation needs to be made in a specialized manufacturing unit.

Lozenge. The advantages and disadvantages of the lozenge are very similar to that of the pastille (Table 5). In cancer patients the eradication of AGNB and yeasts by SDD lozenges has been shown by Spijkervet et al. [41] to take up to 3 weeks, therefore comparing poorly with eradication rates of 3–4 days that have been achieved by the use of SDD paste in ICU patients. One explanation for these differing eradication rates would be that patients on the ICU are unconscious, permitting proper application of sticky paste, whilst patients with head and neck cancer suck their lozenges four times daily and eat normal, unsterilized food. Poor compliance within this group of patients, a lower standard of personal hygiene, and an altered oropharyngeal anatomy may also contribute to the longer eradication times.

Lozenges, when sucked will take approximately 15 min to dissolve *in vivo*. Hence they do not achieve the same length of contact time with the buccal mucosa as the paste or gel, and this is therefore another factor contributing to poorer eradication rates. These results would suggest a need for new formula-

Table 5. Formula for SDD lozenge [42]

Antibiotic mixture	
Amphotericin B powder	10 mg
Colistin sulfate BP	2 mg
Tobramycin sulfate USP	1.6 mg
Basic mixture	
Citric acid	40 mg
Calcium diphosphate	150 mg
Saccharine	795 mg

Shelf life: 3 months

To prepare SDD lozenges, two powder mixtures are prepared. After sieving of the powders, the total mixture is mixed in a turbula mixer (90 rpm) for 15 min. The total powder mixture is then moistened with 25 ml of water and thereafter 25 ml of sodium carboxymethylcellulose (low viscosity) is added. Further mixing then takes place for 10 min, after which the moistened powder is dried for a minimum of 4 h at 40°C. The dried mixture is then mashed through a 0.75-mm sieve and the resultant granulate is then sieved further through a 0.4-mm sieve in order to eliminate the fine powder. Prior to the final tableting stage the granulate is mixed with 0.5% magnesium stearate and 2.5% talc, in the turbula mixer for 2 min

tions to be developed, in order to allow a more protracted and hence more effective delivery of the antimicrobials to the buccal mucosa of ambulant patients.

Gel. The gel is an improvement on the paste in that it is more palatable, much easier to remove, and does not dry the oropharyngeal mucosa [35] (Table 6). The efficacy of this formulation appears to be equal to that of the paste [35]. Patient acceptability with the gel is high and therefore compliance is better. The gel is also sugar free. The gel presents problems, however, in that it is difficult to produce and at present its long-term stability is unknown [36].

Gastrointestinal Tract

Decontamination of the gut is not difficult. Most ICU patients have gut stasis, there is good contact time between antimicrobials and organisms and it can be demonstrated by surveillance culture that decontamination of the esophagus, stomach, and small intestine occurs within 3 days [35, 43]. However, in order to clear PPMs from the large intestine there must be gut motility. Due to this controlling factor, decontamination of the colon and rectum may therefore be longer and may take up to 7 days. A formulation for use in the gastrointestinal

Table 6. Formula for SDD gel 2% [39]

Sodium carboxymethylcellulose (Blanose)	10 g
Glycerol BP	60 ml
Methylhydroxybenzoate	600 mg
Concentrated peppermint water BP	10 ml
Distilled water	200 ml
Amphotericin B powder	6 g (adjusted for potency)
Colistin sulfate BP	6 g
Tobramycin sulfate USP	6 g

Shelf life: 1 month
Refrigerate
A gel base is prepared from sodium carboxymethylcellulose, propylene glycol, or glycerol and methylhydroxybenzoate solution. Peppermint water is added for flavor; 2% by weight of each of amphotericin B, colistin sulfate, and tobramycin sulfate are stirred into the cold gel base and the resulting SDD gel is packed into aluminium tubes using a syringe and tube to aid filling
Colistin sulfomethate sodium has been used in the gel in some centers where a "stringy" texture has been noted when using the sulfate. This method involves the use of the commercial powder for injection (Colomycin injection, manufactured by Pharmax)

tract should therefore ideally release the antimicrobials in the terminal ileum and provide high concentrations of these antimicrobials in the colon and rectum [36]. The product should also be easy to use, acceptable to patients, and have good pharmaceutical stability [36].

To date only oral suspensions and solutions have been used (Tables 7–10). Although Crome [36] in 1989 suggested that research was progressing into the development of colon-positioned release tablets/capsules for use in conscious patients, this research does not appear to have led to the availability or widespread use of these preparations [44]. We have used colonic coated colistin capsules only once [37] in conscious, immunocompromised patients who had functioning guts. The aim of colonic coated preparations is that they should allow release of the capsule contents at a pH of approximately 7–7.2, resulting in disintegration in the ascending colon. The resultant local delivery of antibacterial agents into the colon is thought to achieve fecal flora suppression [45] and by bypassing the esophagus and stomach, gastrointestinal side effects, such as nausea and vomiting, should be reduced.

The widespread use of the oral solutions and suspensions in PICU therefore continues. The advantages of these products being that they are stable [39], easy to produce, and can be given via a nasogastric tube, and are therefore suitable to give to an unconscious patient [36]. Problems with poor taste, however, particularly of colistin, may decrease compliance in conscious patients. In neonates, vomiting and other gastrointestinal problems have been seen, particularly if concentrated solutions are administered to an empty stomach [46]. The osmolality of amphotericin suspension is high, approximately 2,000 mosmol/l

Table 7. Formula for amphotericin suspension 100 mg/ml [39]

Amphotericin B powder	500 g (adjusted for potency)
Sodium citrate BP	25 g
Sodium carboxymethylcellulose (Blanose)	12.5 g
Veegum K	25 g
Citric acid monohydrate	5.95 g to adjust pH to 5.5
Saccharin solution BPC	7 ml
Lycassin	750 ml
Nipasept	6,5 g
Concentrated peppermint water BP	125 ml
Distilled water	to 5,330 g

Shelf life: 6 months
A suspension is prepared with sodium carboxymethylcellulose (Blanose) as suspending and thickening agent, distilled water and Lycassin as the sweetener. Veegum K (hydrated magnesium aluminum silicate) is then added as the anticaking agent. Amphotericin B powder is added gradually to this mixture, stirring after each addition. Nipasept used as a preservative is dissolved in the concentrated peppermint water and then added to the suspension. Peppermint water is added to mask the metallic taste of amphotericin. Finally saccharin solution is added to improve palatability and citric acid monohydrate to adjust the pH of the suspension to 5.5. The remaining water is then added to make up to the final weight

Table 8. Formula for colistin oral solution 100 mg base (3 Munits) in 1 ml [37]

Colistin sulfate powder Ph.Eur	15 g
Nipasept sodium powder	150 mg
Orange syrup BP	10 ml
Purified water	to 100 ml

1.5 g colistin sulfate ≡ 1 g colistin base
Shelf life: 1 month
Refrigerate
Colistin for SDD is prescribed as base
The solution is prepared by dissolving colistin sulfate powder in purified water, using orange syrup as flavoring and Nipasept as the preservative
[A commercial preparation of colistin is available (Colomycin) from Forest. It contains 250,000 units of colistin in 5 ml and is stable for 2 weeks when reconstituted]

N.J. Reilly, A.J. Nunn, K. Pollock

Table 9. Formula for tobramycin sulfate oral solution 120 mg in 1 ml [37] (containing tobramycin base 80 mg in 1ml)

Tobramycin sulfate powder USP	1,200 mg
Orange syrup BP	1 ml
Preserved distilled water	to 10 ml

120 mg tobramycin sulfate ≡ 80 mg tobramycin base

Shelf life: 2 weeks
Store at room temperature.
Tobramycin for SDD is prescribed as base
A solution is prepared with tobramycin sulfate in preserved distilled water using orange syrup for flavoring

Table 10. Formula for preserved distilled water [39]

Nipasept 0.12%	24 g
Absolute alcohol	200 ml
Glacial acetic acid	to pH 4–6
Distilled water	to 20 l

Shelf life: 1 year

compared with an osmolality of approximately 430 mosmol/l with a 25 mg/ml colistin solution and 60 mosmol/l with a 20 mg/ml solution of tobramycin sulfate. Because hyperosmolar medications have been associated with an increased incidence of necrotizing enterocolitis [46], it is recommended that all three PTA ingredients should be diluted in water. Observers have also suggested that PTA may delay gastric emptying/absorption of feeds, and the binding of colistin and tobramycin by food proteins is a factor known to reduce the lethal intestinal antibiotic levels required for eradication of AGNB [29]. This interference with food has been shown to be the reason for SDD failure when oral contaminated feeds were given to a premature neonate [29]. On our PICU we recommend that SDD doses should be administered 30 min before feeds and not with feeds [33].

Although there are a limited number of commercially available products that could be used for SDD, problems with pack sizes, expiry dates, and strengths of the commercial products mean that most ICUs prefer to use extemporaneously prepared products on their patients. For example, colistin syrup is available commercially at a strength of 250,000 units in 5 ml (Colomycin, Forest). This means that to give a dose of 3,000,000 units (≡100 mg) for a patient over 12 years of age, 60 ml would be required per dose, i.e., 240 ml/day.

The same dose using an extemporaneously prepared 100 mg/ml colistin oral solution would equate to a volume of 1 ml, i.e., 4 ml/day. Amphotericin suspension is another example of a problem encountered with a commercial product. Although the strength of the licensed product, Fungilin (Squibb) at 100 mg/ml is equivalent to the extemporaneously prepared product, Fungilin is only available in 12-ml bottles and therefore is very inconvenient for a 5 ml four times a day dose that would be required for a patient over 12 years. Another disadvantage with Fungilin is that once opened the manufacturers advise that the suspension should be discarded after 4 days.

Costs of Decontaminating Agents

Formal cost-benefit analyses of SDD in ICU patients have not been performed. In theory successful prevention of infection may make the ICU more cost-effective, in that reduced infection rates secondary to SDD may lead to a shorter patient stay on ICU, lower ICU costs, parenteral antibiotic usage, and microbiology laboratory costs [30]. It has not been firmly established whether these potential savings offset the additional costs that the SDD regimen incurs through the use of non-absorbable antimicrobials, systemic antimicrobials, and additional microbiological cultures [47]. Hence, despite 54 randomized controlled trials and nine meta-analyses including two recent analyses suggesting that using the full concept of SDD leads to a 22% reduction in mortality [15, 16], the routine use of SDD in ICUs remains controversial [47, 48].

The average costs for the drugs used in the PTA regimen using products prepared by a specialist hospital manufacturing unit are listed in Table 11 and the costs of commercially available preparations in Table 12. The cost of treating a patient over 12 years of age using the available commercial products and products manufactured in the hospital manufacturing unit are also compared.

Tables 11 and 12 show that the cost of SDD can be substantially reduced if preparations for SDD are manufactured in the hospital pharmacy [50]. Due to the commercial unavailability of a tobramycin oral solution and an SDD gel, it would not be possible to follow the PTA regimen without the provision of hospital-made products. Although the daily cost of the licensed amphotericin suspension is actually less than the hospital-prepared product, the small pack size of only 12 ml makes this product impractical for routine use on a busy ICU.

One factor that may make it difficult for a hospital pharmacy to begin manufacturing preparations for SDD regimes is sourcing the "raw ingredients" necessary to make the products. Table 13 therefore provides useful information to overcome this problem.

Table 11. Costs of hospital preparations (March 2004)

Drug	Supplier	Pack size	Cost (£)	Total daily dose >12 years	Cost/day (£)
Amphotericin 100 mg/ml suspension	Western Infirmary, Glasgow	100 ml	21.85	2,000 mg	4.37
Colistin solution 100 mg/ml	Alder Hey Hospital, Liverpool	100 ml	41.50	400 mg	1.66
Tobramycin solution 80 mg/ml	Alder Hey Hospital, Liverpool	100 ml	97.0	320 mg	3.88
SDD gel	Western Infirmary, Glasgow	5 g	7.50	A pea-sized application four times a day	1.5
SDD paste	Western Infirmary, Glasgow	5 g	10.0	A pea-sized application four times a day	2.0
SDD pastilles	Western Infirmary, Glasgow	28	14.0	1 pastille four times a day	2.0

Table 12. Costs of commercially available preparations (March 2004) [49]

Drug	Supplier	Pack size	Cost (£)	Total daily dose >12 years	Cost/day (£)
Colomycin Syrup (colistin sulfate 250,000 units/5 ml)	Forest	80 ml	3.71	400 mg (≡12,000,000 units)	11.13
Colomycin tablets (colistin sulfate 1.5 million unit tablets)	Forest	50	62.18	400 mg (≡12,000,000 units	9.95
Fungilin suspension (amphotericin 100 mg/ml)	Squibb	12 ml	2.31	2,000 mg	3.84
Fungilin tablets (amphotericin 100 mg tablets)	Squibb	56	8.32	2,000 mg	2.97
Fungilin lozenges (amphotericin 10-mg lozenges)	Squibb	60	3.95	1 lozenge four times a day	0.26

Table 13. Possible sources of ingredients

Ingredient	Supplier
Sodium carboxymethylcellulose (Blanose), Sodium benzoate	E. Merck and Lipha, Hunter Boulevard, Magna Park, Lutterworth, Leics, LE17 4XN, UK Tel.: 0800 22 33 44
Amphotericin B powder Tobramycin sulfate powder USP Colistin sulfate powder Ph.Eur.	Fahrhaus Pharma Hamburg, Germany Tel: 00 49 40 61 17 18 19 Fax 00 49 40 61 17 18 18
Glycerol BP, citric acid monohydrate, liquid paraffin	Thornton and Ross Ltd. Linthwaite Laboratories, Huddersfield HD7 5QH, UK Tel.: 01484 842 217
Methylhydroxybenzoate BP	J.M. Loveridge plc. Southampton, UK Tel.: 02380 228411 Fax: 02380 639836

Conclusion

Although the application of the SDD concept to intensive care medicine has been proven to reduce ICU-related morbidity and mortality and in spite of a recent publication validating SDD as an evidence-based medicine maneuver [51], the SDD approach is still not widely used on ICUs. Reasons for this may include:

1. SDD is contrary to the traditional concept that prophylaxis creates resistance.
2. A primacy of opinion over evidence.
3. Opinion leaders control the medical media.
4. SDD formulations are not marketed by the pharmaceutical industry.
5. There is little physician-pharmaceutical industry interaction to stimulate industry interest in manufacturing SDD products.

In the current climate, with a lack of commercial products, the necessary extemporaneous production of SDD formulations must be undertaken by a pharmacy department that is able to commit to the additional workload that this entails. This means that at present the formulation and supply role of the hospital pharmacist is vital in order to facilitate the application of the SDD concept to clinical practice.

References

1. Silvestri L, van Saene HKF, Gullo A (1997) Selective decontamination of the digestive tract in critically ill patients: a pathogenesis-based infection control method. Care Crit Ill 13:227–232
2. van Saene HKF, Damjanovic V, Murray AE, de la Cal MA (1996) How to classify infections in intensive care units—the carrier state, a criterion whose time has come? J Hosp Infect 33:1–12
3. Morar P, Makura Z, Jones A, Baines P, Selby A, Hughes J, van Saene HKF (2000) Topical antibiotics on tracheostoma prevents exogenous colonization and infection of lower airways in children. Chest 117:513–518
4. Gray J, Gossain S, Morris K (2001) Three-year survey of bacteremia and fungemia in a pediatric intensive care unit. Pediatr Infect Dis J 20:416–421
5. Richards MJ, Edwards JR, Culver DH, Gaynes RP (1999) Nosocomial infections in pediatric intensive care units in the United States. Pediatrics 103:1–7
6. Singh-Naz N, Sprague BM, Patel KM, Pollack MM (2000) Risk assessment and standardised nosocomial infection rate in critically children. Crit Care Med 28:2069–2075
7. Patel JC, Mollitt DL, Pieper P, Tepas JJ (2000) Nosocomial pneumonia in the pediatric trauma patient: a single center's experience. Crit Care Med 28:3530–3533
8. Albers MJIJ, Mouton JW, Tibboel D (2001) Colonization and infection by *Serratia* species in a paediatric surgical intensive care unit. J Hosp Infect 48:7–12
9. Ruza F, Alvarado F, Herruzo R, Delagado MA, Garcia S, Dorao P, Goded F (1998) Prevention of nosocomial infection in a pediatric intensive care unit (PICU) through the use of selective digestive decontamination. Eur J Epidemiol 14:719–727
10. Zobel G, Kuttnig M, Graubbauer HM, Semmelrock HJ, Thiel W (1991) Reduction of colonization and infection rate during pediatric intensive care by selective decontamination of the digestive tract. Crit Care Med 19:1242–1246
11. Smith SD, Jackson RJ, Hannakan CJ, Wadowsky RM, Tzakis AG, Rowe MI (1993) Selective decontamination in pediatric liver transplants. Transplantation 55:1306–1309
12. Barret JP, Jeschke MG, Herndon DN (2001) Selective decontamination of the digestive tract in severely burned pediatric patients. Burns 27:439–445
13. Herruzo-Cabrera R, Garcia Gonzalez JI, Garcia-Magan P, Del Rey-Calero JD (1994) Nosocomial infection in a neonatal intensive care unit and its prevention with selective intestinal decolonisation. Eur J Epidemiol 10:573–580
14. van Saene HKF, Stoutenbeek CP, Miranda DR, Zandstra DF, Homan van der Heide JN (1984) A new strategy for infection control in an intensive care unit: a prospective two-year study in cardiac surgery babies. In: Kinderchirugie Kongressberichte. Surgery in infancy and childhood. Hippokrates Verlag Stuttgart 1985, pp. 168–175
15. Liberati A, D'Amico R, Pifferi S et al (2004) Antibiotic prophylaxis to reduce respiratory tract infections and mortality in adults receiving intensive care [Cochrane Review]. In: The Cochrane Library, Issue 1, Chichester, UK, John Wiley & Sons Ltd
16. Nathens AB, Marshall JC (1999) Selective decontamination of the digestive tract in surgical patients. A systematic review of the evidence. Arch Surg 134:170–176
17. Sarginson RE, Taylor N, Reilly N et al (2004) Infection in prolonged pediatric critical illness: A prospective four-year study based on knowledge of the carrier state. Crit Care Med 32:839–847.
18. Stoutenbeek CP, van Saene HKF, Miranda DR, Zandstra DF (1984) The effect of selective decontamination of the digestive tract on colonization and infection rate in mul-

tiple trauma patients. Intensive Care Med 10:185–192

19. Baxby D, van Saene HKF, Stoutenbeek CP, Zandstra DF (1996) Selective decontamination of the digestive tract: 13 years on, what it is, and what it is not. Intensive Care Med 22:699–706

20. Silvestri L, Mannucci F, van Saene HKF (2000) Selective decontamination of the digestive tract: a life-saver. J Hosp Infect 45:185–190

21. Sganga G, Gangeri G, Castagneto M (1998) The gut: a central organ in the development of multiple organ system failure. In: van Saene HKF, Silvestri L, de la Cal MA (eds) Infection control in the intensive care unit. Springer-Verlag, Milan, pp 257–268

22. Pierro A, van Saene HKF, Donnell SC, Hughes J, Ewan C, Nunn AJ, Lloyd DA (1996) Microbial translocation in neonates and infants receiving long-term parenteral nutrition. Arch Surg 131:176–179

23. Pierro A, van Saene HKF, Jones MO, Brown D, Nunn AJ, Lloyd DA (1998) Clinical impact of abnormal gut flora in infants receiving parenteral nutrition. Ann Surg 227:1–7

24. van Saene HKF, Stoutenbeek CP, Hart CA (1991) Selective decontamination of the digestive tract (SDD) in intensive care patients: a critical evaluation of the clinical, bacteriological and epidemiological benefits. J Hosp Infect 18:261–277

25. van Saene HKF, Martin MV (1990) Do microorganisms play a role in irradiation mucositis? Eur J Clin Microbiol Infect Dis 9:861–863

26. Stoutenbeek CP (1988) Topical antibiotic regimen. In: van Saene HKF, Stoutenbeek CP, Lawin P, Ledingham IM (eds) Infection control by selective decontamination. Springer-Verlag, Berlin Heidelberg New York, pp 95–101

27. Markowsky SJ, Sinnott JT, Houston SH (1993) Selective decontamination of the digestive tract in intensive care patients. Infect Dis Newslett 12:49–56

28. Rogers CJ, van Saene HK, Suter PM, Horner R, L'E Orme M (1994) Infection control in critically ill patients: effects of selective decontamination of the digestive tract. Am J Hosp Pharm 51:631–648

29. van Saene HKF, Stoutenbeek CP, Faber-Nijholt R, van Saene JJM (1992) Selective decontamination of the digestive tract contributes to the control of disseminated intravascular coagulation in severe liver impairment. J Pediatr Gastroenterol Nutr 14:436–442

30. Gomez EC, Markowsky SJ, Rotschafer JC (1992) Selective decontamination of the digestive tract in intensive care patients: review and commentary. Ann Pharmacother 26:963–976

31. Ramsay G (1988) Endotoxaemia in multiple organ failure: a secondary role for SDD? In: van Saene HKF, Stoutenbeek CP, Lawin P, Ledingham IM (eds) Infection control by selective decontamination. Springer-Verlag, Berlin Heidelberg New York, pp 135–142

32. Hofstra W, De Vries-Hospers HG, Van der Waaij D (1982) Concentrations of amphotericin B in faeces and blood of healthy volunteers after the oral administration of various doses. Infection 10:223–227

33. Alder Hey, Royal Liverpool Children's NHS Trust. Anti-infective Guidelines, 1999

34. Feron B, Adair CG, Gorman SP, McClurg B (1993) Interaction of sucralfate with antibiotics used for selective decontamination of the gastrointestinal tract. Am J Hosp Pharm 50:2550–2553

35. Boom S, Ramsay G (1991) Selective decontamination of the digestive tract. Theoretical and practical recommendations. Drugs 42:541–550

36. Crome D (1989) Pharmaceutical technology in selective decontamination. In: van Saene HKF, Stoutenbeek CP, Lawin P, Mc A Ledingham I (eds) Infection control by selective decontamination. Springer Verlag, Berlin Heidelberg New York, pp 109–112

37. Data on file. Royal Liverpool Children's Hospital NHS Trust, Alder Hey, Liverpool, UK
38. van Saene HKF, Nunn AJ, Stoutenbeek CP (1995) Selective decontamination of the digestive tract in intensive care patients. Br J Hosp Med 54:558–561
39. Data on file. Western Infirmary, Glasgow, UK
40. Symonds RP, McIlroy P, Khorrami J, Paul J, Pyper E, Alcock SR, McCallum I, Speekenbrink ABJ, McMurray A, Lindemann E, Thomas M (1996) The reduction of radiation mucositis by selective decontamination antibiotic pastilles: a placebo-controlled double-blind trial. Br J Cancer 74:312–317
41. Spijkervet FKL, van Saene HKF, van Saene JJM, Panders AK, Vermey A, Mehta DM, Fidler V (1991) Effect of selective elimination of the oral flora on mucositis in irradiated head and neck cancer patients. J Surg Oncol 46:167–173
42. Data on file. Organon, Oss, The Netherlands
43. Occhipinti DJ, Itokazu G, Danziger LH (1992) Selective decontamination of the digestive tract as an infection control measure in intensive care unit patients. Pharmacotherapy 12:50S-63S
44. van Saene JJM (1990) Colonic delivery of polymyxin E and four quinolones for flora suppression. PhD Thesis, University of Groningen, PAL, Amsterdam
45. Poth EJ (1957) Critical analysis of intestinal antisepsis. JAMA 1163:1317–1322
46. Jew RK, Owen D, Kaufman D, Balmer D (1997) Osmolality of commonly used medications and formulas in the neonatal intensive care unit. Nutr Clin Pract 12:158–163
47. Bonten MJ, Kullberg BJ, Van Dalen R, Girbes AR, Hoepelman IM, Hustinx W, Meer JW van der, Speelman P, Stobberingh EE, Verbrugh HA, Verhoef J, Zwaveling JH (2000) Selective digestive decontamination in patients in intensive care. The Dutch Working Group on Antibiotic Policy. J Antimicrob Chemother 46:351–362
48. Kollef MH (2000) Opinion: the clinical use of selective digestive decontamination. Crit Care 4:327–332
49. British National Formulary, no 42, September 2001. British Medical Association and the Royal Pharmaceutical Society of Great Britain
50. Sanchez Garcia M, Cambronero Galache JA, Lopez Diaz J, Cerda Cerda E, Blasco JR et al (1998) Effectiveness and cost of selective decontamination of the digestive tract in critically ill intubated patients. Am J Respir Crit Care Med 158:908–916
51. Collard HR, Saint S (2001) Prevention of ventilator-associated pneumonia. Making health care safer: a critical analysis of patient safety practices. AHRQ Publication 01-E058. www.ahrq.gov

Chapter 28

Antimicrobial Resistance: a Prospective 5-year Study

H.K.F. van Saene, N. Taylor, N.J. Reilly, P.B. Baines

Pathophysiology

Nowadays a major clinical problem facing the intensive care team is antimicrobial resistance [1]. We believe that the focus of studies should be directed to the clinical aspects of the antimicrobial resistance problem as opposed to concentrating upon molecular-biological mechanisms of antimicrobial resistance.

There are several stages in the development of the carriage of antimicrobial resistant micro-organisms [2]. Firstly, it has only been recently learnt that illness severity is the most important independent risk factor for the carriage of abnormal, often resistant, bacteria [3]. Healthy individuals have innate mechanisms that clear abnormal bacteria. Unhealthy individuals carry abnormal micro-organisms in the throat and gut and, where present, skin lesions. The predominant site of carriage of abnormal bacteria is the gut.

Secondly, for carriage of abnormal flora to occur, the patient must have been exposed to the abnormal micro-organisms. Patients may either carry abnormal flora on admission (import) [4] or the flora may have been normal on admission and then abnormal micro-organisms are acquired whilst on the unit (acquisition) [5].

Thirdly, following exposure, ill patients may develop carriage, i.e., persistent presence in the throat and/or gut. Healthy individuals do not become sustained carriers of abnormal flora [6, 7].

Finally, abnormal carriage inevitably leads to overgrowth of abnormal flora in the critically ill patients [8]. Drugs including opiates, histamine 2 [H_2]-receptor antagonists, and antimicrobials promote overgrowth in reducing peristalsis [9], increasing the gastric pH >4 [10, 11], and via the suppression of the normal indigenous mainly anaerobic flora [12] required to control abnormal flora, respectively.

Digestive tract (gut) overgrowth, defined as $\geq 10^5$ colony forming units of abnormal bacteria per milliliter of saliva, gastric fluid, and feces, represents a serious problem in the intensive care unit (ICU) for three reasons: (1) overgrowth is required for the carriage of a resistant mutant amongst the sensitive population [13]; (2) overgrowth is required for the endogenous super-colonization/infection of the individual patient [14]; (3) overgrowth of resistant micro-organisms promotes dissemination throughout the unit via the hands of carers [15].

These four features, disease severity, exposure, carriage, and subsequent overgrowth, are the reasons why the ICU is the epicenter of the resistance problem [1]. Of the four important factors involved in bacterial resistance, only two are modifiable, namely bacterial carriage and overgrowth.

Traditional Approach to Antimicrobial Resistance

The traditional approach is based on two pillars, restriction of parenteral antibiotics and hygiene including handwashing and isolation.

Restriction of Solely Parenteral Antimicrobials

There is evidence relating antimicrobial usage to emerging resistance [16]. Carriage in the throat and gut and colonization of internal organs, by potentially pathogenic micro-organisms (PPM), are not treated. Only infection is treated (parenterally) to limit the use of antibiotics. Despite widespread attempts to limit the use of systemic antibiotics, over 70% of all patients who stay more than 3 days on the ICU will receive them [17].

There are two approaches to controlling antibiotic usage. These include increasing the specificity of the diagnosis of pneumonia, 30% of all ICU infections, by invasive techniques and scheduled changes of antibiotic classes. The "pneumonia" rate is halved using invasive strategies compared with non-invasive methods [18]. Two randomized trials have demonstrated that diagnosing pneumonia less frequently in this fashion is not associated with a reduction in mortality [19, 20]. A French randomized trial of 413 patients compared 204 patients managed invasively with protected brush specimens with 209 patients managed non-invasively with tracheal aspirates [19]. They failed to show any survival benefit at 28 days (30.9% versus 38.8%, $P=0.10$) using restrictive antibiotic prescribing policies. A Spanish randomized trial of 77 patients, comparing an invasive diagnostic approach ($n=39$) with a non-invasive tracheal aspirate method ($n=38$), found that the 30-day outcome of pneumonia was not influenced (38% versus 46%, $P=0.46$) by the techniques used for microbial investigation [20]. Additionally, both trials evaluated the emergence of antimicrobial resistance as a secondary endpoint. In the French trial the proportions of resistant isolates obtained from lower airway secretions were similar in both invasive (61.3%) and non-invasive (59.8%) groups, despite significantly less use of antibiotics in the invasive group. The Spanish trial reported identical high isolation rates of 58.3% of resistant bacteria, methicillin-resistant *Staphylococcus aureus* (MRSA) and *Pseudomonas aeruginosa* in both groups.

Strategies that recommend manipulating in-hospital antibiotic use have been suggested to reduce the likelihood of emergence of resistance in the critically ill patient. One such strategy is to schedule a rotation of antibiotics. This strategy entails a regimented preference for a specific antibiotic in a given environment over a fixed period, after which preference is switched to an alternative agent with a similar spectrum of activity. The assumption underlying this strategy is that the exposure to each antibiotic in the schedule is sufficiently short to preclude the emergence of significant populations of micro-organisms resistant to any one of them.

The evidence to support this recommendation is sparse and the data are conflicting [21, 22]. In a cardiac ICU, 6 months of ceftazidime administration was followed by 6 months of ciprofloxacin administration and a comparison was made [21]. Although not true cycling (the prior regimen was not reused, and the effect of a full cycle was not tested), this study suggests that scheduled changes in classes of antibiotics may reduce infection with resistant aerobic Gram-negative bacilli (AGNB). There was a significant reduction in the incidence of pneumonia due to resistant AGNB (4% versus 0.9%, $P=0.013$). The non-randomized design is a fundamental flaw confirmed by the difference in the etiology of the causative agents. During ceftazidime treatment there was an outbreak of intrinsically resistant *Serratia*, in addition there were five viral and three *Aspergillus* pneumonias, i.e., 15 of 41 pneumonias were inappropriately treated by ceftazidime. During ciprofloxacin treatment there 22 pneumonias in total, only 1 of which was viral. The difference in pneumonia is no longer significant when comparing the appropriately treated pneumonias, i.e., 26 and 21. In a neonatal ICU, a monthly rotation of gentamicin, piperacilin-tazobactam, and ceftazidime was compared with unrestricted antibiotic use between two geographically separated teams (rotation versus control team) [22]. In total 10.7% of infants on the rotation team versus 7.7% on the control team carried resistant AGNB in the throat and gut. There was no difference in the incidence of infections, morbidity, and mortality. Proponents and antagonists of antibiotic cycling agree that there are many difficult and complex methodological issues surrounding the use of antibiotic cycling. Factors potentially determining the effectiveness of antibiotic cycling include endemic rates of carriage with particular AGNB and their mechanisms of antibiotic resistance, the transmission dynamics of particular AGNB in a specific unit, the population dynamics of the unit staff, the composition and duration of the antibiotic regimens, compliance with antibiotic cycling, and concurrent infection control practices to limit transmission of resistant AGNB. There is limited information on which to base decisions of how long each antibiotic regimen should be used and how many regimens should be cycled.

Hygiene

The classic study of Semmelweis showed the survival benefit of hand disinfection [23]. In women admitted for delivery, the absolute mortality from child bed fever was significantly reduced by 8% following the implementation of handwashing with chlorinated lime, compared with a historical control of physicians who did not wash their hands. There is one randomized controlled trial (RCT) evaluating hygiene including personal protective equipment such as gloves and gowns and hand hygiene in two surgical ICUs as the ICU was the randomization unit [24]. Standard care was administered in the same way in the two units. The same medical staff always administered care but did not mix between units. In one unit, all personnel and visitors donned gowns and gloves before entering the ventilated patient's room; handwashing was required before entry and on leaving the room (test unit). In the control unit all health care workers utilized standard precautions including handwashing and gloves. Remarkably, the incidence of pneumonia was significantly higher in the test group compared with the control group (36.4% versus 19.5%, $P=0.02$). There was no difference in mortality. Surprisingly, there are no RCTs showing that significantly fewer ICU patients die when health care workers adhere to hand disinfection practices alone.

Conclusion

The policy of sole use of parenteral antimicrobials has failed to control resistance. In general, resistance to a new antibiotic emerges within 2 years of general use. We believe that this experience is due to the common denominator of ignoring the gut in all three maneuvers of restricted antibiotic use, cycling of antibiotics, and handwashing. The major source of the gut is left intact allowing resistant mutants to emerge and cause superinfections and subsequent outbreaks.

Selective Digestive Decontamination. The Addition of Enteral to Parenteral Antibiotics

As a development of the underlying concepts, outlined above, that ill patients will develop overgrowth of abnormal flora, which is exacerbated by the administration of parenteral antibiotics that disregard the normal indigenous flora, the approach of selective digestive decontamination (SDD) has four components [25]:

1. twice weekly microbiological surveillance of throat and gut flora;
2. eradication of overgrowth with appropriate enteral non-absorbable antimicrobials
3. pre-1980s parenteral antimicrobials that respect the ecology are used for therapy when necessary for a maximum period of 5 days
4. high standards of hygiene to control transmission of resistant PPM.

In the most extensive meta-analysis of SDD, covering trials over a 10-year period, antibiotic resistance was not a clinical problem [26]. However, antibiotic resistance is a long-term evolutionary issue. Five SDD trials prospectively evaluated resistance for 2, 2.5, 4, 6, and 7 years [27–31]. No increase in the rate of superinfections due to resistant bacteria could be demonstrated. The latest trial, evaluating SDD in about 1,000 patients, had significantly fewer carriers of multi-resistant AGNB in the patients receiving SDD than in the control group [32].

One should remember that the principal aim of SDD is the selective eradication of both oropharyngeal and gastro-intestinal carriage of abnormal AGNB. Thus, SDD not only eliminates a prime source of endogenous infection, but also profoundly influences the balance of forces associated with the emergence of resistance. In principle, the enteral agents polymyxin and tobramycin must exert considerable selective pressure for resistance. However, the combination of very high enteral bactericidal antibiotic levels in saliva and feces, the use of synergistic antibiotic mixtures, and the maintenance of colonization resistance creates a unique environment that has proven strikingly successful in preventing overgrowth of resistant mutants amongst the target micro-organisms.

SDD, by design, is not active against MRSA. Six RCTs, conducted in ICUs where MRSA was endemic at the time of the study, showed a trend towards higher MRSA infection rates in patients receiving SDD [33–38]. These observations suggest that the parenteral and enteral antimicrobials of the SDD protocol, i.e., cefotaxime and polymyxin E, tobramycin and amphotericin B, may cause selection and overgrowth of MRSA in the throat and gut. Under these circumstances SDD requires the addition of oropharyngeal and enteral vancomycin.

Two studies, using 2 g of a 4% vancomycin gel or paste and 2 g of vancomycin solution added to the non-absorbable polymyxin/tobramcyin/amphotericin B component of SDD, demonstrated the prevention and the eradication of carriage and overgrowth of abnormal MRSA [14, 39]. Subsequent MRSA infection, transmission, and outbreaks were controlled. Using this protocol, the ICU becomes and remains free from MRSA. Severe infections, including MRSA pneumonia and septicemia, were significantly reduced using enteral vancomycin in two RCTs [40, 41].

The concern that SDD promotes vancomycin-resistant enterococcus (VRE) carriage and infection has been investigated in two American ICUs with endemic VRE and the incidence of both carriage and infection due to VRE was low and similar in test and control groups [42, 43]. The addition of enteral vancomycin to SDD is required to control MRSA in ICUs with endemic MRSA, and two recent RCTs report that SDD with enteral vancomycin did not increase the incidence of VRE carriage and infection [44, 45]. SDD, combined with enteral vancomycin throughout the treatment on ICU, was evaluated in four European studies, two Spanish studies [14, 39] and two Italian studies [40, 41]. Despite VRE imported into one of the Spanish units, no change in the use of non-absorbable vancomycin and SDD was required, as rapid and extensive spread did not occur over a 4-year period [14]. VRE was not isolated in any of the other three studies [39–41]. Recent literature shows that parenteral antibiotics that do not respect the patient's gut ecology rather than high doses of enteral vancomycin promote the emergence of VRE in the gut [46, 47].

Conclusion

The virtual absence of a resistance problem is due to the eradication of resistant PPM carried in the alimentary canal following the shift from solely systemic antimicrobials towards the combination of parenteral and enteral antimicrobials.

How to Monitor Antimicrobial Resistance

Surveillance cultures of the throat and rectum are not popular amongst many microbiologists. Although the rationale for SDD is based on the detection of abnormal carrier states using surveillance cultures, SDD can still be used in their absence. The effect of SDD treatment on morbidity and mortality was independent of the use of surveillance cultures in the most recent meta-analysis [48]. In seven RCTs, surveillance cultures were not obtained. If the microbiology department is unable to provide a service based on surveillance cultures, SDD infection prophylaxis is still feasible and supported by evidence.

To monitor antimicrobial resistance, we believe that surveillance cultures of the throat and gut are indispensable to detect carriage of resistant PPM at an 'early' stage, before infection due to resistant PPM develops [4, 5].

Resistance During SDD: a 5-Year Prospective Study

Surveillance cultures of the throat and rectum combined with enteral antimicrobials as part of SDD were introduced in the pediatric ICU at Alder Hey Children's Hospital (Liverpool, UK) as an integral part of clinical practice. In this 20-bedded pediatric ICU, the antibiotic policy consists of using pre-1980s antimicrobial agents that respect ecology. Prophylaxis in cardiac and general surgery included three doses of peri-operative teicoplanin/netilmicin and cefotaxime/metronidazole, respectively. Emperical therapy was based on cefotaxime and/or gentamicin for 5 days. Children showing oropharyngeal and/or intestinal overgrowth of abnormal AGNB, yeasts, and MRSA received enteral polymyxin E, tobramycin, amphotericin B, or nystatin, and vancomycin, respectively, throughout their treatment on the pediatric ICU. Surveillance cultures of the throat and rectum were obtained on admission, and afterwards twice weekly to detect the abnormal carrier state. Diagnostic samples were obtained on clinical indication only.

A total of 1,551 children (median age 113 days, paediatric index of mortality score 0.063, stay 8 days) accounted for 1,836 admissions, corresponding to 22,962 patient days. Of these 40% were medical, 38% cardiac surgical, and 22% general surgical. For all but 5 months, enteral antimicrobials were more commonly used than the individual parenteral agents. SDD was administered during 976 of the 1,836 (53%) admissions. Glycopeptide use combined with the aminoglycoside netilmicin (or gentamicin) was consistent throughout the 5 years at between 20% and 30%, reflecting cardiac surgical prophylaxis. Systemic antifungals were administered to 46 patients over 5 years. Throughout the 5-year study, carriage of resistant AGNB or MRSA was not detected in 75% of the patients. A total of 20% and 5% were identified as carriers of ceftazidime- and of tobramycin-resistant AGNB, respectively. The three main representatives of ceftazidime-resistant AGNB were *Enterobacter*, *Citrobacter*, and *Pseudomonas* species, whilst *Klebsiella* and again *Pseudomonas* species were prominent amongst the tobramycin-resistant AGNB. The resistant bacterium was present in the admission flora in 60% of the cases. MRSA carriage was uncommon (2.5%). Over the 5 years, 90% of children were clear of resistant bacteria at the time of unit discharge. The monthly density of children who carried resistant bacteria was always less than 4 patients during the 5-year period (Fig. 1). Figure 2 shows the monthly density of all infected children and of the children infected with resistant bacteria. There are five peaks corresponding to the respiratory syncytial virus winter/spring season. An outbreak involving 15 children was experienced in the winter 2002/2003 [49]. The monthly density of children with infections due to resistant bacteria was always lower than 2. There were 73 children (4.7%) with a total of 153 infections due to resistant bacteria

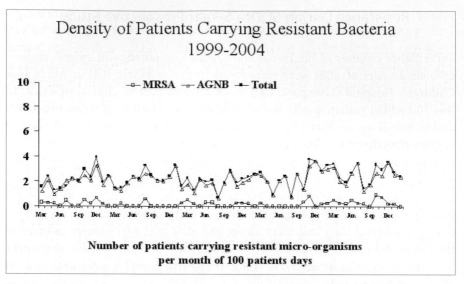

Fig. 1. Density of patients carrying aerobic Gram-negative bacteria (AGNB) resistant to ceftazidime and/or tobramcyin, and/or carrying methicilin-resistant *Staphylococcus aureus* (MRSA). The density defined as the number of patients per month of 100 patient days remained consistently low. Monthly, between 2 (0.71 density) and 16 patients (3.90 density) with carriage of resistant microbes were present on the pediatric intensive care unit (ICU)

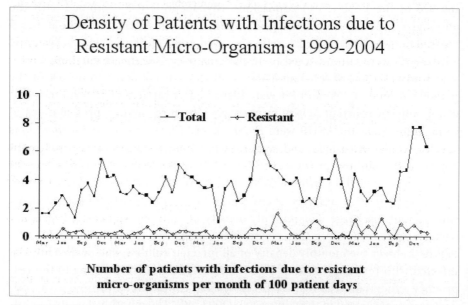

Fig. 2. The density of patients infected with resistant bacteria per 100 patient days in rela-tion to the total number of patients infected. The infected patient density varied between 0 and 1.65 (4 patients) monthly. The total density increased in the winter months reflecting the seasonal distribution, including the 297 viral infections in 272 patients

on the pediatric ICU over a period of 5 years. The main problems were exogenous wound infections due to *Pseudomonas* species, AGNB resistant to ceftazidime, and MRSA in a particular subset of children with severe burns. Although only 8 severely burnt children (8/73=11%) had resistant infections, they were responsible for 63 (63/153=41%) of all infections due to resistant bacteria.

Conclusion

The ICU is the epicenter of the resistance problem. The use of solely parenteral antibiotics, whether restricted or not, maintains an abnormal population of bacteria amongst which resistance is encouraged. The eradication of the reservoir of abnormal bacteria located in the gut has been shown to be effective in significantly reducing morbidity, mortality, and resistance [25, 48].

References

1. Archibald L, Philips L, Monnet D et al (1997) Antimicrobial resistance in isolates from inpatients and outpatients in the United States: increasing importance of the intensive care. Clin Infect Dis 24:211–215
2. Baines PB, Meyer J, de la Cal MA (2001) Antimicrobial resistance in the intensive care unit: the use of oral non-absorbable antimicrobials may prolong the antibiotic era. Curr Anaesth Crit Care 12:41–47
3. Chang FY, Singh N, Gayowski T et al (1998) *Staphylococcus aureus* nasal colonization in patients with cirrhosis: prospective assessment of association with infection. Infect Control Hosp Epidemiol 19:328–332
4. D'Agata EMC, Venkataraman L, De Girolami P et al (1999) Colonisation with broad-spectrum cephalosporin-resistant Gram-negative bacilli in intensive care units during a non-outbreak period: prevalence, risk factors and rate of infection. Crit Care Med 27:1090–1095
5. Garrouste-Orgeas M, Marie O, Rouveau M et al (1996) Secondary carriage with multi-resistant *Acinetobacter baumannii* and *Klebsiella pneumoniae* in an adult ICU-population: relationship with nosocomial infections and mortality. J Hosp Infect 34:279–289
6. Chambers ST, Steele C, Kunin CM (1987) Enteric colonisation with antibiotic resistant bacteria in nurses working in intensive care units. J Antimicrob Chemother 19:685–693
7. Cookson B, Peters B, Webster M et al (1989) Staff carriage of epidemic methicillin-resistant *Staphylococcus aureus*. J Clin Microbiol 27:1471–1476
8. van Saene HKF, Taylor N, Donnell SC et al (2003) Gut overgrowth with abnormal flora: the missing link in parenteral nutrition-related sepsis in surgical neonates. Eur J Clin Nutr 57:548–553
9. Husebye H (1995) Gastro-intestinal motility disorders and bacterial overgrowth. J Intern Med 237:419–427
10. Reusser P, Zimmerli W, Scheiddeger D et al (1989) Role of gastric colonization in noso-

comial infections and endotoxemia: a prospective study in neurosurgical patients on mechanical ventilation. J Infect Dis 160:414–421

11. Reusser P, Gyr K, Scheidegger D et al (1990) Prospective endoscopic study of stress erosions and ulcers in critically ill neurosurgical patients: current incidence and effect of acid-reducing prophylaxis. Crit Care Med 18:270–274

12. van Saene HKF, Stoutenbeek CP, Geitz JN et al (1988) Effect of amoxicillin on colonization resistance in human volunteers. Microb Ecol Health Dis 1:169–177

13. Blazquez J (2003) Hypermutation as a factor contributing to the acquisition of antimicrobial resistance. Clin Infect Dis 37:1201–1209

14. de la Cal MA, Cerda E, van Saene HKF et al (2004) Effectiveness and safety of enteral vancomycin to control endemicity of methicillin-resistant *Staphylococcus aureus* on a medical/surgical intensive care. J Hosp Infect 56:175–183

15. Crossley K, Landesmann B, Zaske D (1979) An outbreak of infections caused by strains of *Staphylococcus aureus* resistant to methicillin and aminoglycosides. II. Epidemiology studies. J Infect Dis 139:280–287

16. Austin DJ, Kristinsson KG, Anderson RM (1999) The relationship between the volume of antimicrobial consumption in human communities and the frequency of resistance. Proc Nat Acad Sci U S A 96:1152–1156

17. Rangel-Frausto MS, Pittet D, Costigan M et al (1995) The natural history of the systemic inflammatory response syndrom (SIRS): a prospective study. JAMA 273:117–123

18. Cook D, Guyatt G, Marshall J et al (1998) A comparison of sucralfate and ranitidine for the prevention of upper gastro-intestinal bleeding in patients requiring mechanical ventilation. N Engl J Med 338:791–797

19. Fagon JY, Chastre J, Wolff M et al (2000) Invasive and non-invasive strategies for management of suspected ventilator-associated pneumonia. A randomised trial. Ann Intern Med 132:621–630

20. Ruiz M, Torres A, Ewig S et al (2000) Non-invasive versus invasive microbial investigation in ventilator-associated pneumonia: evaluation of outcome. Am J Respir Crit Care Med 162:119–125

21. Kollef MH, Vlasnik Jon, Sharpless L et al (1997) Scheduled change of antibiotic classes. A strategy to decrease the incidence of ventilator-associated pneumonia. Am J Respir Crit Care Med 156:1040–1048

22. Toltzis P, Dul MJ, Hoyen C et al (2002) The effect of antibiotic rotation on colonisation with antibiotic-resistant bacilli in a neonatal intensive care unit. Pediatrics 110:707–711

23. Semmelweis IP (1861) Die Aetiologie, der Begriff und die Prophylaxis des Kindbettfiebers. Pest, Hartleben

24. Koss WG, Khalili Th M, Lemus JF et al (2001) Nosocomial pneumonia is not prevented by protective contact isolation in the surgical intensive care unit. Am Surg 67:1140–1144

25. Zandstra DF, van Saene HKF (2001) Selective decontamination of the digestive tract as infection prevention in the critically ill. Does it lead to resistance? Minerva Anestesiol 67:292–297

26. D'Amico R, Pifferi S, Leonetti C et al (1998) Effectiveness of antibiotic prophylaxis in critically ill adult patients: systematic review of randomised controlled trials. BMJ 316:1275–1285

27. Hammond JMJ, Potgieter PD (1995) Long-term effects of selective decontamination on antimicrobial resistance. Crit Care Med 23:637–645

28. Stoutenbeek CP, van Saene HKF, Zandstra DF (1987) The effect of oral non-absorbable antibiotics on the emergence of resistant bacteria in patients in an intensive care

unit. J Antimicrob Chemother 19:513–520

29. Lingnau W, Berger J, Javorsky F et al (1998) Changing bacterial ecology during a five year period of selective intestinal decontamination. J Hosp Infect 39:195–206

30. Leone M, Albanese J, Antonini F et al (2003) Long-term (6-year) effect of selective digestive decontamination on antimicrobial resistance in intensive care, multiple-trauma patients. Crit Care Med 31:2090–2095

31. Tetteroo GWM, Wagenvoort JHT, Bruining HA (1994) Bacteriology of selective decontamination: efficacy and rebound colonisation. J Antimicrob Chemother 34:139–148

32. Jonge E de, Schultz MJ, Spanjaard L et al (2003) Effects of selective decontamination of digestive tract on mortality and acquisition of resistant bacteria in intensive care: a randomised controlled trial. Lancet 362:1011–1016

33. Ferrer M, Torres A, Gonzalez J et al (1994) Utility of selective digestive decontamination in mechanically ventilated patients. Ann Intern Med 120:389–395

34. Gastinne H, Wolff M, Delatour F et al (1992) A controlled trial in intensive care units of selective decontamination of the digestive tract with non-absorbable antibiotics. N Engl J Med 326:594–599

35. Hammond JMJ, Potgieter PD, Saunders GL et al (1992) Double-blind study of selective decontamination of the digestive tract in intensive care. Lancet 340:5–9

36. Lingnau W, Berger J, Javorsky F et al (1997) Selective intestinal decontamination in multiple trauma patients: prospective, controlled trial. J Trauma 42:687–694

37. Verwaest C, Verhaegen J, Ferdinande P et al (1997) Randomised, controlled trial of selective digestive decontamination in 600 mechanically ventilated patients in a multi disciplinary intensive care unit. Crit Care Med 25:63–71

38. Wiener J, Itokazu G, Nathan C et al (1995) A randomised, double-blind, placebo-controlled trial of selective digestive decontamination in a medical/surgical intensive care unit. Clin Infect Dis 20:861–867

39. Silvestri L, Milanese M, Oblach L et al (2002) Enteral vancomycin to control methicillin-resistant *Staphylococcus aureus* outbreak in mechanically ventilated patients. Am J Infect Control 30:391–399

40. Sanchez M, Mir N, Canton R et al (1997) The effect of topical vancomycin on acquisition, carriage and infection with methicillin-resistant *Staphylococcus aureus* in critically ill patients. A double-blind, randomised, placebo-controlled study (abstract). 37th ICAAC, 1997 Toronto, Canada, p 310

41. Silvestri L, van Saene HKF, Milanese M et al (2004) Prevention of MRSA pneumonia by oral vancomycin decontamination. Eur Respir J 23:921–926

42. Arnow PM, Carandang GC, Zabner R et al (1996) Randomised controlled trial of selective bowel decontamination for prevention of infections following liver transplantation. Clin Infect Dis 22:997–1013

43. Hellinger WC, Yao SD, Alvarez S et al (2002) A randomised, prospective, double-blind evaluation of selective bowel decontamination in liver transplantation. Transplantation 73:1904–1909

44. Bergmans DC, Bonten MJ, Gaillard CA et al (2001) Prevention of ventilator-associated pneumonia by oral decontamination: a prospective, randomized, double-blind, placebo-controlled study. Am J Respir Crit Care Med 164:382–388

45. Krueger WA, Lenhart FP, Neeser G et al (2002) Influence of combined intravenous and topical antibiotic prophylaxis on the incidence of infections, organ dysfunctions, and mortality in critically ill surgical patients: a prospective, stratified, randomized, double-blind, placebo-controlled clinical trial. Am J Respir Crit Care Med 166:1029-1037

46. Stiefel U, Paterson DL, Pultz NJ et al (2004) Effect of increasing use of piperacillin/tazobactam on the incidence of vancomycin-resistant enterococci in four academic medical centers. Infect Control Hosp Epidemiol 25:380–383

47. Salgado CD, Giannetta ET, Farr BM (2004) Failure to develop vancomycin-resistant *Enterococcus* with oral vancomycin treatment of *Clostridium difficile*. Infect Control Hosp Epidemiol 25:413–417
48. Liberati A, D'Amico R, Pifferi S et al (2004) Antibiotic prophylaxis to reduce respiratory tract infections and mortality in adults receiving intensive care. Cochrane Review. In: The Cochrane Library, Issue 1. Wiley, Chichester, UK
49. Thorburn K, Kerr S, Taylor N et al (2004) RSV outbreak in a paediatric intensive care unit. J Hosp Infect 57:194–201

Chapter 29

ICU-Acquired Infection: Mortality, Morbidity, and Costs

J.C. Marshall, K.A.M. Marshall

Introduction

Nosocomial infection is a common complication of critical illness [1]. Ambiguities in diagnostic criteria and variation in patient demographics render reliable estimates of its prevalence imprecise, but infection is generally reported to complicate the course of between a quarter and a half of all intensive care unit (ICU) admissions [2–4], and to be associated with increased morbidity, mortality, and costs. ICU-acquired infection, however, is not a random complication, but rather one that affects the sickest and most vulnerable of patients, and has been considered by many to be not so much a cause of morbidity as a reflection of the state of being critically ill [5, 6].

Decisions about optimal strategies for the prevention and management of ICU-acquired infection hinge on assumptions about the attributable morbidity and costs of such infections, assumptions that are only tenuously grounded in robust data. The adoption of strategies to prevent nosocomial infection presupposes that these infections produce excess morbidity or generate increased costs of care; the decision to treat nosocomial infections assumes that eradication of infection will improve clinical status and so reduce morbidity to the patient. These assumptions, self-evident on initial inspection, require closer scrutiny. This chapter will review the concepts of attributable morbidity, mortality, and costs of nosocomial ICU-acquired infection, with the objective of providing an informed basis for clinical decision-making.

Outcome Analyses: Methodological Considerations

Estimation of the impact of nosocomial infection on an outcome—whether mortality, morbidity, or cost—is a complex process, whose conclusions are critically dependent on assumptions made by the investigator, on the variables considered in constructing the analytic model, and, in the case of cost analyses, whose perspective is being considered—the patient, the hospital, or the society.

Crude and Attributable Mortality

ICUs concentrate a variety of life-sustaining technologies with the explicit objective of intervening to avert death. The implication, therefore, appears to be that mortality is an unequivocal measure of the success or failure of ICU care. However, a moment's reflection reveals the limitations inherent in such an assumption. First, mortality as an outcome measure is time dependent: while 1 hour survival might be an appropriate measure of the effectiveness of an intervention during cardiac arrest, successful treatment for cancer is generally measured as 5-year survival. The duration of survival that best defines success or failure in the ICU is unclear. Regulatory agencies have adopted the philosophy that 28-day mortality is the best measure of the effectiveness of novel mediator-directed therapies [7]. However, a patient who dies in the ICU after 47 days can hardly be considered a treatment success, whereas another patient who survives an acute illness to be discharged from hospital on the 13th day, but who dies when struck by a car while heading home does not really represent a treatment failure.

Secondly, mortality is of variable importance to ICU patients and their families [8]. Critical illness is often a complication of other diseases, developing in an already compromised host. For the elderly patient whose health has been failing, death may be less a concern than the prospect of institutionalization and loss of independence. Finally, for the patient with multiple co-morbid conditions, it may be very difficult to ascribe mortality to a specific condition. Is pneumonia that develops in the patient admitted with congestive heart failure, diabetes, and advanced chronic obstructive pulmonary disease the cause of death, or simply a reflection of the further deterioration of a tenuous state of health? The concept of attributable mortality attempts to define the incremental increase in mortality that results from the disease process of interest or the decrement in mortality that occurs as the consequence of an intervention.

The most reliable method of defining the attributable mortality of nosocomial ICU-acquired infection is by means of a randomized control trial of an intervention that reduces the risk of infection or that attenuates its severity. The technique of randomization ensures that patient characteristics and health care interventions that might independently impact on outcome—both those that are known and those that are unknown—are roughly equally distributed between the two populations. Since the only variable that differs systematically between the two populations is the experimental intervention, documentation of differential survival between the study populations implicates the intervention as the cause of that difference.

Clinical trials are costly and time-consuming, and alternate approaches have been used to derive estimates of attributable morbidity from observational data. The technique of logistic regression analysis relates an outcome (survival or death) to a number of potential explanatory factors (infection, acute severity of illness, pre-morbid health status, etc). A univariate analysis is generally performed first, to identify those variables that are associated with the outcome of interest. Those that are found to be predictive of outcome (a p value of 0.10 is typically chosen for this analysis) are then entered into a stepwise analysis that identifies the independent determinants of outcome by adjusting for the strongest prognostic variable to determine the independent contribution of the next most potent predictor variable. The process is then repeated until none of the remaining variables is significantly related to the outcome of interest. The conclusions drawn from such an analysis depend on the potential explanatory variables chosen, which in turn reflect the assumptions and biases of the investigator. For example, although the adequacy of antibiotic therapy is commonly considered as a potential explanatory variable for adverse outcome in nosocomial infection, the corollary—the effect of the administration of unnecessary antibiotics—is not, thus potentially biasing the analysis towards the conclusion that use of broad-spectrum antibiotics is an important determinant of outcome.

Another approach to quantifying attributable mortality entails the use of a matched cohort study. Each patient with the risk factor of interest is matched to a contemporaneous control with similar baseline characteristics, but lacking the risk factor. If we are interested in the attributable mortality of bacteremia, for example, we might match each patient with bacteremia with a control patient whose age, gender, and admission APACHE II score was the same as our case. Such an approach can only control for the variables used in matching, and may overestimate the attributable outcome because of the unrecognized influence of variables that are not used in the matching process. In our example, we would not be matching for events that occurred following ICU admission that might modify mortality risk, such as the development of renal failure or the need for prolonged mechanical ventilation. The use of a sensitivity analysis—altering the assumptions associated with the use and weighting of discrete variables—can increase one's confidence in the conclusions reached [9].

A variation on this technique was employed by Connors et al. [10] to estimate the mortality attributable to the use of a Swan Ganz catheter. Recognizing that there was considerable variability in the use of the catheter from one unit to the next, the authors developed a propensity score that reflected the factors that predicted use of the catheter in those units where it was used frequently. Patients in low-use units were then matched by propensity score and the mortality of the two groups was compared. Their conclusion was that use of the right heart catheter was associated with an attributable increase in mortality of

24%. Once again, however, the conclusion is potentially biased by those variables that are not included in the matching process.

The most reliable method of quantifying outcomes attributable to a particular risk factor, however, is by means of a randomized controlled trial. In an adequately powered study, randomization controls for both known and unknown confounding factors, by distributing them equally between the two groups. Other methods of estimating the impact of a factor such as infection on outcome must be interpreted with caution [11].

Cost analyses

Some general comments on economic analysis are in order prior to a consideration of the differing approaches to estimating the costs of therapy. Costs are inherently difficult to calculate. The cost of an intervention includes both *explicit costs*—the costs expended to achieve the outcome desired—and *implicit costs*—the potential revenues that are not realized as a result of the decision that is made. For example, an intervention that increases survival for an individual patient may increase ICU costs by limiting the admission of a less seriously ill patient who might have consumed fewer resources, and brought in greater revenues from a payer. Usually, such implicit costs are not incorporated into analyses of the costs of medical therapy, for their perspective is not that of the patient, but of the payer. Implicit costs, however, have a potent impact on decisions regarding whether a particular patient or population of patients will be cared for at a given institution, and so shape patterns of the delivery of care within the health system. Explicit costs include *fixed costs*—those such as staffing or building maintenance—that are incurred regardless of the specific intervention—and *variable costs*—those such as the costs of drugs, operative procedures, and radiological investigations that depend on the specific decisions made for a particular patient.

Four types of economic analysis are typically employed to compare treatments (Table 1) [12]. *Cost minimization* analysis proceeds from the assumption that two interventions result in comparable outcomes, and seeks, by enumerating the spectrum of costs associated with each alternative, to identify the one that results in the lowest costs. The units of analysis are monetary units—dollars, Euros, etc. *Cost benefit* analysis considers both the costs and the outcome in monetary units, and so must assign a specific dollar value to the outcome to be achieved—the cost of a life or other clinical outcome—to create meaningful comparisons. *Cost-effectiveness* analysis considers the costs generated per unit of clinical benefit, for example, the cost per life saved or episode of pneumonia prevented. Finally, *cost utility* analysis uses a weighted measure of outcome—

Table 1. Types of economic analyses (adapted from reference [12])

Type of study	Numerator (costs)	Denominator (outcome)	Comments
Cost minimization	Dollars	None	Compares costs of two or more therapies without consideration of consequences
Cost benefit	Dollars	Dollars	Converts clinical effects into associated costs
Cost-effectiveness	Dollars	Measure of clinical efficacy	Expresses costs in terms of outcome of intervention (e.g., cost per case of pneumonia prevented)
Cost utility	Dollars	Quality-adjusted life years	Expresses costs relative to a standardized estimate of benefit and so allows comparisons of differing therapies

quality adjusted life years—to express costs incurred for a comparable degree of clinical benefit. This strategy permits comparison of the costs of very divergent therapies—for example, transplantation of the liver with prevention of ventilator-associated pneumonia. Utilities reflect the value placed on an outcome by patients and are developed using techniques such as a standard gamble, time tradeoff, or through the administration of a questionnaire. Each approach recognizes that patient-centered values represent a compromise between the outcome achieved and the adverse consequences of the interventions required to achieve that outcome. While a cost utility analysis provides the most relevant measure of costs related to patient-centered outcomes, utilities are difficult to measure and are dependent on a number of highly subjective assumptions.

The Attributable Mortality of ICU-Acquired Infection

The most compelling evidence that nosocomial ICU-acquired infection is responsible for increased morbidity and mortality derives from randomized controlled trials of selective decontamination of the digestive tract (SDD). The most recent meta-analysis of 6,922 patients enrolled in randomized trials of SDD documented a significant reduction in mortality from 29% to 24% in patients receiving the prophylactic regimen, in association with a reduction in the odds ratio for developing pneumonia to 0.35 (95% confidence interval 0.29–0.41) [13].

While it is possible that the benefits of the intervention arose for reasons other than the prevention of subsequent nosocomial infection (for example, the treatment of occult community acquired infection or a reduction in the absorption of endotoxin from the gastrointestinal tract), the most plausible interpretation of these data is that nosocomial infection is responsible for a relative increase in the risk of ICU mortality of 22% (an absolute 5% increase from a baseline risk of 24%). For surgical patients, a population in which co-morbid diseases are less prevalent, the relative risk reduction is even greater [14], consistent with the hypothesis that the attributable morbidity and mortality of infection is greatest in those patients with minimal concomitant risk factors for an adverse outcome.

Attributable mortality is highly population dependent: for patient populations with minimal co-morbidity, the signal attributable to an acute event is relatively greater than it is for patient populations with significant co-morbidities. Thus prophylactic strategies such as SDD show their greatest benefit in patients with no significant pre-morbid illness and acute physiological derangement that is of only mild-to-moderate degree. Available estimates of the attributable mortality of common ICU-acquired infections are summarized in Table 2.

Table 2. Attributable mortality of nosocomial infection in the intensive care unit (ICU)

Type of infection	Attributable mortality
Bloodstream infection	0%–50%
Primary bacteremia	20%
Catheter-related bacteremia	12%
Secondary to nosocomial infection	55%
Ventilator-associated pneumonia	20%–30%
Urinary tract infection	5%

Bloodstream Infections

A cohort study of primary bloodstream infections in ICU patients found an overall incidence of 1%, increasing to 4%, or 4.0 infections per 1,000 catheter-days, in patients with central venous catheters [15]. Similar figures have been reported for pediatric patients. Gray et al. [16] found an incidence of nosocomial bloodstream infection of 25 per 1,000 ICU admissions, or 6.8 per 1,000 bed-days. Crude mortality for patients with bloodstream infection was higher (26.5% vs. 8.1%), however, 87% of patients with these infections had significant underlying disease [16]. The mortality associated with ICU-acquired bacteremia, however, is higher in adults, with rates ranging from 43% to 53% [15, 17–19]. Pre-morbid illness, reflected, for example, in a "do not resuscitate" order, is an important independent predictor of mortality. However, bacteremia was also an independent risk factor for death in a study of 1,052 patients with severe sepsis or septic shock [20].

A French study of more than 2,000 critically ill patients reported that bacteremia occurs in 5% of patients who remain in the ICU for longer than 48 h. When the episode of bacteremia was judged to be primary (no obvious focus), the excess mortality attributable to the event was 20%, whereas catheter-related bacteremia led to an excess mortality of 11.5%. When it was judged as secondary nosocomial bloodstream infection, the excess mortality attributable to the bacteremia was estimated to be 55%, and patients remained in the ICU for a median of 9.5 days longer [21]. In contrast, a study of 2,076 episodes of infection in surgical patients, employing logistic regression analysis to control for the potentially confounding influences of co-morbidities, concluded that although associated with critical illness and death, bacteremia is not independently predictive of outcome, but rather a surrogate measure of underlying severity of illness [22]. Digiovine et al. [23], in a study of primary bacteremia in ICU patients, reported that when stratified by illness severity, bacteremic patients did not experience a higher mortality risk, although the length of ICU stay was extended by a median of 5 days [23]. Our own work suggests that when patients are stratified by the clinical severity of the inflammatory response, bacteremia per se does not contribute to adverse outcome, but may, paradoxically, be associated with a superior outcome [3].

Several studies have attempted to evaluate the impact of bacteremia with particular pathogens on ICU outcome. Harbarth et al. [24] evaluated 1,835 episodes of Gram-negative bacteremia in Swiss hospitals, and found that bacteremia caused by *Klebsiella spp.* or by *Pseudomonas aeruginosa*, but not by multi-resistant organisms, was associated with an elevated risk of death. Blot et al. [25] matched 53 patients with *P. aeruginosa* bacteremia to 106 controls based on APACHE II score and diagnosis. Hospital mortality was higher for cases (62.3% vs. 47.2%), but APACHE proved to be the only predictor of survival in a multivariate analysis. These investigators performed a similar study of 73 critically ill patients with candidemia, and found that although candidemia was associated with a prolonged ICU and hospital stay, it did not increase the mortality risk, which was determined primarily by age, acute illness severity, and pre-existing underlying disease [26]. In contrast, they found that bacteremia with methicillin-resistant *S. aureus* carried a significantly elevated attributable mortality rate of 23.4% [27].

Ventilator-Associated Pneumonia

Fagon et al. [28] evaluated the impact of ventilator-associated pneumonia on ICU outcome. They demonstrated a crude mortality rate of 52.4% for 328 patients developing pneumonia, significantly higher than the 22.4% ICU mortality experienced by the 1,650 patients who did not develop pneumonia. The APACHE II score, number of failing organs, presence of pneumonia, development of nosocomial bacteremia, presence of significant underlying disease, and admission from another ICU were all independently associated with adverse outcome by logistic regression analysis. Similarly, a French case-control study suggested that ventilator-associated pneumonia was responsible for a twofold increase in mortality and a 5-day prolongation of ICU stay [29]. A Canadian study found that pneumonia was associated with an increased length of stay and a trend towards an increased mortality [9]. In contrast, a Spanish study of 1,000 consecutive ICU admissions found that the development of ventilator-associated pneumonia increased the length of stay, but not the mortality rate, of ventilated ICU patients [30]. This conclusion was also reached by a French matched case-control study, which showed rates of ventilator-associated pneumonia to be comparable in patients who died while in the ICU compared with those who survived, when matched on the basis of a panel of risk factors for adverse outcome [31]. A study of pneumonia complicating the course of acute respiratory distress syndrome reported that the development of ventilator-associated pneumonia increases the duration of mechanical ventilation, but does not adversely impact on patient survival [32].

Pooled data from a systematic review suggest that the development of ventilator-associated pneumonia results in an increased ICU length of stay of 4 days and an attributable mortality of 20%–30% [33].

Other Nosocomial Infections

There is little available evidence regarding the attributable morbidity and mortality of other nosocomial infections in critically ill patients. Urinary tract infections, although relatively common, are generally thought to be of only modest clinical significance. For example, an Argentinian study reported that catheter-related infections, the most common ICU-acquired infection (comprising 32% of all infections), carry an attributable mortality of 25%, and are associated with an excess length of stay of 11 days. Ventilator-associated pneumonia (25% of all nosocomial infections) was associated with a 35% attributable mortality and a prolongation of ICU stay of 10 days. In contrast, urinary tract infections (23% of infections) had a 5% attributable mortality and an increased length of ICU stay of 5 days [34].

Conclusions

Estimates of the attributable mortality of the two most common nosocomial ICU-acquired infections—bacteremia and ventilator-associated pneumonia—

are highly variable, varying with the study methodology, the country of origin, and the criteria used to define an optimal control population. The most commonly used techniques of analysis—matched cohort studies or population studies using multivariate techniques to control for potential confounders—yield estimates that likely overestimate the true attributable morbidity, for they are unable to completely eliminate the effects of unmeasured confounders. Moreover, inherent uncertainty in the diagnostic criteria used to define nosocomial infections introduces substantial uncertainty into the estimate of attributable outcome. Estimates of attributable morbidity are generally limited to estimates of prolongation of ICU stay. These, however, uniformly indicate an increased burden of illness resulting from the development of infection.

Because of the uncertainty and bias inherent in retrospective studies, the most reliable estimates of the attributable mortality are those deriving from prospective randomized trials of interventions to prevent infection. Pooled data from trials of SDD suggest a 5% absolute and a 22% relative attributable mortality associated with ICU-acquired infection [13]. Even this estimate, however, must be interpreted with caution, for it is not possible to determine whether the increased risk arises from the infection or from the additional interventions undertaken to treat that infection. The distinction is subtle, but important. Two randomized controlled trials of antibiotic minimization strategies in the ICU both demonstrated that antimicrobial resistance is minimized [35] and mortality reduced [36] when explicit diagnostic and therapeutic approaches are used to minimize antibiotic exposure in the patient with suspected ventilator-associated pneumonia.

The Costs of Nosocomial Infection

Reliable estimates of the costs of an ICU complication such as nosocomial infection are difficult to determine for the same reasons that attributable outcomes are difficult to estimate. However, if we adopt the plausible assumption that there is at least some degree of mortality and morbidity attributable to the development of a nosocomial infection, it follows that interventions that can prevent infection can reduce that toll: whether they are worth the cost is the domain of cost-effectiveness analysis.

Cost-effectiveness analysis is predicated on the assumption that an intervention has an effect, and reflects the tradeoff that must be made between the cost of an intervention and the extent to which clinical benefit is achieved. In Fig. 1, the cost-effectiveness of a variety of ICU therapies is presented. Increasing cost is represented on the y axis, increasing benefit on the x axis. Obviously the ideal therapy would be one that reduced costs, while bringing

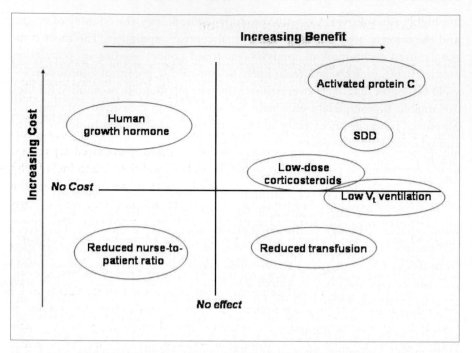

Fig. 1. The relationship between cost and clinical effectiveness. Increasing costs are represented on the *y* axis, increasing clinical benefit on the *x* axis. Examples shown are approximations of the incremental cost associated with increased (or reduced) clinical benefit

increased benefit to the patient, the situation reflected in the lower right quadrant of the graph, and exemplified by the use of a lower transfusion threshold in the anemic critically ill patient [37]. An intervention such as the use of activated protein C brings clinical benefit, but at a substantial cost [38], while the use of growth hormone increases costs and morbidity [39], and so is clearly undesirable. It will be appreciated that ascertainment of the net costs and benefits is challenging, and that the results are both qualitative and potentially controversial.

The perspective of the analysis also differs, depending upon whether the primary effect of the intervention is to treat a disease or to prevent its occurrence. If we assume that measures taken to prevent a disease will have few or no consequences on long-term health-related quality of life, but that the treatment of a disease will not necessarily restore a patient to his or her full pre-morbid state of health, then the tradeoff in prevention is the cost of the intervention against the percentage of patients who might develop the complication. The tradeoff for a therapeutic measure is the cost of the intervention against the predicted improvement in health-related quality of life. The former is a cost-effectiveness analysis, the latter, a cost-utility analysis.

Costs of ICU-Acquired Infection

Several authors have attempted to generate estimates of the costs associated with infection in critically ill patients. Angus et al. [40] used administrative data to generate an estimate that there are approximately 750,000 new cases of severe sepsis (sepsis in association with organ dysfunction) in the United States each year, and that the total costs attributable to these are 16.7 billion dollars annually. However, these estimates include cases of community acquired sepsis and sepsis developing in patients who are not in an ICU, and they fail to include the costs of episodes of nosocomial ICU-acquired infection that do not meet the criteria for severe sepsis. Brun-Buisson et al. [41] found that the costs of sepsis in association with ICU-acquired infection were three times higher than those incurred when sepsis was present at the time of ICU admission. The total costs were approximately 40,000 Euros for each patient developing sepsis in the ICU. Nosocomial infection complicating community-acquired sepsis increased costs by 2.5 times. These observations mirror those of a British study that found a fivefold increase in costs when patients developing sepsis after the 2nd day of their ICU stay were compared with patients admitted with a diagnosis of sepsis [42]. Thus the prevention of nosocomial infection in the ICU has the potential to significantly impact on the costs of ICU care.

Nosocomial Bacteremia

Pittet et al. [43] reported that nosocomial bloodstream infections complicate the course of 3% of patients admitted to an ICU and prolong both the ICU and hospital stay, generating costs of approximately U.S. $ 40,000 per survivor. Similar estimates have been derived by others. Digiovine et al. [23], for example, found that although nosocomial bloodstream infection in the ICU did not increase mortality, it was associated with increased direct costs of U.S. $ 34,508 per episode, while Dimick et al. (unpublished) suggested that catheter-related bloodstream infection in the ICU results in increased total hospital costs of U. S. $ 56,167 per case.

Two analyses have concluded that the use of antibiotic-coated catheters is cost-effective in the prevention of nosocomial bloodstream infections [44, 45]. However, the conclusion is highly dependent on the estimate of the efficacy of such catheters, and intrinsic limitations in the design of the studies evaluating them limit the estimate of their benefits [46].

Ventilator-Associated Pneumonia

Warren et al. [47] estimated the attributable cost of an episode of ventilator-associated pneumonia in the United States to be approximately U.S. $ 12,000.

Because a variety of prophylactic strategies have been shown to be effective in preventing ventilator-associated pneumonia [48], and because these are generally relatively inexpensive to institute, the prevention of ventilator-associated pneumonia is readily demonstrable to be cost-effective. Zack et al. [49], for example, showed that the institution of a comprehensive preventive program resulted in a 57.6% reduction in rates of ventilator-associated pneumonia, and in cost savings of as much as U.S. $ 4 million/year. Other strategies such as minimizing intubation through the use of non-invasive positive pressure ventilation [50] and reducing the frequency of ventilator circuit changes [51] are also cost-effective.

Infection with Antibiotic-Resistant Organisms

Independent of the site of infection, nosocomial infection with resistant organisms is associated with increased costs [52]. Chaix et al. [53] undertook a case-control study of patients with methicillin-resistant *S. aureus*, and reported that the attributable costs of such infections were $9275 per episode. An infection control program that could lower transmission by 14% or more was calculated to be cost-effective. Infection with *Enterobacter spp.* resistant to third-generation cephalosporins was associated with an attributable charge of U.S. $ 29,379 per case [54]. Divergent conclusions have been drawn with respect to infection with vancomycin-resistant enterococci (VRE). While one matched cohort study suggested an 11% increase in mortality and increased hospital costs of more than U.S. $ 20,000 per case of VRE infection [55], a second study using stepwise logistic regression analysis failed to demonstrate that such infections were associated with either attributable morbidity or increased costs [56].

Because indiscriminate antibiotic use is a risk factor for the emergence of resistance, implementation of restrictive antimicrobial prescribing practices can not only reduce costs, but also limit the development of resistance in an ICU environment [35, 57].

The Costs of Effective Treatment

Our focus has been on infectious complications that are amenable to prevention, in no small part because there are few proven effective therapies for infection in the ICU. Thus, although it is widely believed that specific antimicrobial therapy, adequate surgical source control, and the spectrum of supportive measures that comprise ICU care will improve clinical outcome, the attributable effect of any of these in the patient with infection is unknown, and therefore cost-utility analyses are impossible.

The recent approval of activated protein C for the treatment of patients with severe sepsis has provided the first opportunity for cost-utility analyses in critically ill infected patients. Treatment with activated protein C has been shown in a cohort of patients with severe sepsis to reduce mortality by 6.1%, but at a cost of approximately U.S. $ 7,000 per course of therapy. Two independent analyses of the cost-effectiveness of activated protein C show a favorable profile when it is used in the sickest patients. Manns et al. [38] calculated the cost per life-year gained to be U.S. $ 27,936 for all patients in the cohort, while Angus et al. [58] suggested that the cost-utility of activated protein C is U.S. $ 48,800 per quality-adjusted life year.

Conclusions

The development of nosocomial infection in the critically ill patient results in increased morbidity and significantly increases the costs of care. Although the magnitude of both effects is difficult to know with certainty, it is clear that measures that can prevent nosocomial infection in the critically ill patient can both reduce costs and improve clinical outcomes (Table 3). More rigorous evaluation of the economic impact of these is needed.

Table 3. Proven and promising strategies to reduce the morbidity and cost of ICU-acquired infection

Strategy	Examples
Prevent abnormal colonization	Selective digestive tract decontamination Minimize antibiotic exposure Enteral feeding
Reduce device-related infection	Antibiotic-coated catheters Non-invasive ventilation Coated endotracheal tubes or Foley catheters Reduced frequency of ventilator circuit changes
Prevent aspiration	Semi-recumbent positioning

References

1. National Nosocomial Infections Surveillance System (NNIS) System Report, data summary from January 1992 to June 1992, issued August 2002. Am J Infect Control 30:458–475
2. Richards MJ, Edwards JR, Culver DH et al (1999) Nosocomial infections in medical intensive care units in the United States. National Nosocomial Infections Surveillance System. Crit Care Med 27:887–892
3. Marshall JC, Sweeney D (1990) Microbial infection and the septic response in critical surgical illness. Sepsis, not infection, determines outcome. Arch Surg 125:17–23

4. Ponce de Leon-Rosales SP, Molinar-Ramos F, Dominguez-Cherit G, Rangel-Frausto MS, Vazquez-Ramos VG (2000) Prevalence of infections in intensive care units in Mexico: a multicenter study. Crit Care Med 28:1316–1321

5. Fagon JY, Novara A, Stephan F, Girou E, Safar M (1994) Mortality attributable to nosocomial infections in the ICU. Infect Control Hosp Epidemiol 15:428–434

6. Nathens AB, Chu PTY, Marshall JC (1992) Nosocomial infection in the surgical intensive care unit. Infect Dis Clin North Am 6:657

7. Schwieterman W, Roberts R (1997) FDA perspective on study design for therapies for severe sepsis. Sepsis 1:69

8. Patrick DL, Pearlman RA, Starks HE, Cain KC, Cole WG, Uhlmann RF (1997) Validation of preferences for life-sustaining treatment: implications for advance care planning. Ann Intern Med 127:509–517

9. Heyland DK, Cook DJ, Griffith L, Keenan SP, Brun-Buisson C (1999) The attributable morbidity and mortality of ventilator-associated pneumonia in the critically ill patient. Am J Respir Crit Care Med 159:1249–1256

10. Connors AF Jr, Speroff T, Dawson NV, Thomas C, Harrell FE Jr, Wagner D et al (1996) The effectiveness of right heart catheterization in the initial care of critically ill patients. JAMA 276:889–918

11. Asensio A, Torres J (1999) Quantifying excess length of postoperative stay attributable to infections: a comparison of methods. J Clin Epidemiol 52:1249–1256

12. Second American Thoracic Society Workshop on Outcomes Research (2002) Understanding costs and cost-effectiveness in critical care. Am J Respir Crit Care Med 165:540–550

13. Liberati A, D'Amico R, Pifferi S et al (2004) Antibiotic prophylaxis to reduce respiratory tract infections and mortality in adults receiving intensive care [Cochrane Review]. In: The Cochrane Library, Issue 1, Chichester, UK, John Wiley & Sons Ltd

14. Nathens AB, Marshall JC (1999) Selective decontamination of the digestive tract in surgical patients. Arch Surg 134:170–176

15. Warren DK, Zack JE, Elward AM, Cox MJ, Fraser VJ (2001) Nosocomial primary bloodstream infections in intensive care unit patients in a non-teaching community medical center: a 21-month prospective study. Clin Infect Dis 33:1329–1335

16. Gray J, Gossain S, Morris K (2001) Three-year survey of bacteremia and fungemia in a pediatric intensive care unit. Pediatr Infect Dis J 20:416–421

17. Jamal WY, El-Din K, Rotimi VO, Chugh TD (1999) An analysis of hospital-acquired bacteraemia in intensive care unit patients in a university hospital in Kuwait. J Hosp Infect 43:49–56

18. Crowe M, Ispahani P, Humphreys H, Kelley T, Winter R (1998) Bacteraemia in the adult intensive care unit of a teaching hospital in Nottingham, UK, 1985-1996. Eur J Clin Microbiol Infect Dis 17:377–384

19. Pittet D, Thievent B, Wenzel RP, Li N, Auckenthaler R, Suter PM (1996) Bedside prediction of mortality from bacteremic sepsis. A dynamic analysis of ICU patients. Am J Respir Crit Care Med 153:684–693

20. Brun-Buisson C, Doyon F, Carlet J, Dellamonica P, Gouin F, Lepoutre A et al (1995) Incidence, risk factors, and outcomes of severe sepsis and septic shock in adults. A multicenter prospective study in intensive care units. JAMA 274:968–974

21. Renaud B, Brun-Buisson C, ICU-Bacteremia Study Group (2001) Outcomes of primary and catheter-related bacteremia. A cohort and case-control study in critically ill patients. Am J Respir Crit Care Med 163:1584–1590

22. Raymond DP, Pelletier SJ, Crabtree TD, Gleason TG, Pruett TL, Sawyer RG (2001) Impact of bloodstream infection on outcomes among infected surgical inpatients. Ann Surg 233:549–555

23. Digiovine B, Chenoweth C, Watts C, Higgins M (1999) The attributable mortality and costs of primary nosocomial bloodstream infections in the intensive care unit. Am J Respir Crit Care Med 160:976–981

24. Harbarth S, Rohner P, Auckenthaler R, Safran E, Sudre P, Pittet D (1999) Impact and pattern of gram-negative bacteraemia during 6 y at a large university hospital. Scand J Infect Dis 31:163–168

25. Blot S, Vandewoude K, Hoste E, Colardyn F (2003) Reappraisal of attributable mortality in critically ill patients with nosocomial bacteraemia involving *Pseudomonas aeruginosa*. J Hosp Infect 53:18–24

26. Blot SI, Vandewoude KH, Hoste EA, Colardyn FA (2002) Effects of nosocomial candidemia on outcomes of critically ill patients. Am J Med 113:480–485

27. Blot SI, Vandewoude KH, Hoste EA, Colardyn FA (2002) Outcome and attributable mortality in critically ill patients with bacteremia involving methicillin-susceptible and methicillin-resistant *Staphylococcus aureus*. Arch Intern Med 162:2229–2235

28. Fagon J-Y, Chastre J, Vuagnat A, Trouillet J-L, Novara A, Gilbert C (1996) Nosocomial pneumonia and mortality among patients in intensive care units. JAMA 275:866–869

29. Bercault N, Boulain T (2001) Mortality rate attributable to ventilator-associated nosocomial pneumonia in an adult intensive care unit: a prospective case-control study. Crit Care Med 29:2303–2309

30. Rello J, Quintana E, Ausina V, Castella J, Luquin M, Net A et al (1991) Incidence, etiology, and outcome of nosocomial pneumonia in mechanically ventilated patients. Chest 100:439–444

31. Bregeon F, Ciais V, Carret V, Gregoire R, Saux P, Gainnier M et al (2001) Is ventilator-associated pneumonia an independent risk factor for death? Anesthesiology 94:554–560

32. Markowicz P, Wolff M, Djedaini K, Cohen Y, Chastre J, Delclaux C et al (2000) Multicenter prospective study of ventilator-associated pneumonia during acute respiratory distress syndrome. Am J Respir Crit Care Med 161:1942–1948

33. Cook D (2000) Ventilator associated pneumonia: perspectives on the burden of illness. Intensive Care Med 26 [Suppl 1]:S31–S37

34. Rosenthal VD, Guzman S, Orellano PW (2003) Nosocomial infections in medical-surgical intensive care units in Argentina: attributable mortality and length of stay. Am J Infect Control 31:291–295

35. Singh N, Rogers P, Atwood CW, Wagener MM, Yu VL (2000) Short-course empiric antibiotic therapy for patients with pulmonary infiltrates in the intensive care unit. A proposed solution for indiscriminate antibiotic prescription. Am J Respir Crit Care Med 162:505–511

36. Fagon J-Y, Chastre J, Wolff M, Gervais C, Parer-Aubas S, Stephan F et al (2000) Invasive and noninvasive strategies for management of suspected ventilator-associated pneumonia. A randomized trial. Ann Intern Med 132:621–630

37. Hebert PC, Wells G, Blajchman MA, Marshall J, Martin C, Pagliarello G et al (1999) A multicentre randomized controlled clinical trial of transfusion requirements in critical care. N Engl J Med 340:409–417

38. Manns BJ, Lee H, Doig CJ, Johnson D, Donaldson C (2002) An economic evaluation of activated protein C treatment for severe sepsis. N Engl J Med 347:993–1000

39. Takala J, Ruokonen E, Webster NR, Nielsen MS, Zandstra DF, Vundelinckx G et al (1999) Increased mortality associated with growth hormone treatment in critically ill adults. N Engl J Med 341:785–792

40. Angus DC, Linde-Zwirble WT, Lidicker J, Clermont G, Carcillo J, Pinsky MR (2001) Epidemiology of severe sepsis in the United States: analysis of incidence, outcome, and associated costs of care. Crit Care Med 29:1303–1310

Marshall

Marshall

41. Brun-Buisson C, Roudot-Thoaval F, Girou E, Grenier-Sennelier C, Durand-Zaleski I (2003) The costs of septic syndromes in the intensive care unit and influence of hospital-acquired sepsis. Intensive Care Med 29:1464–1471
42. Edbrooke DL, Hibbert CL, Kingsley JM, Smith S, Bright NM, Quinn JM (1999) The patient-related costs of care for sepsis patients in a United Kingdom adult general intensive care unit. Crit Care Med 27:1760–1767
43. Pittet D, Tarara D, Wenzel RP (1994) Nosocomial bloodstream infection in critically ill patients. Excess length of stay, extra costs, and attributable mortality. JAMA 271:1598–1601
44. Shorr AF, Humphreys CW, Helman DL (2003) New choices for central venous catheters: potential financial implications. Chest 124:275–284
45. Marciante KD, Veenstra DL, Lipsky BA, Sainst S (2003) Which antimicrobial impregnated central venous catheter should we use? Modeling the costs and outcomes of antimicrobial catheter use. Am J Infect Control 31:1–8
46. McConnell SA, Gubbins PO, Anaissie EJ (2003) Do antimicrobial-impregnated central venous catheters prevent catheter-related bloodstream infection. Clin Infect Dis 37:65–72
47. Warren DK, Shukla SJ, Olsen MA, Kollef MH, Hollenbeak CS, Cox MJ et al (2003) Outcome and attributable cost of ventilator-associated pneumonia among intensive care unit patients in a suburban medical center. Crit Care Med 31:1312–1317
48. Kollef MH (1999) The prevention of ventilator-associated pneumonia. N Engl J Med 340:627–634
49. Zack JE, Garrison T, Trovillion E, Clinkscale D, Coopersmith CM, Fraser VJ et al (2002) Effect of an education program aimed at reducing the occurrence of ventilator-associated pneumonia. Crit Care Med 30:2407–2412
50. Sinuff T, Cook DJ (2003) Health technology assessment in the ICU: noninvasive positive pressure ventilation for acute respiratory failure. J Crit Care 18:59–67
51. Kotilainen HR, Keroack MA (1997) Cost analysis and clinical impact of weekly ventilator circuit changes in patients in intensive care unit. Am J Infect Control 25:117–120
52. Niederman MS (2001) Impact of antibiotic resistance on clinical outcomes and the cost of care. Crit Care Med 29 [Suppl]:N114–N120
53. Chaix C, Durand-Zaleski I, Alberti C, Brun-Buisson C (1999) Control of endemic methicillin-resistant *Staphylococcus aureus*: a cost-benefit analysis in an intensive care unit. JAMA 282:1745–1751
54. Cosgrove SE, Kaye KS, Eliopoulos GM, Carmeli Y (2002) Health and economic outcomes of the emergence of third-generation cephalosporin resistance in *Enterobacter species*. Arch Intern Med 162:185–190
55. Carmeli Y, Eliopoulos G, Mozaffari E, Samore M (2002) Health and economic outcomes of vancomycin-resistant enterococci. Arch Intern Med 162:2223–2228
56. Pelz RK, Lipsett PA, Swoboda SM, Diener-West M, Powe NR, Brower RG et al (2002) Vancomycin-sensitive and vancomycin-resistant enterococcal infections in the ICU: attributable costs and outcomes. Intensive Care Med 28:692–697
57. Bantar C, Sartori B, Vesco E, Heft C, Saul M, Salamone F et al (2003) A hospitalwide intervention program to optimize the quality of antibiotic use: impact on prescribing practice, antibitoic consumption, cost savings, and bacterial resistance. Clin Infect Dis 37:180–186
58. Angus DC, Linde-Zwirble WT, Clermont G, Ball DE, Basson BR, Ely EW et al (2003) Cost-effectiveness of drotrecogin alfa (activated) in the treatment of severe sepsis. Crit Care Med 31:1–11

Chapter 30

Evidence-Based Medicine in the Intensive Care Unit

A. PETROS, K.G. LOWRY, H.K.F. VAN SAENE, J.C. MARSHALL

Introduction

Evidence-based medicine (EBM) is the conscientious, explicit, and judicious use of current best evidence in making decisions about the care of the individual patient. It means integrating individual clinical expertise with the best-available external clinical evidence from systematic research [1]. EBM asks questions, finds and appraises the relevant data, and uses that information for everyday clinical practice. This is done by formulating a clear clinical question from a patient's problem, searching the literature for relevant clinical articles, evaluating the evidence for its validity and usefulness, and then implementing useful findings into clinical practice.

The central pillar of EBM is the randomized controlled trial (RCT), defined as a clinical trial that involves at least one test treatment and one control treatment, concurrent enrollment and follow-up of the test- and control-treated groups, and in which the treatments to be administered are selected by a random process, such as the use of a random-numbers table. However, often sample sizes are too small to assess endpoints such as mortality and then one needs a systematic review of the literature and a meta-analysis using quantitative methods.

The outcome of these processes enables the evidence to be classified into five levels and this subsequently facilitates the development of five grades of recommendations with regard to treatment options. For a maneuvre to receive a grade A recommendation it needs at least two studies providing level 1 evidence supporting the intervention. Large prospective RCTs with unequivocal results and a very low risk of bias or a meta-analysis with low risk of bias provide level 1 evidence. In contrast non-randomized and historically controlled studies as well as case reports, uncontrolled studies, and expert opinion are classified as level 4 and 5 evidence, allowing only a grade E recommendation.

We screened the intensive care unit (ICU) literature using these EBM principles for maneuvres that may impact on infectious morbidity and mortality. We have classified the most common maneuvres according to levels of evidence and grades of recommendations (Table 1).

Table 1. Levels of evidence and grades of recommendations

Level	Description
1	Large prospective randomized controlled clinical trial with unequivocal results and very low risk of bias; A meta-analysis with a low risk of bias
2	Small prospective randomized controlled clinical trial with unclear results and moderate to high risk of bias; A meta-analysis with a moderate to high risk of bias
3	A prospective randomized controlled clinical trial but not performed in the appropriate patient group; A non-randomized but controlled clinical trial in the correct patient population Cohort studies and patient controlled studies
4	A non-randomized and historically controlled study
5	Case reports Uncontrolled studies Expert opinion

Grade	Description
A	A maneuvre can be recommended if supported by at least two level 1 studies
B	A maneuvre can be recommended if supported by one level 1 study
C	A maneuvre can be recommended if supported only be level 2 studies
D	Supported by at least one level 3 study
E	Only supported by studies rated at level 4 and 5

The Five Traditional Infection Control Maneuvres

Hand Washing, Isolation, Protective Clothing, Care of Equipment and Environment

Hand hygiene has never been shown to control pneumonia or reduce mortality in ventilated patients in a randomized trial. The efficacy of hand hygiene in reducing the incidence of infection has been studied in six non-randomized and two randomized trials [2–9] (Table 2). In only four of these studies was

Table 2. Studies into the effect of hand hygiene on the incidence of nosocomial infections including pneumonia

Author	Year	Study design	Endpoint	Outcome: infectious morbidity	Evidence
Casewell and [2] Phillips	1977	Sequential	Patients with *Klebsiella*	Significant reduction in patients carriers and infected with *Klebsiella* Effect on pneumonia not mentioned	Level 4
Massanari and [3] Hierholzer	1984	Cross-over	Overall infections	Significant reduction of nosocomial infection on some ICUs. Effect on pneumonia not mentioned	Level 4
Maki [4]	1989	Sequential, comparative	Overall infections	Significant reduction of nosocomial infection on some ICUs. Effect on pneumonia not mentioned	Level 4
Simmons et al. [5]	1990	Prospective, retrospective control	Infected patients	No effect on pneumonia	Level 4
Doebbeling [6] et al.	1992	Cross-over	Infected patients	Significant reduction of nosocomial infection on some ICUs. No effect on pneumonia	Level 4
Webster et al. [7]	1994	Sequential	MRSA carriage	Control of MRSA outbreak. Significant reduction of nosocomial infections	Level 4
Koss et al. [8]	2001	RCT	Patients with pneumonia	No effect on pneumonia	Level 2
Slota et al.[9]	2001	RCT	Infected patients	No difference	Level 2

RCT, randomized controlled trial

pneumonia the endpoint and in none did hand washing have any impact. The only study that demonstrated an impact on mortality of hand hygiene was the cohort study of Semmelweis in 1861 [10]. This classic study showed the survival benefit of hand disinfection. In women admitted for delivery, the mortality from child bed fever was significantly reduced from 11.40% to 3.04 % following the implementation of hand washing with chlorinated lime, compared with an historical control group of doctors who did not wash their hands. This study is often referred to as the prime evidence for the effectiveness of hand disinfection. The recent experience with the corona virus infection causing severe acute respiratory syndrome (SARS) in Toronto demonstrates that rigorous implementation of the traditional infection control measures can control an outbreak of a high-level pathogen similar to *Streptococcus pyogenes* seen 150 years ago in Vienna [11].

There are no data available on the effect of isolation, protective clothing, care of equipment, and environment on the rate of bacterial pneumonia and the associated mortality in ventilated patients.

The five traditional infection control measures target the control of transmission of micro-organisms via the hands of carriers. They are important but their impact should not be overestimated. An optimal infection control policy can only reduce infections due to micro-organisms acquired on the unit, i.e., secondary endogenous and exogenous infections. They fail to influence primary endogenous infections due to micro-organisms present in the admission flora. This type of infection is the major infection problem on the ICU varying between 60% and 85% (Chapter 5).

Non-Antibiotic Interventions as Infection Control Maneuvres

Positional therapy. Severely ill patients who require ventilation are often treated in the supine position. This leads to segmental collapse, basal atelectasis, and impaired clearance of secretions. These factors increase the risk of pneumonia. Treating a patient in a specialized rotating bed in which the patient is continuously rotated from -40° +40° around their longitudinal axis could theoretically help in the prevention of pneumonia.

There is one positive meta-analysis of six RCTs [12–14] showing a significant reduction in pneumonia in patients who received rotational therapy, thereby supporting kinetic therapy as an infection control maneuvre. Of the six studies, five were performed in surgical or neurological patients. The sixth trial in which there was no reduction in pneumonia was performed in non-surgical ICU patients. A further more recent RCT in a mixed ICU population does not support the conclusion of the meta-analysis. Rotation therapy requires special beds, which may be associated with increased costs.

Semi-recumbent position. Although in general the throat has been considered as the internal source of potential pathogenic micro-organisms (PPM) causing pneumonia, some people believe that aspiration of PPM carried in the stomach may play a role in the pathogenesis of pneumonia, the so-called stomach-lung route [15]. Based upon this concept, ventilating patients in a semi-recumbent position is thought to have a beneficial effect on reducing the incidence of reflux and aspiration from the stomach, whereby pneumonia in ventilated patients could be prevented. This maneuvre has been investigated in two RCTs [16, 17] (Table 3). The first study shows that ventilating patients in a semi-recumbent position leads to a significant reduction in pneumonia. Mortality rates, however, were identical in both test and control group. However, patients who underwent abdominal or neurosurgery, patients with refractory shock, and patients who were readmitted to ICU within 1 month were excluded. The second RCT, only published in abstract form, failed to confirm these results. There was no difference in pneumonia rate or mortality.

Sub-glottic drainage. Stasis of saliva contaminated with potential pathogens above the cuff of the endotracheal tube increases the risk of aspiration pneumonia. The removal and prevention of this salivary stasis using continuous aspiration via a specially designed endotracheal tube is thought to prevent pneumonia. The intervention of sub-glottic drainage has been evaluated in four RCTs [18–21] (Table 3). Three studies were performed in a mixed ICU population requiring ventilation for >72 h and the fourth study in cardiac surgery patients. The results of these trials are not consistent. Two studies showed a significant reduction in pneumonia, the other two failed to show any impact on pneumonia during ventilation. A meta-analysis of the four studies shows a significantly reduced relative risk of pneumonia due to sub-glottic drainage [relative risk (RR) 0.49 (0.39–0.73)]. There was no difference in mortality in test and control groups in any of the studies. Although the specially designed tubes and suction equipment are expensive, this technique has been suggested to be cost effective on theoretical grounds only [22]. Recent work indicates that sub-glottic drainage causes severe tracheal mucosal damage at the level of the suction port [23].

Immunomodulation

Enteral feeding. Total parenteral nutrition has been shown to be harmful in terms of higher infection rates and liver impairment [24, 25]. This prompted the desire to enterally feed the ICU patient as quickly as possible because it is thought to be essential for the gut anatomy and physiology, in order to prevent loss of mucosa integrity and subsequent translocation. In addition, several nutrients added to the enteral feed have been shown to influence immunologi-

Table 3. Randomized controlled trials into the effect of non-antibiotic interventions on the pneumonia rate and mortality in ventilated patients. RCT=randomised controlled trial; RR=relative risk (95% confidence intervals)

Maneuvre	Author	Year	Study design	n	Pneumonia	Mortality	Evidence
Rotation therapy	Choi and Nelson [12]	1992	Meta-analysis of 6 studies	419	RR 0.50 p=0.002	No difference	Level 1
	Traver et al. [14]	1995	RCT	103	RR 0.62 p=0.21	RR 0.62 p=0.21	Level 1
Semi-recumbent position	Drakulovic et al. [16]	1999	RCT	86	RR 0.24 p=0.003	RR 0.62 p=0.21	Level 1
	Van Nieuwen -hoven et al. [17]	2002	RCT	221		No difference	Level 1
Subglottic suction drainage	Mahul et al.[18]	1992	RCT	145	RR 0.46 (0.23-0.93)	RR 1.14 (0.62-2.07)	Level 1
	Valles et al. [19]	1995	RCT	190	RR 0.56 (0.31-1.01)	RR 1.07 (0.70-1.65)	Level 1
	Kollef et al. [20]	1999	RCT	343	RR 0.61 (0.27-1.40)	RR 0.86 (0.30-2.42)	Level 1
	Smulders et al. [21]	2002	RCT	150	RR 0.25 (0.07-0.85)	RR 1.2 (0.55-2.61)	Level 1

cal and inflammatory responses in humans. There are two recent meta-analyses on immunonutrition in the critically ill [26, 27] (Table 4). Both show a significant reduction in overall infection rates, although they do not specifically consider pneumonia. There was no reduction in mortality in either of the meta-analyses. Surgical patients seemed to benefit more than medical. In two more recent large RCTs, mortality rates were significantly higher in the subgroup that received immunonutrition. Some have speculated that added arginine might have been detrimental to the immune system [28, 29].

Steroids. High doses of steroids given to septic patients are thought to be beneficial for three reasons [30–34]. Steroids effectively suppress generalized inflammation due to micro-organisms and their toxins. They have been shown to significantly reduce septic shock and early mortality within 72 h. They significantly reduce mortality caused by particular invasive infections, including meningitis, typhoid, and *Pneumocystis carinii* pneumonia. The major perceived side effects of high-dose steroids are the associated immune suppression and subsequent risk of super-infections. Indeed the two meta-analyses show a trend towards increased mortality from secondary infection in patients receiving steroids [30, 31]. The next logical step would be to combine steroids with selective decontamination of the digestive tract (SDD), whereby the perceived harmful effects of steroids could be abolished. In that way the early survival benefit from steroids could be preserved by keeping the patient free from secondary infections using SDD.

Anti-inflammatory mediators. Almost 60 RCTs have tested the hypothesis that modulation of the endogenous host inflammatory response can improve survival for patients with a clinical diagnosis of sepsis. The results have been frustrating and no new agent has been introduced into clinical practice [35].

Pooled data from studies using a monoclonal antibody to neutralize tumour necrosis factor demonstrate a statistically significant 3.5% reduction in mortality. In aggregate, the three completed studies using recombinant interleukin-1 (IL-1) receptor antagonists to neutralize IL-1 also showed an absolute mortality reduction of 5%. Zeni et al. [36] showed that the combined results of all completed trials, independent of the therapeutic agents employed, demonstrate a statistically significant 3% overall reduction in 28-day all-cause mortality. It is questionable whether this small clinical benefit is sufficiently important to justify clinical use of these therapies, given the costs and potential toxicity of the agents involved.

Immunoglobulins. Polyclonal intravenous immunoglobulins (IVIG) significantly reduce mortality and can be used as an extra treatment option for sepsis and septic shock [37]. Overall mortality was reduced in patients who received polyclonal IVIG [n=492, RR=0.64, 95% confidence interval (CI) 0.51–0.80]. For the

Table 4. Randomized controlled trials into the effect of non-antibiotic interventions on the general infection rate and mortality in ventilated patients. RCT=randomized controlled trial; RR=relative risk (95% confidence intervals)

Maneuvre	Author	Year	Study design	n	Infection rate	Mortality	Evidence
Immunonutrition	Beale et al. [26]	1999	Meta-analysis of 12 studies	1482	RR 0.67 (0.50-0.89) p=0.006	RR 0.05 (0.78-1.41) p=0.76	Level 1
	Heyland et al. [27]	2001	Meta-analysis of 22 studies	2419	RR 0.66 (0.54-0.80)	RR 1.1 (0.93-1.31)	Level 1
Steroids	Cronin et al. [30]	1995	Meta-analysis o of 9 RCTs	1232	No difference	RR 1.13 (0.99-1.29)	Level 1
	Lefering and Neugebauer [31]	1995	Meta-analysis of 10 RCTs	1329	No difference	Difference in mortality -0.2% (-9.2 - 8.8)	Level 1
	Bollaert et al. [32]	1998	RCT	41	No difference	Difference in mortality 31% (1-61)	Level 1
	Briegel et al. [33]	1999	RCT	40	No difference	No difference	Level 1
	Annane et al. [34]	2002	RCT	300	No difference	Significant reduction	Level 1

two high-quality trials on polyclonal IVIG the RR for overall mortality was 0.30, but the CI was wide (95% CI 0.09–0.99, n=91). However, all the trials were small and the totality of the evidence is insufficient to support a robust conclusion of benefit. Adjunctive therapy with monoclonal IVIG remains experimental. This is level 2 evidence prompting a grade C recommendation for usage.

Activated protein C. Drotrecogin α (activated), or recombinant human activated protein C, is thought to have anti-inflammatory, anti-thrombotic, and profibrinolytic properties. There is one large RCT of 1,690 patients in which the mortally rate was 30.8% in the placebo group and 24.7% in the drotrecogin α group. This translates into an absolute reduction in risk of death of 6.2% (P=0.05). The incidence of serious bleeding was higher in the drotrecogin α (activated) group than the placebo group [38]. This is level 1 evidence and grade B recommendation.

Low Tidal Volume

An RCT of 861 patients concluded that by using lower tidal volumes (6 ml/kg) during mechanical ventilation compared with traditional tidal volumes (12 ml/kg) mortality was lower (31.0% vs. 39.8%, P=0.007) [39]. This is an absolute mortality reduction of 8.8% (95% CI 2.4–15.3) and 11 patients need to receive low tidal volume ventilation to save 1 life.

Glucose Control

In 1,548 patients, intensive insulin therapy reduced mortality during intensive care from 8.0% to 4.6% (P<0.04) [40]. When blood glucose levels were maintained below 6.1 mmol/l, there was an absolute mortality reduction of 3.7% (95% CI 1.3–6.1), which translates into 27 patients needing insulin therapy to prevent 1 death (Table 5).

Table 5. Effect of intervention on reduction in mortality

Intervention	Relative risk [95% CI]	Absolute mortality reduction [95% CI]	No. needed to treat	Grade of recommendation
Low tidal volume [39]	0.78 [0.65 to 0.93]	8.8 [2.4 to 15.3]	11	B
Activated protein C [38]	0.80 [0.69 to 0.94]	6.1 [1.92 to 10.4]	16	B
Intensive insulin [40]	0.40 [0.36 to 0.82]	3.7 [1.3 to 6.1]	27	B
Steroids [34]	0.90 [0.74 to 1.09]	6.4 [-4.8 to 17.6]	16	B
Selective decontamination [42]	0.65 [0.49 to 0.85]	8.1 [3.1 to 13.0]	12	A

Antibiotic Intervention

Selective decontamination of the digestive tract. The philosophy of SDD has been discussed in Chapters 9 and 14. The efficacy of SDD has been studied in 54 RCTs. There are nine meta-analyses of RCTs on SDD. All the meta-analyses show that rates of infection, particularly pneumonia, were significantly reduced. This was independent of the method used to diagnose pneumonia. The full four-component protocol of SDD in a mixed ICU population requiring a minimum of 72 h of ventilation has been analysed in 17 studies [41]. The application of the full four-component protocol reduces morbidity due to pneumonia by 65% and mortality by 22%.

In the latest SDD trial, the randomization was between ICUs and not patients as in all previous trials [42]. This study of approximately 1,000 patients is the largest single study yet undertaken. The primary endpoint was mortality as opposed to infectious morbidity. The risk of mortality was significantly reduced to 0.6 (0.4–0.8) in the unit where SDD was administered to all patients. In the previous 53 trials, the patient had been the 'randomization unit' therefore half the population in the respective ICUs was not decontaminated. Therefore it is possible that the control patients, although not receiving SDD, benefited from the intervention as they were exposed to a lower risk of microbial acquisition and carriage, infection, and subsequent mortality. This 'dilution risk' due to the control group being present with decontaminated patients at the same time in the same unit is termed 'contamination bias'. The design of the latest trial has avoided this type of bias and may explain the highest reported mortality reduction to date, an 8% absolute reduction in mortality. Recently a second RCT of large sample size found an identical 8% mortality reduction [43], meaning that only 12 patients need to receive SDD to prevent 1 death.

The main concern of the liberal use of antibiotics is the emergence of resistance. Antimicrobial resistance and subsequent super-infections emerge within 2 years of the launch of any new parenteral antibiotic [44]. When the enteral antibiotics polymyxin and tobramycin are added and successful decontamination achieved, organisms that may become resistant to the parenteral antibiotic in the gut are eradicated (Chapter 28). In the most recent meta-analysis of 36 trials comprising 6,922 patients covering a period of more than 15 years of clinical investigation, neither super-infections nor outbreaks with multi-resistant bacteria were observed [41]. The Agency for Health Research and Quality of the US Department for Health and Human Services reports that SDD using regular surveillance cultures and applying paste and suspension is cheap and easy to implement [45]. The cost-effectiveness of SDD is not properly assessed [46–49], but costs can hardly be a major concern for a maneuvre of 6 Euros a day that reduces pneumonia by 65 % and mortality by 22% without antimicrobial resistance emerging in unselected ICU patients.

Conclusion

Currently there are five maneuvres that control mortality, all published within the last 3 years, in the twenty-first century (Table 6). Four have been assessed in only one RCT in specific subsets. The only maneuvre with a Grade A recommendation from the Agency for Health Research and Quality of the US Department for Health and Human Services [45] that is applicable to all types of patients is SDD. In addition, only SDD controls resistance, which is becoming the major issue for this century.

Table 6. Analysis of the literature and grading of evidence, and recommendations for the control of morbidity and mortality due to infection in ventilated patients on ICU

	Reduced infection		Reduced mortality	
	Level of evidence	Grade of recommendation	Level of evidence	Grade of recommendation
Non-antibiotic interventions				
Handwashing/isolation/ protective clothing/ care of equipment and environment	5	E	4	E
Positioning				
Rotation therapy	none	none	none	none
Semi-recumbent position	none	none	none	none
Subglottic secretion drainage	none	none	none	none
Immunomodulation				
• Immunonutrition	1	A	none	none
• Steroids	none	none	1	B
• Immunoglobulins	none	none	2	C
• Activated protein-C	none	none	1	B
• Anti-inflammatory modulators	none	none	1	C
Low tidal volume	none	none	1	B
Intensive insulin	none	none	1	B
Antibiotic interventions *Selective Decontamination of Digestive tract (4 component)*	1	A	1	A

References

1. Sackett DL, Rosenberg WMC, Gray JAM, Haynes RB, Richardson WS (1996) Evidence-based medicine: what it is and what it isn't. BMJ 312:71–72
2. Casewell M, Philips I (1977) Hands as route of transmission for *Klebsiella* species. BMJ 2:1315–1317
3. Massanari RM, Hierholzer J (1984) A cross-over comparison of antiseptic soaps on nosocomial infection rates in the intensive care units. Am J Infect Control 12:247–248
4. Maki DG (1989) The use of antiseptics for handwashing by medical personnel. J Chemother 1 [Suppl 1]:3–11
5. Simmons B, Bryant J, Neiman K et al (1990) The role of handwashing in prevention of endemic intensive care unit infections. Infect Control Hosp Epidemiol 11:589–594
6. Doebbeling RN, Stanley G, Sheetz CT et al (1992) Comparative efficacy of alternative handwashing agents in reducing nosocomial infections in intensive care units. N Engl J Med 327:88–93
7. Webster J, Faogali JL, Cartwright D (1994) Elimination of methicillin-resistant *Staphylococcus aureus* from a neonatal intensive care unit after handwashing with tricloson. J Paediatr Child Health 30:59–64
8. Koss WG, Khalili TM, Lemus JF et al (2001) Nosocomial pneumonia is not prevented by protective contact isolation in the surgical intensive care unit. Am Surg 67:1140–1144
9. Slota M, Green M, Farley A et al (2001) The role of gown and glove isolation and strict handwashing in the reduction of nosocomial infection in children with solid organ transplantation. Crit Care Med 29:405–412
10. Semmelweis IP (1861) Die Aetiologie, der Begriff und die Prophylaxis des Kindbettfiebers. Pest, Hartleben
11. Peiris JS, Yuen KY, Osterhaus AD, Stohr K (2003) The severe acute respiratory syndrome. N Engl J Med 349:2431–2441
12. Choi SC, Nelson LD (1992) Kinetic therapy in critically ill patients: combined results based on meta-analysis. J Crit Care 7:57–62
13. Summer WR, Curry P, Haponik EF et al (1989) Continuous mechanical turning of intensive care unit patients shortens length of stay in some diagnostic-related groups. J Crit Care 4:45–53
14. Traver GA, Tyler ML, Hudson LD et al (1995) Continuous oscillation: outcome in critically ill patients. J Crit Care 10:97–103
15. Craven DE, Steger KA (1996) Nosocomial pneumonia in mechanically ventilated patients: epidemiology and prevention in 1996. Semin Respir Infect 11:32–53
16. Drakulovic MB, Torres A, Bauer TT et al (1999) Supine body position as a risk factor for nosocomial pneumonia in mechanically ventilated patients: a randomised trial. Lancet 354:1851–1858
17. van Nieuwenhoven CA, van Tiel FH, vandenbroucke-Grauls C et al (2002) The effect of semi-recumbent position on development of ventilator-associated pneumonia (VAP) (abstract). Intensive Care Med 27 [Suppl 2]:S285
18. Mahul P, Auboyer C, Jaspe R et al (1992) Prevention of nosocomial pneumonia in intubated patients: respective role of mechanical subglottic secretions drainage and stress ulcer prophylaxis. Intensive Care Med 18:20–25
19. Valles J, Artigas A, Rello J et al (1995) Continuous aspiration of subglottic secretions in preventing ventilator-associated pneumonia. Ann Intern Med 122:179–186
20. Kollef MH, Skubas NJ, Sundt TM (1999) A randomised clinical trial of continuous

aspiration of subglottic secretions in cardiac surgery patients. Chest 116:1339–1346

21. Smulders K, van der Hoeven H, Weers-Pothoff I et al (2002) A randomised clinical trial of intermittent subglottic secretion drainage in patients receiving mechanical ventilation. Chest 121:858–862

22. Shorr AF, O'Malley PG (2001) Continuous subglottic suctioning for the prevention of ventilator-associated pneumonia: potential economic implications. Chest 119:228–235

23. van Saene HKF, Ashworth M, Petros AJ et al (2004) Do not suction above the cuff. Crit Care Med 32:2160–2162

24. Alverdy JC, Laughlin RS, Wu L (2003) Influence of the critically ill state on host-pathogen interactions within the intestine: gut-derived sepsis redefined. Crit Care Med 31:598–607

25. Donnell SC, Taylor N, van Saene HK, Magnall VL, Pierro A, Lloyd DA (2002) Infection rates in surgical neonates and infants receiving parenteral nutrition: a five-year prospective study. J Hosp Infect 52:273–280

26. Beale RJ, Bryg DJ, Bihari DJ (1999) Immunonutrition in the critically ill. A systematic review of clinical outcome. Crit Care Med 27:2799–2805

27. Heyland DK, Novak F, Drover JW et al (2001) Should immunonutrition become routine in critically ill patients? A systematic review of the evidence. JAMA 286:944–953

28. Bertolini G, Iapichino G, Radrizzani D, Facchini R, Simini B, Bruzzone P, Zanforlin G, Tognoni G (2003) Early enteral immunonutrition in patients with severe sepsis: results of an interim analysis of a randomized multicentre clinical trial. Intensive Care Med 29:834–840

29. Heyland DK, Samis A (2003) Does immunonutrition in patients with sepsis do more harm than good? Intensive Care Med 29:669–671

30. Cronin L, Cook DJ, Carlet J et al (1995) Corticosteroid treatment for sepsis: a critical appraisal and meta-analysis of the literature. Crit Care Med 23:1430–1439

31. Lefering R, Neugebauer EAM (1995) Steroid controversy in sepsis and septic shock: a meta-analysis. Crit Care Med 23:1294–1303

32. Bollaert PE, Charpentier C, Levy B et al (1998) Reversal of late septic shock with supraphysiologic doses of hydrocortisone. Crit Care Med 26:645–650

33. Briegel J, Forst H, Haller M et al (1999) Stress doses of hydrocortisone reverse hyperdynamic septic shock: a prospective, randomised, double-blind, single-center study. Crit Care Med 27:723–732

34. Annane D, Sebille V, Charpentier C, Bollaert PE et al (2002) Effect of treatment with low doses of hydrocortisone and fludrocortisone on mortality in patients with septic shock. JAMA 288:862–871

35. Marshall J (2000) Clinical trials of mediator-directed therapy in sepsis: what have we learned? Intensive Care Med 26:575–583

36. Zeni F, Freeman B, Natanson C (1997) Anti-inflammatory therapies to treat sepsis and septic shock: a reassessment. Crit Care Med 25:1095–1100

37. Alejandria MM, Lansang MA, Dans LF, Mantaring JBV (2000) Intravenous immunoglobulin for treating sepsis and septic shock (Cochrane Review). In: The Cochrane Library, Issue 3. Oxford Update Software

38. Bernard GR, Vincent JL, Laterre PF et al (2001) Efficacy and safety of recombinant human activated protein C for severe sepsis. N Engl J Med 344:699–709

39. The Acute Respiratory Distress Syndrome Network (2000) Ventilation with lower tidal volumes as compared with traditional tidal volumes for acute lung injury and the acute respiratory distress syndrome. N Engl J Med 342:1301–1308

40. van den Berghe G, Wouters P, Weekers F, Verwaest C, Bruyninckx F, Schetz M, Vlasselaers D, Ferdinande P, Lauwers P, Bouillon R (2001) Intensive insulin therapy in

the critically ill patients. N Engl J Med 345:1359–1367

41. Liberati A, D'Amico R, Pifferi S, Torri V, Brazzi L (2004) Antibiotic prophylaxis to reduce respiratory tract infections and mortality in adults receiving intensive care [Cochrane Review]. In: The Cochrane Library, Issue 1, Chichester, UK. John Wiley & Sons Ltd

42. de Jonge E, Schultz MJ, Spanjaard L et al (2003) Effects of selective decontamination of digestive tract on mortality and acquisition of resistant bacteria in intensive care: a randomised controlled trial. Lancet 362:1011–1016

43. Krueger WA, Lenhart FP, Neeser G, Ruckdeschel G, Schreckhase H, Eissner HJ, Forst H, Eckart J, Peter K, Unertl KE (2002) Influence of combined intravenous and topical antibiotic prophylaxis on the incidence of infections, organ dysfunctions, and mortality in critically ill surgical patients: a prospective, stratified, randomized, double-blind, placebo-controlled clinical trial. Am J Respir Crit Care Med 166:1029–1037

44. van Saene HK, Petros AJ, Ramsay G, Baxby D (2003) All great truths are iconoclastic: selective decontamination of the digestive tract moves from heresy to level 1 truth. Intensive Care Med 29:677–690

45. Collard HR, Saint S (2001) Preventive practices for ventilator-associated pneumonia. In: Shojania KG, Duncan BW, McDonald KM, Wachter RM (eds) Making health care safer: a critical analysis of patient safety practices. Evidence Report, Technology Assessment No 43. Agency for Health Care Research and Quality, publication 01-E058. Rockville, MD, Agency for Healthcare Research and Quality

46. Rocha LA, Martin MJ, Pita S, Paz J, Seco C, Margusino L, Villanueva R, Duran MT (1992) Prevention of nosocomial infections in critically ill children by selective decontamination of the digestive tract. A randomized double blind placebo-controlled study. Intensive Care Med 18:398–404

47. Korinek AM, Laisne MJ, Nicolas MH, Raskine L, Deroin V, Sanson-Lepors MJ (1993) Selective decontamination of the digestive tract in neuro-surgical intensive care unit patients. A double-blind, randomized, placebo-controlled study. Crit Care Med 21:1468–1473

48. Stoutenbeek CP, van Saene HKF, Zandstra DF (1996) Prevention of multiple organ system failure by selective decontamination of the digestive tract in multiple trauma patients. In: Faist E, Baue AE, Schildberg FW (eds) The immune consequences of trauma, shock and sepsis—mechanisms and therapeutic approaches. Pabst, Lengerich, pp 1055–1066

49. Sanchez-Garcia M, Cambronero-Galache JA, Lopez Diaz J, Cerda Cerda E, Rubio Blasco J, Gomez Aquinaga MA, Nunez Reiz A, Rogero Marin S, Onoro Canaveral JJ, Sacristan del Castillo JA (1998) Effectiveness and cost of selective decontamination of the digestive tract in critically ill intubated patients. Am J Respir Crit Care Med 158:908–916

Subject Index

Abnormal
 carriage 3-31, 16, 17, 24, 25, 69, 81, 176, 577, 593
 flora 16, 19, 23-25, 30, 41, 42, 73, 171-173, 178, 180, 211, 239-241, 519, 593, 596
 hospital microorganisms 430
AIDS, acquired immunodeficiency syndrome 495-510
Acquisition 346, 484, 515, 593, 630
AGNB, aerobic Gram-negative bacilli 289, 316, 330, 415, 417, 420, 424, 425, 429, 430, 432, 439, 442, 445-449, 577, 578, 581, 582, 586, 595, 597, 599
Aminoglycosides 358-360
Amphotericin B 297, 300, 394, 426, 440, 441, 445, 447, 457, 458, 464, 465, 506, 507, 519, 524, 525, 577-579, 597, 599
Antimicrobial resistance 56, 57, 126, 177, 179, 241, 242, 300, 305, 307, 323, 358, 442, 593-595, 598, 613, 630
Antiretroviral therapy 495-497, 501, 502
Artificial nutrition 551, 552, 554, 556

Beta-lactams 29, 91-94, 303, 121-125, 128, 132, 134, 138, 139, 141, 172, 234-236, 238, 262, 265-267, 250, 256, 264, 266, 268, 270-272, 276, 250, 284, 285, 359, 459
 penicillins 357, 358
 cephalosporins 138, 357, 360, 369
 combined with beta-lactamase inhibitors 358
Bladder infection 420, 516, 526
Blood and body fluids 197, 198, 482-487
Blood stream infection 243, 337-350, 417, 419-421, 516, 525, 558, 610, 615

Bone marrow transplant patients 459, 460, 465
Bronchitis patients 421, 430
Burn patients 127, 197, 430, 437-440, 448, 558

Carriage 242, 248, 249, 283-285, 289, 251, 253-255, 257, 259-261, 263, 265-267, 269, 272-276, 280, 281, 286-290, 294, 295, 299, 301, 303-305, 307-309, 313, 329, 330, 415-417, 432, 437, 438, 458, 515, 519, 526-529, 575-578, 580, 581, 593, 594, 597-599, 630
 abnormal 3-31, 16, 17, 24, 25, 69, 81, 176, 577, 593
 normal 577
Carrier state 4-6, 10, 25, 29, 31, 38, 39, 50, 61, 63-67, 73, 75, 79, 82-84, 171-173, 175, 196, 200-202, 206, 207, 238-240, 242, 281, 283, 289, 292, 295, 297, 299, 300, 329, 418, 440, 515, 577, 598, 599
Catheter-related infections 611, 612, 615
Cefotaxime 299-303, 357, 360, 369, 370, 381, 401, 424, 426, 441, 442, 446, 447, 518-526, 597, 599
Central nervous system infection 5, 363, 440, 489, 496, 506
Cephradine 99, 100, 136-138, 172, 232, 233, 238, 239, 423, 426, 518, 521, 522, 528
Chronic obstructive pulmonary disease (see COPD)
Ciprofloxacin 108, 177, 203, 232-235, 238, 270, 272, 276, 278, 290, 300-302, 318, 328, 329, 408, 595
Classification of microorganisms 316, 318, 379, 380, 387, 405, 418, 540

CMV, cytomegalovirus 456-458, 460, 464, 486, 487, 496, 502, 508

Colistin 440, 447, 577, 579, 584-587
   polymyxin E 441, 445, 446, 519, 524, 526, 577, 578, 597, 599

Colonization 5, 7, 9, 19, 37-46, 50, 51, 55, 56, 58, 81, 83, 78, 79, 131-134, 156, 166, 201, 214-216, 218, 219, 221, 222, 236, 238-241, 248, 258, 259, 263, 264, 441, 445, 447, 458, 464, 515, 576, 577, 581, 594, 597

Community or normal microorganisms 319, 329, 330, 339, 343, 348, 349, 362, 371, 418, 439, 448

COPD, chronic obstructive pulmonary disease 280, 430, 441-444, 449

Cryptococcal disease 506, 507

CSF, cerebrospinal fluid 362-367, 369-371, 460, 506-509

Culture methods 73-87
   dilution series 78
   four quadrant method combined with enrichment broth 76, 77

Cystitis 54, 405, 406, 408, 422, 577

Dalfopristin + quinopristin 120, 121, 126

Defense 6, 8, 15, 19, 21, 23, 24, 26, 27, 29, 30, 37, 41-45, 73, 124, 232, 325, 339, 383, 401, 500, 577

Diagnostic samples 5, 7, 9, 37-40, 45, 46, 64, 74, 75, 78, 79, 81, 82, 84, 201-203, 205, 331, 421, 458, 518, 520, 522, 524, 526, 528, 599

DIC, disseminated intravascular coagulation 347, 540, 541

Dilution series 78

Direct contact 199, 477, 486, 487

Disseminated intravascular coagulation (see DIC)

Early onset pneumonia (see pneumonia)

Endemicity 30, 181, 203, 290, 526

Endocarditis 106, 119, 122, 125, 238, 337-339, 349-351, 353, 357-362, 365, 371, 372, 497

Endotoxin 18, 25-29, 31, 93, 118, 122, 123, 142-144, 174, 178, 179, 234, 381, 462, 542, 553, 566-568, 570, 610
   gut 25, 26, 28, 29, 31, 178, 330, 578
   throat 25, 28, 29, 31, 329, 330

Enteral antimicrobials 170-173, 175, 176, 178, 179, 181, 182, 240, 241, 299, 300, 307, 330, 448, 526, 599

Exogenous infections 7, 61, 64, 66-69, 79,

82-84, 178, 181, 200-202, 207, 300, 330, 420, 515, 519, 575, 576, 624

Fluoroquinolones 29, 91, 92, 108-111, 116, 121-123, 126-140, 165, 172, 177, 234, 235, 238, 286, 287, 317, 360, 459

Four quadrant method combined with enrichment broth 76, 77

Gentamicin 30, 98, 104-108, 117, 127, 141, 142, 174-178,232-234, 238, 256, 257, 262, 264, 265, 276, 280, 300, 353, 357-360, 370-372, 422-426, 440, 445, 446, 461, 519, 522, 525, 595, 599

Glutamine 550, 552, 556-559

Glycopeptide(s) 116, 117, 123, 125, 174, 282, 357, 424

Grades of recommendations 621, 622

Gut endotoxin 25, 26, 28, 29, 31, 178, 330, 578

HAART, highly active anti-retroviral therapy 495, 497, 501, 502

Hand hygiene 68, 82, 84, 180, 191, 193-196, 206, 214, 215, 221, 263, 299, 528, 596, 622, 624

Hemofiltration 537-547

High level pathogens 7, 418

HIV, Human immunodeficiency virus 482, 484, 485, 495-510

Hospital or abnormal microorganisms 4, 56

Human immunodeficiency virus (see HIV)

Hyperglycemia 559

KS, Kaposi sarcoma 496, 497, 502

ICU, intensive care unit 313-318, 324-330, 338-349, 369, 380, 390, 418, 429, 430, 432, 438-442, 444-448, 455-465, 469, 474-482, 485-490, 496-499, 515, 516, 524-529, 540, 541, 557, 565, 568-570, 575-577, 582, 583, 587, 589, 594-599, 601-617, 622, 624, 625, 630

Immunonutrition 627

Import 76, 179, 242, 593

Indigenous flora 8, 16, 19, 21-23, 40, 51, 53, 54, 56, 173, 174, 231, 232, 418, 430, 528, 553, 578, 596

Inflammation
   markers 241, 362, 364, 368, 381, 383, 420-422, 474, 521, 523, 549, 553, 554, 557, 559, 566, 568-570, 578, 627

Intra-abdominal infections 346, 516
Intrinsic pathogenicity 54-56, 62, 66, 418
Isolation 12, 39, 50, 52, 53, 80, 82, 84, 191,
    195, 198, 201, 206, 214, 215, 255, 257, 265,
    269, 271, 275, 279, 281, 286, 288, 323, 325,
    346, 421, 439, 474, 481, 483, 486, 488, 490,
    524-526, 555, 594, 595, 622, 624
Late onset pneumonia (see pneumonia)
Level of evidence 193, 194, 321, 621-623,
    626, 628, 629, 631
Linezolid 91, 92, 119-121, 124, 358
Liver transplant patients 39, 40, 179, 429,
    430, 444-446, 449, 461, 464
Low level pathogens 8, 383, 418, 523, 525
Lower airway infection 8, 62, 64, 82, 83,
    178, 201, 240, 243, 304, 315, 330, 417-420,
    438, 575, 576

Mediastinitis 279, 391-394
Meningitis 96, 99, 101, 106, 122, 127, 137,
    162, 283, 257, 261, 263, 337, 339, 351, 357,
    362-372, 496, 506, 507, 627
Metabolism 22, 109, 113-115, 160, 550, 569
Microorganisms 39, 130, 135, 191, 417, 434,
    542, 543
    classification 316, 318, 379, 380, 387, 405,
        418, 540
    community or normal 319, 329, 330, 339,
        343, 348, 349, 362, 371, 418, 422, 429,
        439, 448
    hospital or abnormal 4, 56, 330, 430, 456,
        487, 575, 576
    potentially pathogenetic microorga-
        nisms 171-187, 515-533, 575-592
Migration 8, 12, 21, 22, 27, 44, 45, 178, 214,
    405, 577
MRSA, methicillin-resistant Staphylococcus
    aureus 237, 317, 323, 342, 419, 420, 457,
    464, 526-528, 595, 597, 599, 601
Mucosal injury 566

Nervous system infection 469, 488
NICU, neonatal intensive care unit 415-425,
    469, 476, 478, 481, 482, 487
NNRTIs, non-nucleoside reverse transcripta-
    se inhibitors 501
Normal
    carriage 577
    community microorganisms 15-36, 49-
        60, 315-335
    flora 15, 21-23, 40, 132, 134, 197, 232, 291,

    429, 518, 554
Nystatin 39, 165, 173-177, 181, 239, 261, 291,
    299, 300, 424, 445, 446, 461, 464, 599

Osteomyelitis 106, 107, 111, 122, 127
Outbreaks 58, 81, 130, 171, 173, 181, 198,
    199, 203, 205, 231, 247-249, 282-292, 416,
    469, 474, 476-482, 488, 490, 597, 630
Overgrowth 5, 6, 9, 17-19, 22, 23, 27-31, 38,
    39, 42, 45, 66, 69, 73-76, 78-81, 83, 132, 157,
    171-176, 178-182, 201, 202, 232, 239, 291,
    299, 419, 448, 449, 515, 523, 524, 526, 528,
    553, 578, 593, 594, 596, 597, 599

Pancreatitis patients 24, 25, 33, 41, 45, 64,
    238, 242, 302, 385, 429, 430, 432, 434, 437,
    448, 503
Parenteral antimicrobials 29, 45, 172, 179,
    236, 239, 240, 232, 233, 299, 303, 307, 330,
    430, 448, 519, 594-597
Pathogenesis 38, 39, 66, 81, 142, 201, 205,
    248, 282, 283, 285, 287, 288, 290, 316, 317,
    363, 386, 415, 419, 420, 499, 515, 553, 566-
    568, 571, 625
Pathogens 21, 99, 111, 115, 116, 125, 128,
    130, 131, 134, 155, 163, 289, 292, 299, 300,
    316, 317, 323-330, 341-343, 346-349, 362-
    365, 383, 404, 416, 418, 426, 439, 442, 445,
    456, 458, 460, 463-465, 486, 519-525, 553,
    554, 577, 611, 625
    low level 8, 62, 65, 66, 181, 299, 383, 523,
        525
    high level 7, 62, 299, 316, 418
    potential 10, 37, 39, 40, 45, 55, 62, 75, 76,
        130, 134, 180, 182, 175, 235, 237-242,
        291, 416, 418, 420, 426, 519, 520, 526,
        554, 577, 625
Patient care environment 624
Patient care equipment 624
PCP, Pneumocystis carinii pneumonia 496-
    498, 503, 504, 506, 509
PCR, polymerase chain reaction 474, 476,
    480-482, 486-489, 503, 508, 542-545
Peritonitis 106, 125, 166, 379-384, 421, 458,
    516, 523, 524, 542
Personal protective equipment 84, 197, 596,
    622, 624
    gloves 196, 474, 476, 488
    gowns 196, 474, 476, 596
    aprons 196, 480
Pharmacist 206, 231, 575, 576, 579, 580, 589

PICU, paediatric intensive care unit 416-422, 426, 469, 474, 481, 575-578, 581, 586

PIs, protease inhibitors 501

PML, progressive multifocal leukoencephalopathy 496, 502, 508

Pneumocystis carinii (*see PCP*)

Pneumonia 31, 41, 49, 57, 74, 76, 98, 99, 106, 107, 110, 113, 116, 118, 125, 130, 131, 178, 203, 204, 222, 224, 225, 287, 251, 255, 257, 259, 270, 271, 273, 275, 276, 300, 305, 306, 315-332, 337-340, 349, 350, 364, 397, 421, 437-449, 460, 464, 470, 474-477, 496-503, 506, 509, 510, 515-523, 529-542, 567-569, 577, 594-597, 606, 617, 622-627, 630
    early onset 316, 317, 439
    late onset 316, 317, 439, 448
    ventilator-associated 55, 204, 213, 223, 276, 315, 337, 542, 567, 569, 609, 611, 612, 615, 616

Polyenes 178, 232, 235-237, 239, 240

Polymyxins 98, 118, 132, 134, 143, 173, 174, 178, 232, 235-237, 240, 282

Prevention 27, 38, 39, 62, 68, 69, 131, 167, 171, 178, 182, 221, 222, 224-227, 236, 240, 241, 263, 297-299, 324, 337, 422, 426, 430, 444, 455, 459, 464, 465, 474, 476, 480, 497, 519, 528, 559, 567, 569-571, 587, 597, 605, 609, 610, 614-616, 624, 625

Primary endogenous infections 63, 64, 68, 82, 84, 178, 200, 201, 236, 238, 239, 330, 429, 430, 438, 448, 516, 575, 624

Respiratory viruses 456

Samples 38-40, 54, 63, 74, 75, 133, 177, 202, 285
    diagnostic 5, 7, 9, 37-40, 45, 46, 64, 74, 75, 78, 79, 81, 82, 84, 201-203, 205, 331, 421, 458, 518, 520, 522, 524, 526, 528, 599
    surface 75, 202
    surveillance 30, 38-40, 63, 64, 73-75, 78, 79, 81-84, 176-178, 201-203, 205-207, 238, 242, 300

SDD, selective decontamination of the digestive tract 5, 8, 10, 31, 45, 68, 83, 84, 119, 172-182, 203, 204, 206, 238-241, 260, 261, 297-300, 303-305, 307, 326, 388, 422, 424-426, 438, 440, 441, 445-449, 457, 460, 462-465, 519-521, 523, 524, 526, 528, 529, 567, 569-571, 575-589, 597-611, 613, 627, 630, 631
    gel 578

    paste 581, 582
    pastille 581, 582
    lozenge 582
    solution 575-592
    suspension 524

Secondary endogenous infections 51, 64, 66, 82, 78, 178, 201, 207, 239, 297, 300, 330, 418, 515, 575

Sepsis 3, 10, 11, 28, 40, 45, 130, 131, 142, 193, 194, 196, 200, 213, 215, 217, 219, 220, 277, 315, 324, 332, 350, 361, 366, 369, 381, 388, 390, 391, 395, 417, 420, 437, 481, 496, 497, 523, 537-544, 549, 551, 553, 557, 559, 566, 567, 627
    severe 10, 11, 344-346, 348, 349, 367, 383, 498, 538-544, 611, 615-617

Septic shock 142, 344-346, 394, 406, 496, 498, 523, 524, 537, 540-542, 552, 611, 627

Septicaemia 537

Sinusitis 11, 96, 363, 366, 509, 520, 521

SIRS, systemic inflammatory response syndrome 344, 421, 537, 540-545, 549, 553, 578

Stress ulceration 569

Surface samples 75, 202

Surveillance
    samples 30, 38-40, 63, 64, 73-75, 78, 79, 81-84, 176-178, 201-203, 205-207, 238, 242, 300, 329, 420, 518, 522, 526, 527
    of infection 191-211
    of carriage 202
    of infection and of carriage 191-211

Throat endotoxin 329, 330

Tobramycin 10, 31, 64, 79, 98, 104-107, 117, 127, 141-143 , 173-179, 232, 234, 235, 237-239, 241, 264, 266, 267, 285, 299, 300, 303, 307, 404, 440, 441, 445-447, 457, 464, 519, 524, 526, 577, 578, 586, 587, 597, 599, 630

Toxoplasmosis 114, 496, 507-509

Tracheitis 11, 421

Translocation 11, 18, 27-29, 31, 44, 45, 74, 80, 133, 178, 299, 381, 419, 420, 432, 448, 459, 464, 523, 577, 625

Transmission 12, 58, 67-69, 74, 76, 81, 84, 171, 179-182, 191, 194-200, 202, 205, 206, 214, 222, 239, 248, 250, 252, 254, 256, 258, 260, 262, 264, 266, 268, 270, 272, 274, 276, 278, 280, 282, 285, 287, 291, 300, 329, 415, 416, 469, 474, 479-485, 488, 489, 500, 528, 569, 576, 595, 597, 616

Transmural migration or translocation 45,
178
Trauma patients 29, 41, 55, 224, 316, 438-
441, 448

Urinary tract infection 12, 44, 49, 106, 110,
204, 205, 213, 227, 287, 250, 315, 349, 405,
422, 445, 456, 525, 526, 542, 577, 612
Vancomycin 30, 42, 57, 84, 116-120, 124-

126, 131, 145, 146, 172-178, 180-182, 175,
196, 232, 235, 237-242, 256, 257, 267, 280,
286, 299, 300, 307, 318, 329, 357-360, 370,
394, 404, 460, 524-527, 597-599
VRE, vancomycin-resistant enterococci 342,
598, 616

Wound infections 236, 392, 422, 445, 524, 577